Focus on Health

Eleventh Edition

Dale B. Hahn, Ph.D.

Wayne A. Payne, Ed.D.

Ellen B. Lucas, Ph.D.

All of Ball State University
Muncie, Indiana

Special Edition

1 2 3 4 5 6 7 8 9 0 STA STA 15 14 13

ISBN-13: 978-0-07-782801-1
ISBN-10: 0-07-782801-1

Learning Solutions Consultant: Judson Harper
Associate Project Manager: Christian Marty

Brief Contents

Contents

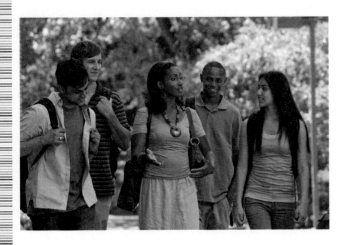

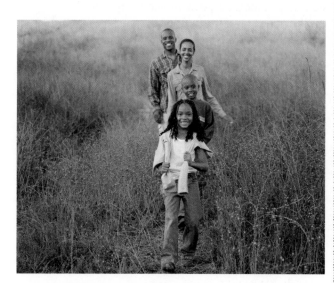

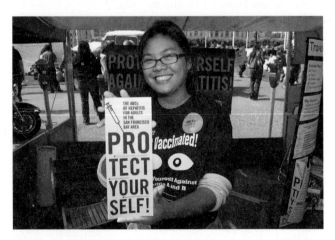

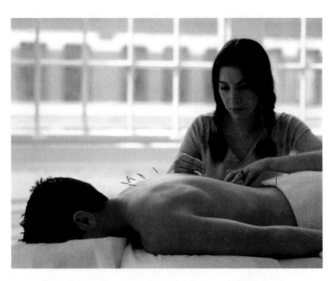

Boxes in Text

Building Media Literacy Skills

Changing for the Better

Learning from Our Diversity

Discovering Your Spirituality

Special Topics

Preface

As a health educator, you already know that personal health is one of the most exciting courses a college student will take. Today's media-oriented college students are aware of the critical health issues of the new millennium. They hear about environmental issues, substance abuse, sexually transmitted infections, fitness, and nutrition virtually every day. The value of the personal health course is its potential to expand students' knowledge of these and other health topics. Students will then be able to examine their attitudes toward health issues and modify their behavior to improve their health and perhaps even prevent or delay the onset of certain health conditions.

Focus on Health accomplishes this task with a carefully composed, well-documented text that addresses the health issues most important to both instructors and students. As health educators, we understand the teaching issues you face daily in the classroom and have written this text with your concerns in mind.

Updated Coverage: New and Expanded Topics

As experienced health educators and authors, we know how important it is to provide students with the most current information available. The eleventh edition of *Focus on Health* has been thoroughly updated with the latest information, statistics, and findings. A summary of notable changes for each chapter follows.

Chapter 1

- New life-related terms: span, expectancy, course, style, and fable
- New information on Generation Z
- New figures depicting the reciprocal relationships between health, role fulfillment, and adult developmental tasks, at each adult life stage
- New section on personalized medicine and regenerative medicine
- Revised information from the Pew Forum on religion and public life

Chapter 2

- Updated statistics and data throughout
- New "Learning from Our Diversity" box on regional, socioeconomic, and racial differences in psychological health

- New section on mindfulness
- New box on cyberviolence

Chapter 3

- Updated statistics and data throughout
- New "Learning from Our Diversity" box on stress-prone personalities
- New section on the type D personality type

Chapter 4

- Updated statistics and data throughout
- Updated section on physical activity guidelines for Americans
- New Table 4.3 on osteoporosis risk factors

Chapter 5

- Updated statistics and data throughout
- New information on the FDA's "smart choice" food labeling program
- Revised information on USDA dietary guidelines

Chapter 6

- Updated statistics and data throughout
- New box on health halo foods
- New information on weight loss drugs Qnexa, lorcaserin hydrochloride, and Contrave

Chapter 7

- Updated statistics and data throughout
- New box on energy drinks
- New section on bath salts
- New sections on Salvia divinorum and K2 or Spice

Chapter 8

- Updated statistics related to tobacco use (principally cigarette smoking) in the United States
- New information on non-daily smokers
- New identified genetic markers for nicotine dependency
- New section on cigarette smoking and cognitive decline (dementia)
- New information on prenatal exposure to second-hand tobacco smoke
- New information on nicotine vaccine development

Chapter 9

- Updated statistics and data throughout

Chapter 10

- Updated cancer data related to site of development and deaths
- New cancer treatment protocols: advances and disappointments
- New information on metabolic syndrome and the development of type 2 diabetes mellitus (Small Steps, Big Rewards program)
- New information on advancements in the understanding and diagnosis of Parkinson's and Alzheimer's disease

Chapter 11

- New information on illnesses caused by antibiotic-resistant bacteria
- New section on stem cell research and the role of parthenotes
- Revised section on immunization schedules (by age groups), American immunization status, immunizations and autism, and new vaccines
- New information on nosocomial infections, monitoring staff via "germ cops"
- New information regarding the diagnosis and treatment of Lyme disease
- New medications and immunizations for hepatitis B and C
- New section on bed bugs

Chapter 12

- Updated statistics and data throughout
- New box on "Don't Ask, Don't Tell"
- New section on sexting
- New section on stalking
- New section on same-sex marriage

Chapter 13

- Updated data and statistics throughout
- New section on extended-cycle pills

- New information on male birth control pills
- New information on emergency contraception
- New section on Adiana sterilization

Chapter 14

- New section on physician use of social media
- New section on patient-centered medical care
- New section on the placebo effect
- New information on medical careers: need versus employment opportunities
- New information on direct-to-consumer marketing (DTC)
- Revised section on palliative care
- New information on paying for medical care and the American health care system's world ranking

Chapter 15

- Updated data and statistics throughout
- New box on cell phone safety and distracted driving
- New information on cyberstalking
- New information on bullying

Chapter 16

- Updated data and statistics throughout
- New information on exposure to dangerous indoor air pollutants
- New information on BPA
- New information on air toxics hotspots
- New section on ionizing radiation
- New information on reducing human population growth
- New box on "too clean" environmental effects

Chapter 17

- Updated data and statistics throughout
- New information on near-death experiences
- New information on living wills
- New information on the Five Wishes directive

Visual Walk-Through

Building Media Literacy Skills

These boxes take a critical look at media sources of health information, helping students get the most out of health information.

Discovering Your Spirituality

These boxes highlight the spiritual dimension of health and its effect on overall wellness.

Changing for the Better

These unique question-and-answer boxes show students how to put health concepts into practice, beginning with a real-life question, followed by helpful tips and practical advice for behavior change.

Learning from Our Diversity

These boxes expose students to alternative viewpoints and highlight what we can learn from the differences that make us unique.

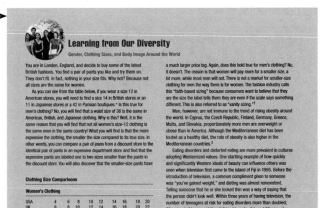

Learning from Our Diversity

Gender, Clothing Sizes, and Body Image Around the World

You are in London, England, and decide to buy some of the latest British fashions. You find a pair of pants you like and try them on. They don't fit. In fact, nothing in your size fits. Why not? Because not all sizes are the same for women.

As you can see from the table below, if you wear a size 12 in American stores, you will need to find a size 14 in British stores or an 11 in Japanese stores or a 42 in Parisian boutiques.* Is this true for men's clothing? No, you will find that a waist size of 38 is the same in American, British, and Japanese clothing. Why is this? Well, it is the same reason that you will find that not all women's size-12 clothing is the same even in the same country! What you will find is that the more expensive the clothing, the smaller the size compared to its true size. In other words, you can compare a pair of jeans from a discount store to the identical pair of pants in an expensive department store and find that the expensive pants are labeled one to two sizes smaller than the pants in the discount store. You will also discover that the smaller-size pants have

a much larger price tag. Again, does this hold true for men's clothing? No, it doesn't. The reason is that women will pay more for a smaller size, a lot more, while most men will not. There is not a market for smaller-size clothing for men the way there is for women. The fashion industry calls this "faith-based sizing" because consumers want to believe that they are the size the label tells them they are even if the scale says something different. This is also referred to as "vanity sizing."†

Men, however, are not immune to the trend of rising obesity around the world. In Cyprus, the Czech Republic, Finland, Germany, Greece, Malta, and Slovakia, proportionately more men are overweight or obese than in America. Although the Mediterranean diet has been touted as a healthy diet, the rate of obesity is also higher in the Mediterranean countries.‡

Eating disorders and distorted eating are more prevalent in cultures adopting Westernized values. One startling example of how quickly and significantly Western ideals of beauty can influence others was seen when television first came to the island of Fiji in 1995. Before the introduction of television, a common compliment given to someone was "you've gained weight," and dieting was almost nonexistent. Telling someone that he or she looked thin was a way of saying that the person did not look well. Within three years of having television, the number of teenagers at risk for eating disorders more than doubled; 74 percent of teens said they felt too big or too fat, and 62 percent reported that they had been dieting in the past month.§

[...] States and oth[...] societies, the cult[...]

Clothing Size Comparisons

Women's Clothing

USA	4	6	8	10	12	14	16	18	20
UK	6	8	10	12	14	16	18	20	22
Russia	40	42	44	46	48	50	52	54	56
Spain	34	36	38	40	42	44	46	48	50

Special Topics

These boxes encourage students to delve into a particular topic or closely examine an important health issue.

Should You Take a Dietary Supplement?

Half of Americans take a dietary supplement for health, weight management, and athletic performance enhancement, spending $23 billion on them in 2009. But what are the risks? Dietary supplements do not have to have clinical trials to prove their safety or effectiveness and are not subject to regulation by the FDA. Due to the lack of quality control, supplements have been routinely found to contain metals, pesticides, high amounts of selenium and chromium, and prescription drugs. People have reported problems with breathing, liver failure, kidney failure, stroke, high blood pressure, heart attacks, joint pain, diarrhea, hair loss, finger- and toenails falling off, skin turning blue, whites of eyes turning yellow, and fatigue. Fatalities have been associated with taking dietary supplements as well.

Consumer Reports, along with the Natural Medicines Comprehensive Database, developed a list of the most dangerous supplements, ones they say should be avoided due to lack of safety and to adverse side effects. They are aconite, bitter orange, chaparral, colloidal silver, coltsfoot, comfrey, country mallow, germanium, greater celadine, kava, lobelia, and yohimbe. They have been associated with liver damage, kidney damage, heart failure, cancer, respiratory problems, and death.

If you do take a dietary supplement, be a cautious and informed consumer. Look for the "USP Verified" mark on the product indicating that the manufacturer has voluntarily undergone quality control testing by U.S. Pharmacopeia. USP is a nonprofit, private

standard-setting authority that verifies the quality, purity, and potency of the product.

You can check out a list of verified products at www.uspverified.org. If the promises seem too good to be true, they probably are. It is illegal for dietary supplement companies to claim that their product can prevent, treat, or cure any disease other than ones caused by nutrient deficiencies. Be sure to tell your doctor or pharmacist if you are taking any dietary supplements to avoid negative interactions with prescription medications. If you experience any problems, consult your doctor immediately.

Source: Dangerous supplements, *Consumer Reports*, September 2010.

Talking Points

Interspersed throughout each chapter, this feature offers students opportunities to start a dialogue about specific health-related issues and situations.

TALKING POINTS Which fast-food restaurants are your favorites? Are you surprised at any of the information in this chapter regarding your favorite meals? Will you change your order next time you visit a fast-food restaurant?

Personal Assessments

Each chapter ends with at least one Personal Assessment that helps capture students' attention, serves as a basis for introspection and behavior change, and provides suggestions for carrying the applications further.

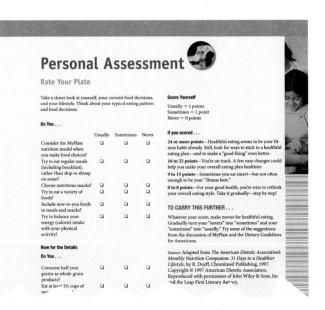

Personal Assessment

Rate Your Plate

Take a closer look at yourself, your current food decisions, and your lifestyle. Think about your typical eating pattern and food decisions.

Do You . . .

	Usually	Sometimes	Never
Consider the MyPlate nutrition model when you make food choices?	☐	☐	☐
Try to eat regular meals (including breakfast), rather than skip or skimp on some?	☐	☐	☐
Choose nutritious snacks?	☐	☐	☐
Try to eat a variety of foods?	☐	☐	☐
Include new-to-you foods in meals and snacks?	☐	☐	☐
Try to balance your energy (calorie) intake with your physical activity?	☐	☐	☐

Now for the Details

Do You . . .

Consume half your grains as whole-grain products?	☐	☐	☐
Eat at least 2½ cups of ve[...]	☐	☐	☐

Score Yourself

Usually = 2 points
Sometimes = 1 point
Never = 0 points

If you scored . . .

24 or more points—Healthful eating seems to be your fitness habit already. Still, look for ways to stick to a healthful eating plan—and to make a "good thing" even better.

16 to 23 points—You're on track. A few easy changes could help you make your overall eating plan healthier.

9 to 15 points—Sometimes you eat smart—but not often enough to be your "fitness best."

0 to 8 points—For your good health, you're wise to rethink your overall eating style. Take it gradually—step by step!

TO CARRY THIS FURTHER . . .

Whatever your score, make moves for healthful eating. Gradually turn your "nevers" into "sometimes" and your "sometimes" into "usually." Try some of the suggestions from the discussion of MyPlate and the Dietary Guidelines for Americans.

Source: Adapted from *The American Dietetic Association's Monthly Nutrition Companion: 31 Days to a Healthier Lifestyle*, by R. Duyff, Chronimed Publishing, 1997. Copyright © 1997 American Dietetic Association. Reproduced with permission of John Wiley & Sons, Inc and the Leap First Literary Agency.

Focus on Health in Loose-Leaf Format

McGraw-Hill has done a considerable amount of research with college students, not only asking them questions about how they study and use course materials, but also using ethnographic research tools to observe how they study. Based on what we heard from students, we are introducing *Focus on Health* in a three-hole-punched, loose-leaf format that offers these advantages:

- Light and easy to carry
- Engaging and relevant to their own lives
- Inexpensive
- Supported by digital activities that help them learn and succeed in their course

Would you still like your students to have a bound book? You will be able to order one through our CREATE system. While you're at it, you can pull out any of the chapters of the book you don't assign. This ensures that students are purchasing only the content that is being assigned to them, making the book 100 percent relevant to your course, more affordable for students, and lightweight and portable.

CREATE, Because Customization Matters

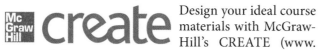 Design your ideal course materials with McGraw-Hill's CREATE (www.mcgrawhillcreate.com). Rearrange or omit chapters, combine material from other sources, and/or upload your syllabus or any other content you have written to make the perfect resource for your students. Search thousands of leading McGraw-Hill textbooks to find the best content for your students, then arrange it to fit your teaching style. You can even personalize your book's appearance by selecting the cover and adding your name, school, and course information. When you order a CREATE book, you receive a complimentary review copy. Get a printed copy in three to five business days or an electronic copy (eComp) via e-mail in about an hour.

Register today at www.mcgrawhillcreate.com, and craft your course resources to match the way you teach.

Instructor and Student Online Resources

The Online Learning Center (www.mhhe.com/hahn11e) includes valuable teaching and learning tools such as assessment tools, classroom presentations, practice quizzes, and updated reference materials.

Acknowledgments

While producing textbooks for nearly three decades, we realize that it takes many talented, dedicated people to develop, write, and publish successful books. For this eleventh edition of *Focus on Health,* we again used the professional expertise and writing talents of a team of three contributing authors, all professors at Ball State University. Lenny Kaminsky, Ph.D., professor of Exercise Science and coordinator of the Clinical Exercise Physiology and Adult Physical Fitness programs, took on the task of revising and updating Chapter 4, "Becoming Physically Fit," and Chapter 9, "Enhancing Your Cardiovascular Health." Robert Pinger, Ph.D., professor emeritus in the Department of Physiology and Health Science, revised Chapter 15, "Preventing Injuries." David LeBlanc, professor of Biology, revised Chapter 16, "The Environment and Your Health." We thank these experienced contributors for their professional dedication to this book and their personal commitment to the health of college students with whom they work on a daily basis.

Focus on Health has benefited from the expert knowledge and helpful suggestions of many people. We are grateful for their participation in this edition:

Zuzana Bic, California State Polytechnic University–Pomona
Sheri Bollinger, Northampton Community College
Jan Dowell, Prairie State College
Stephanie Duguid, Copiah Lincoln Community College
Keri Kulik, Indiana University of Pennsylvania–Indiana
Helene Washington, Black Hawk College

The sponsoring editor for this eleventh edition of *Focus on Health* is Chris Johnson. Chris is also the executive editor for Health and Human Performance at McGraw-Hill Higher Education. With his good sense of humor, his vision and level-headed thinking, we hope to work with him on many future book projects.

New to this edition is our developmental editor, Lynda Huenefeld. We have known Lynda for many years, but have never worked with her so closely on a book project. Lynda deserves a lot of praise for her editorial efforts on this comprehensive book. She is a great communicator and wonderful problem-solver, with a knack for finding quick consensus on thorny issues. We are indeed thankful for having Lynda as the person most closely attached to this edition.

On the production end of this textbook, we have three people that particularly stand out: Holly Irish, Tom Briggs, and Melanie Field. Holly was our production editor. Her duties were to oversee the entire production end of this project. Although we did not have day-to-day contact with Holly, we knew that our revised manuscript was being carefully watched over by Holly's experienced eyes. Thank you for coordinating this massive effort, Holly.

Tom Briggs worked with us for the first time as our manuscript editor. In this capacity, he made certain that all of the text revisions, updated sections, and new information fit well together in the chapters. Much of the clarity of this manuscript is due to Tom's watchful eyes. Thank you, Tom for your ability to work well with all of us.

We were quite fortunate to have Melanie Field serve as our production manager. Melanie has worked on many of our recent book projects and she is a gem. She knows how to juggle the many tasks that come with working with multiple authors and contributors, the permissions editor, the manuscript editor, the book designers, the proofreaders, the compositors, and the printers. We think of Melanie as a head chef in a five-star restaurant, working behind the scenes to produce a product that will be remembered for years. Thank you, Melanie.

Finally, we would like to thank our families for their continued support and love. More than anyone else, they know the energy and dedication it takes to write and revise textbooks. To them we continue to offer our sincere admiration and loving appreciation.

1
Shaping Your Health

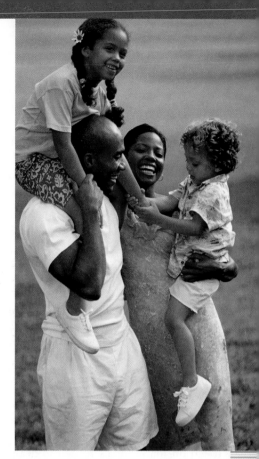

What Do You Know About Health and Wellness?

1. Life expectancy is a measure of the quality of life. True or False?

2. Society holds developmentally oriented expectations for young adults, but not for middle-aged and older adults. True or False?

3. Traditional definitions of health and approaches to health care are strongly influenced by concerns related to morbidity and mortality. True or False?

4. Males' shorter life expectancy, compared with that of females, results almost completely from males' greater genetic weakness. True or False?

5. Changing a health behavior, such as quitting smoking, is primarily a matter of willpower. True or False?

6. A holistic perception of health is a perception totally focused on the structure and function of the body. True or False?

7. Personalized medicine is a field that uses new understandings of the human genome to identify predispositions for future conditions. True or False?

Check your answers at the end of the chapter.

"Take care of your health, because you'll miss it when it's gone," younger people hear often from their elders. This simple and heartfelt advice is given in the belief that young people take their health for granted and assume that they will always maintain the state of health and wellness they now enjoy. Observation and experience should, however, remind all of us that youth is relatively brief, and health is always changing.

How do you imagine your life in the future? Do you ever think about how your health allows you to participate in meaningful life activities—and what might happen if your health is compromised? Consider, for example, how your health affects the following activities:

• Your ability to pursue an education or career
• Your opportunities to socialize with friends and family

- The chance to travel—for business, relaxation, or adventure
- The opportunity to meet and connect with new people
- The ability to conceive or the opportunity to parent children
- Your participation in hobbies and recreational activities
- Your enjoyment of a wide range of foods
- The opportunity to live independently

Intertwined with the concept of health is the concept of quality of life—the sense that you are living your life well. Psychologists routinely ask older adults if they feel satisfied with their lives and if they would do anything differently if they were able to go back and make changes. It is less common for young adults to be asked if they feel they are living their lives well and if they are satisfied with their lives.

In this chapter we do ask these questions. We explore the many factors that go into quality of life, including the ability to complete age-appropriate tasks (like those listed above) and the ability to fulfill age-appropriate roles. We touch on many topics related to health and well-being, ranging from society's expectations for people at every stage of life, to the different perspectives on health care prevalent in American society, to the varied dimensions of health and wellness. Toward the end of the chapter, we draw together these diverse threads into a comprehensive definition of health that reflects the complexity and promise of what it means to be well.

First, though, let's consider some important concepts relevant to the study of health and wellness for people at all stages of life.

- **Life span** is the maximum number of years that humans are capable of living. Regardless of such factors as access to health care and individual health-related choices, there seems to be a limit to the human life span. This maximum appears to be about 120 years, although it is rare for a person to reach this age.
- **Life expectancy** is the average number of years that members of a cohort can expect to live. (A *cohort* is a group of people who share a particular experience or time lived together, such as people who are undergraduates between 2008 and 2012.) The life expectancy of someone born in 1980 in the United States is (on average) 73.7 years; for someone born in 1990, it is 75.4 years; and for someone born in 2000, it is 76.8 years. Many factors affect life expectancy, which varies by sex, race and ethnicity, and geographical region, with white women living the longest, along with people who live in Hawaii! Some people worry that the current state of the American people's health,

especially the high rates of overweight and obesity, may lead to a decline in life expectancy for the first time in our history.

Another measure, called health-adjusted life expectancy, reflects the number of years individuals can expect to live independently and without limitations on activities. Whereas life expectancy reflects quantity (years) of life, health-adjusted life expectancy reflects quality of life.

- **Life course** is the path that people follow through life, or a road map or blueprint of that path. Life course is shaped by the various developmental tasks and roles that society expects of people at each chronological life stage. It is also strongly influenced by the historical and sociocultural context in which people live—particularly those events that occur as individuals pass from adolescence into early adulthood. For example, people who came of age in a post-9/11 world have very different experiences than those who came of age a decade earlier. Events and phenomena like the Great Depression of the 1930s, the counterculture of the 1960s, or the recession that began in 2007–2008 have a powerful impact on the chances, choices, and life outcomes of an individual, a cohort, or even a generation.
- **Lifestyle** is a personalized version of the life course of a cohort or generation. Lifestyle is also the expression of an individual's behavioral choices, such as eating a healthy diet or incorporating physical activity into daily life. Lifestyle is a major factor in a person's quality of life.
- **Life fable** is the "story" of a person's life, as written and directed by that person. It is the picture you have in your head about your life. Periodically, you make additions, subtractions, and modifications to your life fable, as circumstances change and expectations come true or fall by the wayside. Ultimately, you will be the final critic of your life fable—the one who answers questions like these: Have I had a high quality of life? Have I lived my life well?

How do these concepts play into your life? As a college student, you are living out some of the developmental tasks and roles that society expects of people in your life stage. We turn now to a brief examination of these expectations and how they are related to quality of life.

Adult Developmental Expectations

The general period of young adulthood (ages 18–39) is often divided into subgroups: early young adulthood (18–24), middle young adulthood (25–33), and later young adulthood (34–39). **Traditional-age students** are early young adults in this schema (ages 18–24). **Nontraditional-age students** are students of all other ages—middle young adults, later young adults, and individuals in middle or older adulthood. For more on nontraditional-age students, see the box "Back to the Future: Nontraditional-Age Students Enrich the College Experience" on page 8).

Earlier we described *life course* as a path through life shaped by the developmental tasks—predictable areas of growth and development—that society expects of people at each life stage. Of course, people's lives are also shaped by other factors, including their genetics, biology, and inborn temperament and personality traits; their early experiences; and the limitations and opportunities associated with the historical and sociocultural events of their lifetimes. People are also unique and have a fair measure of latitude in how they choose to traverse their life course, as implied in the term *lifestyle*.

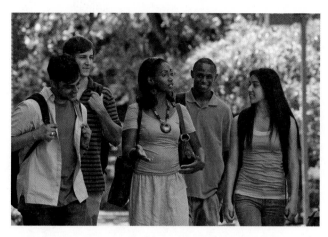

Developmental tasks for young adults include establishing independence from their families, assuming more responsibility for themselves and others, and nurturing intimate relationships, while playing the roles of student and friend.

Young Adult Developmental Expectations

Growth and development do not end with the maturation of the body. Instead, the focus shifts to the development of attitudes that foster the assumption of an increasing array of roles, the ability to engage in the behaviors required for role fulfillment, a recognition of the sense of well-being stemming from such engagement, and continued progress in meeting society's developmental expectations. In this section we consider society's expectations for young adults (Figure 1-1). In the following sections we briefly consider the developmental tasks of middle adulthood and older adulthood.

Forming an Initial Adult Identity As emerging adults, most young people want to present a personally satisfying initial adult identity as they transition from adolescence into early young adulthood. Internally they are constructing perceptions of themselves as the adults they wish to be; externally they are formulating the behavioral patterns that will project this identity to others. Completion of this first developmental task is necessary for young adults to establish a foundation on which to successfully accomplish role undertakings, and nurture their identity during the later stages of adulthood.

TALKING POINTS What does being an adult mean to you at this point? How would you explain this to your best friend?

Establishing Independence Society anticipates that, by the time their college education is completed, younger adults should be moving away from dependent relationships that existed between themselves and their earlier socializers, particularly with their home and their adolescent peer group. Travel, new relationships, military service, marriage, and, of course, college studies have been the traditional avenues for disengagement from the family. Each involves new or modified roles that require and foster greater resourcefulness.

That said, for today's traditional-age students, and perhaps for many nontraditional-age students, the recession that began in 2007–2008 has altered in significant ways their ability to disengage from their families. The inability to secure substantial employment has forced

---

Key Terms

life span The maximum number of years that humans are capable of living.

life expectancy The average number of years that members of a cohort can expect to live.

life course The path that people follow through life, or a road map or blueprint of that map.

lifestyle A personalized version of the life course of an individual, cohort, or generation.

life fable The "story" of a person's life, as written and directed by that person.

traditional-age students College students between the ages of 18 and 24.

nontraditional-age students An administrative term used by colleges and universities for students who, for whatever reason, are pursuing undergraduate work at an age other than that associated with the traditional college years (18–24).

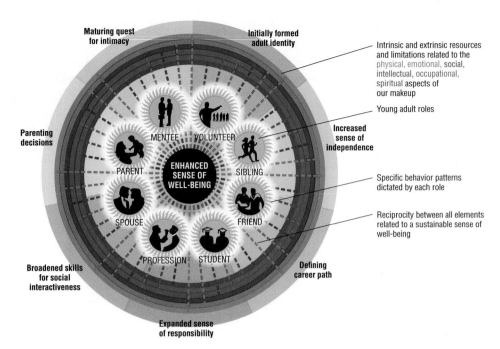

Figure 1-1 Young Adult
Developmental Tasks and Roles

Maturing quest
for intimacy

Initially formed
adult identity

Intrinsic and extrinsic resources
and limitations related to the
physical, emotional, social,
intellectual, occupational,
spiritual aspects of
our makeup

Young adult roles

Parenting
decisions

Increased
sense of
independence

MENTEE   VOLUNTEER

PARENT   ENHANCED
SENSE OF
WELL-BEING   SIBLING

Specific behavior patterns
dictated by each role

SPOUSE   FRIEND

Reciprocity between all elements
related to a sustainable sense of
well-being

PROFESSION   STUDENT

Broadened skills
for social
interactiveness

Defining
career path

Expanded sense
of responsibility

many to return home and seek financial support from parents in order to sustain a sense of independence until a more sustainable form of independence can be achieved.

Assuming Responsibility Our society's third developmental expectation for traditional-age college students is that these young adults will assume increasing levels of responsibility. Traditional-age students have a variety of opportunities, both on and off campus, to begin the process of becoming responsible for themselves and for other individuals, programs, and institutions. Central at this time is the need to assume increasing levels of responsibility in one's movement through the academic curriculum and for one's own and others' health.

Broadening Social Skills The fourth developmental task for early young adults is to broaden their range of appropriate and dependable social skills. Adulthood ordinarily involves "membership" in a variety of groups that range in size from a marital pair to a multiple-member community group or a multinational corporation. These memberships require the ability to function in many different social settings, with an array of people, and in many roles. Accomplishing this task particularly requires that young adults refine their skills in communication, listening, and conflict management. As communication is redefined by digital media, however, some people wonder if there will be a decline in communication skills overall and in face-to-face interactions in particular.

Nurturing Intimacy The task of nurturing intimacy usually begins in early young adulthood and

continues, in various forms, through much of the remainder of life. Persons of traditional college age can experience intimacy in a more mature sense, centered on deep and caring relationships, than was true during adolescence. Dating relationships, close and trusting friendships, and mentoring relationships are the arenas in which mature intimacy will take root. From a developmental perspective, what matters is that we have quality relationships involving persons with whom we share our most deeply held thoughts, feelings, and aspirations as we attempt to validate our own unique approach to life. Young adults who are unwilling or unable to create intimacy can develop a sense of emotional isolation.

Obtaining Entry-Level Employment and Developing Parenting Skills In addition to the five developmental tasks just addressed, two other areas of growth and development are applicable to young adults, but they may come into focus more gradually. They include obtaining entry-level employment within the field of one's academic preparation and developing parenting skills.

For nearly three-quarters of a century (thanks in part to the GI Bill after World War II), the majority of students have pursued a college education in anticipation that its completion would open doors (entry-level opportunities) in particular professions or fields of employment. In many respects these forms of employment meet needs beyond those associated purely with money. Employment of this nature provides opportunities to build new skills that expand upon those learned in academic majors, to undertake new forms of responsibility beyond those available on campus, and to play a more diverse set of roles, including colleague, supervisor, mentor, mentee, or partner. And today, more so than in the past, intimate relationships often have their origin in the workplace.

Although Americans are having fewer children than in past generations, parenting-related decisions and skills are often important components of the young adulthood years. Decisions regarding parenting (both biological and adoptive) involve important questions regarding age for the onset of parenting, number of children, and intervals between subsequent children, as well as the manner in which parenting will be undertaken and the role it will play relative to the overall aspirations of the adults involved. The decision not to have children may also be made, at least in preliminary form, at this time.

Middle Adulthood Developmental Expectations

Expectations for adults in middle adulthood include, among others, achieving generativity and reassessing and concluding the plans of young adulthood (Figure 1-2).

Achieving Generativity In a very real sense, people in middle adulthood are asked to do something they have not been expected to do previously. As a part of their development as unique people, they are expected to "pay back" society for the support it has given them. Most people in middle adulthood begin to realize that the collective society, through its institutions (families, schools, churches), has been generous in its support of their growth and development and that it is time to replenish these resources.[1, 2] Younger and older people may have needs that middle-aged people can best meet. By meeting the needs of others, people in middle adulthood can fulfill their own needs to grow and develop.

Generativity, a term introduced into the field of adult emotional development by psychologist Erik Erikson,[3] reflects a process in which the emotional maturation needs of middle-aged people interact with society's need to support its most vulnerable members—its children and older adults, particularly the infirm and the frail.

The process of repaying society for its support is structured around familiar types of activities. Developmentally speaking, people in middle adulthood are able to select the activities that best use their abilities to contribute to the good of society.

The most traditional way in which people in middle adulthood repay society is through parenting. Children, with their potential for becoming valuable members of the next generation, need the support of people who recognize the contribution they can make. As they extend themselves outward on behalf of the next generation, they ensure their own growth and development. In a similar fashion, their support of aging parents and institutions that serve older adults provides another means to express generativity.

For people who possess artistic talent, generativity may be accomplished through the pleasure brought to others. Volunteer work serves as another avenue for generativity. Most people in middle adulthood also express generativity through their jobs by providing quality products or services and thus contribute to the well-being of those who desire or need these goods and services.

Figure 1-2 Middle Adulthood Developmental Tasks and Roles

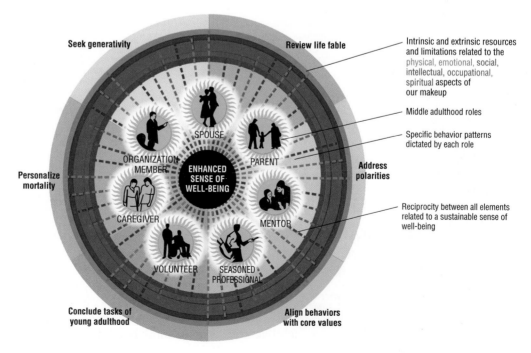

Reassessing the Plans of Young Adulthood People in middle adulthood must also begin coming to terms with the finality of their eventual death (see the box "Why Men Die Young"). In conjunction with doing this, they often feel compelled to take time to think about the goals for adulthood they formulated 25 or more years previously. Their dreams are thus revisited. This reassessment constitutes a second developmental task of people in middle adulthood.

By carefully reviewing the aspirations they had as young adults, middle-aged people can more clearly study their short- and long-term goals. Specifically, strengths and limitations that were unrecognizable when they were young adults are now more clearly seen. The inexperience of youth is replaced by the insights gained through experience. A commitment to quality often replaces the desire for quantity during the second half of the life cycle. Time is valued more highly because it is now seen in a more realistic perspective.

Older Adulthood Developmental Expectations

Expectations for adults in older adulthood include accepting the physical changes of aging, maintaining a high level of physical function, and establishing a sense of integrity (Figure 1-3).

Accepting the Changes of Aging The general decline associated with older adulthood is particularly serious between the seventh and ninth decades. Physically, emotionally, socially, intellectually, and occupationally, older adults must accept at least some decline. For example, a person may

no longer be able to drive a car, which could in turn limit participation in social activities. Even a spiritual loss may be encountered at those times when life seems less humane. A developmental task to be accomplished by the older adult is to accept the nature and extent of these changes.

Maintaining Functionality Because each segment of the life cycle should be approached with the fullest level of involvement possible, the second developmental task of the older adult is to maintain as much functionality in each segment as possible, particularly those that support independence.

For areas of decline in which some measure of reversal is possible, older adults are afforded an opportunity to seek *rehabilitation*. Whether through a self-designed and individually implemented program or with the aid of a skilled professional, older adults can bring back some function to a previously higher level.

The second approach, often used in combination with rehabilitation, is *remediation,* whereby an alternative to the area of loss is introduced, such as a hearing aid. By using alternative resources, function can often be restored.

For a growing number of older adults, rehabilitation and remediation are rarely necessary because of the high level of health that they enjoy. For most, only minor modifications are necessary to enjoy full independence.

Establishing a Sense of Integrity The third major developmental task that awaits older adults is to establish their sense of integrity, or a sense of wholeness, concerning the journey that may be nearly complete. The elderly must look back over their lives to see the value in what they were able to accomplish. They must address these

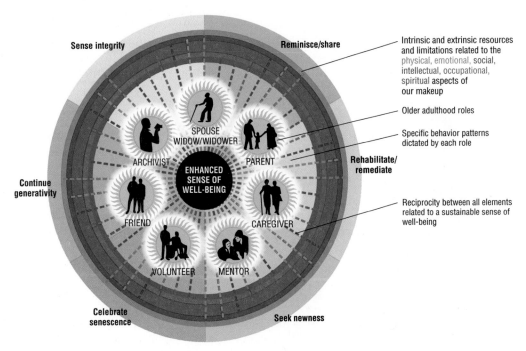

Figure 1-3 Older Adulthood Developmental Tasks and Roles

Why Men Die Young

The extra longevity of women in our society is well established. In fact, the difference in life expectancy for male and female infants born today is projected to be 80 years for females but only 75 for males. This five-year difference has commonly been attributed to genetic factors. However, new evidence demonstrates that this discrepancy may be affected more by male behavior than by genetic traits.

Men outrank women in all of the top 15 causes of death except for Alzheimer's disease. Men's death rates are twice as high for suicide, homicide, and cirrhosis of the liver. In every age group, American males have poorer health and higher risk of mortality than do females. Common increased risks include the following:

• More men than women smoke.

• Men are twice as likely to be heavy drinkers and to engage in other risky behaviors such as abusing drugs and driving without a seatbelt.

• More men work in dangerous settings than women do, and men account for 90 percent of on-the-job fatalities.

• More men drive SUVs that are rollover prone and suffer fatalities in motorcycle accidents.

Perhaps some of these increased risks are associated with deep-seated cultural beliefs, which reward men for taking risks and facing danger head-on. This "macho" attitude seems to extend to the care that men take of their own physical and mental health. Women are twice as likely to visit their doctor on an annual basis and explore preventive medical treatments than are men. Men are more likely to ignore symptoms and less likely to schedule checkups or seek follow-up treatment. Psychologically, men tend to internalize their feelings or stressors, or even self-medicate to deal with stress, while women tend to seek psychological help. Almost all stress-related diseases are more common in men.

In the final analysis, men and women alike must be responsible for their own health and well-being. By making sound choices regarding diet, exercise, medical care, and high-risk behaviors, both genders can attempt to maximize the full potential of their life expectancy.

simple but critical questions: Would I do it over again? Am I satisfied with what I managed to accomplish? Can I accept the fact that others will have experiences to which I can never return?

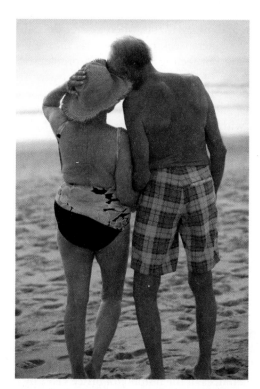

Accepting the physical changes of aging while maintaining a high level of functionality is a key developmental task for older adults.

If older adults can answer these questions positively, then they will feel a sense of wholeness, personal value, and worth. Having established this sense of integrity, they will believe that their lives have had meaning and that they have helped society.

Since they have already experienced so much, many older adults have no fear of death, even though they may fear the process of dying. Their ability to come to terms with death thus reinforces their sense of integrity.

Like all the other developmental tasks, this critical area of growth and development is a personal and, thus, a unique experience. Older adults must assume this last developmental task with the same sense of purpose they used for earlier tasks. When older adults can feel this sense of integrity, their reasons for having lived will be more fully understood.

Roles and Their Reciprocal Relationship to Developmental Tasks

Throughout life individuals are assigned or selected to assume a variety of roles and, in doing so, to assume the behavioral patterns that accompany (and define) these roles. Depending on the life stage, we experience the majority of the following roles: being a child, a sibling, a grandchild, a student, a peer group member, a team member, an employee, a significant other, a parent, an employer, a mentee or mentor, a neighbor, a community member, a grandparent, and so on. These roles are played out both privately and publicly, and they have a reciprocal relationship with the major developmental tasks of

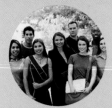

Learning from Our Diversity

Back to the Future: Nontraditional-Age Students Enrich the College Experience

To anyone who's visited a U.S. college campus in the last 20 years, it's abundantly clear that the once typical college student—White, middle class, between the ages of 18 and 24—is not always a majority on campus. In most institutions of higher learning, today's student body is a rich tapestry of color, culture, language, ability, and age. Wheelchair-accessible campuses roll out the welcome mat for students with disabilities; the air is filled with the music of a dozen or more languages spoken by students from virtually every part of the world; students in their 60s chat animatedly with classmates young enough to be their grandchildren.

Of all the trends that are changing the face of college enrollment in the United States, perhaps the most significant is the increasing diversity in the age of students now on campus. Older students today are both a common and welcome sight in colleges and universities across the country. Many women cut short their undergraduate education—or defer graduate school—to marry and raise children. Divorcees, widows, and women whose children are grown often return to college, or enroll for the first time, to prepare for professional careers. And increasingly, both men and women are finding it desirable, if not

essential, to further their education as a means of either keeping their current job or qualifying for a higher position.

Just as children are enriched by the knowledge and experience of their grandparents and other older relatives, so too is today's college classroom a richer place when many of the seats are filled by students of nontraditional age. Without being didactic or preachy, older students can provide valuable guidance and direction to younger classmates who may be uncertain of their career path, or who may be wrestling with decisions about marriage and parenthood. In doing so, nontraditional-age students can gain helpful insights about young people's feelings, attitudes, challenges, and aspirations.

Among the many important benefits of today's increasingly diverse college campus, surely one of the most significant is the enhanced opportunity for intergenerational communication and understanding made possible by the growing numbers of students of nontraditional age.

In your classes, how would you characterize the interactions between traditional-age students and those of nontraditional age? In what ways are they enriching one another's college experience?

---

each life stage. For example, the development of an initial adult identity may influence and be influenced by the occupational role you are able to assume. Or, as a second example, a midlife adult's growth in generativity will be influenced by her role as a parent and her pending role of a grandparent. For those in older adulthood, the interplay of earlier developmental expectations and requirements associated with roles once (or still) played may be the basis for answers to the questions posed toward the end of life: Have I played my roles well? Was my life well lived? Am I entitled to feel a sense of life satisfaction and the feeling of well-being that accompanies it?

 TALKING POINTS You are in charge of a campus event for students of various ages from several cultural groups. How would you go about finding out what would make the event attractive to students with backgrounds different from your own?

Current Definitions of Health and Approaches to Health Care

As noted at the beginning of this chapter, developmental tasks and roles cannot be carried out without some measure of good health. Ideas about what constitutes *health* have changed over the years, and many of these ideas are reflected in the various approaches to health care prevalent in our society today. We consider these approaches next.

Episodic Health Care

The vast majority of Americans use the services of professional health care providers during periods (*episodes*) of illness and injury, that is, when we are "unhealthy." We consult providers, seeking a diagnosis that will explain why we are not feeling well. Once a problem is identified, we expect to receive effective treatment from the practitioners that will lead to our recovery (the absence of illness) and thus a return to health. If we are willing to comply with the care strategies prescribed by our practitioners, we should soon be able to define ourselves as "healthy" once again.

The familiarity of episodic health care is evident in the 994 million times that Americans visited physicians during 2009.[4] Although some of these visits were for preventive health care (see discussion in the following section), the vast majority were in conjunction with illness. When viewed according to racial group, approximately 46.2 percent of Whites, 46.8 percent of Blacks, 44.3 percent of Hispanics/Latinos, 50.1 percent of American Indians or Alaskan Natives, 50.6 percent of Asians, and 41.4 percent of multiracial persons made at least one to three visits to the office of a primary care physician. When viewed collectively, 13.2 percent of all Americans over the age of 18 made 10 or more visits.

Differences in the number of office visits by race are most likely related to a combination of factors, including differences in the types and extent of illnesses within specific racial groups, health insurance or ability to pay for health care services, proximity to services, availability of dependable transportation, and personal and cultural practices related to illness.

Of the many office visits made in 2009, women were more likely to visit physicians than were men, and infants and persons over 65 were twice as likely to visit physicians than were older children, adolescents, and adults under age 65.

When office visits are viewed in terms of the types of physicians visited, primary care physicians (general medicine, family practice, general internal medicine, pediatrics, and gynecology) accounted for the majority of visits while surgeons and other specialists accounted for the remainder. Usually, surgeons and specialists become involved in a patient's care only after a referral from a primary care physician.

Preventive/Prospective Medicine

Simple logic would seem to suggest that it makes more sense to prevent illness than to deal with it through episodic health (medical) care. This philosophy characterizes **preventive, or prospective, medicine**. Unfortunately, however, many physicians say they have little time to practice preventive medicine because of the large number of episodically sick people who fill their offices every day.

When physicians do practice preventive or prospective medicine, they first attempt to determine their patient's level of risk for developing particular conditions. They make this assessment by identifying **risk factors** (and **high-risk health behaviors**) with a variety of observational techniques and screening tests, some of which may be invasive (taking tissues from the body such as a biopsy or blood draw). Additionally, an important tool in assessing risk is an accurate family health history, something that over one-third of all adults cannot adequately provide to their health care providers.[5] So important is a health history that the federal government has established a website to assist us in becoming familiar with our family's health history (www.hhs.gov/familyhistory).[6] Certainly, if you identify any of the leading causes of death in your family health history, they should be shared with your primary care physician.

It is disconcerting to report that important medical information, including laboratory reports, comprehensive drug inventories, and family health histories, is often missing from medical files. A 2003 study involving primary care physician medical records suggests that perhaps one out of every seven patient files is missing information important to providing comprehensive health care.[7]

Once they have identified levels of risk in patients, health practitioners try to lower those risk levels through patient education, lifestyle modification, and, when necessary, medical intervention. Continued compliance on the part of the patients should result in a lower level of risk that will continue over the years. Note that preventive medicine is guided by practitioners, and patients are expected to be compliant with the directions they are given.

Although preventive medical care appears to be a much more sensible approach than episodic care is in reducing **morbidity** and **mortality**, third-party payers (insurance plans) traditionally have not provided adequate coverage for these services. Managed health care plans that earn a profit by preventing sickness, such as health maintenance organizations, or HMOs (see Chapter 14), should be much more receptive to the concept and practice of preventive medicine.

In recent years the belief that preventive or prospective medical care can reduce the incidence of chronic illnesses, and thus reduce the likelihood of premature death, has been clouded by conflicting results from studies involving prevention-oriented changes in lifestyle, including, among others, dietary practices, exercise protocols, smoking cessation, weight management strategies, the use of hormone supplementation, and the inclusion of spiritual practices in daily routines. This inconsistency in effectiveness is seen by many experts as being largely a methodological problem in research study design. However, when viewed from a cost-benefit perspective, there is now some concern that preventive (prospective) medicine may be less cost effective than treating some chronic conditions in a more episodic manner.[8, 9] Regardless, when successful, this form of health care provides people with a personal sense of **empowerment** that is always a useful resource for leading a healthy, productive, and satisfying life.[10]

In their efforts to prevent and treat chronic illnesses, the scientific and medical fields have most recently moved into two new areas: personalized medicine and

Key Terms

preventive/prospective medicine Physician-centered medical care in which areas of risk for chronic illnesses are identified so that they might be lowered.

risk factor A biomedical index such as serum cholesterol level or a behavioral pattern such as smoking associated with a chronic illness.

high-risk health behavior A behavioral pattern, such as smoking, associated with a high risk of developing a chronic illness.

morbidity Pertaining to illness and disease.

mortality Pertaining to death.

empowerment The nurturing of an individual's or group's ability to be responsible for their own health and well-being.

regenerative medicine. **Personalized medicine** uses the newly established understanding of the human genome and associated technology to identify genetic markers that suggest predispositions for future illnesses. With such knowledge, focused planning can be implemented, even if no successful intervention or cure currently exists. Such knowledge can also be used to determine the treatment that may be most effective in a particular patient.[11]

A second emerging form of medical care is **regenerative medicine,** which uses stem cell technology to grow replacement body tissues and structures. In recent years a wide array of tissues and structures have been fabricated, including an outer ear, portions of corneas, skin, dental materials, and a urinary bladder. Tissue engineering holds promise for the future, but applications are limited by the extreme complexity of major organs and organ systems.[12]

Health Promotion—Personal and Collective Empowerment

High-level health is more likely to be obtained and maintained by people who have been exposed to the knowledge, behaviors, and attitudes required in adopting a health-enhancing approach to living. Whether these "tools" for better health are sought out by an individual or developed by a group of people working as a "learning community," they become the resources reflected in the term *empowerment*. Empowered persons, individually or collectively, are now active participants in their own health enhancement quest. Health promotion specialists have played an active role in leading people in this process.

Individually Oriented Health Promotion Throughout the United States, YMCA/YWCA-sponsored wellness programs, commercial fitness clubs, and corporate fitness centers offer risk-reduction programs under the direction of qualified instructors, many of whom are university graduates in disciplines such as exercise science, wellness management, and **health promotion.** Using approaches similar to those employed in preventive medicine, these nonphysician health professionals attempt to guide their clients toward activities and behaviors that will lower their risk of chronic illness. Unlike preventive medicine, with its sometimes invasive assessment procedures and medication-based therapies, health promotion programs are not legally defined as medical practices and thus do not require the involvement of physicians. In addition, the fitness focus, social interaction, and healthy lifestyle orientation these programs provide tend to mask the emphasis on preventing chronic illness that would be the selling point of such efforts if they were undertaken as preventive medicine. In fact, it is likely that people receiving health promotion

in these settings do not recognize it as such. Rather, they are very often submitting to assessments and listening to health-related information only as incidental parts of personal goals, such as losing weight, preparing for their first marathon, or simply meeting friends for lunch-hour basketball.

Group-Oriented Health Promotion In addition to the practices just described, a group-oriented form of health promotion is offered in many communities. This approach to improving health through risk reduction is directed at empowering community groups, such as church congregations or neighborhood associations, so they can develop, operate, and financially sustain their own programs with little direct involvement of health promotion specialists. Most often these community-based programs are initially funded by small governmental grants and, upon becoming self-funded, may have very small costs per person served. For example, one particular program, "Shape Up Somerville," was able to improve the nutritional quality of the local school's lunch program in a sustainable and cost-effective manner.[13]

Empowerment programs have produced positive health consequences for groups that traditionally have been underserved by the health care system, such as minority populations. Once such people are given needed information, inroads into the political process, and skills for accessing funding sources, they become better able to plan, implement, and operate programs tailored to their unique health needs.

Wellness

In recent years, the focus of the health care system has expanded to include **wellness.** Practitioners describe wellness as a process of extending information, counseling, assessment, and lifestyle-modification strategies, leading to a desirable change in the recipients' overall lifestyle, or the adoption of a wellness lifestyle. Once adopted, the wellness lifestyle produces a sense of well-being that in turn enables recipients to unlock their full potential (see the box "Factors That Influence Health and Well-Being").

Although wellness appears to differ from episodic health care, preventive/prospective medicine, and health promotion because of its lack of interest in morbidity and mortality, in practice wellness programs are not all that different from other kinds of health care. Wellness programs, as carried out on college campuses, in local hospital wellness centers, and in corporate settings, routinely transmit familiar health-related information and engage in the same risk-reduction activities that characterize preventive/prospective medicine and health promotion. The wellness movement would appear to

Factors That Influence Health and Well-Being

Research conducted by Canadian Ronald Labonte identified four arenas from which conditions beneficial to higher-level health and a sense of well-being arose. The conclusion was that when these conditions were experienced simultaneously, they led to an enhanced quality of life, higher levels of functioning, and a sense of well-being. Although not conducted in this country, the research would most likely be applicable to health and wellness in the United States.

Protective Factors

Healthy conditions and environments	Psychosocial factors	Effective health services	Healthy lifestyles
Safe physical environments	Participation in civic activities and social engagement	Provision of preventative services	Decreased use of tobacco and drugs
Supportive economic and social conditions	Strong social networks	Access to culturally appropriate health services	Regular physical activity
Regular supply of nutritious food and water	Feeling of trust	Community participation in the planning and delivery of health services	Balanced nutritional intake
Restricted access to tobacco and drugs	Feeling of power and control over life decisions		Positive mental health
Healthy public policy and organizational practice	Supportive family structure		Safe sexual activity
Provision for meaningful, paid employment	Positive self-esteem		
Provision of affordable housing			

Quality of life, functional independence, well-being

Source: Labonte R, *A Community Development Approach to Health Promotion: A Background Paper on Practice Tensions, Strategic Models, and Accountability Requirements for Health Authority Work on the Broad Determinants of Health,* Health Education Board of Scotland, Research Unit on Health and Behaviour Change, University of Edinburgh, Edinburgh, 1998. © NHS Health Scotland, 1998.

---

be health promotion being carried out under a different label.

In short, all the approaches to health care considered here—episodic health care, preventive/prospective health care, health promotion, and wellness—are concerned with morbidity and premature mortality (curing or managing illness and extending life) and thus reinforce our traditional definitions of health. Our *health care system* is in fact a *medical care system*. If a true health care system were to exist, it would have to be much more broadly based and less medically oriented. This proposition is discussed in more detail at the end of the chapter.

A Federal Program to Improve the Health of the American People

Health care professionals are not the only ones with concerns about health and health care; the government is also involved. It is well known that the American people face numerous health-related challenges. Among them are the adult-onset chronic conditions that constitute the leading causes of death in the United States, including heart disease, cancer, stroke, and diabetes. In response

to these concerns, the U.S. government has launched the Healthy People initiative, setting national health goals focused on preventing disease and improving people's quality of life.[14] The latest version, *Healthy People 2020,* was released in 2010. The report envisions "a society in which all people live long, healthy lives" and proposes

Key Terms

personalized medicine Uses the newly established understanding of the human genome and associated technology to identify genetic markers that suggest predispositions for future illnesses.

regenerative medicine Uses stem cell technology to grow replacement body tissues and structures.

health promotion A movement in which knowledge, practices, and values are transmitted to people for use in lengthening their lives, reducing the incidence of illness, and feeling better.

wellness A process intended to aid individuals in unlocking their full potential through the development of an overall wellness lifestyle.

the eventual achievement of the following broad national health objectives:

- *Eliminate preventable disease, disability, injury, and premature death.* This objective involves activities such as taking more concrete steps to prevent diseases and injuries among individuals and groups, promoting healthy lifestyle choices, improving the nation's preparedness for emergencies, and strengthening the public health infrastructure.

- *Achieve health equity, eliminate disparities, and improve the health of all groups.* This objective involves identifying, measuring, and addressing health differences between individuals or groups that result from a social or economic disadvantage.

- *Create social and physical environments that promote good health for all.* This objective involves implementing health interventions at many different levels (such as anti-smoking campaigns by schools, workplaces, and local agencies), improving the situation of undereducated and poor Americans by providing a broader array of educational and job opportunities, and actively developing healthier living and natural environments for everyone.

- *Promote healthy development and healthy behaviors across every stage of life.* This objective involves taking a cradle-to-grave approach to health promotion by encouraging disease prevention and healthy behaviors in Americans of all ages.

As can be seen, the Healthy People initiative is a broadly conceived health promotion campaign with a focus on curing, managing, and preventing disease and extending life, as well as improving the quality of life for all Americans.

Improving Health Through Planned Behavior Change

Although some health concerns can be successfully addressed through local, state, or national efforts such as those just outlined, most are ultimately based on the willingness and ability of persons to change aspects of their own behavior. However, for many people health-related behavior change proves difficult or even impossible to make.

Why Behavior Change Is Often Difficult

Several factors can strongly influence a person's desire to change high-risk health behaviors, including these:

1. A person must know that a particular behavioral pattern is clearly associated with (or even causes) a particular health problem. For example: cigarette smoking is the primary cause of lung cancer.
2. A person must believe (accept) that a behavioral pattern will make (or has made) him susceptible to this particular health problem. For example: my cigarette smoking will significantly increase my risk of developing lung cancer.
3. A person must recognize that risk-reduction intervention strategies exist and that should she adopt these in a compliant manner she too will reduce her risk for a particular health condition. For example: smoking-cessation programs exist, and following such a program could help me quit smoking.
4. A person must believe that benefits of newly adopted health-enhancing behaviors will be more reinforcing than the behaviors being given up. For example: the improved health, lowered risk, and freedom from dependence resulting from no longer smoking are better than the temporary pleasures provided by smoking.
5. A person must feel that significant others in his life truly want him to alter his high-risk health behaviors and will support his efforts. For example: my friends who are cigarette smokers will make a concerted effort to not smoke in my presence and will help me avoid being around people who smoke.

When one or more of these conditions is not in place, the likelihood that persons will be successful in reducing health-risk behaviors is greatly diminished.

The Transtheoretical Model of Health Behavior Change

The process of behavioral change unfolds over time and progresses through defined stages. James Prochaska, John Norcross, and Carlo DiClemente outlined six predictable stages of change. They studied thousands of individuals who were changing long-standing problem behaviors such as alcohol abuse, smoking, and gambling. While these people used different strategies to change their behavior, they all proceeded through six consistent stages of change in the process referred to as the **Transtheoretical Model of Health Behavior Change.**[15]

Precontemplation Stage   The first stage of change is called *precontemplation*, during which a person is not thinking about making a change and may not be aware there is a problem. For example, during this phase a smoker might have just started smoking, may be unaware of the serious health risks, or may not realize he or she is addicted.

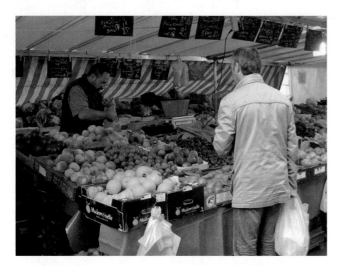

People can improve their health through planned behavior change. As part of a plan to improve his eating habits, this man shops for healthy foods.

Contemplation Stage   For many, however, progress toward change begins as they move into a *contemplation* stage, during which they might develop the desire to change but have little understanding of how to go about it. Typically they see themselves taking action within the next six months. For example: when the semester is finished and my stress level is lower, I'll start the stop-smoking program that I have material about.

Preparation Stage   Following the contemplation stage, a *preparation* stage begins, during which change begins to appear to be not only desirable but possible as well. A smoker might begin making plans to quit during this stage, setting a quit date for the very near future (a few days to a month) and perhaps enrolling in a smoking-cessation program. For example: this is the last weekend of my "smoking career"—on Monday I plan to get started.

Action Stage   Plans for change are implemented during the *action* stage, during which changes are made and sustained for a period of about six months.

Maintenance Stage   The fifth stage is the *maintenance* stage, during which new habits are consolidated and practiced for an additional six months. For example: I think that I'm almost home, but I better continue paying attention to my maintenance plan for a bit longer—returning to the bar scene too soon could be my downfall.

Termination Stage   The sixth and final stage is called *termination,* which refers to the point at which new habits are well established, and so efforts to change are complete.

Health: More Than the Absence of Illness

What exactly is health? Is it simply the absence of disease and illness, as Western medicine has held for centuries—or is it something more?

Rather routinely, national news magazines (and other media) feature articles describing advances in modern medicine. These articles describe vividly in words and images the impressive progress being made in fields such as drug research, gene manipulation, robotic-aided surgery, and the role of diet in health. Because of articles like these that relate health to medical care, most of us continue to hold to our traditional perception of health as (1) the virtual absence of disease and illness (low levels of morbidity) and (2) the ability to live a long life (reduced risk of mortality). However, in striving to be fully "health educated" in the new century, perhaps we need to consider a much broader definition that more accurately reflects the demands associated with becoming functional and satisfied persons as we transition through each adult stage of life—*young adulthood, middle adulthood,* and, finally, *older adulthood.* With this in mind, look forward to another definition of health—one that recognizes the importance of the more familiar definitions of health but is focused on the requirements of a life well lived.

The Multiple Dimensions of Health

Earlier in the chapter we promised to give you a new definition of health that would be less focused on morbidity (illness) and mortality (death) than most others are. However, before we present that new definition, we introduce here a *multidimensional concept of health* (**holistic health**)—a requirement for any definition of health that moves beyond the cure/prevention of illness and the postponement of death.

Although our modern medical care community too frequently acts as if the structure and the function of the physical body are the sole basis of health, common experience supports the validity of a holistic nature to health. In this section we examine six components, or dimensions, of health, all interacting in a synergistic manner allowing us to engage in the wide array of daily role-related activities (see Figures 1-1, 1-2, and 1-3).

Physical Dimension

Most of us have a number of physiological and structural characteristics we can call on to aid us in accomplishing the wide array of activities that characterize a typical day and, on occasion, a not-so-typical day. Among these physical characteristics are our body weight, visual ability, strength, coordination, level of endurance, level of susceptibility to disease, and powers of recuperation. In certain situations the physical dimension of health may be the most important. This importance almost certainly is why traditional medicine for centuries has equated health with the design and operation of the body.

Emotional Dimension

We also possess certain emotional characteristics that can help us through the demands of daily living. The emotional dimension of health encompasses our ability to see the world in a realistic manner, cope with stress, remain flexible, and compromise to resolve conflict.

For young adults, growth and development often give rise to emotional vulnerability, which may lead to feelings of rejection and failure that can reduce productivity and satisfaction. To some extent we are all affected by feeling states, such as anger, happiness, fear, empathy, guilt, love, and hate. People who consistently try to improve their emotional health appear to enjoy life to a much greater extent than do those who let feelings of vulnerability overwhelm them or block their creativity.

Social Dimension

A third dimension of health encompasses social skills and cultural sensitivity. Initially, family interactions, school experiences, and peer group interactions foster development in these areas, but future social interactions will demand additional skills development and refinement of already existing skills and insights. In adulthood, including young adulthood, the composition of the social world changes, principally because of our exposure to a wider array of people and the expanded roles associated with employment, parenting, and community involvement.

The importance of the social dimension of health, in terms of a sense of well-being, cannot be understated. Most succinct is the declining number of confidants that the typical American possesses. Whether called "friends," "best friends," or "trusted friends," these may

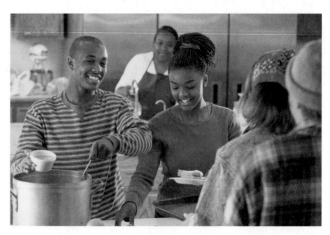

Community service—such as volunteering at a homeless shelter—can be a way to express personal values and nurture the spiritual dimension of health.

be the most important persons in one's social environment. Today one out of every four American adults has no one to play this important role. In the absence of someone to confide in, both on a regular basis and during times of conflict, stress is often more frequent, of greater intensity, longer in duration, and eventually damaging to all of the dimensions of health.

Increasingly, questions are being raised regarding the ramifications of social networking.[16] As today's early young adults (and some older adults) respond positively to adding yet another person to their list of "cyberfriends," information once reserved for trusted friends is potentially placed in the hands of hundreds of other people. Academics question whether this medium, capable of reaching so many, will prove powerfully healthful or, perhaps, will serve as a detriment to sustaining traditional relationships, thus increasing the stress of living in the twenty-first century.

Intellectual Dimension

The abilities to process and act on information, clarify values and beliefs, and exercise decision-making capacity rank among the most important aspects of total health. For many college-educated persons, the intellectual dimension of health may prove to be the most important and satisfying of the six. The ability to analyze, synthesize, hypothesize, and then act on new information enhances the quality of life in multiple ways.

Spiritual Dimension

The fifth dimension of health is the spiritual dimension. Although certainly it includes religious beliefs and practices, many young adults would expand it to encompass more diverse belief systems, including relationships with other living things, the nature of human behavior, and the need and willingness to serve others (see the box "How Does Spirituality Affect Your Life?"). All are important components of spiritual health.

The extent to which the American public professes a personal relationship with God or some form of supernatural power source is frequently assessed by the academic community. In a study by sociologists at Baylor University, which used data supplied by the Pew Research Center, interesting findings emerged. Analysis of these data indicated that approximately 93 percent of the adults sampled attended services or participated in activities focusing on religion or the enhancement of spiritual understanding. Further, among those who reported believing in God, four prevailing perceptions of God's nature emerged—an authoritarian God, a benevolent God, a critical God, or a distant God.[17] These perceptions to a large extent influence the nature of the believers' relationship with God—and perhaps their daily relationships with others within the home, school, and community. Further, believers' views of God's personality would also affect their views on important questions regarding issues such as gay marriage, the role of faith-based programs in the delivery of government-financed services, abortion, and stem cell research—and even the question of whose side God is on during times of war. Subsequent study of the original interviews and a more recent second group of interviews found that respondents were nearly equally divided on the God-view they held—28 percent identified with the authoritative God view, 22 percent with the benevolent God view, 21 percent with the critical God view, and 34 percent with the distant God view; 5 percent of the sample were atheist or agnostic.[18] A 2007 study of young adults ages 18–29 reported that living a very religious life was identified as important by 15 percent of those interviewed. Being a good parent, having a happy marriage, helping others, and owning a home were ranked higher.[19]

For those persons for whom a theist-based perception of life's meaning is repugnant, lacking in validity, or just not of importance, other paths could be capable of providing a sense of meaning of and direction for living. Typically college and university campuses are excellent arenas for finding programs, sources of information, and kindred spirits devoted to spiritual growth in the absence of a religious orientation.

Occupational Dimension

In today's world employment and productive efforts play an increasingly important role in how we perceive ourselves and how we see the "goodness" of the world in which we live. In addition, the workplace serves as both a testing ground for and a source of life-enhancing skills. In our place of employment, we gain not only the financial resources to meet our demands for both necessities and luxuries but also an array of useful skills such

Discovering Your Spirituality

How Does Spirituality Affect Your Life?

Spirituality or faith can include religious practice, but it can also be quite distinct from it. Spirituality is the most fundamental stage in the human quest for the meaning of life. It's a developing focus of the total person that gives purpose and meaning to life.

By the time people reach college age, their spirituality or faith may have already placed them in uncomfortable situations. Taking seriously their responsibility for their own commitments, lifestyles, beliefs, and attitudes, they've had to make some difficult personal decisions. This demands objectivity and a certain amount of independence. It requires finding a balance between personal aspirations and a developing sense of service to others. Finally, actual behavioral choices can be conflicted by religiously related issues. The following examples depict such situations:

- A newly developing dating relationship that triggers religiously based intolerance on the part of one partner's parents
- The momentary uncertainty of wishing your professors either Merry Christmas or, rather, the more secular Happy Holidays, or saying nothing at all
- A decision to fast for Ramadan, or to set it aside, in fear that midday lethargy could negatively affect your energy level during the days on which you have your fullest schedule of classes
- Being the only Jewish student attending a small, church-affiliated, college

as conflict resolution, experiences in shared responsibility, and intellectual growth that can be used to facilitate a wide range of nonemployment-related interactions. In turn, the workplace is enhanced by the healthfulness of the individuals who contribute to its endeavors.

Environmental Dimension

Some academics would add to the dimensions just discussed an *environmental dimension*. If this dimension is defined on the basis of land, air, and water, then it might be an additional dimension to consider. However, should the environmental dimension be extended to include all that is material and metaphysical surrounding each individual, such a concept seems beyond the scope of this chapter. Thus, we have elected not to expand the number of holistic dimensions of health beyond those traditionally discussed.

A New Definition of Health

Now that we have considered a wide range of topics and themes related to health and well-being, we are ready to propose a new definition of health. This new view is far less centered in morbidity and mortality concerns than are the traditional concepts of health drawn from episodic and preventive/prospective medicine, health promotion, and even wellness. The definition that we propose takes into account a full range of factors and considerations, and it distinguishes between *what health is for* (its role) and *what health is* (its composition).

The role of health in our lives is very similar to the role of a car. Much as a car (or other vehicle) takes us to places we need to be, good health enables us to accomplish the activities that transition us into and through the developmental tasks associated with each stage of adulthood and allows us to fulfill role requirements.

The composition of health can be seen as being more than simply having a body free of illness and apparently destined for a long life. Rather, the composition of health is that of a collection of resources, from each dimension of health, determined to be necessary for the successful accomplishment of activities that you need or want to do. Some of these needed resources are already within you (intrinsic), whereas others need to come from outside (extrinsic). Regardless of their origin, however, these resources must be directed toward the behaviors that lead to the fulfillment of role-required behavioral patterns. To recognize what resources are needed, you must be a student of society's expectations for persons of your age, such as those developmental tasks identified for early, middle, and older adulthood, and the role-related behavioral patterns that ensure both role functionality and, eventually, your claim to task mastery. Successful completion of a decades-long trip through life requires that the predictable expectations of society have been called to your attention so that your own unique approach to meeting these expectations is both personally satisfying and deemed adequately functional by society.

By combining the role of health with the composition of health, we are able to arrive at a new definition of **health:** a reflection of the ability to use and apply both the intrinsic and extrinsic resources related to each dimension of our holistic makeup to (1) participate fully in the activities that sustain role fulfillment, (2) foster the mastery of developmental expectations, and (3) experience a sense of well-being as we evaluate our progress through life.

Standards by which people measure their progress through life often include their own predetermined aspirations, performance demonstrated by comparable others (often peers or older siblings), the expectations of significant others (parents, employers, spouses), standards held by societal institutions, available demographic standards (starting salary, size and cost of first home), or even for some, God's expectations. Regardless, this comparative process often forms the nature of our "sense of well-being" and later in life, after a final self-assessment, "a sense of life satisfaction based on a life well-lived."

Key Terms

health A reflection of the ability to use and apply both the intrinsic and extrinsic resources related to each dimension of our holistic makeup to (1) participate fully in the activities that sustain role fulfillment, (2) foster the mastery of developmental expectations, and (3) experience a sense of well-being as we evaluate our progress through life.

Taking Charge of Your Health

- Complete the Comprehensive Health Assessment on pages 19–28. Develop a plan to modify your behavior in the areas in which you need improvement.

- Take part in a new spiritual activity, such as meditating, creating art or music, or attending a religious service.

- To promote the social dimension of your health, try to meet one new person each week during the semester.

- Choose one developmental task you would like to focus on, such as assuming responsibility, and plan the steps you can follow to progress in this area.

- Volunteer to be an assistant in a community service program, such as a literacy project or a preschool program.

SUMMARY

- Each life stage involves a set of personal developmental tasks that are common to all people yet may be undertaken differently by each individual. Young adulthood is characterized by five key developmental tasks: forming an initial adult identity, establishing independence, assuming responsibility, broadening social skills, and nurturing intimacy.
- Developmental tasks of middle adulthood include achieving generativity and reassessing the plans of young adulthood. Developmental tasks of older adulthood include maintaining functionality and establishing a sense of integrity.
- When we seek the services of medical care practitioners because of symptoms of illness or disease, we are said to be seeking episodic health care.
- Preventive/prospective medical care attempts to minimize the incidence of illness and disease by identifying early indicators of risk to bring them under control.
- Individual-centered health promotion involves risk-reduction activities similar to those used in preventive medical care, except that the techniques cannot be invasive and are directed by professionals who are not physicians. Its most visible emphasis tends to be on fitness and body composition.
- Group-centered health promotion involves the empowerment of individuals collectively so that they can organize and participate in their own health promotion activities.
- The wellness model emphasizes living a wellness lifestyle that leads to a sense of well-being.
- The Healthy People initiative is a U.S. government program that sets national health goals.
- A decision to change a health behavior is often difficult to make because of the multiplicity of factors underlying the maintenance of the high-risk behavior.
- Health behavior change requires movement through a multistaged process, including precontemplation, contemplation, preparation, action, maintenance, and termination.
- Current multidimensional definitions of health may include many or all of the following dimensions: physical, emotional, social, intellectual, spiritual, and occupational.
- Our new definition of health includes the role of health and the composition of health. The role of health is to enable individuals to participate in the activities that transition them into and through the developmental tasks associated with each stage of adulthood and allow them to fulfill role requirements. The composition of health is the intrinsic and extrinsic resources on which individuals can draw to participate fully in their own growth and development.

REVIEW QUESTIONS

1. What is meant by the terms *life span, life expectancy, life course, lifestyle,* and *life fable?*
2. What are the five developmental tasks of young adulthood, and how can the accomplishing of one influence the accomplishing of any of the remaining four?
3. What is implied by the statement "growth and development are predictable yet unique"?
4. What is the most likely route that midlife adults will take in their quest for a sense of generativity?
5. What are morbidity and mortality, and how are they involved in the more traditional definitions of health?
6. In preventive/prospective medical care, who determines a person's level of risk and decides what risk-reduction techniques should be implemented?
7. What does the term *empowerment* mean, and how would it appear as a component of a group-centered community-based health promotion program?
8. What factors could underlie the inability or unwillingness of persons to change their health behavior?
9. What are the six stages that persons pass through as they consider and then attempt to change their health behavior?
10. What are the most frequently included dimensions of a holistically centered definition of health?
11. What is meant by the role of health? The composition of health?
12. How does our definition of health differ from traditional definitions?
13. Why is it necessary to understand developmental expectations and their relationship to roles before we can answer the question "Are you healthy (resourceful) enough to . . . ?"

ANSWERS TO THE "WHAT DO YOU KNOW?" QUIZ

1. False   2. True   3. True   4. False   5. False   6. False   7. True

Visit the Online Learning Center (**www.mhhe.com/hahn11e**), where you will find tools to help you improve your grade, including practice quizzes, key terms flashcards, audio chapter summaries for your MP3 player, and many other study aids.

SOURCE NOTES

1. Whitbourne SK, Sneed JR, Sayer A. Psychosocial development from college through midlife: A 34-year sequential study. *Developmental Psychology,* 45(5), 1328–1340, 2009.
2. Cox KS, Wilt J, Olson B, et al. Generativity, the Big Five, and psychosocial adaptation in midlife. *Journal of Personality,* 78(4), 1185–1208, 2010.
3. Erikson EH. *The Life Cycle Completed* (extended ed.) New York: Norton, 1998.
4. Table 80. National Health Interview Survey, Family Core and Sample Adult Questionnaire (2009), CDC/NCHS. *Health, United States 2009 Web Update.* www.cdc.gov/nchs/nhis.htm.
5. Roper Center for Public Opinion Research (for Pfizer Women's Health), University of Connecticut. Adults know their family history. *USA Today,* May 30, 2000, p. 5D.
6. *U.S. Surgeon General's Family History Initiative.* Washington, DC: U.S. Department of Health and Human Services, 2004. www.hss.gov/familyhistory/download.html.
7. Smith PC, et al. Missing information during primary care visits. *Journal of the American Medical Association,* 293(5), 567–571, 2005.
8. Cohen T, Neumann P, Weinstein M. Does preventive care save money? Health economics and the presidential candidates. *New England Journal of Medicine,* 358(7), 661–663, 2008.
9. Fielding J, Husten C, Richland J. Does preventive care save money? *New England Journal of Medicine,* 368(26), 2847, 2008.
10. McKenzie JF, Nelger BL, Thackeray R. *Planning, Implementing, and Evaluating Health Promotion Programs: A Primer* (5th ed.). San Francisco: Benjamin Cummings, 2009.
11. Bloss CS, Schork NJ, Topol EJ. Effect of direct-to-consumer genome-wide profiling to assess disease risk. *New England Journal of Medicine,* 364(6), 524–534, 2011.
12. Rustad KC, Sorkin M, Longaker NT, et al. Strategies for organ level tissue engineering. *Organogenesis,* 6(3), 151–157, 2010.
13. Goldberg JP, Collins JJ, Folta SC, et al. Retooling food service for early elementary school students in Somerville, Massachusetts: the Shape Up Somerville Experience. *Prevention of Chronic Disease,* 6(3), A103, 2009.
14. U.S. Department of Health and Human Services, 2011. *Healthy People.* www.healthypeople.gov.
15. Prochaska JO, Norcross J, DiClemente C. *Changing for Good: A Revolutionary Six-Stage Program for Overcoming Bad Habits and Moving Your Life Positively Forward.* New York: Harper Paperbacks, 1995.
16. Rosen C. Virtual friendships and the new narcissism. *The New Atlantis,* 17, 15–31. Summer 2007.
17. *American Piety in the 21st Century: New Insights to the Depths and Complexity of Religion in the U.S.* Baylor Institute for Studies of Religion, Baylor University, September 2006. www.baylor.edu/isreligion/index.[jp?id=40634.
18. Froese P, Barder C. *America's Four Gods: What We Say About God—and What That Says About Us.* New York: Oxford University Press, 2010.
19. Pew Forum on Religion and Public Life. *Religion Among the Millennials. U.S. Religious Landscape Report.* February 2010. www.religious.pewforum.org/report-religious-landscape-study-full/pdf.

Comprehensive Health Assessment

Now that you have read the first chapter, complete the following Comprehensive Health Assessment. We strongly suggest that you retake this assessment after you have completed your health course. Then compare your responses in each section of the assessment. Have your scores improved?

Social and Occupational Health	Not true/ rarely	Somewhat true/ sometimes	Mostly true/ usually	Very true/ always
1. I feel loved and supported by my family.	1	2	3	(4)
2. I establish friendships with ease and enjoyment.	1	(2)	3	4
3. I establish friendships with people of both genders and all ages.	1	(2)	3	4
4. I sustain relationships by communicating with and caring about my family and friends.	1	2	(3)	4
5. I feel comfortable and confident when meeting people for the first time.	1	(2)	3	4
6. I practice social skills to facilitate the process of forming new relationships.	1	(2)	3	4
7. I seek opportunities to meet and interact with new people.	1	(2)	3	4
8. I talk with, rather than at, people.	1	2	3	(4)
9. I am open to developing or sustaining intimate relationships.	1	2	3	(4)
10. I appreciate the importance of parenting the next generation and am committed to supporting it in ways that reflect my own resources.	1	2	(3)	4
11. I recognize the strengths and weaknesses of my parents' child-rearing skills and feel comfortable modifying them if I choose to become a parent.	1	2	(3)	4
12. I attempt to be tolerant of others whether or not I approve of their behavior or beliefs.	1	2	(3)	4
13. I understand and appreciate the contribution that cultural diversity makes to the quality of living.	1	2	(3)	4
14. I understand and appreciate the difference between being educated and being trained.	1	2	3	(4)
15. My work gives me a sense of self-sufficiency and an opportunity to contribute.	1	2	(3)	4
16. I have equal respect for the roles of leader and subordinate within the workplace.	1	2	(3)	4
17. I have chosen an occupation that suits my interests and temperament.	1	2	(3)	4
18. I have chosen an occupation that does not compromise my physical or psychological health.	1	2	3	(4)
19. I get along well with my coworkers most of the time.	1	2	(3)	4
20. When I have a disagreement with a coworker, I try to resolve it directly and constructively.	1	2	(3)	4

POINTS _60_

Social and Psychological Health	Not true/ rarely	Somewhat true/ sometimes	Mostly true/ usually	Very true/ always
1. I have a deeply held belief system or personal theology.	1	2	3	(4)
2. I recognize the contribution that membership in a community of faith or spirituality can make to a person's overall quality of life.	1	2	3	(4)
3. I seek experiences with nature and reflect on nature's contribution to my quality of life.	1	2	(3)	4
4. My spirituality is a resource that helps me remain calm and strong during times of stress.	1	2	(3)	4
5. I have found appropriate ways to express my spirituality.	1	2	(3)	4
6. I respect the diversity of spiritual expression and am tolerant of those whose beliefs differ from my own.	1	2	(3)	4
7. I take adequate time to reflect on my own life and my relationships with others and the institutions of society.	1	2	(3)	4
8. I routinely undertake new experiences.	1	(2)	3	4
9. I receive adequate support from others.	1	2	(3)	4
10. I look for opportunities to support others, even occasionally at the expense of my own goals and aspirations.	1	2	(3)	4
11. I recognize that emotional and psychological health are as important as physical health.	1	2	3	(4)
12. I express my feelings and opinions comfortably, yet am capable of keeping them to myself when appropriate.	1	2	(3)	4
13. I see myself as a person of worth and feel comfortable with my own strengths and limitations.	1	(2)	3	4
14. I establish realistic goals and work to achieve them.	1	2	(3)	4
15. I understand the differences between the normal range of emotions and the signs of clinical depression.	1	2	3	(4)
16. I recognize signs of suicidal thoughts and am willing to intervene.	1	2	(3)	4
17. I regularly assess my own behavior patterns and beliefs and would seek professional assistance for any emotional dysfunction.	1	(2)	3	4
18. I accept the reality of aging and view it as an opportunity for positive change.	1	2	3	(4)
19. I accept the reality of death and view it as a normal and inevitable part of life.	1	2	3	(4)
20. I have made decisions about my own death to ensure that I die with dignity when the time comes.	1	(2)	3	4

POINTS _62_

Stress Management	Not true/ rarely	Somewhat true/ sometimes	Mostly true/ usually	Very true/ always
1. I accept the reality of change while maintaining the necessary stability in my daily activities.	1	2	(3)	4
2. I seek change when it is necessary or desirable to do so.	1	2	(3)	4
3. I know what stress-management services are offered on campus, through my employer, or in my community.	1	2	3	(4)
4. When necessary, I use the stress-management services to which I have access.	(1)	2	3	4

Comprehensive Health Assessment—*continued*

	Not true/ rarely	Somewhat true/ sometimes	Mostly true/ usually	Very true/ always
5. I employ stress-reduction practices in anticipation of stressful events, such as job interviews and final examinations.	1	2	(3)	4
6. I reevaluate the ways in which I handled stressful events so that I can better cope with similar events in the future.	1	2	(3)	4
7. I turn to relatives and friends during periods of disruption in my life.	1	2	3	(4)
8. I avoid using alcohol or other drugs during periods of stress.	1	(2)	(3)	4
9. I refrain from behaving aggressively or abusively during periods of stress.	1	2	3	(4)
10. I sleep enough to maintain a high level of health and cope successfully with daily challenges.	1	2	(3)	4
11. I avoid sleeping excessively as a response to stressful change.	1	2	(3)	4
12. My diet is conducive to good health and stress management.	1	(2)	3	4
13. I participate in physical activity to relieve stress.	1	2	(3)	4
14. I practice stress-management skills, such as diaphragmatic breathing and yoga.	(1)	2	3	4
15. I manage my time effectively.	1	2	(3)	4

POINTS 43

Fitness	Not true/ rarely	Somewhat true/ sometimes	Mostly true/ usually	Very true/ always
1. I participate in recreational and fitness activities both to minimize stress and to improve or maintain my level of physical fitness.	1	(2)	3	4
2. I select some recreational activities that are strenuous rather than sedentary in nature.	1	2	(3)	4
3. I include various types of aerobic conditioning activities among the wider array of recreational and fitness activities in which I engage.	1	(2)	3	4
4. I engage in aerobic activities with appropriate frequency, intensity, and duration to provide a training effect for my heart and lungs.	1	(2)	3	4
5. I routinely include strength-training activities among the wider array of fitness activities in which I engage.	1	(2)	3	4
6. I routinely vary the types of strength-training activities in which I participate in order to minimize injury and strengthen all of the important muscle groups.	1	(2)	3	4
7. I do exercises specifically designed to maintain joint range of motion.	1	(2)	3	4
8. I believe that recreational and fitness activities can help me improve my physical health and my emotional and social well-being.	1	2	3	(4)
9. I include a variety of fitness activities in my overall plan for physical fitness.	1	(2)	3	4
10. I take appropriate steps to avoid injuries when participating in recreational and fitness activities.	1	(2)	3	4
11. I seek appropriate treatment for all injuries that result from fitness activities.	1	(2)	3	4

	Not true/ rarely	Somewhat true/ sometimes	Mostly true/ usually	Very true/ always
12. I believe that older adults should undertake appropriately chosen fitness activities.	1	2	3	(4)
13. My body composition is consistent with a high level of health.	1	2	(3)	4
14. I warm up before beginning vigorous activity, and I cool down afterward.	1	(2)	3	4
15. I select properly designed and well-maintained equipment and clothing for each activity.	1	2	(3)	4
16. I avoid using performance-enhancing substances that are known to be dangerous and those whose influence on the body is not fully understood.	1	2	3	(4)
17. I sleep seven to eight hours daily.	1	2	(3)	4
18. I refrain from using over-the-counter sleep-inducing aids.	1	2	3	(4)
19. I follow sound dietary practices as an important adjunct to a health-enhancing physical activity program.	1	(2)	3	4
20. My current level of fitness allows me to participate fully and with reasonable comfort in my daily activities.	1	2	(3)	4

POINTS _53_

Nutrition and Weight Management

	Not true/ rarely	Somewhat true/ sometimes	Mostly true/ usually	Very true/ always
1. I balance my caloric intake with my caloric expenditure.	(1)	2	3	4
2. I obtain the recommended number of servings from each of the newly adopted "food plate."	(1)	2	3	4
3. I select a wide variety of foods from each area on the "food plate."	(1)	2	3	4
4. I understand the amount of a particular food that constitutes a single serving.	1	2	3	(4)
5. I often try new foods, particularly when I know them to be healthful.	(1)	2	3	4
6. I select breads, cereals, fresh fruits, and vegetables in preference to pastries, candies, sodas, and fruits canned in heavy syrup.	1	(2)	3	4
7. I limit the amount of sugar that I add to foods during preparation and at the table.	1	(2)	3	4
8. I examine food labels to determine the presence of trans fats (trans-fatty acids) and select foods free of these fats.	(1)	2	3	4
9. I select primarily nonmeat sources of protein, such as peas, beans, and peanut butter, while limiting my consumption of red meat and high-fat dairy products.	(1)	2	3	4
10. I consume an appropriate percentage of my total daily calories from protein.	1	(2)	3	4
11. I select foods prepared with unsaturated vegetable oils while reducing consumption of red meat, high-fat dairy products, and foods prepared with lard (animal fat) or butter.	(1)	2	3	4
12. I carefully limit the amount of fast food that I consume during a typical week.	1	(2)	3	4
13. I consume an appropriate percentage of my total daily calories from fat.	(1)	2	3	4
14. I select nutritious foods when I snack.	1	(2)	3	4
15. I limit my use of salt during food preparation and at the table.	1	2	(3)	4

Comprehensive Health Assessment—*continued*

	Not true/ rarely	Somewhat true/ sometimes	Mostly true/ usually	Very true/ always
16. I consume adequate amounts of fiber.	(1)	2	3	4
17. I routinely consider the nutrient density of individual food items when choosing foods.	(1)	2	3	4
18. I maintain my weight without reliance on over-the-counter or prescription diet pills.	1	2	3	(4)
19. I maintain my weight without reliance on fad diets or liquid weight loss beverages.	1	2	3	(4)
20. I exercise regularly to help maintain my weight.	1	(2)	3	4

POINTS 37

Alcohol, Tobacco, and Other Drug Use	Not true/ rarely	Somewhat true/ sometimes	Mostly true/ usually	Very true/ always
1. I abstain or drink in moderation when offered alcoholic beverages.	1	2	3	(4)
2. I abstain from using illegal psychoactive (mind-altering) drugs.	1	2	3	(4)
3. I do not consume alcoholic beverages or psychoactive drugs rapidly or in large quantities.	1	2	3	(4)
4. I do not use alcohol or psychoactive drugs in a way that causes me to behave inappropriately.	1	2	3	(4)
5. My use of alcohol or other drugs does not compromise my academic performance.	1	2	3	(4)
6. I refrain from drinking alcoholic beverages or using psychoactive drugs when engaging in recreational activities that require strength, speed, or coordination.	1	2	3	(4)
7. I refrain from drinking alcoholic beverages while participating in occupational activities, regardless of the nature of those activities.	1	2	3	(4)
8. My use of alcohol or other drugs does not generate financial concerns for myself or for others.	1	2	3	(4)
9. I refrain from drinking alcohol or using psychoactive drugs when driving a motor vehicle or operating heavy equipment.	1	2	(3)	4
10. I do not drink alcohol or use psychoactive drugs when I am alone.	1	2	(3)	4
11. I avoid riding with people who have been drinking alcohol or using psychoactive drugs.	1	2	(3)	4
12. My use of alcohol or other drugs does not cause family dysfunction.	1	2	3	(4)
13. I do not use marijuana.	1	2	3	(4)
14. I do not use hallucinogens.	1	2	3	(4)
15. I do not use heroin or other illegal intravenous drugs.	1	2	3	(4)
16. I do not experience blackouts when I drink alcohol.	1	2	3	(4)
17. I do not become abusive or violent when I drink alcohol or use psychoactive drugs.	1	2	3	(4)
18. I use potentially addictive prescription medication in complete compliance with my physician's directions.	1	2	3	(4)
19. I do not smoke cigarettes.	1	2	3	(4)
20. I do not use tobacco products in any other form.	1	2	3	(4)
21. I minimize my exposure to secondhand smoke.	1	(2)	3	4

	Not true/ rarely	Somewhat true/ sometimes	Mostly true/ usually	Very true/ always
22. I am concerned about the effect that alcohol, tobacco, and other drug use is known to have on developing fetuses.	1	2	3	(4)
23. I am concerned about the effect that alcohol, tobacco, and other drug use is known to have on the health of other people.	1	2	3	(4)
24. I seek natural, health-enhancing highs rather than relying on alcohol, tobacco, and illegal drugs.	1	2	(3)	4
25. I take prescription medication only as instructed, and I use over-the-counter medication in accordance with directions.	1	2	3	(4)

POINTS __94__

Disease Prevention

	Not true/ rarely	Somewhat true/ sometimes	Mostly true/ usually	Very true/ always
1. My diet includes foods rich in phytochemicals.	1	2	(3)	4
2. My diet includes foods rich in folic acid.	1	2	(3)	4
3. My diet includes foods that are good sources of dietary fiber.	1	2	(3)	4
4. My diet is low in dietary cholesterol.	1	(2)	3	4
5. I follow food preparation practices that minimize the risk of foodborne illness.	1	2	3	(4)
6. I engage in regular physical activity and am able to control my weight effectively.	1	(2)	(3)	4
7. I do not use tobacco products.	1	2	3	(4)
8. I abstain from alcohol or drink only in moderation.	1	2	3	(4)
9. I do not use intravenously administered illegal drugs.	1	2	3	(4)
10. I use safer sex practices intended to minimize my risk of exposure to sexually transmitted diseases, including HIV and HPV.	1	2	3	(4)
11. I take steps to limit my risk of exposure to the bacterium that causes Lyme disease and to the virus that causes hantavirus pulmonary syndrome.	1	2	(3)	4
12. I control my blood pressure with weight management and physical fitness activities.	1	2	(3)	4
13. I minimize my exposure to allergens, including those that trigger asthma attacks.	1	2	(3)	4
14. I wash my hands frequently and thoroughly.	1	2	3	(4)
15. I use preventive medical care services appropriately.	1	2	(3)	4
16. I use appropriate cancer self-screening practices, such as breast self-examination and testicular self-examination.	1	2	(3)	4
17. I know which chronic illnesses and diseases are part of my family history.	1	2	3	(4)
18. I know which inherited conditions are part of my family history and will seek preconceptional counseling regarding these conditions.	1	2	(3)	4
19. I am fully immunized against infectious diseases.	1	2	3	(4)
20. I take prescribed medications, particularly antibiotics, exactly as instructed by my physician.	1	2	3	(4)

POINTS __68__

Comprehensive Health Assessment—*continued*

Sexual Health

	Not true/ rarely	Somewhat true/ sometimes	Mostly true/ usually	Very true/ always
1. I know how sexually transmitted diseases are spread.	1	2	3	(4)
2. I can recognize the symptoms of sexually transmitted diseases.	1	2	(3)	4
3. I know how sexually transmitted disease transmission can be prevented.	1	2	3	(4)
4. I know how safer sex practices reduce the risk of contracting sexually transmitted diseases.	1	2	3	(4)
5. I follow safer sex practices.	1	2	3	(4)
6. I recognize the symptoms of premenstrual syndrome and understand how it is prevented and treated.	1	(2)	3	4
7. I recognize the symptoms of endometriosis and understand the relationship of its symptoms to hormonal cycles.	1	(2)	3	4
8. I understand the physiological basis of menopause and recognize that it is a normal part of the aging process in women.	1	2	(3)	4
9. I understand and accept the range of human sexual orientations.	1	(2)	3	4
10. I encourage the development of flexible sex roles (androgyny) in children.	1	(2)	3	4
11. I take a mature approach to dating and mate selection.	1	2	3	(4)
12. I recognize that marriage and other types of long-term relationships can be satisfying.	1	2	3	(4)
13. I recognize that a celibate lifestyle is appropriate and satisfying for some people.	1	2	(3)	4
14. I affirm the sexuality of older adults and am comfortable with its expression.	1	2	3	(4)
15. I am familiar with the advantages and disadvantages of a wide range of birth control methods.	1	2	3	(4)
16. I understand how each birth control method works and how effective it is.	1	2	3	(4)
17. I use my birth control method consistently and appropriately.	1	2	3	(4)
18. I am familiar with the wide range of procedures now available to treat infertility.	1	2	3	(4)
19. I accept that others may disagree with my feelings about pregnancy termination.	1	2	3	(4)
20. I am familiar with alternatives available to infertile couples, including adoption.	1	2	3	(4)

POINTS _69_

Safety Practices and Violence Prevention

	Not true/ rarely	Somewhat true/ sometimes	Mostly true/ usually	Very true/ always
1. I attempt to identify sources of risk or danger in each new setting or activity.	1	(2)	3	4
2. I learn proper procedures and precautions before undertaking new recreational or occupational activities.	1	(2)	3	4
3. I select appropriate clothing and equipment for all activities and maintain equipment in good working order.	1	2	(3)	4
4. I curtail my participation in activities when I am not feeling well or am distracted by other demands.	1	2	3	(4)
5. I repair dangerous conditions or report them to those responsible for maintenance.	1	2	(3)	4

	Not true/ rarely	Somewhat true/ sometimes	Mostly true/ usually	Very true/ always
6. I use common sense and observe the laws governing nonmotorized vehicles when I ride a bicycle.	1	2	③	4
7. I operate all motor vehicles as safely as possible, including using seat belts and other safety equipment.	1	2	3	④
8. I refrain from driving an automobile or boat when I have been drinking alcohol or taking drugs or medications.	1	2	3	④
9. I try to anticipate the risk of falling and maintain my environment to minimize this risk.	1	2	③	4
10. I maintain my environment to minimize the risk of fire, and I have a well-rehearsed plan to exit my residence in case of fire.	1	2	3	④
11. I am a competent swimmer and could save myself or rescue someone who was drowning.	①	2	3	4
12. I refrain from sexually aggressive behavior toward my partner or others.	1	2	3	④
13. I would report an incident of sexual harassment or date rape whether or not I was the victim.	1	2	3	④
14. I would seek help from others if I were the victim or perpetrator of domestic violence.	1	2	3	④
15. I practice gun safety and encourage other gun owners to do so.	1	2	3	④
16. I drive at all times in a way that will minimize my risk of being carjacked.	1	2	3	④
17. I have taken steps to protect my home from intruders.	1	2	③	4
18. I use campus security services as much as possible when they are available.	1	②	3	4
19. I know what to do if I am being stalked.	1	2	③	4
20. I have a well-rehearsed plan to protect myself from the aggressive behavior of other people in my place of residence.	1	2	3	④

POINTS _51_

Health Care Consumerism	Not true/ rarely	Somewhat true/ sometimes	Mostly true/ usually	Very true/ always
1. I know how to obtain valid health information.	1	2	③	4
2. I accept health information that has been deemed valid by the established scientific community.	1	2	③	4
3. I am skeptical of claims that guarantee the effectiveness of a particular health care service or product.	1	2	3	④
4. I am skeptical of practitioners or clinics who advertise or offer services at rates substantially lower than those charged by reputable providers.	1	2	③	4
5. I am not swayed by advertisements that present unhealthy behavior in an attractive manner.	1	2	3	④
6. I can afford proper medical care, including hospitalization.	①	2	3	4
7. I can afford adequate health insurance.	1	②	3	4
8. I understand the role of government health care plans in providing health care to people who qualify for coverage.	1	2	③	4
9. I know how to select health care providers who are highly qualified and appropriate for my current health care needs.	①	2	3	4
10. I seek a second or third opinion when surgery or other costly therapies are recommended.	1	2	③	4

Comprehensive Health Assessment—*continued*

	Not true/ rarely	Somewhat true/ sometimes	Mostly true/ usually	Very true/ always
11. I have told my physician which hospital I would prefer to use should the need arise.	①	2	3	4
12. I understand my rights and responsibilities as a patient when admitted to a hospital.	①	2	3	4
13. I practice adequate self-care to reduce my health care expenditures and my reliance on health care providers.	1	2	3	④
14. I am open-minded about alternative health care practices and support current efforts to determine their appropriate role in effective health care.	1	2	③	4
15. I have a well-established relationship with a pharmacist and have transmitted all necessary information regarding medication and use.	1	2	③	4
16. I carefully follow labels and directions when using health care products, such as over-the-counter medications.	1	2	3	④
17. I finish all prescription medications as directed, rather than stopping use when symptoms subside.	1	2	3	④
18. I report to the appropriate agencies any providers of health care services, information, or products that use deceptive advertising or fraudulent methods of operation.	1	②	3	4
19. I pursue my rights as fully as possible in matters of misrepresentation or consumer dissatisfaction.	1	②	3	4
20. I follow current health care issues in the news and voice my opinion to my elected representatives.	①	2	3	4

POINTS 52

Environmental Health

	Not true/ rarely	Somewhat true/ sometimes	Mostly true/ usually	Very true/ always
1. I avoid use of and exposure to pesticides as much as possible.	1	2	③	4
2. I avoid use of and exposure to herbicides as much as possible.	1	2	3	④
3. I am willing to spend the extra money and time required to obtain organically grown produce.	①	2	3	4
4. I reduce environmental pollutants by minimizing my use of the automobile.	1	②	3	4
5. I avoid the use of products that contribute to indoor air pollution.	1	②	3	4
6. I limit my exposure to ultraviolet radiation by avoiding excessive sun exposure.	1	②	3	4
7. I limit my exposure to radon gas by using a radon gas detector.	1	②	3	4
8. I limit my exposure to radiation by promptly eliminating radon gas within my home.	1	②	3	4
9. I limit my exposure to radiation by agreeing to undergo medical radiation procedures only when absolutely necessary for the diagnosis and treatment of an illness or disease.	1	2	③	4
10. I avoid the use of potentially unsafe water, particularly when traveling in a foreign country or when a municipal water supply or bottled water is unavailable.	1	2	3	④
11. I avoid noise pollution by limiting my exposure to loud noise or by using ear protection.	1	2	③	4

	Not true/ rarely	Somewhat true/ sometimes	Mostly true/ usually	Very true/ always
12. I avoid air pollution by carefully selecting the environments in which I live, work, and recreate.	(1)	2	3	4
13. I do not knowingly use or improperly dispose of personal care products that can harm the environment.	1	2	(3)	4
14. I reuse as many products as possible so that they can avoid the recycling bins for as long as possible.	(1)	2	3	4
15. I participate fully in my community's recycling efforts.	1	2	(3)	4
16. I encourage the increased use of recycled materials in the design and manufacturing of new products.	1	(2)	3	4
17. I dispose of residential toxic substances safely and properly.	1	2	(3)	4
18. I follow environmental issues in the news and voice my opinion to my elected representatives.	(1)	2	3	4
19. I am aware of and involved in environmental issues in my local area.	(1)	2	3	4
20. I perceive myself as a steward of the environment for the generations to come, rather than as a person with a right to use (and misuse) the environment to meet my immediate needs.	1	(2)	3	4

POINTS 45

YOUR TOTAL POINTS 634

Interpretation

770 to 880 points—Congratulations! Your health behavior is very supportive of high-level health. Continue to practice your positive health habits, and look for areas in which you can become even stronger. Encourage others to follow your example, and support their efforts in any way you can.

550 to 769 points—Good job! Your health behavior is relatively supportive of high-level health. You scored well in several areas; however, you can improve in some ways. Identify your weak areas and chart a plan for behavior change, as explained at the end of Chapter 1. Then pay close attention as you learn more about health in the weeks ahead.

330 to 549 points—Caution! Your relatively low score indicates that your behavior may be compromising your health. Review your responses to this assessment carefully, noting the areas in which you scored poorly. Then chart a detailed plan for behavior change, as outlined at the end of Chapter 1. Be sure to set realistic goals that you can work toward steadily as you complete this course.

Below 330 points—Red flag! Your low score suggests that your health behavior is destructive. Immediate changes in your behavior are needed to put you back on track. Review your responses to this assessment carefully. Then begin to make changes in the most critical areas, such as harmful alcohol or other drug use patterns. Seek help promptly for any difficulties that you are not prepared to deal with alone, such as domestic violence or suicidal thoughts. The information you read in this textbook and learn in this course could have a significant effect on your future health. Remember, it's not too late to improve your health!

TO CARRY THIS FURTHER . . .

Most of us can improve our health behavior in a number of ways. We hope this assessment will help you identify areas in which you can make positive changes and serve as a motivator as you implement your plan for behavior change. If you scored well, give yourself a pat on the back. If your score was not as high as you would have liked, take heart. This textbook and your instructor can help you get started on the road to wellness. Good luck!

2

Achieving Psychological Health

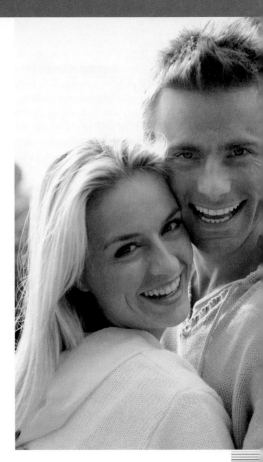

What Do You Know About Psychological Health?

1. Psychological health has been associated with having a good sense of humor. True or False?

2. Self-esteem is the highest level of psychological health on Maslow's hierarchy of needs. True or False?

3. Pessimists tend to live longer than optimists do. True or False?

4. It has been proven that personality is influenced more by heredity than by environment. True or False?

5. Mental disorders are the leading cause of disability in the United States. True or False?

6. Middle-aged individuals have a higher risk of suicide than the elderly or young people. True or False?

7. Schizophrenia is a mental disorder that involves having dissociative identity disorder. True or False?

Check your answers at the end of the chapter.

Defining Psychological Health

The terms *emotional wellness* and *psychological health* have been used interchangeably to describe how people function in the affective and cognitive realms of their lives. **Psychological health** relates to how people express their emotions; cope with stress, adversity, and success; and adapt to changes in themselves and their environment, as well as to cognitive functioning—the ways people think and behave in conjunction with their emotions. You will learn more about psychological health in this chapter.

When you apply the resources from the multiple dimensions of health (Chapter 1) in ways that allow you to direct your growth, assess deeply held values, deal effectively with change, and have satisfying relationships with others, you are psychologically healthy. Research in the area of health psychology has shown that there is a mind-body connection in which biological, psychological, and social factors interact to influence health or illness. This is referred to as the **biopsychological model.** [1] We know that one's psychological state has a significant effect on physical health: Stress, depression, and anxiety have been associated with how the immune system responds and can impair physical health. For example, studies

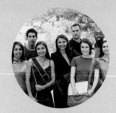
have shown that terminally ill cancer patients who had good psychological health lived longer lives and reported having a higher quality of life than did other cancer patients.[2] Psychological health has diminished in college students over the past few years. Only 52 percent of college students rated their emotional health "above average or high," a drop from 64 percent from the past year.[3] More students are struggling with depression, anxiety, attention deficit disorder, and other problems than their predecessors. We will discuss these psychological disorders and others later in the chapter. Psychological health does not refer just to your emotional state but also to your cognitive and social functioning.

Psychological health has also been associated with developing and maintaining a positive **self-concept,** positive **self-esteem,** and a high level of **emotional intelligence.** However, as you will see, psychological health is much more than just the absence of mental illness.

Characteristics of Psychologically Healthy People

Psychologically healthy people are not perfect. They have their share of problems, flaws, and mistakes. However, it is how they perceive themselves and how they cope with their stress and problems that separates them from unhealthy individuals.

Psychologically healthy people

- Accept themselves and others
- Like themselves
- Appropriately express the full range of human emotions, both positive and negative
- Give and receive care, love, and support
- Accept life's disappointments
- Accept their mistakes

- Express empathy and concern for others
- Take care of themselves
- Trust others as well as themselves
- Establish goals, both short and long term
- Can function both independently and interdependently
- Lead a health-enhancing lifestyle that includes regular exercise, good nutrition, and adequate sleep

Normal Range of Emotions

How many feelings are people capable of expressing? Happy, sad, fearful, and angry are the four primary

---

Key Terms

psychological health A broadly based concept pertaining to cognitive functioning in conjunction with the way people express their emotions; cope with stress, adversity, and success; and adapt to changes in themselves and their environment.

biopsychological model A model that addresses how biological, psychological, and social factors interact and affect psychological health.

self-concept An individual's internal picture of himself or herself; the way one sees oneself.

self-esteem An individual's sense of pride, self-respect, value, and worth.

emotional intelligence The ability to understand others and act wisely in human relations and to measure how well one knows one's emotions, manages one's emotions, motivates oneself, recognizes emotions in others, and handles relationships.

emotions that humans universally feel. These emotions are considered to be hardwired into human neuroanatomy for survival. Permutations of these four primary emotions result in our capacity to express about 100 different emotions, such as feeling frustrated, although cultural differences do exist[4] (see the box "Regional, Socioeconomic, and Racial Differences in Psychological Health"). There is some debate about whether thoughts influence feelings or feelings cause us to think and behave a certain way. However, the most accepted view is that the way we think can directly change how we feel about an event or a situation. Thus, you can change your feelings about something by changing your perspective about a situation. Life has its ups and downs, and the concept of the "normal range of emotions" reflects these changes. It is when emotions fluctuate to an extreme level up and down, aren't expressed appropriately, or are out of control and overwhelming that people can become psychologically unhealthy.

Self-Esteem

What is self-esteem? How do you know when someone is lacking in self-esteem? Most people answer this question by saying that they define positive self-esteem as

- Having pride in yourself
- Treating yourself with respect
- Considering yourself valuable, important, worthy
- Feeling good about yourself
- Having self-confidence, being self-assured
- Accepting yourself

People with low levels of self-esteem tend to allow others to mistreat them, don't take care of themselves, and have difficulty being by themselves. In addition, they have little self-confidence and so avoid taking risks and have trouble believing that other people care about them. People with low self-esteem tend to take things personally, are sometimes seen as "overly sensitive" and perfectionistic, criticize themselves and others, and believe that they can't do anything right. These individuals tend to have a pessimistic outlook on life and see themselves as undeserving of good fortune. We explore the concepts of optimism and pessimism as they relate to psychological health in a later section of this chapter.

People with low self-esteem also have a poor self-concept, meaning that their internal picture of themselves, how they see themselves, is very negative. Because of this poor self-concept, people with low self-esteem are more vulnerable to allowing others to mistreat or abuse them, and fail to be assertive. Many psychological problems have their underpinnings in low self-esteem, including eating disorders, substance abuse, depression, and anxiety disorders.

Where do we get our self-esteem? Most people would say from their parents, teachers, peers, siblings, religious institutions, and the media. While these factors certainly can positively or negatively affect our self-concept and self-esteem, they are all *external* factors. We don't have much control over other people, but we do have control over what we internalize or accept as true about ourselves. Self-concept refers to our *internal* self-perception. If our self-esteem and self-concept were based solely on external factors, then we would need only to change our environment and the people around us to raise our self-esteem. This is the reason that people tend to tell themselves, "If I just made more money, had a nicer car, were married, or had a more prestigious job, I would feel better about myself." This situation can become a vicious cycle, leaving the person always seeking more and being perpetually unsatisfied with him- or herself. This can also lead to perfectionism and not accepting yourself.

Self-esteem is not an all-or-none commodity. Most people have varying degrees of self-esteem, depending on their stage of development, events in their lives, and their environment.[5]

Emotional Intelligence

A third aspect of psychological health is the degree of emotional intelligence you possess. Emotional intelligence refers to "the ability to understand others and act wisely in human relations."[6] Furthermore, emotional intelligence can be broken down into five main domains:

- *Knowing your emotions.* This is considered to be the cornerstone of emotional intelligence and relates to how much self-awareness and insight you have. How quickly you are able to recognize and label your feelings as you feel them determines the level of your emotional intelligence.
- *Managing your emotions.* This relates to how you appropriately express your feelings and cope with your emotions. People who have trouble coping with anxiety, distress, and failures tend to have lower levels of emotional intelligence.
- *Motivating yourself.* People who can motivate themselves tend to be more highly productive and independent than are those who rely on external sources for motivation. The more you can self-motivate and engage in goal-directed activities, the higher your emotional intelligence.
- *Recognizing emotions in others.* Another aspect of emotional intelligence is the degree of empathy you have, or how sensitive you are to the feelings of others and how you relate to other people.
- *Handling relationships.* The more interpersonally effective you are and the more you are able to negotiate conflict and build a social support network, the more emotional intelligence you possess.

Of course, people have differing levels of emotional intelligence and may have higher levels in one domain than in another. People with high overall levels of emotional intelligence tend to take on leadership roles, are confident and assertive, express their feelings directly and appropriately, feel good about themselves, are outgoing, and adapt well to stress.[6]

Personality

There is some debate about how much control people actually do have over their psychological health. A general consensus is that two factors, **nature** and **nurture,** influence psychological health, but there are differing views on how much each contributes to our psychological makeup. *Nature* refers to the innate factors we are born with that genetically determine our degree of psychological health. *Nurture* is the effect that the environment, people, and external factors have on our psychological health.[7] We all know some people who are high strung or anxious by nature and others who are cheerful and naturally outgoing. We seem to be born with a predisposition toward a certain psychological health, which is often similar to our parents'. "She is serious like her father" and "He is funny like his mother" are remarks people may make alluding to this genetic link. Environmental factors, such as social relationships, family harmony, financial resources, job and academic concerns, living situations or events, and even the weather, can influence your personality.

Maslow's Hierarchy of Needs

Abraham Maslow has been among the significant contributors to the understanding of personality and psychological health. Central to Maslow's contribution to twentieth-century American psychological thought was his view of psychological health in terms of the individual's attempt to meet inner needs, what he called the *hierarchy of needs* (see Figure 2-1).[8]

Maslow's theory is a positive, optimistic theory of human behavior. He believed that people are motivated to grow and fulfill their potential, referring to this phenomenon as **self-actualization.** He described self-actualization as "the need to become more and more what one is, to become everything that one is capable of becoming."[8] Maslow differentiated between two categories of needs: **basic needs** and **metaneeds.** Basic needs, physiological needs, safety and security, belonging and love, and esteem needs are the deficiency needs and are essential and urgent. Metaneeds come into play once the basic needs are met and include spirituality, creativity, curiosity, beauty, philosophy, and justice. Maslow's hierarchy of needs is arranged with the basic needs on the bottom, as they are the most fundamental and powerful

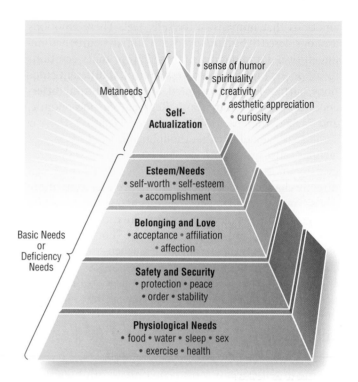

Figure 2-1 Maslow's Hierarchy of Needs Once basic needs are met, metaneeds such as creativity, spirituality, and justice come into play.

Source: Maslow, AH, Frager, RD (Ed.), Fadiman, J (Ed.), *Motivation and Personality,* 3rd ed. © 1987.

needs. Lower-level needs must be met before the next level of needs can be satisfied. Maslow believed that the fulfillment of metaneeds is necessary for one to become a completely developed human being. Left unfulfilled, people can become cynical, apathetic, and lonely.[9]

Maslow arrived at this model by examining people whom he considered to be exceptionally healthy, people he defined as having developed to their fullest potentials. People whom Maslow identified as self-actualized included Albert Einstein, Albert Schweitzer, Eleanor Roosevelt, and Abraham Lincoln. He perceived these people to share similar personality characteristics, such as being comfortable with themselves, having a strong ethical and moral code of conduct, and being innovative, compassionate, altruistic, goal oriented, and internally motivated.[9]

Spiritual Health

Having a sense of purpose, direction, and awareness is a dimension of spiritual health. This aspect of psychological health also refers to how well we integrate our beliefs and values with our behavior. People with spiritual health seek meaning and purpose in their lives and have a deep appreciation for a sense of unity and community (see the box "Mindfulness" on page 34). Spiritual health also includes one's morals, ethics, intrinsic values, and beliefs.

It also refers to an awareness and appreciation of the vastness of the universe, and a recognition of a dimension beyond the natural and rational, involving perhaps a belief in a force greater than oneself.[10] People who incorporate spirituality into their lives reported better psychological coping, increased well-being, increased satisfaction with life, lower anxiety and fewer depressive symptoms, less hostility and anger, and greater happiness in general.[11] Similarly, spirituality has also been related to better physical health. Studies have shown that no matter how spirituality was defined or measured, it has a positive effect on reducing coronary heart disease, high blood pressure, stroke, and cancer, and increasing life expectancy.[12]

As a resource for the spiritual dimension of health, spirituality provides a basis on which a belief system can mature and an expanding awareness of life's meaning can be fostered. In addition, spirituality influences many of the experiences that you will seek throughout life and tempers your emotional response to these experiences.

In nearly all cultures, spirituality provides individuals and groups with rituals and practices that foster a sense of community—"a community of faith." In turn, the community nurtures the emotional stability, confidence, and sense of competence needed for living life fully.[13]

Creative Expression

Another characteristic of people who have developed their psychological health is creativity. Allowing yourself to express your thoughts, feelings, and individuality in a creative manner entails having self-confidence, self-esteem, and flexibility. Confidence and self-esteem are essential so that you feel free to share your creative side with others and don't feel embarrassed by your creativity. Children can easily do this when they draw a picture or make up a dance and say, "Look at me. Look at what I made." However, as we age, some of us become inhibited and don't allow ourselves to be creative or to share this part of ourselves. If you don't exercise your creative side, it can atrophy, just as unexercised muscles do.

What are some resources that you might need to develop to foster your creativity?

- *Nonconformity.* Creative individuals aren't terribly concerned about what other people think of them. They are willing to risk looking foolish or proposing ideas that are divergent from others' ideas or traditional ways of thinking.

- *Independence.* Highly creative people tend to work well alone and sometimes prefer this to working in a group. As children, they often were encouraged to solve problems on their own rather than having someone do it for them.

- *Motivation.* Creative people are motivated by intrinsic rather than external rewards, meaning they like to be creative for their own pleasure, not to please others or because it is expected of them. They enjoy creativity for creativity's sake alone, not to reap rewards or praise from others.

- *Curiosity.* Creative people have a wide range of interests and a broad base of knowledge. They are open to new experiences and question things that other people ignore or take for granted.

- *Persistence.* This is one of the most important traits of a creative person. As Thomas Edison said, "Genius is one-tenth inspiration and nine-tenths perspiration." Persistence requires not giving up when your first efforts are not successful and continually thinking of new ways of doing something, problem solving, or thinking "outside of the box."[14]

Some people reviewing the preceding list may recognize many of these characteristics as being already well developed in their own personalities. Others may not have demonstrated some of the traits listed, and the traits may appear far beyond their reach. Nevertheless, most people can increase their creativity by giving themselves permission to be creative. Some people state, "I'm not a creative person," and yet they haven't explored that part of their personality, perhaps since childhood. There are many avenues of creativity, and the first step is to experiment, to be open and spontaneous. In this way, you can gain greater psychological health from accessing your inner strengths and resources.

Keys to Psychological Health

Most people have the opportunity to function at an enhanced level of psychological well-being. This state is often achieved by improving certain skills and abilities,

---

Key Terms

nature The innate factors that genetically determine personality traits.

nurture The effects that the environment, people, and external factors have on personality.

self-actualization The highest level of psychological health, at which one reaches his or her highest potential and values truth, beauty, goodness, faith, love, humor, and ingenuity.

basic needs Deficiency needs that are viewed as essential and fundamental, including physiological, safety and security, belonging and love, and esteem needs.

metaneeds Secondary concerns, such as spirituality, creativity, curiosity, beauty, philosophy, and justice, that can be addressed only after the basic needs are met.

---

including improving verbal and nonverbal communication, learning to use humor effectively, developing better conflict resolution skills, and taking an optimistic approach to life. This section explores each of these facets of psychological health.

Develop Communication Skills

Verbal Communication   Communication can be viewed in terms of your role as sender or receiver. In sending messages, you can enhance the effectiveness of your *verbal* communication in several ways. First, take time before speaking to understand what needs to be said. For example, does the audience/listener need information, encouragement, humor, or something else? Focus on the most important thoughts and ideas. Talk *with,* rather than *at,* the listener to encourage productive exchanges. Begin verbal exchanges on a positive note, and maintain a positive environment. Use "minimal encouragers," such as short questions, to gain feedback. Avoid using sarcasm, which can be destructive to communication. Recognize when other forms of communication, such as e-mail messages or handwritten notes, would be better for transmitting information or ideas.

You also need to be a skilled listener. First, listen attentively to hear everything that is being said. If you aren't sure of what he or she is saying, stop the speaker at certain points and ask him or her to repeat or rephrase the information. Focus on what is being said and not on what you want to say next. Ask for clarification and summarize what you think you heard the speaker say to ensure you have received the message accurately. Also try to focus on one main topic and don't go off on tangents.

Nonverbal Communication   Strengthening your nonverbal communication skills can also enhance your psychological health. Nonverbal communication is what is communicated by your facial expressions, body posture, tone of voice, movements, and even the way you breathe—such as when you sigh or yawn. Nonverbal communication is a very powerful and sometimes more important aspect of the message than what is verbally communicated, especially when the verbal communication appears untrustworthy or vague.[15] In fact, people use information from facial cues more than any other source. Facial cues, particularly from the eyes, are attended to more than any other type of nonverbal communication, even when information from other sources—such as from hand and body movements—may provide a more accurate picture of what the person is feeling. The following suggestions can enhance your nonverbal communication skills:

- *Facial expressions.* Facial expressions have been cited as one of the most important sources of nonverbal communication in terms of a person's emotional state. When people speak with their eyebrows raised, they tend to be seen as more animated, excited, and happy. Flushing of one's face can indicate embarrassment, and crinkling one's nose can mean that you don't like something. Facial expressions are inborn and not culturally learned as previously believed.[16] Every part of your face can communicate some type of emotional reaction.

- *Eye contact.* Maintaining eye contact is an important component of positive nonverbal communication, while looking away or shifting your eyes can be read as seeming dishonest. But don't stare—five to seven seconds seems to be the maximum amount of time of eye contact before the person begins to feel scrutinized.

- *Personal space.* There are cultural differences in how much personal space or distance is comfortable and acceptable when sitting or standing next to another person. For example, Americans' personal space—about 3 to 4 feet for a casual conversation—tends to be much greater than that of Arabs or Italians but less than for Japanese or Britons. Gender, age, and degree of familiarity are other factors that can determine the amount of personal space you are comfortable having between you and another person.

- *Body posture.* Assertiveness is equated with people who carry themselves with their head up and shoulders back and who maintain eye contact. Folded arms, crossed legs, and looking away from the speaker can indicate defensiveness and rejection.

Managing Conflict Communication can be especially challenging when there is a conflict or disagreement. Emotions such as anger, hurt, and fear might alter your ability to communicate as effectively as you would like. Various techniques are available for managing angry or upset people or conflictual situations:

- *Listen to and acknowledge the other person's point of view, even if it differs from your own.* Sometimes people are so busy thinking of the next thing they want to say that they don't pay attention to what the other person is saying. To ensure that you have heard the person accurately and to let that person know you are listening, repeat back or summarize what you heard, and ask if you misunderstood something that was said.

- *Use assertive communication.* Using "I" statements rather than "you" statements helps to avoid putting people on the defensive and is especially helpful when negotiating conflict or disagreements. Rather than saying "You are inconsiderate," you can say, "I feel upset when you're late and haven't called to let me know."

- *Focus not just on what you say but how you say it.* Pay attention to your tone of voice and speak in a conversational tone. People tend to talk louder because they erroneously think they will be heard if they speak louder. This can result in a shouting match in which neither person hears the other.

- *Acknowledge the other person's feelings.* Use statements like "I can understand why this is so frustrating for you."

- *Watch your body posture.* Don't fold your arms in a closed, defensive posture, maintain eye contact, and be aware of your facial expressions so that you are not conveying hostility nonverbally. Make sure your nonverbal communication matches your verbal communication.

- *Accept valid criticism.* If you made a mistake, admit to it and apologize for whatever you think you did to contribute to the misunderstanding or conflict. This will open the door for the other person to take responsibility for his or her part in the conflict as well.

- *Focus on the problem at hand.* Don't bring up past hurts and problems. If you try to resolve every disagreement you have ever had with this person, you'll just wind up feeling frustrated and overwhelmed, and won't accomplish much. Stay on track by talking about the present situation.

- *Take a team approach.* Engage in mutual problem solving. This alleviates the winner-versus-loser paradigm. Look for areas of compromise and find a middle ground you can both live with.

- *Agree to disagree.* There is probably more than one right answer, and you can agree that you will not persuade the other to change his or her point of view.

- *Agree to discuss this at a later time.* Sometimes the conversation becomes too heated. Some time and distance from the problem can be beneficial. Also ask yourself if this is really important enough to you to continue arguing about the situation.

See Chapter 13 for more on communication in intimate relationships.

Cultivate Your Sense of Humor

Having a sense of humor is another important component of psychological health. Humor helps to put things in their proper perspective, alleviating tension and pain by releasing more endorphins in our bodies. In addition, laughter reduces stress,[17] boosts the immune system,[18] alleviates pain,[19] stabilizes mood,[19] decreases anxiety,[20] enhances communication,[21] and inspires creativity.[22] The research suggests that we need to laugh 30 minutes total per 24-hour period to attain these benefits. This is an easy task for children, who on average laugh 250 times a day, but more challenging for adults, who tend to laugh only 15 times a day.[23] Employers have been putting the benefits of laughter to good use to increase productivity in factories. Factories in India have created "laughing clubs" in which workers laugh together for 20 minutes a day, resulting in less absenteeism and better performance.[24]

Recognizing the humor in everyday situations and being able to laugh at yourself will make you feel better about yourself. People who build humor into their daily lives generally feel more positive, and others enjoy being around them. Some people will say that if they don't laugh about a particular situation, they will cry, and laughing seems the better choice. In fact, humor is viewed as one of the higher-level coping mechanisms, compared to denying the problem, rationalizing or minimizing the problem, or blaming others. Some researchers have suggested that recovery from an injury or illness is enhanced when patients maintain a sense of humor.[25]

Take an Optimistic Approach to Life

One important key to psychological health is the way that you think about and interpret events in your life. For example, if you say "hello" to someone and you don't get a response, do you begin to wonder if that person is angry with you? Or do you surmise that he or she didn't

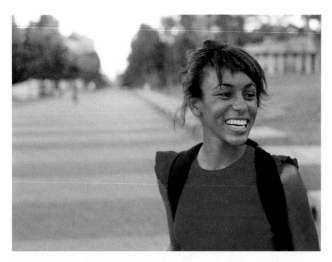

Optimists—those who see the glass as half full—interpret life's events positively and are better able to cope with setbacks and adversity.

hear you or perhaps was distracted? Research shows that having a positive interpretation of life's events, particularly how you cope with adversity, can make a significant difference in terms of your health and academic and work performance as well as how long you will live.[26] Compared with pessimists, optimists tend to

- Contract fewer infectious diseases
- Have better health habits
- Possess stronger immune systems
- Be more successful in their careers
- Perform better in sports, music, and academics

We do know that people can learn to be helpless and ultimately become depressed and even suicidal. Martin Seligman demonstrated the concept of "learned helplessness" in his classic study in which he administered an electric shock to dogs that were harnessed and couldn't escape the shocks. When he moved the dogs to another room, the dogs lay down and whimpered and didn't try to avoid the shocks. But when the dogs were not harnessed and could have easily escaped the shocks by moving to another side of the room, they failed to do so. This reaction has been referred to as **learned helplessness.** The dogs learned that there was nothing they could do to affect their lives, and they lost hope and felt trapped and powerless.[27] We have seen this same phenomenon with humans. College students who took a test and started answering the most difficult questions first performed significantly more poorly on the easier questions as compared to those students who started with the easy questions and then moved on to the harder questions. Interestingly, both groups scored about the same number correct on the more difficult questions. This suggests that when the students expected the test to be hard

and perhaps anticipated failure, they began to feel helpless and their performance declined.[28] Battered women have demonstrated this same sense of powerlessness and helplessness in their inability to escape the abuse they are subjected to by their partners.

If people can learn to be helpless and pessimistic, can they also learn to feel more optimistic, powerful, and in control? Martin Seligman, a prominent psychologist, conducted studies to prove that this is possible; he called this concept **learned optimism.** Learned optimism refers to your explanatory style—in other words, whether you describe the glass as being half full or half empty. Seligman identified three key factors that contribute to having an optimistic or pessimistic perspective.[2]

Permanence The first dimension of learned optimism is **permanence.** Pessimists tend to give up easily because they believe the causes of bad events are *permanent.* They say things like "Nothing ever works out for me," "That won't ever work," or "He's always in a bad mood." Such permanence language—words like *never, always,* and *forever*—implies that these negative situations are not temporary but will continue indefinitely. Optimists tend to use language of temporariness—words like *sometimes, frequently,* and *often*—and they blame bad events on transient conditions. Examples of optimistic language are "It didn't work out this time," "Doing it that way didn't work," and "He's in a bad mood today." Optimists see failure as a small, transitory setback and are able to pick themselves up, brush themselves off, and persevere toward their goals.

Key Terms

learned helplessness A theory of motivation explaining how individuals can learn to feel powerless, trapped, and defeated.

learned optimism An attribution style regarding permanence, pervasiveness, and personalization; how people explain both positive and negative events in their lives, accounting for success and failure.

permanence The first dimension of learned optimism, related to whether certain events are perceived as temporary or long lasting.

pervasiveness The second dimension of learned optimism, related to whether events are perceived as specific or general.

personalization The third dimension of learned optimism, related to whether an individual takes things personally or is more balanced in accepting responsibility for positive and negative events.

Pervasiveness The second aspect of learned optimism is **pervasiveness.** It refers to whether you perceive negative events as universal and generalize them to everything in your life, or you can compartmentalize and keep them defined to the specific situation. Pessimists tend to give universal explanations for their problems, and, when something goes wrong in one part of their lives, they give up on everything. While pessimists would say that they are not good at math, optimists would say that they didn't perform well in that particular class with that type of math. "I'm good at algebra but not as good with geometry."

Personalization The last aspect of learned optimism is determined by whether you blame bad things on yourself or on other people or circumstances. Pessimism and low self-esteem tend to come from **personalization** — blaming oneself and having an internal explanatory style for negative events. An optimist might say, "The professor wrote a very poor exam and that is the reason I received a lower score," whereas the pessimist would say, "I am stupid" or "I didn't study enough." This is different from not taking responsibility for one's actions and blaming other people for your problems or mistakes. The key is to have a balanced perspective and outlook on life. Pessimists tend to give credit to other people or circumstances when good things happen and to blame themselves when bad events occur. For example, a pessimist would say, "That was just dumb luck" rather than taking credit for a success. However, if pessimists fail, they readily blame themselves, saying "I messed up." In contrast, optimists tend to give themselves credit for their accomplishments, saying "I worked hard and did a good job," and they don't belittle themselves when things go wrong.

Seligman conducted many studies to test how an optimistic explanatory style might be useful in daily living. For example, he worked with a swimming team from the University of California, Berkeley, to see how optimism or pessimism might affect their performance. He had their coaches tell the athletes that their times were slower than they actually were. The swimmers were then asked to swim the event again as fast as they could. The performance of the pessimists decreased in their 100-yard event by 2 seconds, the difference between winning the event and finishing dead last. The optimists got faster by 2–5 seconds, again enough to be the difference between losing and winning the race.[2] So how you interpret events, your attribution style, can make a tremendous difference in your eventual success or failure in your endeavors.

Building Optimism So how can you learn to be more optimistic? Albert Ellis developed a cognitive framework, known as the ABC method, that can help you become more positive in how you think and feel about things that happen in your life. When you encounter an event, the "A" part of the formula, you try to make sense out of it and explain what has happened. For example, if you receive a notice from the bank that you have overdrawn your checking account, you start to think, "How did this happen?" These thoughts are associated with your beliefs, the "B" in ABC. You might think, "I'm irresponsible for letting this happen; I can't manage my money." Then you begin to feel bad about yourself, worthless, and upset. Your beliefs affect your feelings, and so you can control your emotions by changing your beliefs and thoughts.[29] If you said, "The bank probably made a mistake" or "I might have added something incorrectly," you will most likely feel much better about yourself and the situation. The "C" aspect is the consequence of the event, how you end up feeling about the situation. When someone feels depressed, he or she feels hopeless, trapped, and powerless. By adopting a more positive way of reframing or thinking about events, you create options, hope, and a strategy for solving problems rather than staying stuck, like the whimpering dogs laying down and putting up with being shocked. In the overdraft scenario, you can generate ideas such as "I need to check with the bank, go over my bank statement, be more careful in recording and calculating my balances, and request overdraft protection to prevent this from becoming a problem again."

Everyone encounters adversity sometime in his or her life. You can become discouraged by these events, blame yourself, and feel hopeless, worthless, and cynical about the world. Or you can be persistent and become stronger by overcoming these obstacles, by having a positive outlook, and by seeing these problems as short-lived, specific, and not as a flaw in your character. When you embrace an optimistic perspective, you will feel more hopeful, stronger, and more confident. You will be able to accept new challenges and take risks in your life. Take the Personal Assessment at the end of the chapter to find your level of optimism and pessimism.

Psychological Disorders

In the course of one year, an estimated 26 percent of Americans suffer from a diagnosable mental disorder.[30] Nearly one-half of Americans will have a diagnosable mental disorder in their lifetime. In addition, mental disorders are the leading cause of disability in the United States for Americans ages 15–44.[31] However, two-thirds of those suffering from psychological disorders do not receive treatment owing to the stigma and cost associated with mental health treatment (see the box "Television Advertisements for Psychological Medications").[32] Overall, minorities and Caucasians share the same prevalence rate of mental disorders; however, there are great disparities in the rate of mental health care for minorities compared with the nonminority population.

While there are over 300 different types of mental illness that can be diagnosed, we will cover three major categories of mental disorders: mood disorders, including depression and bipolar disorder; anxiety disorders; and schizophrenia.[33] We will also briefly discuss attention deficit hyperactivity disorder. Over 450 million people worldwide are affected by mental disorders at any given time, and these numbers are expected to increase in the future.[34]

Mood Disorders

Mood disorders, such as depression, seasonal affective disorder, and bipolar disorder, refer to psychological problems in which the primary symptom is a disturbance in mood.[33] You might perceive someone as moody and be unable to predict if the person will be in a good or bad mood from one day to the next.

Depression   About 1 in 10 Americans suffers some form of depression, with women experiencing **clinical depression** twice as often as men.[35] The incidence of depression starting in childhood and adolescence has recently dramatically increased. We have already begun to see this trend, as the number of college students with depression has doubled over recent years.[36] A survey of 71,860 college students nationwide revealed that 38 percent of students reported feeling so depressed that they had difficulty functioning. Another study found that working can mitigate depression, as full-time workers tended to be less depressed than the unemployed did. With the economic downturn that began in mid-2007, we have seen an increase in the incidence of depression. While depression can develop at any age, the average age of onset is the mid-20s. Figure 2-2 depicts the percentage of adult Americans who reported experiencing major

Key Terms

clinical depression A psychological disorder in which individuals experience a lack of motivation, decreased energy level, fatigue, social withdrawal, sleep disturbance, disturbance in appetite, diminished sex drive, feelings of worthlessness, and despair.

neurotransmitters Chemical messengers that transfer electrical impulses across the synapses between nerve cells.

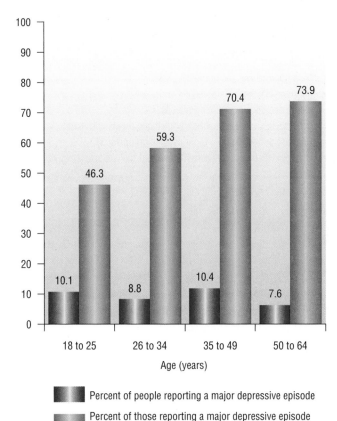

Figure 2-2 Rates of Major Depression and Treatment by Age
Percentage of American adults reporting a major depressive disorder episode and, of this group, the percentage that sought treatment in the year 2004, by age group.

Source: NSDUH Report, Depression Among Adults. Office of Applied Studies, Substance Abuse and Mental Health Services Administration (SAMHSA), November 18, 2008.

depression in 2004, with the 18-to-25 age group being the most prevalent, and 65 and older the least. It also shows that the 50- to 64-year-olds were the most likely to receive treatment for depression, with 18- to 25-year-olds being the least likely.

Symptoms of Depression How can you tell the difference between having the blues and being clinically depressed? The symptoms of depression are as follows:

- Depressed mood most of the day, nearly every day
- Frequent crying
- Withdrawal and isolation from others
- Lack of interest in activities that are typically enjoyable
- Increase or decrease in appetite resulting in significant weight loss or weight gain
- Insomnia, disturbed or restless sleep, or sleeping more than usual

- Feeling tired most of the time, regardless of how much sleep you have had
- Low self-esteem and feelings of hopelessness and worthlessness
- Difficulty concentrating, remembering things, and focusing on a task, and indecisiveness
- Frequent thoughts of suicide

Many people have experienced some of these symptoms at some point in their lives; however, clinically depressed individuals experience most of these symptoms every day and have felt this way for at least two weeks. Most people can find ways to pull themselves out of feeling down, but when you have clinical depression, the normal methods you have used in the past to cope with the blues don't work. Clinical depression can range from mild to severe and can result in significant impairment in functioning, such as not being able to get out of bed to attend classes or go to work or not having the energy or motivation to take care of your basic needs for food, hygiene, and rest. Some depressed people tend to become irritable, negative, and uncommunicative, which can cause greater stress and conflict in their relationships. Depression has been described as constantly having a black cloud over your head and not being able to get out from underneath it no matter what you do. You might want to take the online self-assessment screening at www.depression-screening.org to assess your risk for clinical depression and to access more information on depression.

Causes of Depression There are several causes of or triggers for depression. New research has found a gene variant for depression, gene 5-HTTLPR, that predisposes people to depression.[37] This makes sense as we know that there is a genetic link for depression. If you have a family history of depression or any type of mood disorder, you are more prone to developing a depressive disorder. In fact, rates of depression for a child with a depressed parent are two to four times greater than for children without this type of heredity.[38] While there is no single gene that causes depression, your genetic makeup can make you more vulnerable to depression. **Neurotransmitters** and hormone levels play a major role in the way your brain regulates your mood and emotions. Two neurotransmitters, serotonin and norepinephrine, are often found to be deficient in people with depression. (Chapter 7 includes a detailed discussion of neurotransmitters.)

However, biological processes are not the only explanation for depression. You may have a family history of depression and never develop depressive symptoms. Conversely, you may have no genetic predisposition and still become clinically depressed. Depression can be caused by many psychological factors, such as these:

- Loss of a significant relationship
- Death of a family member or friend

Chapter Two Achieving Psychological Health **39**

- Physical or sexual abuse or assault
- Serious illness or health problems
- Numerous setbacks and problems occurring simultaneously

Having a support system, effective coping strategies, and a positive attributional style can make the difference between succumbing to depression and being protected during stressful and adverse times in our lives (see the box "Reaching Out to Someone Who's Depressed"). Some people turn to the Internet to find increased social involvement and to cope with depression. While it might seem that this would be a helpful way to build your support system and cope with depression, research shows that greater use of the Internet is associated with increasing depression, social isolation, and withdrawal (see the box "A New Problem . . . Cyberbullying").

Treatments for Depression There are many ways to treat depression, but the most effective treatment approach is a combination of counseling and medication.[39] Counseling can help people develop healthy coping skills, learn stress-management strategies, focus on developing an optimistic explanatory style, and improve relationships and social skills. Medications, such as antidepressants, can be helpful in the treatment of depression because they act to increase the serotonin or norepinephrine levels to a normal and functional range. Antidepressants include fluoxetine (Prozac), paroxetine (Paxil), sertraline (Zoloft), mirtazapine (Remeron), venlafaxine (Effexor), escitalopram (Lexapro), citalopram (Celexa), and duloxetine (Cymbalta). It takes four to six weeks for an antidepressant to be fully effective, and there may be side effects such as dry mouth, decreased sex drive, drowsiness, constipation, or diarrhea. Most of these will disappear after two weeks of taking the medication.

Most people take an antidepressant for six months to a year and then are able to taper off of the medication without a recurrence of symptoms. If you have had three separate episodes of depression, recovering from each episode and then relapsing, this can be a sign that your depression is chemically caused and an indication that you may need to continue taking an antidepressant medication long term. Despite FDA "black box" warnings concerning children and adolescents taking antidepressants, the number of 6- to 17-year-olds taking antidepressants has doubled.[40] In 2006, the FDA recommended extending the warning of increased suicidal risk to people taking an antidepressant who are 25 years of age and under.

Herbal supplements, such as St. John's wort, have also been touted as a treatment for depression, although there is some debate as to how effective they truly are. As is the case with all herbal supplements, St. John's wort is not subject to FDA approval, and it has not been put through the clinical trials that prescription medications have undergone to establish therapeutic dose and efficacy. In addition, St. John's wort can negatively interact with other medications such as those used to control HIV infection or to treat heart disease, depression, seizures, cancer, and organ transplant rejection. It can also interfere with the effectiveness of oral contraception.[41]

Exercise and activity level also play a significant role in alleviating and insulating people from depression.

A New Problem . . . Cyberbullying

From YouTube videos showing how to cut, burn, and harm yourself to cyberbullying, some Internet users have turned social networking into a new way to abuse, bully, and humiliate others. In a survey of 43,321 teenagers, 50 percent admitted to being bullied at least once. One of the most heartbreaking stories was that of 18-year-old Tyler Clementi, who was studying violin at Rutgers University. He posted on his Facebook page, "jumping off the gw bridge sorry," after he was shown having sex with another man online. His is not the

only suicide related to cyberbullying. Thirteen-year-old Ryan Halligan committed suicide after he was ridiculed on the Internet. Megan Meier, also 13 years old, hanged herself when she realized her Internet romance was a hoax. While there have always been bullies, cyberbullying takes bullying to a new level of abuse, as millions of people can witness the victim's humiliation and embarrassment, and it can be relived and viewed over and over again.

There is a call out for digital citizenship. We need to remind ourselves that, although

there is a sense of anonymity created by the Internet that can make it easier to reveal information about ourselves and others, the hurt and pain that cyberbullying can cause is very real and lasting.

Sources: Has social networking gone too far? *USA Today*, October 1, 2010; Teens say bullying is widespread. *USA Today*, October 25, 2010.

Again it seems that the endorphin levels and effects on brain chemistry and hormonal levels are part of the explanation for why this is a powerful antidote for depression.[42]

Electroconvulsive therapy (ECT) is another form of treatment for depression, with 100,000 Americans receiving this treatment each year. The procedure involves delivering a 90-volt burst of electricity, equal to the electricity in a 40-watt light bulb, to the brain for about a minute, causing a grand mal seizure. Proponents of ECT claim that shock treatments produce positive treatment effects for depression when no other antidepressant or treatment regimen has worked. Critics of ECT say that it causes brain damage and memory loss, and that the decrease in depressive symptoms is only temporary.[43] ECT can cause short-term memory loss, confusion, and disorientation. However, patients don't have permanent negative cognitive effects.[43]

 TALKING POINTS Have you ever felt depressed? If so, what did you do to cope with these feelings? What did you do that worked or didn't work to make you feel better?

Seasonal Affective Disorder In addition to the types of depression just described, some people may be especially vulnerable to depression on a seasonal basis. **Seasonal affective disorder (SAD)** is a form of depression that develops in relation to the changes in the seasons. While most people with SAD begin to feel increasingly depressed in October and report that their depression lifts in March or April, about one in six SAD sufferers experiences Summer SAD, beginning in May or June and ending in the fall months. Twice as many women as men are affected with SAD.[44] January 24 has been identified as the "most depressing day of the year" due to gloomy, cold weather; increasing debt following the holidays; failed New Years resolutions; and letdown

from the holidays. Research shows that people are happiest on the weekends and that Wednesday is the most depressing day of the week because it is in the middle of the workweek.[45]

SAD seems to be related to environmental factors such as light, temperature, and situational stressors. Weight gain, fatigue, increased sleep, diminished sex drive, and mood swings are some of the symptoms of Winter SAD; agitation, loss of appetite, insomnia, and increased suicidal thoughts are characteristic of Summer SAD. Seasonal depression in the winter seems to be linked to increases in the production of melatonin, a chemical that helps set the brain's daily rhythm, set off by the decrease in light. Antidepressants, counseling, and light therapy have been used to treat SAD. Light therapy for Winter SAD involves sitting in front of a lightbox with about a 10,000-lux-intensity light bulb, housed in a plastic diffusing screen, for 20–90 minutes each day so that the light is falling on the eyes.[44] For Summer SAD, which tends to occur in hotter locales, individuals are instructed to travel to cooler climates, to swim in cool water, and to stay in darkened, air-conditioned rooms.

Suicide Suicide is the third-leading cause of death for young adults 15–24 years old. It is the eleventh leading cause of all deaths in the United States but the second-leading cause of death for college students. More than half of college students reported contemplating suicide at some point in their lives, with 15 percent seriously considering it.[46] Men commit suicide four times more often than women do, and 72 percent of all suicides are

---

Key Terms

seasonal affective disorder (SAD) A type of depression that develops in relation to the changes in the seasons.

---

committed by white men. Suicide occurs most often among middle-aged Americans.[44] However, women are three times more likely than men to attempt suicide, and middle-aged women have seen a significant increase in their rate of suicide over the past decade, with an increase in hanging and suffocation as methods. The suicide rate for women 10–24 years of age increased an alarming 76 percent, the biggest increase in 15 years. Hanging and suffocation were the most common suicide methods for this group. Soldiers ages 20–24 are four times more likely to commit suicide than nonmilitary individuals, and soldiers in all age groups are two times more likely to commit suicide compared to those not in the military. Men tend to employ more violent methods such as shooting themselves, hanging, or jumping from high places, whereas women tend to use slower methods such as overdosing with pills or cutting their wrists, which allow more time for medical intervention. Suicide rates for African Americans have significantly decreased. Asian Americans are one of the lowest-risk groups in terms of ethnicity. The suicide rate for the Hispanic population is higher than for Caucasians and African Americans, a reverse trend from past years. While using a firearm is still the most common method of committing suicide, it has decreased as a method over the years. While most people assume suicides increase in the winter months, actually more suicides occur in summer than during any other season.

Why do people attempt or commit suicide? The majority of suicidal people have depressive disorders and feel helpless and powerless over their lives. They say things like "I just want the pain to stop" and don't see any other options available to them. There are some risk factors associated with suicidal behavior, such as these:

- Little to no support system
- Previous suicide attempts
- Family history of mental illness, including substance abuse
- Family history of suicide
- Problems with drugs or alcohol
- Possession of a firearm
- Exposure to suicidal behavior of others, including through the media

After the economic crisis began in 2007, there was a dramatic increase in calls to suicide hotlines and mental health centers as a result of people losing their jobs, houses, and health care and feeling hopeless because of the poor economy. It is estimated that over 300,000 suicide attempts occur each year in the United States, or more than one every 2 minutes.[47] Eleven hundred of these suicides occur on college campuses. Some people say that suicidal gestures or threats are merely a cry for attention and ignore them. But left ignored, the person may go ahead and take the next step to attempt suicide because no one seems to care. It is always best to take any threats or talk about suicide seriously and act accordingly. What should you do if a friend or family member talks to you about thoughts of suicide? See the box "Dos and Don'ts of Suicide Intervention" for strategies.

Bipolar Disorder Another important mood disorder is **bipolar disorder,** a condition that was previously known as manic depression. *Bipolar* refers to the extreme mood swings individuals with this disorder experience, from feeling euphoric, energetic, and reckless to feeling depressed, powerless, and listless. It is the least common of the mood disorders. Men and women are equally likely to develop this condition, and the average age of onset for the first manic episode typically is in the early to mid-20s. This change in mood or "mood swing" can last for hours, days, weeks, or months, and it is found among all ages, races, ethnic groups, and social classes. The illness tends to run in families and appears to have a genetic link, as it is more likely to affect the children of parents who have the disorder.[33] When one parent has bipolar disorder, the risk to each child is estimated to be 15–30 percent. When both parents have bipolar disorder, the risk increases to 50–75 percent.[48]

We described depression in the previous section. Bipolar disorder involves having both depressive periods and manic episodes. **Mania** is characterized by the following:

- Having excessive energy, needing little sleep
- Experiencing racing thoughts, feeling as though your mind is going 50 mph
- Speaking rapidly, changing from topic to topic quickly in conversation
- Becoming irritable
- Acting impulsively and recklessly—for example, going on spending sprees or having increased involvement in sexual activity, and drug and alcohol use
- Trying to do too much, feeling as though you can accomplish a great deal
- Being easily distracted
- Becoming excitable

> ### Key Terms
>
> **bipolar disorder** A mood disorder characterized by alternating episodes of depression and mania.
>
> **mania** An extremely excitable state characterized by excessive energy, racing thoughts, impulsive and/or reckless behavior, irritability, and proneness to distraction.

The Dos and Don'ts of Suicide Intervention

Do . . .

1. *If possible, stay with the person* until you can get further assistance.
2. *Offer support and assistance.* Tell the person he or she is not alone.
3. *Remain calm.* Talk about the person's feelings of sadness and helplessness.
4. *Encourage problem solving* and taking positive steps.
5. *Emphasize the temporary nature of the problem.* Suicide is a permanent solution to a temporary problem.
6. *Seek help; don't try to handle this problem on your own.* This might involve contacting the person's family, religious advisor, friends, or teachers, or calling a mental health agency for consultation.

7. *Ask the person to promise not to hurt or kill him- or herself.*

Don't . . .

1. *Avoid talking about suicide or dance around the topic.* Talking about suicide doesn't upset people more. In fact, often people who are thinking about killing themselves say it is a relief to talk about it and it helps them to let go of this idea, not pursue it further.
2. *Be judgmental or argumentative.* Now is not the time to debate the morality of suicide—you will lose the debate and possibly the person.
3. *Assume that the person is not serious.* Saying "You're not serious" or "You don't

mean that" may inadvertently encourage the person to show you how serious she or he truly is.
4. *Argue.* Telling a suicidal person that things aren't that bad or that other people have it worse can make the person feel worse about him- or herself and guilty about his or her feelings of unhappiness.
5. *Promise not to tell anyone.* If you keep this promise and something happens to this person, how will you feel?

Many people with bipolar disorder will tell you that they enjoy the "highs" but dread the lows. However, manic behavior can become very destructive because when people are in a manic phase they can accumulate enormous credit card debt, abuse drugs and alcohol, drive recklessly, and often feel invincible. They stay up all night and feel very little need for rest or food, and eventually their bodies can't function and they collapse. Mood stabilizers such as lithium carbonate (Lithobid), anticonvulsant medications such as valproic acid (Depakote), gabapentin (Neurontin), topiramate (Topamax), and lamotrigine (Lamictal), and antipsychotic medications such as aripiprazole (Abilify), along with psychotherapy, have been used to treat bipolar disorder.

Anxiety Disorders

Bill, a very talented and bright 26-year-old, has a promising career as an executive in a large accounting firm. However, he is in jeopardy of losing his job because of his absenteeism and tardiness. He has missed several important meetings with clients and not been able to get his work done on time as a result. It can take him hours to get to work even though he lives 15 minutes away, and sometimes he doesn't go to work even though he is in the car and ready to go. Bill has a routine in the morning that involves checking the windows, doors, iron, stove, and garage door five times to ensure that things are secure and safe. Sometimes he drives off and then returns to the house to check again. He feels a need to turn the handles on doors five times, and if he loses track, he starts all over again.

Susan has been having such severe panic attacks in the car while driving to work that she has needed to pull over. Her heart races, her breathing is labored, and she sometimes feels as though she is having a heart attack and is dying. She is frightened of being in the car alone and having an attack and being unable to get help, or of having an accident. She is beginning to be afraid to leave her house and feels safer at home. She has declined invitations to go out with her friends and goes out only when absolutely necessary. She feels as though she is losing control of her life.

John worries constantly about what other people think of him. When he hears people laughing, he assumes that they are laughing at him. He has trouble having conversations with people because he believes whatever he says will sound stupid and that people will not like him. He also plays conversations over and over in his head when he is trying to go to sleep, thinking about what he should have said and worrying about how people are judging him.

Bill, Susan, and John are all suffering from *anxiety disorders.* While everyone tends to feel nervous or worry about something at some point in their lives, people with anxiety disorders feel anxious most, if not all, of the time. They also feel out of control and powerless to alleviate their anxiety, and they tend to worry about becoming anxious, so their anxiety causes them even greater anxiety. Anxiety is related to fear and is part of daily life. Some anxiety can even be helpful and motivating at times. Anxiety is a physiological, adaptive response to danger or potential threat and can enhance performance and keep us out of harm's way. In Chapter 3 we discuss

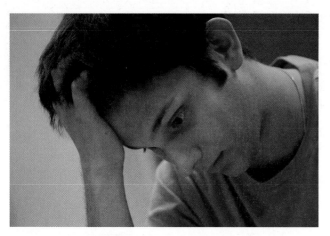

Anxiety is one of the three most frequent problems students report experiencing during college.

the fight or flight response and how the stress response is related to anxiety. Anxiety disorders are differentiated from daily stress as being

- Intense, often debilitating, experiences during which people sometimes think they are going to die
- Long lasting, persisting after the danger or stressful event has passed
- Dysfunctional, causing significant interference in daily functioning

Anxiety disorders include **generalized anxiety disorder (GAD); obsessive-compulsive disorder (OCD),** such as Bill's problem; posttraumatic stress disorder; **panic disorder,** which describes Susan's symptoms; and phobias such as the **social phobia** John suffers from.[49] Approximately 40 million Americans have an anxiety disorder, and women are twice as likely as men to suffer from panic disorder, posttraumatic stress disorder, generalized anxiety disorder, agoraphobia, and other specific phobias.[50] There are no gender differences with obsessive-compulsive disorder or social phobia. There is a genetic component associated with developing an anxiety disorder: Studies suggest that you are more likely to develop one if your parents have one. Environmental stressors and events can be instrumental in whether this predisposition is activated or not.

The treatment for anxiety disorders may involve a combination of medication and counseling. There is some evidence that a deficiency in the neurotransmitter serotonin or a disturbance in metabolizing serotonin is associated with this condition, and taking an antidepressant increases the serotonin levels in the brain. Individuals suffering from anxiety disorders can also benefit from learning stress management, relaxation, and ways of coping with the stress.[49] Exercise, good nutrition, and avoidance of stimulants such as caffeine can also be helpful in alleviating anxiety.

Attention Deficit Hyperactivity Disorder (ADHD)

Once thought to be only a childhood disorder, **attention deficit hyperactivity disorder (ADHD)** is now being diagnosed in record numbers in adults. This increase might be the result of overlooking or misdiagnosing problems in childhood that later are accurately diagnosed in adults. With symptoms that include being fidgety, disorganized, overactive, and easily distracted, a child may be seen as simply misbehaving rather than having a diagnosable disorder. It is often the child with ADHD who is seen as "disruptive" in the classroom and "lazy, stupid, or a daydreamer" by friends and family. Actually, the truth about these individuals is often the opposite: They tend to be highly intelligent, motivated, creative, and energetic individuals.

It is currently estimated that over 15 million Americans suffer from this disorder, affecting males more than females, 3:1. There is strong evidence of a genetic cause for ADHD, although environmental factors can certainly contribute to the problem. One of the landmark studies in ADHD was conducted on adults and showed that there is a difference at the cellular level in energy consumption between the parts of the brain that regulate attention, emotion, and impulse control in people with ADHD compared with those without.[51]

Following are the symptoms often seen in adult ADHD:

- A sense of underachievement, or not meeting one's goals
- Difficulty getting organized
- Chronic procrastination or trouble getting started
- Trouble with following-through and completing tasks
- Many tasks going on simultaneously, switching from one to another
- Easily bored and frequently searching for high stimulation
- Easily distracted, trouble focusing and sustaining attention
- Creative, intuitive, highly intelligent
- Impulsive, doesn't stop to think things through
- Impatient, low tolerance for frustration
- Tendency to worry needlessly and endlessly
- Insecure
- Moody
- Restless
- Tendency toward addictive behavior
- Low self-esteem
- Inaccurate self-concept, unaware of effect on others
- Childhood history of ADHD or presence of symptoms since childhood

Psychological tests such as the Test of Variability of Attention (TOVA) and an IQ test can help substantiate a diagnosis of ADHD. The TOVA tests the subject by flashing different shapes on a screen and quantifying attention, distractibility, and impulsivity based on the subject's responses. The most effective treatment for ADHD involves a multimodal approach: counseling and coaching the individual to provide strategies, techniques, and structure for daily life; education, tools such as daily planners and organizers; goal setting and time management; and medication such as methylphenidate (Concerta, Ritalin), amphetamine-dextroamphetamine (Adderall), atomoxetine (Strattera), and lisdexamfetamine dimesylate (Vyvanse). (These medications are discussed in more detail in Chapter 7.)

Schizophrenia

Schizophrenia is one of the most severe mental disorders; it is characterized by profound distortions in one's thought processes, emotions, perceptions, and behavior. People with schizophrenia experience hallucinations (seeing things that are not there, hearing voices), delusions (believing that they are Jesus, the CIA is after them, or radio waves are controlling their mind), and disorganized thinking (wearing multiple coats, scarves, and gloves on a warm day, shouting and swearing at passersby, maintaining a rigid posture and not moving for hours). The movie *A Beautiful Mind* gives a glimpse into the life of one schizophrenic, John Nash, and how he managed his symptoms.

There are several types of schizophrenia: paranoid, disorganized, catatonic, and undifferentiated. This disabling illness affects 1 percent of the U.S. population, and symptoms typically surface in people in their late teens and early 20s. Men and women are equally likely to develop schizophrenia, and it seems to run in families. Schizophrenia is often confused with dissociative identity disorder (formerly called multiple personality disorder), which is an entirely separate and distinct mental illness. People with dissociative identity disorder display two or more distinct identities or personalities that take control of their lives; people with schizophrenia do not have multiple, separate, enduring personalities.

There are many theories to explain what causes schizophrenia. Some research suggests that heredity accounts for about 80 percent of the cause of schizophrenia, with the other 20 percent due to environmental stressors or situations. Researchers have also identified a number of abnormalities in the brains of diagnosed schizophrenics, including smaller temporal lobes, enlargement of the ventricles, and cerebral atrophy in the frontal lobes. Research is also being done on how the variations in chromosome-22 genes may be linked to schizophrenia. Individuals with schizophrenia also seem to have nearly double the number of dopamine receptors in their brains, leading to the theory that too much dopamine is being released into the brain pathways and causing schizophrenia symptoms. The antipsychotic medications act to block the receptors and prevent the transmission of dopamine, reducing the amount of dopamine in the system that is creating this chemical imbalance.[1]

While there is no cure for schizophrenia, there are antipsychotic medications, such as quetiapine (Seroquel), risperidone (Risperdal), olanzapine (Zyprexa), aripiprazole (Abilify), and ziprasidone (Geodon), that can effectively treat this illness and enable people to live functional, satisfying lives. Psychotherapy can be helpful in developing problem-solving approaches, in addition to identifying stressors and triggers, and early detection of a psychotic episode. Unfortunately, some people with schizophrenia are unable to recognize that they are delusional or irrational, and so do not get treatment or take their medications on a regular basis.

Treatment for Psychological Disorders

Many effective treatments and therapies are available for psychological disorders.

Key Terms

generalized anxiety disorder (GAD) An anxiety disorder that involves experiencing intense and nonspecific anxiety for at least six months, in which the intensity and frequency of worry is excessive and out of proportion to the situation.

obsessive-compulsive disorder (OCD) An anxiety disorder characterized by obsessions (intrusive thoughts, images, or impulses causing a great deal of distress) and compulsions (repetitive behaviors aimed at reducing anxiety or stress that is associated with the obsessive thoughts).

panic disorder An anxiety disorder characterized by panic attacks, in which individuals experience severe physical symptoms. These episodes can seemingly occur "out of the blue" or be triggered by something and can last for a few minutes or for hours.

social phobia A phobia characterized by feelings of extreme dread and embarrassment in situations in which public speaking or social interaction is involved.

attention deficit hyperactivity disorder (ADHD) Inability to concentrate well on a specified task; often accompanied by above-normal physical movement.

schizophrenia One of the most severe mental disorders, characterized by profound distortions in one's thought processes, emotions, perceptions, and behavior. Symptoms may include hallucinations, delusions, disorganized thinking, and a rigid posture or motionlessness.

Chapter Two Achieving Psychological Health

Providers of Treatment   As in other areas of health care, a variety of practitioners treat and manage the mental health conditions described in this chapter. Practitioners may vary in their training and in the specific therapies they use.

Psychiatrists are medical doctors who specialize in treating psychological disorders through the use of biological and medical interventions; they can prescribe drugs and perform procedures such as electroshock therapy. They tend to place less focus on talking about one's problem and to treat more severely and chronically ill patients.

Psychologists have a doctoral-level degree in counselling or clinical psychology and must be licensed by the state. They treat a range of conditions, from relationship problems to severe psychological disorders. Psychologists may use behavioral therapy, problem solving, and other techniques that focus on changing a client's attitudes, behaviors, and patterns of thinking.

Counselors typically have a master's degree in counseling or clinical psychology. Master's-level counselors can be licensed as professional mental health counselors in every state. They specialize in areas such as substance abuse treatment, marriage and family therapy, and vocational rehabilitation.

Social workers have a master's degree in social work and must also be licensed. They provide both mental health services and social services to the community. They typically counsel clients and arrange for services that can help them, including drug rehabilitation, child care, and debt counseling.

Approaches to Treatment   There are hundreds of approaches to treating psychological disorders, and new variations and models continue to develop. Most are based on a few basic therapeutic models, which are briefly summarized as follows:

Psychodynamic therapy focuses on the childhood forces that affect personality development and underlie an individual's current problems. Dynamic therapy is usually long term, intensive, and expensive, and insurance companies might refuse to cover it.

Interpersonal process therapy (IPT) is a relational approach to psychotherapy. It is predicated on the belief that problems are interpersonal in nature and that family experiences have a significant impact on one's sense of self and others. IPT assumes that people reenact their family dynamics in their current relationships. It is the goal of therapy to reenact these same patterns between the client and the therapist and to resolve them in a healthy, effective manner.

Humanistic therapy is based on the belief that people, left to their own devices, will naturally grow in positive and constructive ways. The therapist helps clients unearth their natural potential and gain greater self-awareness and self-acceptance.

Behavior therapy is based on the idea that behavior is learned and so can be unlearned, and that different, more adaptive behavior can be taught. Treatment focuses on behavior change. Behavior therapy may be especially effective for the treatment of anxiety disorders such as phobias.

Cognitive-behavioral therapy focuses on changing an individual's cognitive patterns in order to change his or her behavior and emotional state. The therapist helps clients become aware of their distorted thought patterns and change them through strategies such as cognitive restructuring and thought stopping (see the section "Building Optimism" on page 37 for examples of cognitive restructuring). This type of treatment has been used for many conditions, including anxiety disorders, mood disorders, and eating disorders.

Solution-focused therapy is a goal-oriented approach that helps clients change by looking for solutions rather than dwelling on problems. Clients are encouraged to envision a future in which their problems are no longer a dominant force in their lives. Treatment interventions are designed to reach that goal.

Couples and family therapy includes premarital and marital counseling, conflict mediation, and divorce counseling. Psychological issues that may be addressed include communication and assertiveness skills, sexual disorders, anger management, and blended families.

Group therapy allows clients to overcome a sense of isolation and learn new behaviors in a safe, supportive atmosphere. A small group of people meet regularly with a therapist to focus on a problem they share—such as childhood sexual abuse, eating disorders, or drug abuse. Group members understand one another's experiences and can support one another.

Psychological Health: A Final Thought

As you can see, psychological health involves how your emotions, thoughts, and behavior interplay with one another and with the world around you. There is an important mind-body connection in terms of your psychological health having a significant impact on your physical health, and vice versa. Psychological health is not just the absence of mental illness, and there is a range

---

Key Terms

interpersonal process therapy A relational approach to psychotherapy that suggests problems are interpersonal in nature and family experiences have a significant impact on one's sense of self and others.

or continuum of psychological health. Possessing a positive self-concept, developing high self-esteem, and cultivating an optimistic attitude toward life can promote psychological health and enhance relationships with others. While heredity plays a role in the development of personality and psychological health, environmental factors and stressors seem to have an equally important role. As people age and encounter developmental milestones, they also encounter new challenges, obstacles, and resources in continuing to maintain their psychological health.

Taking Charge of Your Health

- Take the Personal Assessment at the end of this chapter to assess your explanatory style.
- Apply the steps of an optimistic approach to life to a situation in your life.
- Take the online screening assessment for depression, bipolar disorder, anxiety, or

posttraumatic stress disorder at www. dbsalliance.org (look under signs and symptoms then screenings).
- Keep a journal, and each day write down things you like about yourself or feel good about.

- Take a risk and do something you have been wanting to do, such as joining a club, trying a sport, or meeting new people.

SUMMARY

- Psychological health has also been associated with developing and maintaining a positive self-concept, positive self-esteem, and emotional intelligence.
- Two factors, nature and nurture, influence the shaping of personality. *Nature* refers to the innate factors we are born with that genetically determine our personality traits. *Nurture* is the effect that the environment, people, and external factors have on our personality.
- Maslow's theory is a positive, optimistic theory of human behavior. He believed that people are motivated to grow and fulfill their potential, referring to this phenomenon as self-actualization.
- Nonverbal communication is what is communicated by your facial expression, body posture, tone of voice, and movements.

- Having a positive interpretation of life's events, particularly how you cope with adversity, can make a significant difference in terms of your health and academic and work performance, as well as how long you will live.
- Clinical depression can range from mild to severe and can result in significant impairment in functioning.
- The majority of suicidal people have depressive disorders and feel helpless and powerless over their lives.
- Schizophrenia is one of the most severe mental disorders, characterized by profound distortions in one's thought processes, emotions, perceptions, and behavior.

REVIEW QUESTIONS

1. What are three factors that have been associated with psychological health?
2. What are the characteristics commonly demonstrated by psychologically healthy people?
3. What is the definition of *self-esteem,* and how can self-esteem be enhanced?
4. What characterizes people with overall high levels of emotional intelligence?
5. What relationship is there between humor and psychological health?

6. What is nonverbal communication?
7. Describe Maslow's theory of the hierarchy of needs.
8. How can having a positive interpretation of life's events make a significant difference in people's health?
9. How is clinical depression different from having the "blues"?
10. How should you respond to someone threatening or talking about committing suicide?

ANSWERS TO THE "WHAT DO YOU KNOW?" QUIZ

1. True   2. False   3. False   4. False   5. True   6. True   7. False

Visit the Online Learning Center (**www.mhhe.com/hahn11e**), where you will find tools to help you improve your grade including practice quizzes, key terms flashcards, audio chapter summaries for your MP3 player, and many other study aids.

SOURCE NOTES

1. Kosslyn S, Rosenberg R. *Psychology in Context* (3rd ed.). Boston: Pearson, 2006.
2. Seligman M. *Learned Optimism.* New York: Simon & Schuster, 1990.
3. Mental health low in college freshmen. *USA Today,* January 27, 2011.
4. Turner J, Stels J. *The Sociology of Emotions.* New York: Cambridge University Press, 2005.
5. McKay M, Fanning P. *Self-Esteem* (3rd ed.). Oakland, CA: New Harbinger, 1992.
6. Goleman D. *Emotional Intelligence.* New York: Bantam Books, 1997.
7. Baucum D, Smith C. *Psychology: An Introduction* (9th ed.). Belmont, CA: Wadsworth, 2004.
8. Maslow AH. *Motivation and Personality* (2nd ed.). New York: Van Nostrand, 1970.
9. Maslow AH. *The Farthest Reaches of Human Nature.* Magnolia, MA: Peter Smith, 1983.
10. Lefton L, Brannon L. *Psychology* (9th ed.). Boston: Pearson, 2006.
11. Helliwell J, Putnam R. The social context of well-being. *Philosophical Transactions of the Royal Society of London,* B, 359, 1435–1446, 2004.
12. Schnall E. Attend religious services, live longer. *Psychology and Health,* 2008.
13. Deaton A. Income, health, and well-being around the world: evidence from the Gallup World Poll. *Journal of Economic Perspectives,* 22(2), 53–72, 2008.
14. Wade C, Tavris C. *Psychology* (10th ed.). New York: Harper & Row, 2010.
15. Martin LR, Friedman HS. Nonverbal communication and health care. In RE Riggio and RS Feldman (Eds.), *Application of Nonverbal Communication.* Hillsdale, NJ: Lawrence Erlbaum, 2004.
16. Matsumoto D, Willingham B. Spontaneous facial expressions of emotion of congenitally and non-congenitally blind individuals. *Journal of Personality and Social Psychology,* 96(1), 1–10, 2009.
17. Castro B, Eshleman J, Shearer R. Using humor to reduce stress and improve relationships. *Seminar Nurse Management,* 7(2), 90–92, 1999.
18. Berk L, Felten D, Tan S, Bittman B, Westengard J. Modulation of neuroimmune parameters during the eustress of humor associated mirthful laughter. *Alternative Therapies in Health and Medicine,* March 2001.
19. Bennett M, Zeller J, Rosenberg L, McCann J. The effect of mirthful laughter on stress and natural killer cell activity. *Alternative Therapies in Health and Medicine,* March-April 2003.
20. Skinner N, Brewer, N. The dynamics of threat and challenge appraisals prior to stressful achievement events. *Journal of Personality and Social Psychology,* September 2002.
21. Futch A. The effect of sense of humor, defensiveness, and gender on the interpretation of ambiguous messages. *Communication Quarterly,* January 1, 1999.
22. Bennett M, Lengacher C. Humor and laughter may influence health: III laughter and health outcomes. *Evidence-Based Complementary and Alternative Medicine,* March 2008.
23. Santhanam K. Laugh and be well. *The Hindu,* March 12, 2000.
24. Nair M. A documentary: *The Laughing Clubs of India,* 2001.
25. Berk L, et al. Modulation of neuroimmune parameters during the eustress of humor associated mirthful laughter. *Alternative Therapies in Health and Medicine,* 7(2), 67–72, 2001.
26. Barefoot J, Brummett B, Williams R, Siegler I, Helms M, Boyle S, Chapp-Channing N, Mark D. Recovery expectations and long-term prognosis of patients with coronary heart disease. *Journal of Personality and Social Psychology,* 96(1), 2009.
27. Seligman M, Maier S. Failure to escape traumatic shock. *Journal of Experimental Psychology,* 74, 1–9, 1967.
28. Firmin M, Hwang C, Copella M, Clark S. Learned helplessness: the effect of failure on test-taking. *Education,* 124(4), 674–688, 2004.
29. Ellis A. *Reason and Emotion in Psychotherapy.* New York: Lyle Stuart, 1962.
30. Kessler R, Chiu W, Demier O, Walters E. Prevalence, severity, and comorbidity of twelve-month DSM-IV disorders in the National Comorbidity Survey Replication (NCS-R). *Archives of General Psychiatry,* 62(2), 617–627, 2005.
31. U.S. Census Bureau. Population estimates by demographic characteristics. Table 2: Annual estimates of the population by selected age groups and sex for the United States: April 1, 2000 to July 1, 2004. (NC-EST2004-02). www.census.gov/popest/national/asrh/PopulationDivision. June 9, 2005.
32. World Health Organization. The World Health Report 2005: Changing History. Annex table 3: Burden of disease in DALY's by cause, sex, and mortality stratum in WHO regions, estimates for 2003. Geneva: WHO, 2005.
33. American Psychiatric Association. *Diagnostic and Statistical Manual of Mental Disorders* (4th ed.) (DSM-IV-TR). Washington, DC: American Psychiatric Press, 2000.
34. World Health Organization. *Mental Health,* 2005.
35. National Institute of Mental Health, 2010.
36. Dramatic increases seen in college students' mental health problems over the last 13 years. *Journal of Professional Psychology: Research and Practice,* February 2003.
37. Pappas S. Depression gene really exists, new study claims, www.msnbc.com, January 4, 2010.
38. Peterson K. Resilience, talking can help kids beat depression. *USA Today,* June 4, 2002.
39. Depression and anxiety. *Consumer Reports,* July 2010.
40. Americans taking antidepressants doubles. *USA Today,* August 4, 2009.
41. Hypericum Depression Trial Study Group. Effect of *Hypericum perforatum* (St. John's wort) in major depressive disorder: a randomized controlled study. *Journal of the American Medical Association,* 287(14), 1807–1814, 2002.
42. Exercise better than drugs for depression. *British Journal of Sports Medicine,* 35, 114–117, 2001.
43. Rami L, Bernardo M, Boget T, Ferrer J, Portella M, Gil-Verona J, Salamero M. Cognitive status of psychiatric patients under maintenance electroconvulsive therapy: a one-year longitudinal study. *The Journal of Neuropsychiatry and Clinical Neurosciences,* 16, 465–471, 2004.
44. Rosenthal NE. *Winter Blues* (rev. ed.). New York: Guilford Press, 2005.
45. There's a psychological reason you're happiest on the weekends. *USA Today,* January 12, 2010.
46. Half of all college students consider suicide, www.msnbc.com, August 18, 2008.
47. U.S. Suicide Rate Increases. Johns Hopkins Bloomberg School of Public Health, October 21, 2008.
48. McGuffin P, et al. The heritability of bipolar affective disorder and the genetic relationship to univocal depression. *Archives of General Psychiatry,* 60(5), 497–502, 2003.
49. Bourne E. *The Anxiety and Phobia Workbook.* Oakland, CA: New Harbinger, 1995.
50. Kessler RC, Chiu WT, Demler O, Walters EE. Prevalence, severity, and comorbidity of twelve-month DSM-IV disorders in the National Comorbidity Survey Replication (NCS-R). *Archives of General Psychiatry,* 62(6), 617–627, 2005.
51. Hallowell E, Ratey J. *Driven to Distraction.* New York: Simon & Schuster, 1995.

Personal Assessment

What Is Your Explanatory Style?

Instructions: For each statement, circle the response that best fits you.

1. The project you are in charge of is a great success.
   A. I kept a close watch over everyone's work. 1
   B. Everyone devoted a lot of time and energy to it. 0
2. You and your partner make up after a fight.
   A. I forgave my partner. 0
   B. I'm usually forgiving. 1
3. You get lost driving to a friend's house.
   A. I missed a turn. 1
   B. My friend gave me bad directions. 0
4. You were extremely healthy all year.
   A. Few people around me were sick, so I wasn't exposed. 0
   B. I made sure I ate well and got enough rest. 1
5. You forgot your friend's birthday.
   A. I'm not good at remembering birthdays. 1
   B. I was preoccupied with other things. 0
6. Your boss gives you too little time to finish a project, but you get it done anyway.
   A. I am good at my job. 0
   B. I am an efficient person. 1
7. They won't honor your credit card at a store.
   A. I sometimes overestimate how much money I have. 1
   B. I sometimes forget to pay my credit card bill. 0
8. Your car runs out of gas on a dark street late at night.
   A. I didn't check to see how much gas was in the tank. 1
   B. The gas gauge was broken. 0
9. You fail an important examination.
   A. I wasn't as smart as the other people taking the test. 1
   B. I didn't prepare for it well enough. 0
10. You lose your temper with a friend.
    A. My friend is always nagging me. 1
    B. My friend was in a hostile mood. 0
11. You win an athletic contest.
    A. I was feeling unbeatable. 0
    B. I trained hard. 1
12. A friend thanks you for helping her get through a bad time.
    A. I enjoy helping her through tough times. 0
    B. I am good at giving useful advice. 1

Scoring Key

Add together items 3, 5, 7, 8, 9, and 10 to get your B (bad events) score = _____

If you scored:

5 to 6—You tend to be very pessimistic and explain bad things as resulting from something you did or a personal characteristic that is lasting and extends to many areas of your life.

2 to 4—You tend to have an average level of pessimism about negative events.

0 to 1—You tend to be very optimistic and explain bad things as resulting from something someone else did or a circumstance that is temporary and specific to only that situation.

Add together items 1, 2, 4, 6, 11, and 12 to get your G (good events) score = _____

If you scored:

5 to 6—You tend to be very optimistic and explain good things as resulting from something you did or a personal characteristic that is lasting and extends to many areas of your life.

2 to 4—You tend to have an average level of optimism about positive events.

0 to 1—You tend to be very pessimistic and explain good things as resulting from something someone else did or a circumstance that is temporary and specific to only that situation.

TO CARRY THIS FURTHER . . .

How did you score? If your explanatory style tends to be pessimistic, try some of the strategies suggested in Chapter 2 for building optimism. When you encounter adversity, pay attention to your thinking patterns and consciously reframe them to be more positive and more focused on problem solving. Building a more optimistic approach to life can improve many dimensions of your health.

Source: Adapted from M. Seligman, *Learned Optimism.* New York: Pocket Books, 1990.

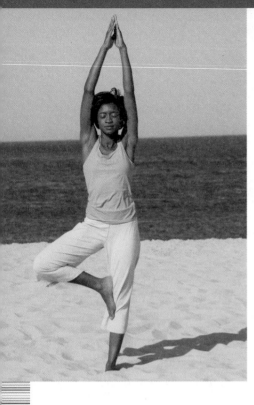

3

Managing Stress

What Do You Know About Managing Stress?

1. Having stress in your life is negative. True or False?

2. Time management is the reason most college students cite for their academic success or failure. True or False?

3. Laughing is important to managing stress. True or False?

4. Different colors, sounds, and smells can affect your stress level. True or False?

5. Breathing is the key to stress management. True or False?

6. You can make up for not sleeping enough during the week by sleeping more on the weekend. True or False?

7. Exposing yourself to stressful situations can sometimes help you reduce your stress. True or False?

Check your answers at the end of the chapter.

What Is Stress?

How do you know when you are stressed? You might experience headaches, stomachaches, or back and neck aches, or you might feel irritable, tired, anxious, and depressed. Some people eat more, while others find eating difficult when they are stressed. **Stress** refers to physiological and psychological responses to a significant or unexpected change or disruption in one's life. It can be brought on by real or imagined factors or events.

Stress was first described in the 1930s by Hans Selye, who observed that patients suffering from a variety of illnesses all showed common symptoms, such as fatigue, appetite disturbance, sleep problems, mood swings, gastrointestinal problems, and diminished concentration and recall. He called this collection of symptoms—this stress disease—stress syndrome, or the **general adaptation syndrome (GAS).** He also described this as "the syndrome of being ill."[1] We will discuss Selye's discovery later in the chapter.

Selye defined stress as "the nonspecific response of the body to any demand whether it is caused by or results in pleasant or unpleasant conditions."[1] Stress can be positive or negative. It is our response to stress—how we manage stress—that makes a difference in terms of how it affects us. Stress resulting from unpleasant events or conditions is called **distress** (from the Greek *dys*, meaning "bad," as in displeasure). Stress resulting from pleasant events or conditions is called **eustress** (from the Greek *eu*, meaning "good," as in euphoria). Both distress and eustress elicit the same physiological responses in the body, as noted in Selye's GAS model.

While stress may not always be negative, our responses to it can be problematic or unhealthy. Both positive and negative stressful situations place extra demands on the body—your body reacts to an unexpected change or a highly emotional experience, regardless of whether this change is good or bad. If the duration of the stress is relatively short, the overall effect is minimal, and your body will rest, renew itself, and return to normal. But, as you will learn in this chapter, experiencing long-lasting stress or multiple stressors simultaneously, and not managing stress effectively can take a toll on your body.

How We Respond to Stress

When we are stressed, we react in specific ways. The stress response is the result of learned and conditioned habits adopted early in life as a way of coping with problems, conflict, and disruptive events. But many of our responses to stress are innate, basic human survival mechanisms with primordial roots. In prehistoric times, the best response to perceived danger, such as seeing a saber-toothed tiger about to attack, was either to fight the animal or to run away. Stress in modern times remains the same except that we are responding to twenty-first-century threats and dangers rather than to saber-toothed tigers. Again, it is not the events that determine how stressed we will feel but our response to these stressors (see the box "Stress-Prone Personalities"). We next discuss the way that this innate stress response affects our modern lives.

Fight or Flight Response

Our response to stress involves many physiological changes that are collectively called the fight or flight response. In situations in which you must react immediately to danger, it is advisable to either fight off the danger or flee. For example, you are walking back from class at night, thinking about all the studying you need to do, and you begin to cross the street. Suddenly, out of nowhere, a car's headlights are coming right at you. Since your best response is probably not to fight the car, you run as fast as you can to the other side of the road. In that split second when you see the car careening toward you, your muscles tense, your heart beats faster, your adrenaline pumps faster and is released at increased levels into your bloodstream, your breathing becomes more shallow and rapid, and your pupils dilate to see the car better.

This is the fight or flight response. Again, all these changes are adaptive and helpful to your survival in getting out of harm's way. In the car example, when you get to the other side of the road and realize that you are okay, your body begins to relax and return to its normal state. You take a deep breath and let out a big sigh of relief. Your muscles may feel even weaker than usual, your breathing may become deeper and heavier than is typical, and you may feel shaky as your body goes from extreme arousal to rapid relaxation. Figure 3-1a depicts the changes from the normal state to an arousal state to a very relaxed state, and then back to normal.

Chronic Stress

Now let's consider a different situation. You have a test in a week that you are very concerned about. It seems to be preoccupying your every waking thought, and you are having trouble sleeping as well. You are worried that you won't perform well on the test, and you really need to do better than you did on your last test. Your parents have been putting a great deal of pressure on you to do better in school in general. Because our bodies respond similarly to perceived or anticipated threats, you can have the same response to things that have and have not yet occurred. In other words, your heart races, your breathing becomes labored, your muscles are tense, your body sweats, and blood flow is constricted to the extremities and digestive organs and increases to the major muscles and your brain. Your body is becoming ready to fight or flee. However, you cannot take any action and make a fight or flight response because nothing has happened yet. You haven't taken the test yet, and even once you have done so, you won't know your grade. So your body remains at this high level of arousal, as depicted in Figure 3-1b.

Remaining in a continued state of physiological arousal for an extended period of time is called chronic stress. This high level of arousal is similar to putting your foot on the accelerator of your car while it is in park and not letting up on the gas pedal. Since the fight or flight response is meant to be a very quick, short-acting response, your body begins to wear down if kept at this physiological state of arousal for too long; eventually, you will begin to feel exhausted. This is also the reason that people cope better with anxiety by

> **Key Terms**
>
> **stress** The physiological and psychological state of disruption caused by the presence of an unanticipated, disruptive, or stimulating event.
>
> **general adaptation syndrome (GAS)** Sequenced physiological responses to the presence of a stressor, involving the alarm, resistance, and exhaustion stages of the stress response.
>
> **distress** Stress that diminishes the quality of life; commonly associated with disease, illness, and maladaptation.
>
> **eustress** Stress that enhances the quality of life.
>
> **stress response** The physiological and psychological responses to positive or negative events that are disruptive, unexpected, or stimulating.
>
> **fight or flight response** The physiological response to a stressor that prepares the body for confrontation or avoidance.
>
> **chronic stress** Remaining at a high level of physiological arousal for an extended period of time; can also occur when an individual is not able to immediately react to a real or a perceived threat.

Chapter Three Managing Stress

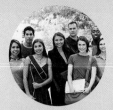

Learning from Our Diversity

Stress-Prone Personalities

Are you someone who has a low stress tolerance? Or are you a thrill seeker who thrives on an adrenaline rush? There has been a great deal of research on how our personalities determine how we react to stress. There are a variety of personality types in relation to stress: types A, B, and D personalities; stress-hardy personalities; helpless-hopeless personalities; survivor personalities; and sensation seekers.

You are probably familiar with the type A and B personalities. Type A individuals feel pressured, are impatient and easily annoyed, talk and move rapidly, and are ambitious and competitive. Type B's are the opposite: relaxed, easygoing, patient. Type A personality has been associated with a higher rate of cardiovascular disease. Type D personalities respond to distress with feelings of depression, loneliness, and negativity and have low self-esteem. Type D personalities also are strongly associated with hypertension and coronary heart disease, are less responsive to treatment, and have a shorter life expectancy.

Stress-hardy individuals seem to share three personality characteristics: commitment, challenge, and control. They demonstrate a strong commitment to their work, family, values, and themselves. They show a sense of resiliency in the face of adversity similar to what is discussed in Chapter 2 concerning optimistic individuals. You can take the Personal Assessment at the end of the chapter to see if you have a stress-hardy personality.

The helpless-hopeless personality type was also discussed in Chapter 2 in relation to learned helplessness. These are people who have low self-esteem and feel powerless to overcome adversity. They readily admit defeat and are negative and pessimistic in their outcome on life. They tend to have an external locus of control and believe that external factors (luck, chance, other people) are stronger determinants than internal factors (self-confidence, faith, intuition) in what happens in their lives. The helpless-hopeless personality tends to have more trouble managing stress effectively and to feel depressed, frustrated, and dissatisfied with life.

Survivor personality types encompass optimism, problem solving, and creativity, responding rather than reacting to stressful situations. Aron Ralston is an example of a survivor. He cut off his right arm with a pocket knife in order to free himself from an 800-pound boulder that had crushed his arm when he was rock climbing. Then he rappelled 80 feet down and hiked miles to his car.

Sensation seekers, or type R (risk taker) personalities, embrace stress rather than run from it. They have several common personality characteristics: They seek adventures and experiences, are uninhibited, and are easily bored. They learn survival skills that they successfully apply to stressful situations. They participate in extreme sports and activities, such as skydiving, rock climbing, and hang gliding, that better prepare them for unexpected stressful events.

Do any of these personality types fit you? Does your personality type help or hinder you in coping with stress?

Source: Seaward B, *Managing Stress* (6th ed.). Sudbury, MA: Jones & Bartlett, 2009.

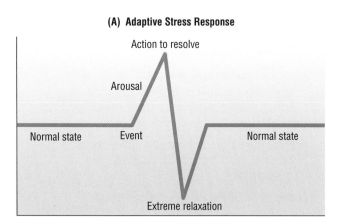

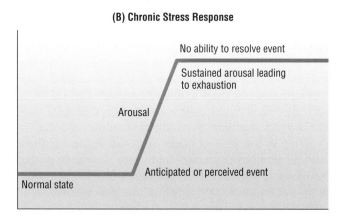

Figure 3-1 Resolving Stress How quickly and effectively you act to resolve stress has a significant effect on how long your body remains at a high level of physiological arousal.

Source: Selye H, *The Stress of Life.* New York: McGraw-Hill, 1984.

taking some action, doing something about whatever they are worried about, rather than stewing about their problems. Thus, the fight or flight response can be triggered inappropriately in response to phobias, irrational beliefs, an overactive imagination, or hallucinations or delusions.

The Three Stages of Stress

Once under the influence of a stressor, people's bodies respond in remarkably similar, predictable ways. For example, when you have to give a speech for a class, your heart rate may increase, your throat may become dry, your palms may sweat, and you may feel lightheaded, dizzy, and nauseous. If an individual lost her or his job or discovered that her or his partner wanted to terminate their relationship, she or he might experience similar sensations. It is clear that different stressors are able to evoke common physical reactions.

Selye described the typical physical response to a stressor in his general adaptation syndrome model discussed earlier in the chapter.[1] Selye stated that the human body moves through three stages when confronted by stressors, as follows.

Alarm Stage

Once exposed to any event that is perceived as threatening or dangerous, the body immediately prepares for difficulty, entering what Selye called the **alarm stage.** These involuntary changes, shown in Figure 3-2, are controlled by the hormonal and nervous systems, and they trigger the fight or flight response. For example, you realize that the final exam you thought was today was actually scheduled for yesterday. You may begin to experience fear, panic, anxiety, anger, depression, and restlessness.[2]

Resistance Stage

The second stage of a response to a stressor is the **resistance stage,** during which the body attempts to reestablish its equilibrium or internal balance. The body is geared for survival, and because staying in the alarm stage for a prolonged amount of time is not conducive to optimal functioning, it will resist the threat or attempt to resolve the problem and reduce the intensity of the response to a more manageable level. Specific organ systems, such as the cardiovascular and digestive systems, become the focus of the body's response.[2] During this phase, you might take steps to calm yourself down and relieve the stress on your body. You might deny the situation, withdraw and isolate yourself from others, and shut down your emotions. Thus, in the previous example, you may not tell anyone about missing the exam, may tell yourself that you don't care about that class anyway, and go back to bed.

Exhaustion Stage

Your ability to move from the alarm stage to a less damaging resistance stage determines the effect that the stressor has on your physical and psychological health. As you gain more control and balance is reestablished, you can begin to recover from the stress.

The length of time, the energy, and the effort required to achieve recovery determines how exhausted your body becomes as a result of the stressor. Of course, the longer your body is under stress and out of balance, the more negative the effects. Experiencing long-term exposure to a stressor or coping with multiple stressors at the same time often results in overloading your system.

Specific organs and body systems that were called on during the resistance stage may not be able to resist a stressor indefinitely. When all the psychological and physical resources we rely on to deal with stress are used up, an **exhaustion stage** results, and the levels of stress-producing hormones such as adrenaline increase again.[2] This is when chronic and serious illnesses can begin to develop, and the individual may even develop clinical depression.

The Effects of Stress

Constant arousal and increased levels of adrenaline in your system will eventually wear down your body's immunological system. As this occurs, you are less able to cope with stress, and so it takes less and less to cause a stress reaction. When you are chronically stressed, it takes very little to frustrate you, and you can feel easily irritated at and stressed by the littlest things. Your body is both psychologically and physically less able to cope with stress. This can compromise your immune system, and you may become ill more easily. It may also take longer for you to recover from illness.

A variety of medical problems have been associated with stress, such as these:

- Cardiovascular problems (heart attacks, strokes, hypertension)
- Gastrointestinal problems (ulcers, irritable bowel syndrome, diarrhea, constipation, diverticulitis)
- Headaches and migraines
- Muscle spasms and cramps
- Sleep disorders
- Anxiety
- Jaw problems (temporomandibular joint [TMJ] syndrome)
- Allergies
- Cancer
- Back pain
- Asthma

(continued on page 55)

> **Key Terms**
>
> **alarm stage** The first stage of the stress response, involving physiological, involuntary changes that are controlled by the hormonal and the nervous systems; the fight or flight response is activated in this stage.
>
> **resistance stage** The second stage of the stress response during which the body attempts to reestablish its equilibrium or internal balance.
>
> **exhaustion stage** The point at which the physical and the psychological resources used to deal with stress have been depleted.

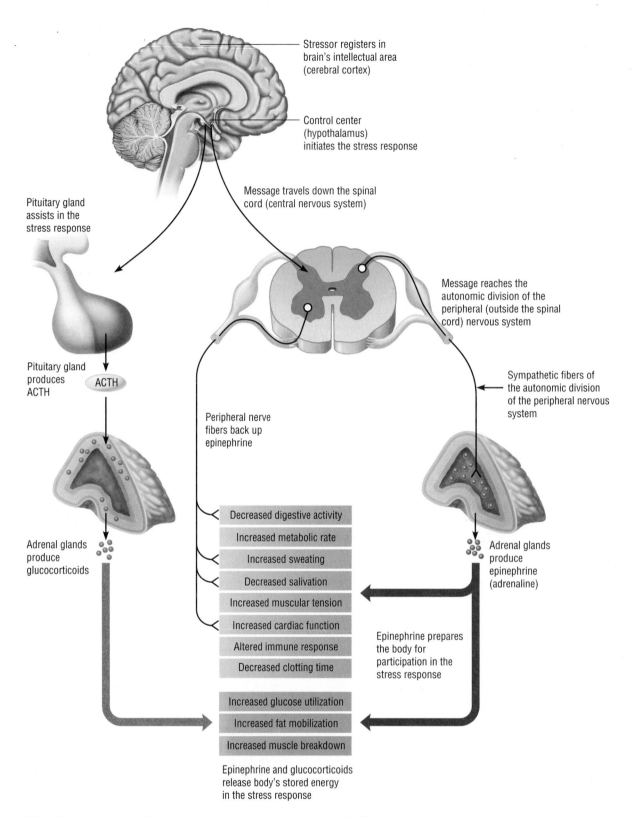

Stressor registers in brain's intellectual area (cerebral cortex)

Control center (hypothalamus) initiates the stress response

Message travels down the spinal cord (central nervous system)

Pituitary gland assists in the stress response

Pituitary gland produces ACTH

ACTH

Message reaches the autonomic division of the peripheral (outside the spinal cord) nervous system

Sympathetic fibers of the autonomic division of the peripheral nervous system

Peripheral nerve fibers back up epinephrine

Adrenal glands produce glucocorticoids

Adrenal glands produce epinephrine (adrenaline)

Decreased digestive activity
Increased metabolic rate
Increased sweating
Decreased salivation
Increased muscular tension
Increased cardiac function
Altered immune response
Decreased clotting time

Epinephrine prepares the body for participation in the stress response

Increased glucose utilization
Increased fat mobilization
Increased muscle breakdown

Epinephrine and glucocorticoids release body's stored energy in the stress response

Figure 3-2 The Stress Response   Physiological reactions to a stressor are controlled by the hormonal and nervous systems.

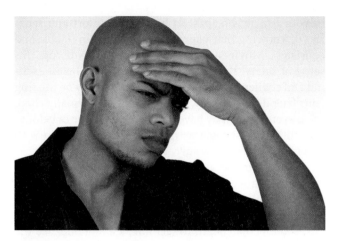

Chronic stress can contribute to headaches, anxiety, insomnia, and many other health problems.

- Kidney disease
- Sexual dysfunction
- Infertility
- Alcoholism and drug abuse

The Immune System and Stress

Corticosteroids are produced in the adrenal cortex as part of the stress response. Cortisol increases the body's fuel supply of carbohydrates, glucose, and fat, which are needed to respond to stress. It is important not to keep these levels elevated for very long, though, as too much cortisol in the system can also act to suppress the immune system. Remember that the stress response is meant to be a rapid, temporary response. Individuals who are chronically stressed are constantly pumping out a high level of corticosteroids, which over time can result in a breakdown of muscle tissues, a decreased number of immune cells, and a diminished inflammatory response. This can render the body less able to defend against bacteria and viruses—a stressed person is more likely to become ill. Hypertension and fluid retention are also associated with constant high levels of corticosteroids. On the other hand, if the level of corticosteroids in your system is too low, you can have an overactive immune system, which can harm healthy cells, resulting in autoimmune diseases such as lupus and rheumatoid arthritis.

Cardiovascular Disease and Stress

Your level of stress also contributes to your risk for developing cardiovascular disease. Chronic stress exposes your body to unhealthy, persistently elevated levels of stress hormones such as adrenaline and cortisol. Studies also link stress to changes in the way blood clots, which increases the risk of heart attack. Job stress, personality factors, and social isolation have all been suggested as factors contributing to cardiovascular disease. For example,

one study found that people who worked more than 60 hours a week were twice as likely to have a heart attack as those working 40 hours a week.[3] High levels of stress can make other risk factors (such as high cholesterol levels or high blood pressure) worse, which in turn increases the chances of developing cardiovascular disease.

Benefits of Stress

As we have said, while too much stress can have a negative effect and cause some serious health problems, a moderate level of stress is positive and beneficial. Stress can be motivating and energizing. Without some stress, many of us may not get much accomplished in our day or even get out of bed! Look at the diagram in Figure 3-3. What do you notice? Too little and too much stress are not helpful. When you are not stressed at all, you can be apathetic and lethargic. When you are too stressed, you are paralyzed with fear, like deer in the headlights. This is referred to as the **Yerkes-Dodson Law,** which uses a bell-shaped curve to demonstrate that there is an optimal

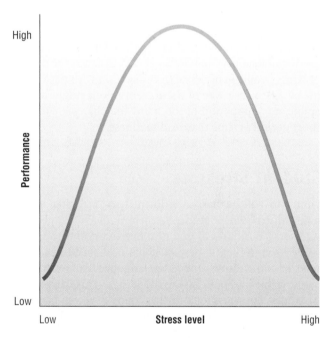

Figure 3-3 The Yerkes-Dodson Law   Too little or too much stress is not helpful, but a moderate level of stress encourages peak performance.

Source: Hebb DO, Drives and the CNS (conceptual nervous system), *Psychological Review*, 62(4), 243–254, 1955.

> **Key Terms**
>
> **Yerkes-Dodson Law**   A bell-shaped curve demonstrating that there is an optimal level of stress for peak performance; this law states that too little or too much stress is not helpful, whereas a moderate level of stress is positive and beneficial.

level of stress for peak performance. This fact holds true for any type of performance, from academic or work activities to music or athletics.[4] Recognizing the appropriate level of stress for your ideal performance level is important in reaching your potential.

Sources of Stress

There are other causes of stress besides experiencing positive or negative events in life. What events or situations trigger stress for you? For some it is financial worries, for others it might be relationship conflict, and for still others it is work-related. Even positive events, such as getting married, starting a new job, or moving to a new place, can be **stressors.** Going on vacation can be stressful as you get things done ahead of time to prepare for being away, pack your bags, spend money on the trip, and completely change your routine. Any type of change in your life has the potential to trigger a stressful response.

Because stress involves a physiological response, it has a direct link to your physical and psychological health. Thomas Holmes and Richard Rahe found direct connections between changes in people's lives and physical illness. They developed a widely used inventory, called the Social Readjustment Rating Scale, to assess the degree of stress people experience in connection with particular life events. While one of these events alone might be tolerable, a combination of too many life changes within a short period of time may lead to illness.[5]

Student Stressors

Going to college has been likened to "crossing into a new culture" where students face unique challenges and stressors.[6] Similarly to going to live in another country, students must learn new customs and traditions, new ways of doing things, and a new language, and must leave comfortable and familiar surroundings. This can lead to a high level of stress for students, many of whom have left their support system behind to live in a place where they know few people. In fact, incoming college freshmen have the highest levels of stress of any entering class. More students are reporting that they are stressed, with 85 percent feeling stressed in their daily lives.[7] In the sections that follow, we cover some of the specific stressors college students face and offer ways to manage these situations.

Interpersonal Stressors

Homesickness   Homesickness is one of the most common problems facing college students—which is understandable given that they are separated from friends and family and learning to live in an entirely new environment.[6] When you are undergoing a great deal of change

in your life, it is helpful to have the comfort and security of knowing that your home base remains stable and consistent. Moving from home to college can disrupt this sense of safety. While the college years can be an exciting and challenging time in your life, you may be missing your friends and family, with whom you normally share these events. You may have also lost your sense of belonging while you struggle with finding a way to fit in with and navigate your new surroundings.

Often homesickness doesn't hit until a few weeks or maybe a month after you have moved, since the first few weeks are filled with unpacking, meeting new people, and participating in social activities. After the dust settles, some people begin to feel lonely and alone. See the box "Overcoming Homesickness" for advice on how to deal with homesickness.

Relationship Problems   Along with homesickness, another common stressor for students is relationship problems. Often students are separated by long distances from their best friends and romantic partners. While it can be difficult to maintain long-distance relationships, it is not impossible. Studies show that the key to effective long-distance relationships is communication.[8] The quality of a long-distance relationship is improved if you both are committed to each other; you can talk openly about your concerns, feelings, and fears; and you can agree on the rules of the relationship, such as talking to other people. In addition, there needs to be a strong level of trust between the partners, since trust is often tested in long-distance relationships. Both of you will change, and you must share these changes so that you can grow together, not apart. Agree on how often you will see each other, and focus on spending high-quality time together.

It can be beneficial to have your friends visit you at college (rather than you going home) so that they can interact with you in your new environment and meet your new friends. Often students feel as though they live in two worlds, home and school, and it can be stressful to negotiate going from one to the other. The more you can connect these two worlds, the less stress you will experience. So it can be helpful to share what you are doing in your day—activities around campus, details of your classes—with your friends and family back home, and ask what they have been doing.

Balancing Work, Home, and School   It is estimated that about two-thirds of students work while going to college, and more students are working full-time to pay tuition. In addition, an estimated 5–10 percent of college students also have children. This, of course, adds stress to a student's life in terms of making time for school, children, work, and household responsibilities (see Figure 3-4). The increase in the number of students who have children is partly a result of a nationwide trend of more women in their mid-20s or older starting or

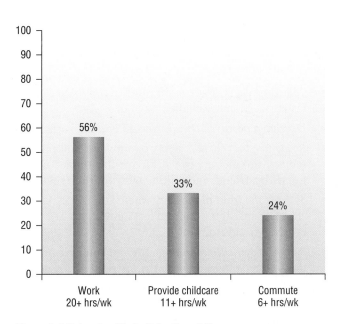

Figure 3-4 Balancing Work, School, and Home

Source: Community College Survey of Student Engagement (CCSSE): High Expectations and High Support. Austin, Texas: The University of Texas at Austin, Community College Leadership Program. © 2008 permission granted for unlimited copying with appropriate citation.

returning to college. In fact, a national study by the University of Michigan showed that the number of full-time female students over 25 years old grew by 500 percent in recent years.[9]

While some campuses offer child care, many do not, which leaves students having to coordinate schedules and juggle responsibilities, causing even more stress. Also, the cost of child care can be exorbitant for some and can certainly add to financial worries. Managing time well and having a strong support system are essential for students with children, particularly single parents. Often there is little to no time available for relaxation, socializing, or exercising, and so employing stress relief strategies can be challenging.

Academic Stressors

How does stress affect learning? Research suggests that people who are highly anxious tend to perform better than others on simple learning tasks but less well than others on difficult tasks, particularly those involving reasoning activities and time-limited tests.[10] When you are more stressed or anxious, you have a diminished ability to concentrate, to recall information, and to engage in problem-solving activities. You may find yourself reading the same page in your textbook over and over again, not knowing what you read.[11]

Suppose you have studied for the test you are about to take and are well prepared. You look at the first test question and suddenly your mind goes blank. The harder you try to think, the more nervous and distressed you feel. You just can't think clearly and feel as though you have some type of mental block—what is happening?

Key Terms

stressors Factors or events, real or imagined, that elicit a state of stress.

One-fifth of students experience these feelings, referred to as **test anxiety.** Exams are one of the greatest sources of stress for college students. The physical sensations associated with test anxiety are similar to those of general anxiety. People suffering from test anxiety make more mistakes on their tests, don't read the test accurately, and tend to make simple mistakes, such as spelling errors or adding something incorrectly. Many don't pace themselves well and have a hard time finishing exams. Test anxiety is a form of performance anxiety—people anticipate that they will perform poorly on the test.[11]

 TALKING POINTS What are some problems with stress described in this chapter that you have experienced?

As we have mentioned, speech anxiety, or fear of public speaking, is one of the most common anxiety disorders. Since students are frequently required to give oral presentations, expected to engage in class discussion, and graded on class participation, this can present a problem for some.

In addition to the basic stress-management techniques outlined in this chapter, the following strategies can be used to cope with speech anxiety:

- *Volunteer to go first.* Anxiety is dealt with best by taking action. Pressure and expectations tend to mount with each person who takes a turn, so you can lessen your stress level by being the first to present. Another advantage is that your performance is judged on its own merit without being compared to anyone else's.

- *Practice in front of a mirror and for your friends.* Solicit feedback: Do you need to slow down or speak louder? Practice will also help you to remember your talk so that you don't read it word for word, which can seem less interesting to your audience.

- *Engage in positive visualization.* Take deep breaths and imagine yourself giving your speech with confidence and receiving positive feedback and compliments about your performance.

- *Vary your presentation style and format.* Use visuals, such as slides, and engage your audience in discussion so that they are an active, not a passive, part of your presentation. This transfers some of the focus from you and removes some pressure too.

Another common stressor for college students is math anxiety. People who suffer from math anxiety feel that they are incapable of performing well in activities and classes that involve math. The incidence of math anxiety among college students has risen significantly over the last decade. Typically, people with math anxiety have the potential to perform well in math, and it is more a psychological, rather than intellectual, problem.

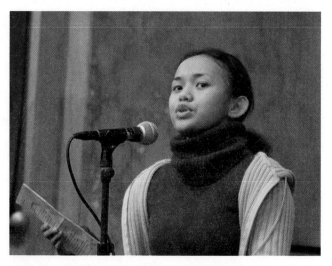

Effective behavioral and psychological interventions exist to treat speech anxiety.

Students who fear math often avoid asking questions to save embarrassment, sit in the back of the classroom, fail to seek help from the instructor, and usually put off studying math until the last moment. All these negative behaviors are intended to reduce the student's anxiety but actually result in more intense anxiety. However, there are a number of strategies that can be used to overcome math anxiety:

- *Take an easier, slower math course* as opposed to a faster-paced, more challenging one.

- *Develop a positive attitude toward math.*

- *Recognize that there is safety in numbers!* You can reduce your anxiety by working with a tutor, studying with a friend, and talking with your instructor.

- *Sit near the front of the class* where you will experience fewer distractions and feel more a part of what is being discussed.

- *Ask for clarification and repetition* if you have questions or can't keep up with the instructor.[12]

- *Review the material.* Research shows that you will remember 50 percent of what you heard in class if you review it immediately after class, but only 20 percent is retained 24 hours later if you didn't review the material right away.[13]

Internal Stressors

We can also generate stress within ourselves by putting too much pressure on ourselves, procrastinating, expecting too much of ourselves, and being self-critical. These **intrapsychic stressors** refer to our internal worries, criticisms, and negative self-talk, which were discussed in Chapter 2. Students say that procrastination, perfectionism, and poor goal setting are common sources of stress in their lives.

Procrastination **Procrastination** means postponing something that is necessary to do to reach a goal.[14] Putting things off is a common problem that plagues students and can cause stress. A survey of college students found that approximately 52 percent of students said their procrastination was causing them problems academically.[15] Procrastination has been viewed as a time-management problem, but it is really more than that, and so time-management strategies tend to be ineffective in resolving this problem. Procrastination is also different from indecision because people can make a decision but have trouble implementing it.

Typically, there is a psychological aspect to procrastination because we tend to delay doing things we don't want to do. Emotions such as anxiety, guilt, and dread often accompany thinking about the task. By putting the dreaded activity off, you can temporarily alleviate your anxiety and discomfort, which is a reinforcing aspect of procrastination. In the short term, procrastination seems to be a good solution and helps you to feel better. However, in the long run, procrastination usually leads to bigger problems and more work. For example, putting off paying your bills may feel good at the moment, but when your electricity is turned off and you have to pay late fees, and your roommates are upset with you because they thought you had paid the bill, your pleasurable feelings will turn sour.

Many people who procrastinate report feeling overwhelmed and anxious. They have difficulty tuning out external stimulation and concentrating on the task at hand. They also worry about how their performance will be judged by others and have perfectionistic standards for themselves. Students who procrastinate tend to perform less well and retain less than students who do not.[16] We discuss perfectionism in the next section.

Perfectionism **Perfectionism** leads to undue stress, because perfection is an unattainable goal. By setting the standard at perfect, you will set yourself up to fail.

Perfectionists tend to be their own worst critic; they are harder on themselves than anyone else is on them, and they are also critical of others. These individuals are described as neat and organized, seeming to "have it all together" and to be able to do more than most people and do it exceptionally well. Often people envy perfectionists because they seem very confident and competent; however, individuals who are perfectionists never feel good enough and often feel out of control in their lives.[17] Perfectionists focus on what they haven't accomplished or haven't done right rather than on what they have completed or have done well. Making mistakes is especially humiliating to perfectionists, and they tend to feel a strong sense of shame and low self-esteem when someone catches them in error. They have difficulty with criticism or any negative feedback because much of their self-esteem is based on being accurate, competent, and the best. While striving to do your best is an admirable quality, expecting to be perfect in everything you do and never making a mistake places a great deal of stress and pressure on you.

Problems with Goal Setting and Time Management

With the rising cost of education, many students feel pressured to earn their degrees as quickly as possible, and this adds another layer of stress for them. Learning for the sake of learning can sometimes seem like a luxury, because earning top grades to get into graduate programs and land well-paying jobs tend to take priority. Research shows that many students drop out of college because they don't know why they are in school, haven't found a direction or major, and feel pressured to either declare a major or quit. In addition, an overwhelming number of students identify time management as the reason for their academic success or failure.[18] Setting priorities and goals, balancing academic life with your social life, and finding time for sleeping, eating, exercising, and working along with studying is an essential aspect of managing your stress effectively, and strategies will be discussed later in this chapter.

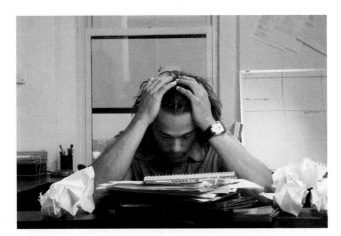

Many people who procrastinate, or "put off" tasks, such as homework, end up feeling overwhelmed or anxious.

> ### Key Terms
>
> **test anxiety** A form of performance anxiety that generates extreme feelings of distress in exam situations.
>
> **intrapsychic stressors** Our internal worries, self-criticisms, and negative self-talk.
>
> **procrastination** A tendency to put off completing tasks until some later time, sometimes resulting in increased stress.
>
> **perfectionism** A tendency to expect perfection in everything one does, with little tolerance for mistakes.

Job Stressors

Americans are spending more time at work than ever. In fact, the United States has overtaken Japan as the industrialized country with the longest working hours. Americans work 350 more hours per year than European workers.[3] What is the cost of these increased work hours? Less leisure time; less time for family, exercise, and sleep; less time for anything else but work! Seventy-five percent of workers stated that they experience job stress or burnout at work. Conflict with coworkers was the number-one source of job stress, followed by unrealistic workloads, tight deadlines, last-minute projects, and difficult bosses.[19]

Many students are stressed about their future and the possibility of finding a job once they graduate. Economic stress has recently become the most commonly experienced source of stress, and many students find that it is taking them an average of 18 months to find a job once they graduate from college. Money and the economy were at the top of the list of stressors for most Americans in a recent survey and have also been linked to an increase in irritability, anger, fatigue, insomnia, and unhealthy eating.[20] Students can also share their parents' stress as they face the possibility of losing their family home and not being able to afford to pay for college; this can place more financial burden on students to cover the costs of college.[21] Financial constraints may force people to find new ways to manage stress because they can't afford to take vacations, go out to eat, shop, go to the movies, or buy a new CD, book or DVD as they did in the past.[22] One particular job, as a soldier in the military, has accounted for a tremendous increase in the number of people experiencing stress and stress-related illnesses.[23]

Environmental Stressors

Light, sounds, smells, air quality, and temperature can all affect your stress level. Some people feel more stressed if their environment is disorganized or messy, and feel a need to clean it up before they can concentrate or relax. As you read in Chapter 2, the amount of light and type of lighting you are exposed to can affect your levels of stress and depression. Artificial light, as well as certain colors, can increase one's stress level. People tend to associate the color red with anger and hostility and gray with depression.[24] Stress has also been linked to being exposed to prolonged, daily noise such as in a factory, at a construction site, or in a crowded room.[25] Air that is too cold or too warm, or that contains mold or pollutants, can be a source of stress. Higher temperatures have been associated with an increase in violence and aggression and decreased concentration and productivity. Situations in which one does not have control over one's environment—such as being stuck in a traffic jam, in line, or in an elevator—can also be stressful. Your stress level might also increase if you don't have control over the noise, temperature level, or appearance of your environment. Advertisers try to increase their audience's stress levels in their ads so they can sell their products, which promise to relieve that stress (see the box "Advertisers May Be Selling You Stress").

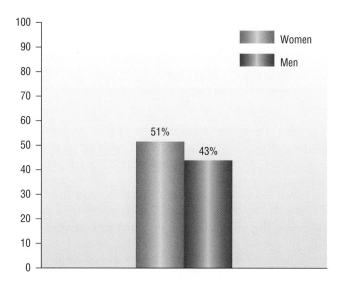

Figure 3-5 Stress and Gender Forty-three percent of men and 51 percent of women feel concerned about their level of stress.

Source: Only half of worried Americans try to manage their stress, *USA Today*, February 23, 2006.

Approaches to Stress Management

The research on how people cope with crisis and stress in their lives has shown that people tend to resolve problems within two weeks of experiencing them. Because stress involves a disruption in equilibrium, and the body does not function well in a chronic state of unbalance, it is human nature to seek a way to alleviate the stress the body is experiencing and return to a steady state. As we discussed previously, our bodies cannot function for very long in a sustained fight or flight response without serious damage, and so a person will naturally strive to make changes to resolve the stress for survival (see Figure 3-5). However, the way that people resolve their problems and alleviate stress may be positive or negative.

A number of negative ways of dealing with stress are quite common and often quite harmful. As indicated in Figure 3-6, some people turn to alcohol and drugs to avoid their problems and numb their feelings, and cigarettes are also cited as a way of relieving stress. Many people use food to comfort themselves. Putting off distasteful tasks and avoiding stressful situations is another negative way of coping with stress. Some people use sleep as a way of escaping their problems, and certainly depression has been associated with not having the ability to effectively manage stress. In the next section, we discuss ways of effectively managing stress.

What are some positive, effective methods for coping with stress? Different strategies and methods for stress management involve the physical, social, environmental, and psychological aspects of your stress. We will review techniques and strategies within each of these dimensions, and you will need to practice and experiment to find the stress-management techniques that are right for you.

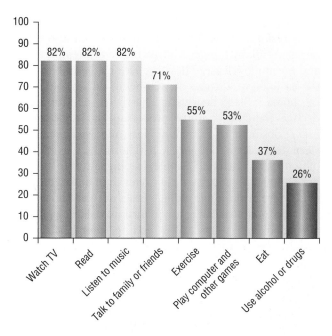

Figure 3-6 How Americans Cope with Stress People have different ways of coping with stress, such as watching TV, reading, listening to music, or playing video games. How do you cope with stress?

Source: Research reveals casual games provide mental balance, stress relief and relaxation, www.realnetworks.com, August 14, 2006; Americans reveal top stressors, how they cope, Mental Health America, www.nmha.org, November 16, 2006.

Physical Aspects of Stress Management

The physical aspects of stress management involve meeting your basic needs for sleep, exercise, and nutrition as was discussed in Chapter 2 under Maslow's hierarchy of needs.[26]

Sleep As with eating, too much sleep or too little is also an ineffective way of managing stress. Most adults require 7–9 hours of sleep a night.[27] Sometimes people get very little sleep during the week and try to "catch up" over the weekend, sleeping 14 hours at a time or taking naps during the day. Sleep is not like a bank account in which you can make deposits and withdrawals, and so getting an average of 7–9 hours a night over a week's time is not the same thing as sleeping this amount each night. Sleep problems are becoming more prevalent. Seventy million Americans have stated that they have problems with sleep.[28]

People also need uninterrupted sleep. Normal **circadian rhythms,** the biological processes related to the 24-hour light/dark cycle, are necessary for normal

> **Key Terms**
>
> **circadian rhythms** The internal, biological clock that helps coordinate physiological processes with the 24-hour light/dark cycle.

sleep and optimal daytime functioning. Our sleep patterns relate to these biological cycles, which also affect our patterns of hunger and eating, body temperature, and hormone release. These cycles must be in harmony for us to have a sense of well-being during our waking hours.[29] Sleep deprivation has been found to cause declines in higher cognitive processing and in the performance of simple tasks, memory loss, and, with prolonged sleep deprivation, temporary psychosis, such as hallucinations and delirium.[30] People sleeping less than 4 hours per night had higher mortality rates than those getting 6 or 7 hours of sleep per night.[31] Research also shows that sleeping too much can result in increased depression and decreased energy levels. Not getting enough sleep has been related to increases in weight, depression, anxiety, cardiovascular disorders, and accidents. Staying awake for more than 24 hours has been compared to having a blood alcohol content over the legal limit. College students who regularly pull all-nighters are said to have a 10-fold deterioration in cognitive performance.[32]

So how do you cope with sleep problems? Americans are turning to prescription medications in alarming numbers. The use of sleeping pills has doubled among 20- to 40-year-olds since 2000.[28] People are using more caffeine and energy drinks to wake up in the morning to compensate for morning grogginess due to hangover effects from sleep aids. Memory lapses, sleepwalking, and dependency have been associated with taking sleep medications. Sleeping pills can interfere with normal brain-wave activity during sleep and cause a rebound effect of increased insomnia when you discontinue taking them.

It is recommended that you develop healthy sleep habits so that you can get enough rest without sedatives and stimulants. Here are some tips for good sleep hygiene:

- *Establish a sleep routine.* Go to bed every night at the same time and wake up at the same time every morning, regardless of how much sleep you actually got.

- *Engage in sleep rituals before bedtime* (just like when you were a child), such as taking a bath before bed, reading a book, or listening to relaxing music.

- *Avoid caffeine use five hours before bedtime.* Also avoid eating two to three hours before bedtime, decrease fluid intake before bedtime, and avoid smoking and drinking alcohol before going to sleep.

- *Don't exercise before you go to sleep* or engage in any stimulating or arousing activities before bedtime.

- *Associate your bed with sleeping.* Don't study, eat, or watch television in bed.

- *If you have been lying in bed for 20 minutes and haven't gone to sleep, get up and do something relaxing* for 30–60 minutes and then try again. Keep getting out of bed after 20 minutes of no sleep and don't return to bed after your scheduled wake-up time.

- *Don't take naps during the day*—this will interfere with your sleep schedule.

- *If you worry while in bed, keep a worry journal* and write in it a few hours before bedtime to get these things out of your head and alleviate stress.[28]

Exercise   Exercise is another physical aspect of stress management. Exercising aerobically at least three times a week for 20–30 minutes has been found to manage stress effectively for several reasons. First, exercising requires you to focus on your breathing and to breathe deeply, the key to stress management. By tensing and releasing the muscles through exercise, you are allowing your body to relax and unwind. Second, exercise can alleviate stress through the release of endorphins, naturally occurring chemicals in the brain. Endorphins help to counter stress, subdue pain, and increase pleasure, which is the reason people talk about the runner's high. Hitting a racquetball against the wall or playing basketball can be a great way to release the frustrations of the day and let go of tension and stress. Aerobic exercise includes walking briskly, running, bicycling, skating, and dancing. The benefits of exercise are further discussed in Chapter 4.

Nutrition   In Chapter 5 you will learn about the nutrients that provide the fuel the body needs to function. When people are stressed, they often skip meals or eat on the run. Since the fight or flight response requires more energy than is normally needed, during stressful times, you must eat a balanced, nutritious diet. Without proper nutrition, the body will begin to break down its own tissues in an effort to obtain the energy required to survive. The immune system can then become compromised, making the body more susceptible to disease. It is not a coincidence that many people who are under a great deal of stress for prolonged periods of time become ill and that regaining their health takes longer than it does for those who are managing their stress well.

As we previously mentioned, people often use food to cope with stress and can overeat, typically eating high-sugar and high-fat foods such as chips, candy, and cookies. Eating too much or too little is not an effective way to manage stress and can eventually lead to serious health problems such as obesity, eating disorders, diabetes, and hypertension.

Mind-Body Approaches

Massage Therapy   Massage therapy helps lower blood pressure and heart rate, increase blood flow, release beta endorphins and toxins, and reduce muscle tightness in the body. Some research has reported that massage therapy is more beneficial for chronic pain, insomnia, and stress management than prescription medications.[33] There is a variety of types of massage, including Swedish, deep-tissue, reflexology, and acupressure. Massage usually involves holding, pressing, and moving across particular stress points in the body to remove stress from these areas.

Acupuncture Acupuncture involves stimulation of anatomical points in the body by a variety of techniques using hair-thin, metallic needles. The goal of acupuncture is to release the energy flow that is blocked in your body and regain balance. The process stimulates endorphins, neurotransmitters, neurohormones, and immune cells.[33]

Ayurvedic Medicine Ayurvedic medicine is the "science of life" and is a holistic approach to stress management. It incorporates yoga, herbs, specific foods and diets, massage, and meditation to manage stress. It is based on the belief that different body types require different diets, herbs, and regimens. Health and disease are seen to be related to the state of imbalance or balance of one's physical and mental states, as well as lifestyle factors.[34]

More research needs to be conducted on how these therapies work and their rate of effectiveness, as well as any adverse side effects. If you want to try an alternative form of medicine, make sure that the people you receive the services from are certified, adequately trained, and knowledgeable about these alternative medicines.

Social Aspects of Stress Management

To manage stress effectively, you must also make time for fun and play. Like exercise, laughter triggers the release of endorphins and requires you to breathe deeply, and so having humor in your life is an essential part of stress management.[35] Research has shown that stress can be related to having inadequate social interactions.[36] Hugs and human contact have also been shown to have a significant effect in reducing the harmful physical effects of stress.[37] Participating in social activities such as social organizations or sports, or just talking with friends can give you the break you need to rest your mind and focus on something other than work (see the box "The Fast-Growing Slow Movement").

Actually, you don't even have to have human contact to reduce stress—just owning a pet can make a difference. Studies have shown that just petting an animal produces calming effects such as lowered blood pressure and decreased heart rate. Cardiac patients who own pets tend to live much longer than those who have no pets.[38]

Environmental Aspects of Stress Management

To effectively manage your stress, you need to take into consideration environmental stressors such as noise level, amount of light, and the aesthetic quality of the space you inhabit. Natural light tends to elevate your mood, and different colors can raise or lower your stress and energy levels. Having plants or photos of friends and family around your living and work space can also alleviate stress.

Smell can also play a significant role in managing stress. As the saying goes, "Stop and smell the roses." Studies have shown that aromatherapy, using different aromas or odors therapeutically, can lower stress levels. When you breathe in these aromas, they send a direct message to your brain via your olfactory nerves, where they can then affect the endocrine and hormonal systems via the hypothalamus. Odors have an amazing effect on our emotional states because they hook into the emotional or primitive parts of our brains. Aromatherapy has been used to relieve pain, promote relaxation and stress relief, loosen tense muscles, soften dry skin, and enhance immunity. So it is wise to pay attention to your aromatic surroundings, because they may affect you much more than you realize.

While social interaction has been shown to lessen the effects of stress, the beneficial effect depends on the type of friends with whom you surround yourself. Spending time with negative, pessimistic people can increase your stress level rather than decrease it. It is more advantageous to surround yourself with positive, optimistic friends.[36] Feeling crowded in a room and not having enough personal space can also lead to an increase in stress.[36] Interestingly, it is not being in crowds itself but how familiar you are with the people and the activity that is taking place, and how much control you feel over your personal space that make the difference. In other words, being in a crowded room filled with your friends during a party feels subjectively different from feeling trapped in a crowded restaurant filled with strangers.

Other important aspects of managing stress in your environment include having meaningful work and challenging and interesting classes. Having work that is stimulating but not beyond your abilities helps to keep your stress response at a moderate, optimal level for performance.

Psychological Aspects of Stress Management

You can also effectively cope with stress by using a variety of cognitive and psychological strategies. There are several different techniques, but as you will see, many are focused on deep breathing, which is the key to managing stress.

Relaxation and Deep Breathing The relaxation response is a powerful weapon in ensuring that you do not remain in the stress response too long. It is effective because it entails the opposite of the stress response. Rather than taking shallow breaths, you need to breathe deeply, inhaling

The Fast-Growing Slow Movement

Our culture has developed an increasing need for speed. We are a fast-paced society, encouraged to eat, work, play, and move faster and faster. Our addiction to speed makes us a slave to time. What is the first thing you look at in the morning when you wake up? The clock, of course. Time tells us what to do when, and how long we have to engage in that activity. We have a need for speed that feeds our thirst for excitement and pumps out more adrenaline.

This pressure to do more in less time also causes stress in our lives. We can never be fast enough; there is never enough time. As Carrie Fisher once said, "Instant gratification takes too long." In order to beat the clock, we are consuming more caffeine and amphetamines and sleeping less. We are eating more fast food and gaining weight. We are working longer hours and taking less time to exercise, socialize, and enjoy leisure activities. The increase in road rage and relationship conflicts, and the general lack of civility in our society have also been linked to our obsession with saving time. Time management and finding ways to do things more efficiently were originally intended to give us more leisure time and reduce the level of stress in our lives, but the opposite has occurred, and we now pay a high price for speed.

There is a new, growing trend in society called the "slow movement." Books such as *In Praise of Slowness* discuss the merits of finding a balance in our lives; becoming more calm, careful, patient, and reflective; and developing real, meaningful connections with people. In fact, the author contends that slower can be better, as we can develop healthier relationships in our work and family life. We can have higher quality in our food, exercise, and other aspects of our lives if we take the time to do things well. Sometimes doing something more slowly can yield faster results, because doing things quickly can result in making mistakes and having to redo things.

We are beginning to see this trend in many facets of life. Yoga and meditation have become increasingly popular, as has the slow food movement. In the United States and around the world, some cities are becoming slow cities—which means these communities have made a commitment to create an environment that helps people slow down. The slow philosophy translates into city ordinances such as banning motorized vehicles from some streets, banning fast-food chains and neon signs, and lowering speed limits. These communities have speed bumps that read "Ready, Set, Relax," and they set aside time for "family focus night" with no school practices, no homework, and no meetings. October 24 has been designated "Take Back Your Time Day" in the United States, because by October 24 each year, Americans have worked as much as Europeans do all year.

How can you begin to break away from the cult of speediness? Here are some tips:

- Don't overschedule yourself.
- Don't multitask; focus on one thing only.
- Take time to play.
- Do nothing; just sit there.
- Meditate or do yoga.
- Make a meal from scratch.
- Eat without watching television, reading, or doing anything else.
- Walk and talk slower than you normally do.
- Don't wear a watch.
- Let someone else go before you in line.
- Don't drink caffeinated beverages.
- Sleep eight hours a night.

Test yourself to see how difficult it is for you to do these things. Do you have trouble relaxing and doing nothing? It is important to note that the slow movement doesn't necessarily mean that we do everything at a snail's pace. Instead, it means finding a balance in our lives. There may be times when it is appropriate to act quickly, to be time oriented, or to multitask. The slow movement suggests only that we take back control of our time and go at our own pace, instead of rushing around all of the time when it may not be necessary and may even be counterproductive.

Sources: Honoré C, *In Praise of Slowness.* New York: HarperCollins, 2004; Worldwide, we seem to have lost the art of doing nothing, *USA Today,* May 16, 2006.

---

to a count of four and exhaling to a count of four while sitting in a comfortable position. As you breathe deeply, your muscles unwind and relax, again the opposite of the stress response. It is generally advised not to cross your legs or arms so that your muscles can relax easily. Blood flows to the extremities, and your heart rate slows. In fact, experienced users of this technique can temporarily lower their breathing rate from a typical rate of 14–18 breaths per minute to as few as 4 breaths per minute. Body temperature decreases, and blood pressure is lowered as well. The entire nervous system is slowed, in direct opposition to its role in the stress response. The key is to focus on your breathing and inner experience and become less aware of your external environment. To help tune out the outside world, close your eyes and let go of the worries and concerns of the day.[39]

To try this technique, take a moment to focus on your breathing, and breathe in for a count of four and out for four. After doing so a few times, tighten your body; clench your hands, teeth, and jaw; close your eyes tightly; and pull your shoulders up while you are still breathing deeply. Are you able to do so? It is virtually impossible to tense your body and breathe deeply because they are mutually exclusive activities. Thus, the relaxation response is the foundation of most of the stress-management techniques described in this chapter. Deep breathing is the fundamental aspect of stress management, and it can also be used to alleviate anger (see the box "The Antidote for Anger . . . Relaxation").

Progressive Muscle Relaxation (PMR) Progressive muscle relaxation involves learning to recognize the

The Antidote for Anger . . . Relaxation

As with the stress response, the key to managing anger is to change how we respond to events and express our anger. So, instead of blowing up, should you just keep your anger inside? No; this can eventually result in an explosion similar to that caused by pressure that builds in a pressure cooker or a shaken soda can. This is the "last straw" kind of anger response. To an observer, you may seem to be overreacting to the particular situation when you are really responding to a multitude of situations and frustrating events. You may take your anger out on an innocent bystander or the dog. Here are some tips on effective, respectful anger management:

- *Relax,* take a deep breath, count to 10.
- *Take a time-out if needed.* Don't continue to engage in a discussion if it is getting too heated.
- *Avoid name calling.* Use "I" language, as was discussed in the previous chapter.
- *Stay connected to the individual* with whom you are speaking. Don't withdraw physically or psychologically unless you need a time-out, and then say this directly.
- *Ask yourself what underlies your anger.* Hurt, guilt, feelings of rejection and shame, and fear of abandonment may

be feelings that you need to express but that come out as anger. Especially for men, anger tends to be a more comfortable emotion to express.

- *Ask yourself if there is a hidden agenda to your anger.* Are you using your anger to control, change, or punish someone? If so, use assertive language instead, and share your thoughts and feelings directly.
- *Speak in a quieter, calmer voice than you typically do.* People tend to speak more loudly than normal in order to get the other person's attention. You may feel that you don't have power or people's attention unless you yell. While anger can be attention grabbing, this kind of attention is probably not what you want. People may tend to yell back, tune you out, or agree with you without meaning it, just to stop the yelling.
- *Choose your battles wisely.* Don't argue every point. Ask yourself, "Is this something that is really important to me and will be as meaningful tomorrow as it is right now for me?"
- *Express your anger in a timely fashion.* Don't wait a week or a month or bring up issues when you have accumulated a bunch of things that have been bothering

you over time. However, it may be more productive to wait until morning to express your anger if you are tired and irritable in the evenings. Another option is to wait and arrange a specific time to talk to avoid rushing through a conversation as you get ready to leave for work or class.

- *Recognize that although it might feel easier or safer to redirect the anger you feel* toward your boss at your best friend or partner, but that doesn't solve your conflict with your boss, and it might create conflict with your friend or partner.

After you have respectfully expressed your anger, make sure you allow time and opportunity for the other person to express his or her feelings. Tell the person you appreciate how he or she listened to you and responded to you. Share other feelings besides the primary ones of hurt and anger, so that the person knows you can be angry with him or her and still care about him or her. Remember that your way of expressing anger and resolving conflict can either be destructive or be a way of connecting with people and improving relationships.

Sources: McKay M, Rogers P, *The Anger Control Workbook.* Oakland, CA: New Harbinger, 2000; Paleg K, McKay M, *When Anger Hurts Your Relationship.* Oakland, CA: New Harbinger, 2001.

---

difference between contracted and relaxed muscles, in order to gain a sense of control over the body and the stress response. PMR enables you to intentionally put certain muscles into a controlled state of relaxation and reduce your overall stress level.

PMR involves placing your body in a comfortable position, sitting or lying down, and concentrating on certain muscle groups. As you inhale, breathing in for a count of four, you contract your muscles, starting with your forehead, and count to four as you exhale and relax your muscles. Continue to clench and relax the muscles, using your breathing to help you to tighten and release, working your way down your body all the way to your feet. Concentrate on the sensations of relaxation and how different they are from the feelings of tension and stress. Fifteen minutes, twice a day, is the recommended schedule. In one to two weeks, you will have mastered the basics and will be aware of which muscles need more

attention in order to relax. You will also be more sensitive to the buildup of tension in your body so that you will be able to decrease your stress level before it becomes overwhelming.

Guided Imagery and Visualization Guided imagery involves having someone describe a beautiful, relaxing scene while you focus on taking deep breaths. While in a comfortable position, in an environment free from interruptions and distractions, you breathe deeply, relax your muscles, and imagine a pleasant scene. The imagery includes all the senses, not just what you see but pleasant smells, sounds, touches, and even tastes. Guided imagery can be self-taught, or you can listen to recordings of narrated scripts.

Visualization is similar to guided imagery, but with the scene being more specifically focused on something you are about to do or want to accomplish, or on some performance or activity that may be causing you distress. Guided imagery and visualization techniques help you change through positive mental images. For example, you might imagine yourself auditioning for a part in a play, seeing yourself reciting your lines effortlessly and flawlessly, and feeling confident and proud of yourself. You are probably already skilled at visualization; unfortunately, we frequently engage in negative visualization but are unaware of doing so. For example, we imagine ourselves making fools of ourselves or making mistakes.

Athletes are trained in using positive visualization to improve their performance and achieve their goals.[39] Positive visualization has also been used in managing pain, especially chronic pain. This technique has been effective in weight management, smoking cessation, insomnia, and for almost any type of behavior change as well.

Meditation   Meditation allows the mind to transcend thought effortlessly when the person concentrates on a focal point. In transcendental meditation, a widely recognized approach to meditation, people repeat a mantra, or a personal word, while using deep-breathing and relaxation techniques. In other forms of meditation, alternative focal points are used to establish the depth of concentration needed to free the mind from conscious thought. Physical objects, music, and relaxing environmental sounds or breathing can be used as focal points. Meditation is also used in yoga.

Hypnosis   Hypnosis is a natural state of mind that occurs spontaneously in nearly every person. It is a trancelike state, similar to those that you experience upon awakening, before falling asleep, or when you are engrossed in thought while performing other tasks—such as driving down a highway—on autopilot. It resembles, but is physiologically distinct from, sleep. It involves a heightened state of suggestibility that creates flexible and intensified attention and receptiveness, and an increased responsiveness to an idea or set of ideas. The focus is on the unconscious rather than on the conscious state of mind, using deep-breathing and relaxation techniques. Hypnosis is perhaps the oldest and most misunderstood type of relaxation technique. It has been given a bad reputation by stage entertainers who use hypnosis to have unsuspecting audience members engage in embarrassing behavior.

It is possible to learn self-hypnosis from a trained professional or participate in hypnosis sessions with a qualified hypnotherapist.

Biofeedback   Biofeedback is a training technique in which people are taught to improve their health and performance by using signals from their own bodies. It

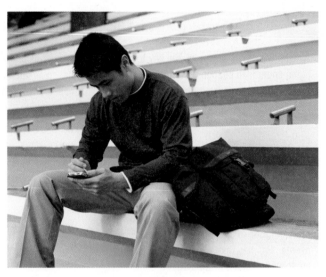

Use of a daily planner is a strategy that can help you manage your time more effectively as well as reduce your stress level.

operates on the premise that individuals can alter their involuntary responses by being "fed back" information either visually or audibly about what was occurring in their bodies. In addition, studies have shown that we have more control over so-called involuntary bodily functions than we once thought possible.

One commonly used device, for example, picks up electrical signals from the muscles and translates the signals into a form that people can detect. This device triggers a flashing light or activates a beeper every time muscles become tense. To slow down the flashing or beeping, you need to relax your tense muscles by breathing more slowly and deeply. People learn to associate sensations from the muscle with actual levels of tension and develop a new, healthy habit of keeping muscles only as tense as is necessary for as long as necessary. After treatment, individuals are then able to repeat this response at will without being attached to the sensors. Other biological functions that are commonly measured and used in a similar way to help people gain control are skin temperature, heart rate, sweat gland activity, and brain-wave activity. People can manage stress by decreasing the physiological components of the stress response.

Cognitive Aspects of Stress Management

Time Management   Managing your time effectively can help you cope with your stress by feeling more in control, having a sense of accomplishment, and having a sense of purpose in your life. Establishing good time-management habits can take two to three weeks. By using specific systems, even the most disorganized persons can make their lives less chaotic and stressful.

Assess Your Habits The first step is to analyze how you are spending your time. What are your most productive and least productive times of day and night? Do you tend to underestimate how long something will take you to complete? Do you waste time or allow interruptions to take you off task? Carrying a notebook with you for a week and writing down how you spend your time might provide you with some insight into the answers to these questions and how you spend your time. You might find that you've been devoting most of your time to less important tasks. Perhaps it is tempting to do your laundry rather than to start writing that term paper, but this may not be the best use of your time.

Use a Planner Keeping a daily planner to schedule your time is the next step in managing your time more effectively. First block off all of the activities that are consistent, regular, weekly activities, such as attending classes, eating meals, sleeping, going to meetings, exercising, and working. Then look at the open, available time remaining. Schedule regular study time, relaxation time, and free time. Remember to schedule your study time during the more productive part of your waking hours. When you have a one-hour block of time, what can you realistically get done in that time? This could be a good time to review your notes from class, pay bills, or get some reading done.

Set Goals and Prioritize Set goals for the week as well as for each day. If something unexpected interferes with your schedule, modify your plans but don't throw out the entire schedule.

Making a to-do list can be helpful, but it is only the first step. Breaking the large tasks into smaller, more manageable pieces and then prioritizing them is the key to effective time management. When you prioritize your tasks, try the "ABC" method of task management. The A tasks are those items that are most urgent and must be done today. The B tasks are those things that are important but, if need be, could wait 24 hours. The C tasks are activities that can easily wait a few days to a week. Don't fall into the C trap, which is when you do the less important tasks because they are quick and can be checked off your list with ease. This can lead to putting off the more important A activities, leaving them until you feel stressed and overwhelmed.[18]

Stress Inoculation Working in a manner similar to a flu shot, stress inoculation involves exposing an individual to specific stressful situations, a little at a time, under controlled, safe conditions. Stress inoculation teaches individuals to relax using deep breathing and progressive muscle relaxation while they are being exposed to stressful situations.

The first step is to construct your personal list of stressful situations, arranging the list from the least to the most stressful items. You learn how to evoke each of these situations in your mind while at the same time focusing on your breathing and relaxing your muscles. The second step is to create an arsenal of stress-coping thoughts, such as "I'm going to be all right," "I've succeeded with this before," and "Getting started is the hardest part, then it will get easier for me." The third step is to practice this *in vivo*, meaning in real-life situations, while using the relaxation and cognitive techniques to minimize the stress response.[40] In addition to stress management, stress inoculation has been helpful in anger management.

Cognitive Self-Talk What we tell ourselves, our self-talk, has a tremendous effect on how well we manage our stress. Stress can be generated from drawing faulty conclusions, misinterpreting things, and expecting the worst. Some people claim that if they expect the worst, they won't feel disappointed or hurt, but in reality, they still feel the pain from their disappointment. We need to be careful about what we expect because we may inadvertently make it happen, a phenomenon referred to as a **self-fulfilling prophecy.** [41] Self-fulfilling prophecies can work for you or against you. If you expect that work will be boring and uninteresting, you will tend to have a negative, unmotivated attitude and will probably have a miserable time. However, if you expect to enjoy yourself at work, you are more likely to go looking for challenges and to have fun.

To change your cognitive distortions, you need to generate some rebuttals to your negative self-statements. This entails finding a middle ground between all-or-nothing thinking by asking yourself what evidence proves that a statement is true and identifying some exceptions to this statement. Look for balance by asking yourself what is the opposite of this negative self-statement. Rather than telling yourself what you *should* do, ask yourself what you *want* to do. Be specific instead of generalizing, and avoid labeling yourself and others. Instead of telling yourself, "I'm lazy," you might say, "I wish I would have studied a few more hours for that test." Stick to the facts without blaming yourself or others. Question yourself as to how you know something is true and if you might be making an assumption or "mind reading." Be mindful of your self-fulfilling prophecies. It may be wiser to acknowledge that you don't know or consider many different possible outcomes rather than to expect the worst.

Key Terms
self-fulfilling prophecy The tendency to make something more likely to happen as a result of one's own expectations and attitudes.

Changing negative self-talk requires time, practice, and patience. We develop these patterns of thinking over years, and they become almost automatic. It takes concentrated effort to be aware of and change negative thinking. Remember that your rebuttals need to be strong, nonjudgmental, and specific. Practice developing more flexible and balanced thinking about people, behavior, and situations.

Conquering Procrastination   Some techniques for combating procrastination involve time management, stress management, assertiveness training, and increasing self-esteem and self-acceptance. Procrastinators tend to both over- and underestimate how much time a task will take. When they underestimate the time, they feel justified in procrastinating because they erroneously believe they have plenty of time to complete the task. When they overestimate the time needed, they are intimidated by the magnitude of the job, feel anxious, and so have trouble getting started. So it is important to give yourself more time than you think you might need for a project and to start earlier than needed in case of unforeseen delays. Breaking the task down into manageable pieces can also make it less daunting.

People also report procrastinating when they feel forced or pressured to do something they don't want to do. Rather than communicating assertively, they rebel by agreeing to do something but constantly put it off, which can be a passive-aggressive way of behaving. They fear the consequences of saying no or not fulfilling their obligations but are also angry about what they perceive as unfair expectations and demands on them. This is when some assertiveness training may be helpful. Finally, increasing self-esteem can solve problems with procrastination because feeling better about yourself relieves you of worrying about what others think of you and having constantly to prove yourself to them. Some people procrastinate because they think they need to do everything perfectly or not at all. With increased self-esteem, you are more accepting of mistakes and don't expect yourself to perform perfectly.

Combating Perfectionism   To help alleviate the stress of perfectionism, base your self-esteem on who you are rather than on what you do. This involves accepting yourself and others unconditionally, including imperfections. Lowering your expectations of yourself and others and aiming for 80 percent rather than 100 percent is another strategy in battling perfectionism. Note what you are doing well and have accomplished rather than what is still left to do. Time-management strategies such as those outlined previously can be useful in managing your expectations of yourself. Push yourself to take risks, and allow yourself to make mistakes. It can be useful to make mistakes on purpose in order to get accustomed to this experience and realize that people still like and accept you and that nothing bad will happen. Relaxation and stress-management techniques such as the ones described at the end of this chapter can also help alleviate the stress that comes with perfectionism. You might want to take the survey at the end of this chapter to assess your level of perfectionism.

As you can see, there are many different aspects to consider in managing stress, as well as its physical, social, environmental, and psychological components. As you think about how you can more effectively manage your stress level, you will need to practice and experiment to find the stress-management techniques most beneficial for you.

 TALKING POINTS Think back to stressful times in your life. What were some positive ways you coped, and what were some negative things you did to cope?

Taking Charge of Your Health

- Prioritize your daily goals in a list that you can accomplish, allowing time for recreational activities.

- Counteract a tendency to procrastinate by setting up imaginary (early) deadlines for assignments and rewarding yourself when you meet those dates.

- Replace a negative coping technique that you currently use, such as smoking, with an effective alternative, such as deep breathing, relaxation exercises, yoga, or exercise.

- List the positive aspects of your life, and make them the focus of your everyday thoughts.

- Take the Hardy Personality Profile at the end of this chapter.

- Determine if you suffer from perfectionism by completing the perfectionism assessment at the end of this chapter.

- Join a yoga, meditation, or exercise class on campus or in the community.

- Assess your sleep routine and incorporate into your sleep habits some of the tips recommended in this chapter.

SUMMARY

- Stress refers to physiological changes your body has in response to a situation, a real or a perceived threat.
- The fight or flight response is a physiological response to perceived, anticipated, or real threat; the heart races, breathing becomes labored, muscles are tense, the body sweats, and blood flow is decreased to the extremities and digestive organs and increased to the major muscles and brain.
- Chronic stress refers to remaining at a high level of physiological arousal for too long and not being able to take immediate, effective action to alleviate the perceived or real threat.
- While too much stress can have a negative effect and cause some serious health problems, a moderate level of stress is positive and beneficial.
- Constant arousal and increased levels of adrenaline in your system will eventually wear down your body's immunological system. You will be less able to cope with stress, and so it takes less and less to cause a stress reaction.
- General adaptation syndrome is a sequenced physiological response to the presence of a stressor, involving the alarm, resistance, and exhaustion stages of the stress response.
- Students can experience unique types of stressors, such as homesickness, relationship problems, test anxiety, speech anxiety, math anxiety, and problems with goal setting, time management, procrastination, and perfectionism.
- An overwhelming number of students identify time management as the reason for their academic success or failure. Setting priorities and goals, balancing academic life with social life, and finding time for sleeping, exercising, eating, and working along with studying are essential aspects of managing stress effectively.
- To effectively manage your stress, you need to take into consideration environmental stressors such as the noise level, amount of light, and aesthetic quality of the space you inhabit. It is equally important to get adequate sleep, exercise, and nutrition.
- Effective psychological tools for managing stress include progressive muscle relaxation, visualization, guided imagery, meditation, hypnosis, biofeedback, stress inoculation, and cognitive self-talk.

REVIEW QUESTIONS

1. What is stress? How is it linked to your physical and psychological health?
2. What is the fight or flight response?
3. What are some of the long-term effects of chronic stress?
4. Describe the Yerkes-Dodson Law.
5. Explain the three stages of the general adaptation syndrome.
6. List at least five unique stressors students can experience.
7. What are some ways to cope with test anxiety? Math anxiety? Speech anxiety?
8. What do an overwhelming number of students identify as the reason for their academic success or failure?
9. List some environmental stressors, and explain how high levels of stress have been linked to environmental factors.
10. Name five psychological tools for stress management and explain how they work.

ANSWERS TO THE "WHAT DO YOU KNOW?" QUIZ

1. False   2. True   3. True   4. True   5. True   6. False   7. True

Visit the Online Learning Center (**www.mhhe.com/hahn11e**), where you will find tools to help you improve your grade including practice quizzes, key terms flashcards, audio chapter summaries for your MP3 player, and many other study aids.

SOURCE NOTES

1. Selye H. *Stress Without Distress*. New York: New American Library, 1975.
2. Selye H. *The Stress of Life*. New York: McGraw-Hill, 1984.
3. Honore C. *In Praise of Slowness*. New York: HarperCollins, 2004.
4. Lefton L, Brannon L. *Psychology* (9th ed.). Boston: Pearson Education, 2006.
5. Holmes T, Rahe R. Social Readjustment Rating Scale. *Journal of Psychosomatic Research*, 11, 1967.
6. Rowh M. *Coping with Stress in College*. New York: College Board Publications, 1989.
7. AP poll: many students stressed, some depressed. *The Post-Journal*, May 22, 2009.
8. Raber M, Dyck G. *Managing Stress for Mental Fitness*. Menlo Park, CA: Crisp Publications, 1993.
9. Vandenbeele J. Affordable care for kids squeezes college students. *The Detroit News*, November 23, 2001.
10. Baucum D, Smith C. *Psychology* (9th ed). Belmont, CA: Wadworth/Thompson Learning, 2004.
11. Newman E. *No More Test Anxiety*. Los Angeles: Learning Skills Publications, 1996.
12. Arem C. *Conquering Math Anxiety: A Self-Help Workbook*. Pacific Grove, CA: Brooks/Cole, 1993.
13. Kahn N. *More Learning in Less Time*. Berkeley, CA: Ten Speed Press, 1992.

14. Roberts M. *Living Without Procrastination*. Oakland, CA: New Harbinger, 2001.
15. Gallagher R, Borg S, Golin A, Kelleher K. The personal, career, and learning skills needs of college students. *Journal of College Student Development* 33(4), 301–310, 1992.
16. Ferrari J, Johnson J, McGown W. *Procrastination and Task Avoidance; Theory, Research and Treatment*. New York: Plenum, 1995.
17. Basco M. *Never Good Enough*. New York: Simon & Schuster, 1999.
18. Lakein A. *How to Get Control of Your Time and Your Life*. New York: New American Library, 1989.
19. Haefner R. Survey: Three in four workers suffer stress on the job. http://msn.careerbuilder.com, May 26, 2006.
20. Health takes a hit as economy creates more stress. *USA Today*, October 7, 2008.
21. Financial worries, other stresses are manifested physically. *USA Today*, September 17, 2008.
22. Economic pain is a nail biter. *USA Today*, October 7, 2008.
23. Iraq vets may suffer depression, stress. *USA Today*, November 13, 2007.
24. Depression comes in shades of gray. *USA Today*, February 10, 2010.
25. Rosenthal NE. *Winter Blues*. New York: Guilford Press, 2005.
26. Maslow AH. *Motivation and Personality* (2nd ed.). New York: Van Nostrand, 1970.
27. Ferber R. *Solve Your Child's Sleep Problems*. New York: Simon & Schuster, 2006.
28. Lack of sleep catches up with today's workforce. *USA Today*, March 3, 2008.
29. Saladin KS. *Anatomy and Physiology: The Unity of Form and Function*. New York: McGraw-Hill, 2001.
30. Davis M, Eshelmar E, McKay M. *The Relaxation and Stress Reduction Workbook*. Oakland, CA: New Harbinger, 2000.
31. Experts: put insomnia to bed quickly. *USA Today*, August 27, 2009.
32. Don't bank on weekend to make up for sleep loss. www.comcast.net/articles/newshealth/2010013/US.MED.Sleep.loss.
33. Pearson N, Johnson L, Nahin R. Insomnia, trouble sleeping and alternative medicine: analysis of the 2002 National Health Interview Survey data. *Archives of Internal Medicine*, 166, 1775–1782, 2006.
34. National Institutes of Health. A closer look at Ayurvedic medicine. *Focus on Complementary Care and Alternative Medicine*, 12(4), Fall 2006.
35. Rentafriend. *Star Press*, June 18, 2010.
36. Seligman M. *Learned Optimism*. New York: Pocket Books, 1992.
37. Human touch may have some healing properties. *USA Today*, September 29, 2008.
38. Allen K, Shykoff BE, Izzo JL Jr. Pet ownership but not ACE inhibitor therapy blunts home blood pressure responses to mental stress. *Hypertension*, 38(4), 815–820, 2001.
39. Fanning P. *Visualization for Change*. Oakland, CA: New Harbinger, 1994.
40. McKay M, Davis M, Fanning P. *Thoughts and Feelings: The Art of Cognitive Stress Intervention*. Oakland, CA: New Harbinger, 2007.
41. Jones RA. *Self-Fulfilling Prophecies*. Hillsdale, NJ: Wiley, 1981.

Personal Assessment

Hardy Personality Profile: Test Your Hardiness

This questionnaire is adapted from the work of Suzanne Kobasa, co-creator of the hardy personality. This inventory is based on 12 questions. In the words of Kobasa, "Evaluating hardiness requires more than a quick test, but this survey will give you an idea of your degree of hardiness." Using a scale of 0–3, estimate your answer for each question. Please answer how you are, not how you would like to be. Then score your answers for Control, Commitment, and Challenge.

0 = strongly disagree
1 = mildly disagree
2 = mildly agree
3 = strongly agree

_____ 1. My best efforts at work/school make a difference.

_____ 2. Trusting to fate/universe is sometimes all I can do in a relationship.

_____ 3. I often wake up each day eager to start, work on, or complete a project.

_____ 4. Viewing myself as a free person tends to promote stress and frustration.

_____ 5. I would be willing to sacrifice financial security in my work if something really challenging came along.

_____ 6. I get stressed when my plans go awry and my schedule is disrupted.

_____ 7. Anybody, from any social demographic, can have an influence on politics.

_____ 8. Without the right breaks, it is difficult to be successful in my field.

_____ 9. I know what I am doing and why I am doing it at work/school.

_____ 10. Becoming close to people makes me feel a sense of obligation to them.

_____ 11. I relish the chance to encounter new situations as an important part of life.

_____ 12. I really don't mind when I have lots of free time with nothing to do.

Scoring

To estimate your level of hardiness, calculate the scores for each component (by adding and subtracting where indicated). A total score of 10–18 indicates a hardy personality, 0–9 suggests moderate hardiness, and a score less than 0 indicates low hardiness.

Control Score = _____

1 _____ + 7 _____
subtract
2 _____ + 8 _____

Commitment Score = _____

3 _____ + 9 _____
subtract
4 _____ + 10 _____

Challenge Score = _____

5 _____ + 11 _____
subtract
6 _____ + 12 _____

Total Hardiness Score _____

Source: Seaward B, *Managing Stress* (6th ed.). Sudbury, MA: Jones & Bartlett, 2009.

Personal Assessment

Am I a Perfectionist?

Below are some ideas that are held by perfectionists. Which of these do you see in yourself? To help you decide, rate how strongly you agree with each of the statements below on a scale from 0 to 4.

0	1	2	3	4
I do not agree		I agree somewhat		I agree completely

_____ 1. I have an eye for details that others can miss.

_____ 2. I can get lost in details and forget the real purpose of the task.

_____ 3. I can get overwhelmed by too many details.

_____ 4. It stresses me when people do not want to do things the right way.

_____ 5. There is a right way and a wrong way to do most things.

_____ 6. I do not like my routine to be interrupted.

_____ 7. I expect a great deal from myself.

_____ 8. I expect no less of others than I expect of myself.

_____ 9. People should always do their best.

_____ 10. I am neat in my appearance.

_____ 11. Good grooming is important to me.

_____ 12. I do not like being seen before I have showered and dressed.

_____ 13. I do not like making mistakes.

_____ 14. Receiving criticism is horrible.

_____ 15. It is embarrassing to make mistakes in front of others.

_____ 16. Sharing my new ideas with others makes me anxious.

_____ 17. I worry that my ideas are not good enough.

_____ 18. I do not have a great deal of confidence in myself.

_____ 19. I'm uncomfortable when my environment is untidy or disorganized.

_____ 20. When things are disorganized, it is hard for me to concentrate.

_____ 21. What others think about my home is important to me.

_____ 22. I have trouble making difficult decisions.

_____ 23. I worry that I may make the wrong decision.

_____ 24. Making a bad decision can be disastrous.

_____ 25. I often do not trust others to do the job right.

_____ 26. I check the work of others to make certain it was done correctly.

_____ 27. If I can control the process, it will turn out fine.

_____ 28. I am a perfectionist.

_____ 29. I care more about doing a quality job than others do.

_____ 30. It's important to make a good impression.

_____ **TOTAL SCORE**

Scoring

Add all 30 items together to get total score. If your score was less than 30, then you are probably not a perfectionist, although you may have a few of the traits. Scores from 31 to 60 suggest mild perfectionism. When you are stressed, your score may be higher. Scores of 61 to 90 suggest moderate perfectionism. This probably means that perfectionism is causing you trouble in some specific areas but is not out of control. Scores higher than 91 suggest a level of perfectionism that could cause you serious problems.

TO CARRY THIS FURTHER . . .

If you scored in the moderate to high range for perfectionism, consider taking some of the steps described in this chapter for combating perfectionism. Allow yourself to take risks and make mistakes. General relaxation strategies can also be helpful in overcoming an unhealthy degree of perfectionism.

Source: Adapted with the permission of The Free Press, a Division of Simon & Schuster Adult Publishing Group, from *Never Good Enough: Freeing Yourself From the Chains of Perfection* by Monica Ramirez Basco, Ph.D. Copyright © 1999 by Monica Ramirez Basco. All rights reserved.

4
Becoming Physically Fit

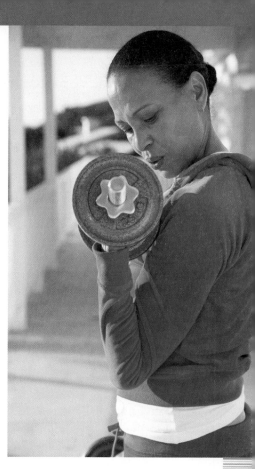

What Do You Know About Exercise and Physical Activity?

1. One of the benefits of endurance (aerobic) exercise training is that it improves both your good (HDL) and bad (LDL) cholesterol. True or False?

2. The old saying "Use it or lose it" is correct when applied to exercise training. True or False?

3. You can estimate your maximum heart rate by subtracting your age from 200. True or False?

4. You will burn more calories in a typical aerobic exercise training session than you will in a typical resistance training session. True or False?

5. Exercise is a subcategory (that is, a specific type) of physical activity. True or False?

6. A person will obtain a greater improvement in aerobic fitness by exercising at higher intensity for a shorter duration compared with a more moderate intensity performed for a longer duration. True or False?

7. Muscle mass declines with age, beginning around age 50. True or False?

Check your answers at the end of the chapter.

For many people, the day begins early in the morning; continues with classes, assignments, study, a job, and/or recreational activities; and does not end until after midnight. This kind of pace demands that one be physically fit. Even a highly motivated college student must have a reasonably well conditioned body to maintain such a schedule.

Okay, let's simplify things a bit. The paragraph above reflects how college health professors might view the value of fitness—it helps people function well enough to cope with their hectic lifestyles. But what motivates students to value **physical fitness?** Quite simply, students say that overall body fitness helps them look and feel better.

Many college students want to look in the mirror and see the kind of body they see in the media: one with well-toned muscles, a trim waistline, and no flabby tissue, especially on the arms and legs. Students become motivated to start fitness programs because they hope that they can build a better body. Through their efforts to do so, students usually start to feel better, both physically and mentally. They realize that change is possible, since they see it happening to their bodies with each passing week. "Go for it" and "Just do it" then become more than just sports marketing phrases; they become reminders that the activities that lead to fitness are a meaningful part of their lives (see the box "Harnessing the Spirit"). Fitness actually becomes fun.

Fortunately, you don't have to be a top-notch athlete to enjoy the health benefits of physical activity. In fact, even a modest increase in your daily **physical activity** level can be rewarding. According to the surgeon general's report on physical activity and health,[1] moderate amounts of physical activity can produce significant health benefits, including lowering the risk of premature death, coronary heart disease, hypertension, colon cancer, and diabetes. Even a variety of simple activities, such as gardening, walking, raking leaves, and dancing, that consistently increase a person's daily activity levels can be helpful for the majority of Americans. The health benefits of fitness can come from regular participation in moderate-intensity **exercise,** such as brisk walking or dancing.[2]

Prior to the 1990s, fitness professionals recommended that people needed to exercise above certain minimal (of time, intensity, and frequency) levels to obtain fitness benefits. Their message was correct; however, many people believed that if they could not meet the minimums, they were obtaining no benefits. Thus, it was viewed as an all-or-none proposition.

In 1995 the American College of Sports Medicine and the Centers for Disease Control and Prevention issued a public health statement, Physical Activity and Public Health.[3] This report, which was updated in 2007,[4] documented that there are clear benefits to 30 minutes a day of moderate-intensity physical activity and suggested that activities such as gardening and housework could be beneficial to health. Another important aspect of this report was that the health benefits could be obtained by accumulating activity throughout the day (for example, three 10-minute bouts of activity: one in the morning, one in the afternoon, and one in the evening).

The surgeon general's report on physical activity and health was issued in 1996 and helped clarify the difference between health benefits and fitness benefits.[2] There are numerous health benefits to regular physical activity. Among these benefits are control of body weight, blood pressure, blood sugar, and cholesterol. The surgeon general also operationalized the amount of activity required to obtain health benefits as 150 kilocalories per day. The report suggested that this could be achieved in a variety of ways (15 minutes of jogging, 30 minutes of walking, or 45 minutes of playing volleyball). Additionally, the report clarified that doing more than this amount would result in additional benefits. In other words, the more activity (dose), the greater the benefits (response).

In 2008 the U.S. Department of Health and Human Services released the first federal policy on physical activity, titled *Physical Activity Guidelines for Americans.*[5] These guidelines provide the most up-to-date, research-supported recommendations about physical activity and health. The major summary points are that substantial health benefits can be derived by performing (1) at least 150 minutes per week of moderate-intensity physical activity or (2) 75 minutes per week of vigorous-intensity physical activity and that (3) additional and extensive health benefits can be derived by increasing to either 300 minutes per week of moderate-intensity activity or 150 minutes per week of vigorous-intensity physical activity. The guidelines also mention that an equivalent combination of moderate and vigorous physical activity can be used. More information about these guidelines can be found at the U.S. Department of Health and Human Services website: http://www.health.gov/PAguidelines/.

Because exercise is a form of physical activity, when one exercises regularly, one gets the same (or greater) health benefits as those who choose to just maintain a regularly active lifestyle. The bonus for those who exercise is that they will also derive physical fitness benefits from their program.

Five Components of Physical Fitness

Physical fitness is characterized by the ability to perform occupational and recreational activities without becoming unduly fatigued and the capacity to handle unforeseen emergencies. The following sections focus on cardiorespiratory endurance, muscular strength, muscular endurance, flexibility, and body composition. These characteristics of physical fitness can be categorized as health-related physical fitness. Other characteristics, such as speed, power, agility, balance, and reaction time, are associated with what would be called performance-related physical fitness. Although the latter type is most important for competitive athletes, it is the former type that has the most relevance to the general population. Thus, this chapter focuses on health-related physical fitness.

Cardiorespiratory Endurance

If you were limited to improving only one area of your physical fitness, which would you choose—muscular strength, muscular endurance, or flexibility? Which would a dancer choose? Which would a marathon runner select? Which would an expert recommend?

The experts, exercise physiologists, would probably say that one fitness dimension is most important for overall health. They regard improvement of your heart, lung, and blood vessel function as the key focal point of a physical fitness program. **Cardiorespiratory endurance** forms the foundation for whole-body fitness.

Cardiorespiratory endurance increases your capacity to sustain a given level of energy production for a prolonged period. It helps your body to work longer and at greater levels of intensity.

Your body cannot always continually produce the energy it needs for short-term activity. Certain activities require performance at a level of intensity that will outstrip your cardiorespiratory system's ability to transport oxygen efficiently to contracting muscle fibers. This oxygen-deprived form of energy production is called **anaerobic** (without oxygen) **energy production,** the type that fuels many intense, short-duration activities. For example, rope climbing, weight lifting for strength, and sprinting are short-duration activities that quickly cause muscle fatigue;

they are generally considered anaerobic activities. The key factor is if the energy demand of the activity exceeds the aerobic energy production capability. Thus, even activities that are typically considered to be aerobic (walking or cycling) can require anaerobic energy if the intensity is high enough.

If you usually work or play at low intensity but for a long duration, you have developed an ability to maintain **aerobic** (with oxygen) **energy production.** As long as your body can meet its energy demands in this oxygen-rich mode, it will not convert to anaerobic energy production. Thus, fatigue will not be an important factor in determining whether you can continue to participate. Marathon runners, serious joggers and cyclists, distance swimmers, and aerobic dancers can perform their chosen activity because of their highly developed aerobic fitness. The cardiorespiratory systems of these aerobically fit people have developed a large capacity to take in, transport, and use oxygen.

Besides allowing you to participate in activities such as those mentioned, aerobic conditioning (cardiorespiratory endurance conditioning) may also provide benefits that affect other dimensions of your life; see the box "Structural and Functional Benefits of Cardiorespiratory (Aerobic) Fitness." It is now well accepted that regular physical activity that produces aerobic fitness will reduce the risk of heart disease, type 2 diabetes, osteoporosis, obesity, depression, and cancer of the breast and colon.[4]

> **Key Terms**
>
> **physical fitness** A set of attributes that people have or achieve that relates to the ability to perform physical activity.[6]
>
> **physical activity** Any bodily movement produced by skeletal muscles that results in energy expenditure.[6]
>
> **exercise** A subcategory of physical activity; it is planned, structured, repetitive, and purposive in the sense that an improvement or maintenance of physical fitness is an objective.[6]
>
> **cardiorespiratory endurance** The ability of the heart, lungs, and blood vessels to process and transport oxygen required by muscle cells so that they can contract over a period of time.
>
> **anaerobic energy production** The body's means of energy production when the necessary amount of oxygen is not available.
>
> **aerobic energy production** The body's means of energy production when the respiratory and circulatory systems are able to process and transport a sufficient amount of oxygen to muscle cells.

Aerobic fitness can help you do the following:

- Complete and enjoy your daily activities.

- Strengthen and increase the efficiency of your heart muscle.

- Increase the proportion of high-density lipoproteins (good cholesterol) in your blood.

- Increase the capillary network in your body.

- Improve collateral circulation, the ability of nearby blood vessels to enlarge and carry blood around a blocked blood vessel.

- Control your weight.

- Stimulate bone growth.

- Cope with stressors.

- Ward off infections.

- Improve the efficiency of your other body systems.

- Bolster your self-esteem.

- Achieve self-directed fitness goals.

- Reduce negative dependence behavior.

- Sleep better.

- Recover more quickly from common illnesses.

- Meet people with similar interests.

- Obtain reduced insurance premiums.

Muscular Strength and Muscular Endurance

Muscular fitness is the term used to represent the capabilities of the skeletal muscles to perform contractions. The capacity of the muscles has two distinct yet integrated characteristics: **muscular strength** and **muscular endurance.** The strength of the muscle is related to its ability to perform at or near its maximum level for a short period of time. The endurance of the muscle is related to its ability to perform at submaximum levels for a long period of time.

Both muscular strength and muscular endurance are essential for your body to accomplish work. Your ability to maintain good posture, walk, lift, push, and pull are familiar examples of the constant demands you make on your muscles to maintain or increase their level of contraction. The stronger you are, the greater your ability to contract muscles and maintain a level of contraction sufficient to complete tasks.

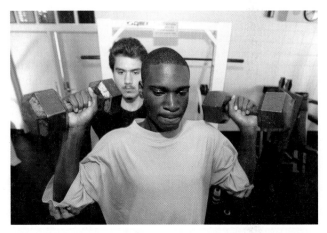

Muscular fitness training has both functional and health benefits. People with good muscular fitness can perform daily tasks more easily and enjoy more recreational activities. Muscular fitness training can also improve body composition.

Flexibility

The ability of your joints to move through their natural range of motion is a measure of your **flexibility.** This fitness trait, like so many other aspects of structure and function, differs from point to point within your body and among different people. Not every joint in your body is equally flexible (by design), and, over the course of time, use or disuse will alter the flexibility of a given joint. Certainly, gender, age, genetically determined body build, and current level of physical fitness affect your flexibility.

Inability to move easily during physical activity can be a constant reminder that aging and inactivity are the foes of flexibility. Failure to use joints regularly will result in a loss of elasticity in the connective tissues and shortening of muscles associated with the joints. Benefits of flexibility include improved balance, posture, and athletic performance and reduced risk of low-back and other joint pain.

Body Composition

Body composition refers to the different components the body is made up of (muscle, bone, fat, water, minerals).[7] Of particular interest to fitness experts are percentages

Key Terms

muscular fitness The ability of skeletal muscles to perform contractions; includes muscular strength and muscular endurance.

muscular strength The component of physical fitness that deals with the ability to contract skeletal muscles to a maximal level; the maximal force that a muscle can exert.

muscular endurance The aspect of muscular fitness that deals with the ability of a muscle or muscle group to repeatedly contract over a long period of time.

flexibility The ability of joints to function through an intended range of motion.

of body fat and fat-free weight. Health experts are especially concerned about the large number of people in our society who are obese and with the loss of muscle as one ages. Increasingly, cardiorespiratory fitness trainers are recognizing the importance of body composition and are including strength-training exercises. (See Chapter 6 for further information about body composition, health effects of obesity, and weight management.)

 TALKING POINTS Which benefits of exercise are most important to you? What would motivate you to become and stay active?

Developing a Personalized Fitness Program

In order to develop a healthy lifestyle, it is important to set goals. The National Institutes of Health suggest that useful goals should be specific, attainable (doable), and forgiving (less than perfect). Knowledge about both the principles and characteristics of exercise training is essential to developing useful goals.

Principles of Training

A personalized exercise program should meet both the needs and the preferences of the individual. The best exercise program is the one that the person will perform regularly. However, there are a number of principles of training that need to be followed for the program to be successful.

The most basic of all the principles of exercise training is *overload*. The objective of exercise is to improve something in the body (such as heart function). To obtain this improvement, the body must be placed under a stress to make it work harder than it is accustomed to. When a body part or system is overloaded in an appropriate manner, that body part undergoes adaptation, increasing the capability of that body part.

A second important principle of training is *specificity*. To produce an adaptation, the exercise must be specific to the outcome that is targeted for improvement. A good example of this can be seen by considering two different types of strength training: isometric and isotonic. Over time, persons who regularly perform isometric exercise will increase their capacity to perform an isometric contraction (they will be able to generate more muscular force without lengthening their muscle); however, their ability to perform muscular contractions throughout the full range of motion will not be improved significantly. In contrast, people who prefer isotonic exercises will increase their ability to perform the muscular contraction throughout the full range of motion.

A third important principle of training is *reversibility* (sometimes referred to as *regression*). This is basically what is meant by the old saying "Use it or lose it." In order for people to maintain the benefits of exercise, they must perform the exercise on a regular basis. The details of how to train will be discussed in the following sections.

Cardiorespiratory Endurance

For people of all ages, cardiorespiratory conditioning can be achieved through many activities. As long as the activity you choose places sufficient demand on the heart and lungs, improved fitness is possible. In addition to engaging in the familiar activities of swimming, running, and cycling, many people today participate in rollerblading, cross-country skiing, brisk walking, and group classes involving dance, kickboxing, or spinning. Regardless of age or physical limitations, you can select from a variety of enjoyable activities that will condition the cardiorespiratory system (see the box "A Different Kind of Fitness"). Complete the Personal Assessment at the end of this chapter to determine your level of fitness.

Many people think that any kind of physical activity will produce cardiorespiratory fitness. Golf, bowling, hunting, fishing, and archery are not considered to be forms of exercise. If performed regularly and for sufficient periods of time, they may enhance your health. However, they do not meet the requirements to be called exercise and would not necessarily lead to improved physical fitness. The American College of Sports Medicine (ACSM), the nation's premier professional organization of exercise physiologists and sport physicians, has well-accepted guidelines for exercise training.[2]

The ACSM's most recent recommendations for cardiorespiratory conditioning were published in 2009. They include four major areas: (1) mode of activity, (2) frequency of training, (3) intensity of training, and (4) duration of training. The ACSM has also made recommendations for muscular fitness and flexibility training. Some have used the acronym FITT to help them remember these four areas. F represents frequency, I represents intensity, T represents time (duration), and T represents type (mode). These recommendations are summarized in the following sections. If you are already exercising regularly, you may wish to compare your existing fitness program with these standards. It would also be valuable to assess your current fitness level (see pages 92–93) and to monitor changes in your fitness level as you change your exercise routine.

Mode of Activity The ACSM recommends that the mode of activity be any continuous physical activity that uses large muscle groups and can be rhythmic and aerobic in nature. Among the activities that generally meet this requirement are continuous swimming, cycling, aerobics, basketball, cross-country skiing, rollerblading,

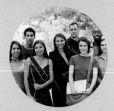

Learning from Our Diversity

A Different Kind of Fitness: Developmentally Disabled Athletes Are Always Winners in the Special Olympics

In America, as in many other countries around the world, physical fitness and athletic prowess carry a high degree of prestige, whereas lack of conditioning and poor sports performance often draw scorn and rejection. As anyone knows who's ever been picked last when sides were being chosen for a schoolyard game, few things are more damaging to youthful self-esteem than being the player nobody wants.

Some of these children blossom into accomplished athletes as they gain coordination or are inspired and guided by caring coaches. Others, lacking strong interest in sports, turn to less physical arenas in which they can excel—drama, debating, music, computers, science.

But what about people who want to be athletes at almost any cost, but who have no realistic hope of attaining the standards of athletic accomplishment set for those in top physical condition? The Joseph P. Kennedy Foundation created an arena in which these athletes could compete when it established the Special Olympics in 1968. Joseph Kennedy was the father of President John F. Kennedy, whose older sister Rosemary was virtually shut away from the world when her family discovered she was mentally disabled. Many people at that time shared the Kennedys' view that the kindest way to treat family members who were developmentally disabled was to "protect" them from stares and whispers by keeping them at home or placing them in institutions or residential facilities. Spearheaded by President Kennedy's sister Eunice

Kennedy Shriver, the Special Olympics was intended to change the old attitudes toward developmentally disabled people by giving them an opportunity to compete at their own level and to celebrate their victories publicly.

Now, over 40 years later, the Special Olympics holds both winter and summer games and boasts participation of more than 1 million developmentally disabled athletes in 140 countries around the world. The games are open to athletes between the ages of 8 and 63, some of whom have proved wrong the specialists who claimed they would never walk, let alone compete internationally. "Mainstream" Olympic champions such as figure-skating silver medalist Brian Orser and a host of well-known entertainers have attended opening-day ceremonies to cheer on and inspire the special athletes.

But medals aren't what the Special Olympics is all about. No matter where a Special Olympian finishes in a contest, he or she is applauded and celebrated for the accomplishment of "running the race" and seeing it through. The oath taken by each participant in the Special Olympics aptly states the credo of this remarkable group of athletes: "Let me win. But if I cannot win, let me be brave in the attempt."

In what ways other than physical conditioning do you think a developmentally disabled person might benefit from participating in the Special Olympics? What can the rest of us learn from these athletes' courage and perseverance?

step training (bench aerobics), hiking, walking, rowing, stair climbing, dancing, and running. Water exercise (water or aqua aerobics) is another popular fitness mode, and it is especially effective for pregnant women and elderly, injured, or disabled people.

Endurance games and activities, such as tennis, racquetball, and basketball, are fine as long as you and your partner are skilled enough to keep the ball in play; walking after the ball will do very little for you. Riding a bicycle is a good activity if you keep pedaling; coasting will do little to improve fitness. Softball and football are generally less than sufficient continuous activities—especially the way they are played by weekend athletes. Again, it is important to note that from a general health perspective, all physical activities are good; however, if fitness is the goal, the frequency, intensity, and duration of the activity are important.

Regardless of which continuous activity you select, it should also be enjoyable. Running, for example, is not for everyone—despite what some accomplished runners say! Find an activity you enjoy. If you need others around you to have a good time, get a group of friends to join you. Vary your activities to keep from becoming bored. You might cycle in the summer, run in the fall, swim in the winter, and play racquetball in the spring.

Frequency of Training **Frequency** of training refers to the number of times per week a person exercises. The ACSM recommends three (vigorous-intensity) to five (moderate-intensity) times per week. For most people, participation in fitness activities more than five times each week does not significantly further improve their level of conditioning. Likewise, an average of only two workouts each week does not seem to produce a measurable improvement in cardiorespiratory conditioning. Thus, although you may have a lot of fun cycling twice each week, do not expect to see a significant improvement in your cardiorespiratory fitness level from doing so.

Intensity of Training How much effort should you put into an activity? Should you run quickly, jog slowly, or swim at a comfortable pace? Must a person sweat profusely to become fit? These questions all relate to **intensity** of effort.

The ACSM recommends that healthy adults exercise at an intensity level of between 64 percent and 91 percent of their maximum heart rate (estimated by subtracting one's age from 220) or 30–85 percent of their heart rate reserve. This level of intensity is called the **target heart rate (THR)** and can be determined using the methods shown in Table 4.1. This rate refers to the minimum number of times your heart needs to contract (beat) each minute to

Table 4.1 Calculation of Target Heart Rate for Exercise Training

Method	Percentage of maximum heart rate (% HR_{max})	Heart rate reserve (HRR)
Information needed	Age and desired training intensity (percent)	Age, resting heart rate (HR), and desired training intensity (percent)
	Age-Predicted Maximal Heart Rate = 220 − age	
Example Calculation	22-year-old, training at 75 percent $(220 - 22) \times .75 = 148$ bpm	45-year-old, resting HR 75 beats per minute (bpm), training at 70 percent $([(220 - 45) - 80] \times .70) + 80 = 150$ bpm

have a positive effect on your heart, lungs, and blood vessels. This improvement is called the *training effect:* Intensity of activity below the THR will be insufficient to make a significant improvement in your fitness level.

Although intensity below the THR will still help you expend calories and thus lose weight, it will probably do little to make you more aerobically fit. However, an intensity that is significantly above your THR will probably cause you to become so fatigued that you will be forced to stop the activity before the training effect can be achieved. For persons who are quite unfit, the 2009 ACSM recommendations suggest intensity levels as low as 30 percent of HRR or 57 percent of % HR_{max}.

Choosing a particular THR between 64 percent and 91 percent of % HR_{max} or 30–85 percent of HRR depends on your initial level of cardiorespiratory fitness. If you are already in relatively good physical shape, you might want to start exercising at 75% HR_{max}. A well-conditioned person needs to select a higher THR for his or her intensity level, whereas a person with a low cardiorespiratory fitness level will still be able to achieve a training effect at a lower THR.

Determining your heart rate is not a complicated procedure. Find a location on your body where an artery passes near the surface of the skin. Pulse rates are difficult to determine by touching veins, which are more superficial than arteries. Two easily accessible sites for determining heart rate are the carotid artery (one on either side of the windpipe at the front of your neck) and the radial artery (on the inside of your wrist, just above the base of the thumb).

Practice placing the front surface of your index and middle fingertips at one of these locations and feeling for a pulse. Once you have found a regular pulse, look at the second hand of a watch. Count the number of beats you feel in a 10-second period and multiply this number by 6. This number is your heart rate. With a little practice, you can become proficient at determining your heart rate.

Duration of Training The ACSM recommends that the **duration** of training be between 20 and 90 minutes of continuous or intermittent aerobic activity. Intermittent activity can be accumulated in 10-minute segments throughout the day. This is especially helpful for persons who cannot take a single large chunk of time during the day to devote to an exercise program.

However, for most healthy adults, the ACSM recommends moderate-intensity activity levels with longer duration times, totaling at least 150 minutes per week. For healthy adults who train at higher intensity levels, the duration of training will likely be shorter, totaling at least 75 minutes per week.[2] Adults who are unfit or have an existing medical condition should check with their fitness instructor or physician to determine an appropriate duration of training.

Muscular Fitness

Recognizing that overall body fitness includes muscular fitness, the ACSM recommends resistance training in its current standards. This training should help develop and maintain a healthy body composition—one with an emphasis on lean body mass. The goal of resistance training is not to improve cardiorespiratory endurance, but to improve overall muscle strength and endurance. For some people (such as individuals with type 2 diabetes), high-intensity resistance training and isometric contractions are not recommended because they can induce a sudden and potentially dangerous increase in blood pressure.

> **Key Terms**
>
> **frequency** The number of exercise sessions per week; for aerobic fitness, three to five days are recommended.
>
> **intensity** The level of effort put into an activity.
>
> **target heart rate (THR)** The number of times per minute the heart must contract to produce a training effect.
>
> **duration** The length of time one needs to exercise at the THR to produce a cardiorespiratory training effect.

Types of Muscular Fitness Exercises and Equipment

Muscular strength can be improved best by training activities that use the **overload principle.** By overloading, or gradually increasing the resistance (load, object, or weight) your muscles must move, you can increase your muscular strength. The following three types of training exercises are based on the overload principle.

In **isometric** (meaning "same length") **exercises,** the resistance is so great that the contracting muscles cannot move the resistant object at all. For example, you could contract your muscles against an immovable object such as a wall. Because of the difficulty of precisely evaluating the training effects, isometric exercises are not usually used as a primary means of developing muscular strength. These exercises should be avoided by people with hypertension and type 2 diabetes.

Isotonic (meaning "same tension") **resistance exercises** are currently the most popular type of strength-building exercises and include the use of traditional free weights (dumbbells and barbells), as well as many resistance exercise machines. People who perform progressive resistance exercises use various muscle groups to move (or lift) specific fixed resistances or weights. Although during a given repetitive exercise the weight resistance remains the same, the muscular contraction effort required varies according to the joint angles in the range of motion. The greatest effort is required at one angle (sticking point) in the range of motion.

Isokinetic (meaning "same speed") **exercises** use mechanical devices that provide resistances that consistently overload muscles throughout the entire range of motion. The resistance moves only at a preset speed, regardless of the force applied to it. For the exercise to be effective, a user must apply maximal force. Isokinetic training requires elaborate, expensive equipment, so the use of isokinetic equipment may be limited to certain athletic teams, diagnostic centers, or rehabilitation clinics. The most common isokinetic machines are Cybex, Orthotron, Biodex, Mini-Gym, and ExerGenie.

Which type of strength-building exercise (machines or free weights) is more effective? Take your choice, since all will help develop muscular strength. Some people prefer machines because they are simple to use, do not require stacking the weights, and are already balanced and less likely to drop and cause injury. Other people prefer free weights because they encourage the user to work harder to maintain balance during the lift. In addition, free weights can be used in a greater variety of exercises than weight machines. There is also a wide variety of types of accessory equipment that can be used for strength training, including stability balls, exercise bands and tubes, inflatable exercise discs, weighted exercise balls ("medicine balls"), and abdominal isolation devices. Many of these exercise accessories are inexpensive enough to be purchased for use at home.

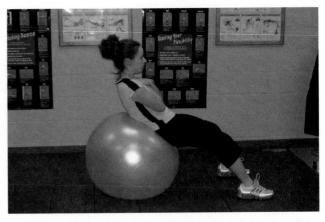

Many types of inexpensive accessory equipment are available for muscular fitness training, including stability balls (shown here), resistance bands, and weighted "medicine" balls.

Muscular endurance can be improved by performing repeated contractions of a less than maximal level. This aspect of muscular fitness is most related to common physical activities (leaf raking, pushing a lawn mower). Although it is not as glamorous as muscular strength, muscular endurance is an important part of muscular fitness.

Amateur and professional athletes often wish to increase the endurance of specific muscle groups associated with their sports activities. This can be achieved by using exercises that gradually increase the number of repetitions of a given movement. However, muscular endurance is not the physiological equivalent of cardiorespiratory endurance. For example, a world-ranked distance runner with highly developed cardiorespiratory endurance and extensive muscular endurance of the legs may not have a corresponding level of muscular endurance of the abdominal muscles.

Frequency, Intensity, and Duration   The resistance training recommended by the ACSM includes two to four sets of 8–12 repetitions (10–15 for adults over age 50) of 8–10 different exercises performed two or three times a week. These exercises should be geared to the body's major muscle groups (legs, arms, shoulders, trunk, and back) and should not focus on just one or two body areas. Isotonic (progressive resistance) or isokinetic exercises are recommended. For the average person, resistance training activities should be done at a moderate to slow speed, use the full range of motion, and not impair normal breathing. With just two sets recommended for each exercise, resistance training is not very time-consuming. The ACSM, however, indicates that three to four sets could provide greater benefits, if time is available.

Flexibility Training

To develop and maintain a healthy range of motion for the body's joints, the ACSM suggests that flexibility exercises be included in one's overall fitness program. Stretching can be done in conjunction with other cardiorespiratory or muscular fitness training or can be performed separately. Note that if flexibility training is done separately, a general warm-up (walking or stationary cycling) should be performed before stretching so that the muscles are warm before they are stretched.

Types of Stretching Exercises   Flexibility can be developed and maintained through a program of regular stretching. Types of stretching exercises include **static stretching,** which involves the slow lengthening of a muscle group, and **ballistic stretching,** which involves repetitive and forceful bouncing movements. For most people, static stretching is the better type, because ballistic stretching carries a higher risk of injury; however, conclusive research evidence for this is lacking.

Frequency, Intensity, and Duration   The ACSM recommends that a flexibility program include stretches for all the major muscle and/or tendon groups. Stretching exercises should be performed at least two to three days per week, but stretching is an activity that can be safely performed daily. Each stretch should extend to a position where you feel mild discomfort—not pain—in the muscle. Slowly extend each stretch and then hold the extended position for 15–60 seconds. Relax and breathe normally during the stretch; do not hold your breath. Repeat each stretch at least four times per training session.

Training Considerations for Body Composition

When training to improve body composition, the goal is to increase muscle (and possibly bone) mass, decrease body fat, or a combination of both. Training to maintain or increase muscle mass was covered earlier in this chapter in the discussion of muscular fitness. It is important to recognize that muscle mass declines with age, beginning sometime after age 35. This loss of muscle mass is called **sarcopenia.** Thus, strength training to maintain the amount and the quality of muscle is a recommended component of adult exercise programs.

Due to the prevalence of obesity, the most common exercise goal related to body composition is to lose body fat. To achieve this, the exercise program should seek to maximize the caloric expenditure. Aerobic exercise activities are the best to produce relatively high rates of energy expenditure for a prolonged period of time. The ACSM recommends that an exercise program should progress to 250–300 minutes of at least moderate-intensity physical activity per week. For some individuals, even more activity (60–90 minutes per day) may be necessary to promote and maintain weight loss. Frequency should be most, if not all, days of the week.

Warm-Up, Conditioning, and Cooldown

Each training session consists of three basic parts: the warm-up, the conditioning, and the cooldown.[2] The warm-up should last 5–10 minutes. During this period, you should begin slow, gradual, comfortable movements related to the upcoming activity, such as walking or slow jogging. All body segments and muscle groups should be exercised as you gradually increase your heart rate. Near the end of the warm-up period, the major muscle groups should be stretched. This preparation helps protect you from muscle strains and joint sprains.

The warm-up is a fine time to socialize. Furthermore, you can mentally prepare yourself for your activity or think about the beauty of the morning sky, the changing colors of the leaves, or the friends you will meet later in the day. Mental warm-ups can be as beneficial for you psychologically as physical warm-ups are physiologically.

The second part of the training session is the conditioning phase, the part of the session that involves improving muscular fitness, cardiorespiratory endurance, and flexibility. Workouts can be tailor-made, but they should follow the ACSM guidelines discussed earlier in this chapter (see Table 4.2).

The third important part of each fitness session, the cooldown, consists of a 5- to 10-minute session of relaxing exercises, such as slow jogging, walking, and stretching. This activity allows your body to cool and return to a resting state. A cooldown period helps reduce muscle soreness.

Key Terms

overload principle   The principle whereby a person exercises at a level above which he or she is normally accustomed to.

isometric exercises   Muscular strength training exercises in which the resistance is so great that the object cannot be moved.

isotonic resistance exercises   Muscular strength training exercises in which traditional barbells and dumbbells with fixed resistances are used.

isokinetic exercises   Muscular strength training exercises in which machines are used to provide variable resistances throughout the full range of motion at a fixed speed.

static stretching   The slow lengthening of a muscle group to an extended stretch; followed by holding the extended position for 15–60 seconds.

ballistic stretching   A "bouncing" form of stretching in which a muscle group is lengthened repetitively to produce multiple quick, forceful stretches.

sarcopenia   A reduction in the size of the muscle fibers, related to the aging process.

Table 4.2 Summary of Exercise Training Recommendations for Each Component of Physical Fitness

	Cardiorespiratory Endurance	Muscular Strength	Muscular Endurance	Flexibility	Body Composition
Mode	Any using large muscle groups in a rhythmic pattern	Free weights, machines, resistive devices	Free weights, machines, resistive devices	Static is usually recommended	Aerobic for fat loss and strength for muscle mass gains
Intensity	64–91% HR$_{max}$ or 40–85% HRR	Amount of weight that can be moved only 8–12 times without rest	Less than maximal	To point of mild to moderate discomfort	Specific to mode of training
Duration	150 minutes per week (moderate intensity), 75 minutes per week (vigorous intensity)	2–4 sets of 8–10 repetitions using major muscle groups	2–4 sets of 8–10 repetitions using major muscle groups	At least 4 repetitions of 15–60 seconds each for all major joints	At least 300 minutes per week
Frequency	3–5 days per week	2–3 days per week	3–5 days per week	2–3 days per week	5–7 days per week

Note: HR$_{max}$ = maximum heart rate; HRR = heart rate range.
Source: Adapted from American College of Sports Medicine.

Exercise and Aging

Exercise throughout the life span is important for health and well-being. Active young adults can continue with their exercise programs into their 30s, 40s, and beyond. Young adults who have been sedentary can increase their level of activity gradually—say, by walking more each day. (See the box "Overcoming Barriers to Being Regularly Active" for advice on getting started on an exercise program.) And it is never too late to start exercising—with some care, physical activity can be an enjoyable part of the daily routine for older adults.

Aging Physically

The period between 45 and 64 years of age brings with it a variety of subtle changes in the body's structure and function. When life is busy and the mind is active, these changes are generally not evident. Even when they become evident, they are not usually the source of profound concern. Your parents, older students in your class, and people with whom you will be working are, nevertheless, experiencing these changes:

- Decrease in bone mass and density
- Increase in vertebral compression
- Degenerative changes in joint cartilage
- Increase in adipose tissue; loss of lean body mass
- Decrease in capacity to engage in physical work
- Decrease in visual acuity
- Decrease in resting energy requirements
- Decrease in fertility
- Decrease in sexual function

For some midlife adults, these health concerns can be quite threatening, especially for those who view aging with apprehension and fear. Some middle-aged people reject these physical changes and convince themselves they are sick. Indeed, hypochondriasis is much more common among midlife people than among young people.

Two medical conditions influenced by physical activity, osteoporosis and osteoarthritis, deserve careful examination and are discussed in following sections.

Exercise for Older Adults

An exercise program designed for younger adults may be inappropriate for older people, particularly those over age 50. Special attention must be paid to matching the program to the interests and abilities of the participants. Often, this is best achieved by having older individuals begin their exercise program under the supervision of a certified exercise professional. The goals of the program should include both social interaction and physical conditioning.

Older adults, especially those with a personal or family history of heart problems, should have a physical examination before starting a fitness program. This examination should include an exercise stress test, an evaluation of all cardiac risk factors, and an evaluation of joint functioning. Participants should learn how to monitor their own cardiorespiratory status during exercise.

Well-designed fitness programs for older adults will include activities that begin slowly, are monitored frequently, and are geared to the enjoyment of the participants.[2] The professional staff coordinating the program should be familiar with the signs of distress (excessively elevated heart rate, nausea, breathing difficulty, pallor, and pain) and must be able to perform CPR and use an automated external defibrillator (AED). Warm-up and cooldown periods should be included. Activities to increase flexibility are beneficial in the beginning and ending segments of the program. Participants should

I've never really been active and can't seem to get started on an exercise program. What can I do?

Barriers to physical activity frequently listed by Americans are lacking time, motivation, and support and finding exercise inconvenient, boring, and unpleasant. Do you find it difficult to be regularly active? Take the quiz at the first InfoLink site listed below to find out your personal barriers. The same site also lists suggestions for overcoming common barriers, including the following strategies:

- *Lack of time.* Monitor your daily activities for a week to identify available time slots. Add physical activity to your daily routine, and select activities that require minimal time. Don't create a complicated exercise program.
- *Lack of energy.* Schedule activity for times in the day or week when you feel energetic, and remind yourself that physical activity will increase your energy level. Try incorporating music into your workouts.
- *Lack of motivation.* Plan ahead by including activity in your daily or weekly schedule. Ask a friend to exercise with you, or join an exercise group or class. Measure your improvement by keeping a log, and reward yourself when you reach fitness goals.
- *Social influences.* Invite friends to exercise with you, and plan enjoyable social activities involving physical activity.

- *Lack of skill.* Select activities requiring no new skills, and exercise with people at the same skill level. Take a class to learn new skills.
- *Fear of injury.* Choose activities involving minimum risk, and learn how to warm up, cool down, and work out in ways that are appropriate to your age, fitness level, and health status.
- *Lack of resources.* Select activities that require minimal facilities or equipment, such as walking or calisthenics. Investigate resources available on your campus.
- *Weather conditions.* Develop a set of regular activities that are always available regardless of weather. Look on outdoor activities that depend on weather conditions as bonus activities.
- *Family obligations.* Exercise with the kids or while the kids are busy playing or sleeping. Trade babysitting time with a friend or neighbor who also has small children.

Source: Centers for Disease Control and Prevention, Physical activity for everyone: making physical activity part of your life—overcoming barriers to physical activity, www.cdc.gov/nccdphp/dnpa/physical/life/overcome.htm.

InfoLinks

www.cdc.gov/nccdphp/dnpa/physical/life/overcome.htm
www.smallstep.gov

wear comfortable clothing and appropriate shoes and should be mentally prepared to enjoy the activities.

A program designed for older adults will largely conform to the ACSM criteria specified in this chapter. Certainly, specific modifications or restrictions to the exercise program may be required due to health concerns that are more frequent in older adults. Also, because of possible joint, muscular, or skeletal problems, certain activities may have to be done in a sitting position. Pain or discomfort should be reported immediately to the fitness instructor.

Fortunately, properly screened older adults will rarely have health emergencies during a well-monitored fitness program. For some older adults, individual fitness activities may be more enjoyable than supervised group activities. Either choice offers important benefits.

Specific Health Concerns

Low-Back Pain   A common occurrence among adults is the sudden onset of low-back pain. Four out of five adults develop this condition at least once in their lifetime, which can be so uncomfortable that they miss work, lose sleep, and generally feel incapable of engaging in daily activities. Many of the adults who have this condition will experience these effects two to three times per year.

Although low-back pain can reflect serious health problems, most low-back pain is caused by mechanical

(postural) problems. As unpleasant as low-back pain is, the symptoms and functional limitations usually subside within a week or two. The services of a physician, physical therapist, or chiropractor are not generally required.

By engaging in regular exercise, such as swimming, walking, and bicycling, and by paying attention to your

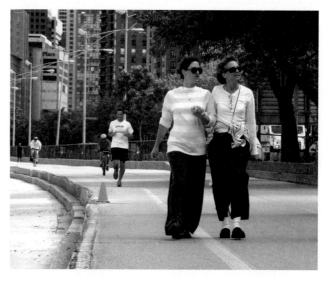

Choosing activities that are safe, convenient, and enjoyable can help people maintain an exercise program throughout the life span.

Table 4.3 Osteoporosis Risk Factors

Nonmodifiable Risk Factors	Lifestyle Factors
• **Age**—This is more common in older people than younger people. • **Sex**—Women have greater risk than men. Many women also lose bone quickly after menopause. However, up to one in four men over the age of 50 will break a bone because of osteoporosis. • **Menopause**—Bone loss increases after menopause. • **Family history**—Heredity and genetics play a major role in osteoporosis. • **Low body weight/being small and thin**—Those with small bones are more likely to have osteoporosis. • **Broken bones or height loss**—People who have broken one or more bones during their adult years may already have osteoporosis and not know it. Broken bones in the spine can cause height loss.	• **Not enough calcium, vitamin D** • **Not enough fruits, vegetables** • **Too much protein, sodium, caffeine** • **Inactive lifestyle** • **Smoking** • **Drinking too much alcohol**

back during bending, lifting, and sitting, you can minimize the occurrence of this uncomfortable and incapacitating condition. Commercial fitness centers and campus recreational programs are starting to offer specific exercise classes geared to muscular improvement in the lower back and abdominal areas.

Osteoporosis **Osteoporosis** is a condition often seen in older middle-aged women. A complete set of risk factors as established by the National Osteoporosis Foundation is shown in Table 4.3. It is not fully understood why menopausal women are so susceptible to the increase in calcium loss that leads to fractures of the hip, wrist, and vertebral column. In 2005, approximately 2 million fractures occurred that were attributable to osteoporosis.[8]

The endocrine system plays a large role in the development of osteoporosis. At the time of menopause, a woman's ovaries begin a rapid decrease in the production of estrogen, one of two main hormones associated with the menstrual cycle. This lower level of estrogen may reduce the conversion of the precursors of vitamin D into the active form of vitamin D, the form necessary for absorbing calcium from the digestive tract. As a result, calcium may be drawn from the bones for use elsewhere in the body.

An important fact to know is that 85–90 percent of one's peak bone mass is obtained by age 20. Thus, it is essential to encourage lifestyle habits that promote bone building in youth. Premenopausal women have the opportunity to build and maintain a healthy skeleton through an appropriate intake of calcium. Depending on age, current recommendations are for an intake of 1,000–1,300 mg of calcium per day. Three to four daily servings of low-fat dairy products should provide sufficient

calcium. Adequate vitamin D must also be in the diet because it aids in the absorption of calcium.

Many women do not take in an adequate amount of calcium. Calcium supplements, again in combination with vitamin D, can be used to achieve recommended calcium levels. It is now known that calcium carbonate, a much-advertised form of calcium, is no more easily absorbed by the body than are other forms of calcium salts.

In premenopausal women, calcium deposition in bone is facilitated by exercise, particularly exercise that involves movement of the extremities. Today, women are encouraged to consume at least the recommended servings from the milk group and engage in regular physical activity that involves the weight-bearing muscles of the legs, such as aerobics, jogging, and walking.

Postmenstrual women who are not elderly can markedly slow the resorption of calcium from their bones through the use of hormone replacement therapy (HRT). When combined with a daily intake of 1,500 mg of calcium, vitamin D, and regular exercise, HRT almost eliminates calcium loss. Women need to work closely with their physicians in monitoring the use of HRT because of continuing concern over the role of HRT and the development of breast cancer and the increased risk of coronary artery disease and stroke.

Osteoarthritis Arthritis is an umbrella term for more than 100 forms of joint inflammation. The most common form is **osteoarthritis.** It is likely that as we age, all of us will develop osteoarthritis to some degree. Often called "wear and tear" arthritis, osteoarthritis occurs primarily in the weight-bearing joints of the knee, hip, and spine. In this form of arthritis, joint damage can occur to bone ends, cartilaginous cushions, and related structures as the years of constant friction and stress accumulate.

The object of current management of osteoarthritis (and other forms) is not to cure the disease but rather to reduce discomfort, slow the progression of the disease, and maintain or improve function in daily activities.[9] Nonsteroidal anti-inflammatory drugs (NSAIDs) are the medications most frequently used to treat osteoarthritis. Loss of excess body weight can also play an important role in reducing symptoms associated with osteoarthritis.

It is now believed that osteoarthritis develops most commonly in people with a genetic predisposition for

Key Terms

osteoporosis A decrease in bone mass that leads to increased incidence of fracture, primarily in postmenopausal women.

osteoarthritis Arthritis that develops with age; largely caused by weight bearing and deterioration of the joints.

excessive damage to the weight-bearing joints. Thus, the condition seems to "run in families." Further, studies comparing the occurrence of osteoarthritis in those who exercise and those who do not demonstrate that regular movement activity may decrease the likelihood of developing this form of arthritis.

Fitness Questions and Answers

Along with the main components of your fitness program, you should think about many additional issues when you start a fitness program.

Should I See My Doctor Before I Get Started?

This issue has probably kept thousands of people from ever beginning a fitness program. The hassle and expense of getting a comprehensive physical examination is an excellent excuse for people who are not completely sold on the idea of exercise. It is highly desirable to have regular checkups as part of your overall health plan. However, the surgeon general has suggested that most adults can safely increase their activity level to a moderate amount without the need for a comprehensive medical evaluation.[1] Individuals with chronic diseases should consult with their physician before increasing their activity level. If more vigorous forms of exercise are desired, then a medical exam is recommended for men over the age of 45 and women over the age of 55. It is also recommended for individuals with more than one risk factor for coronary artery disease or with any other notable health problems. The American College of Sports Medicine also recommends an exercise ("stress") test for these individuals.[2]

What Should I Wear for Exercise?

Clothes for exercise should be comfortable and promote temperature regulation. Loose-fitting attire that does not restrict movement is appropriate. More form-fitting clothing can also be comfortable and nonrestrictive if made from newer materials that promote temperature regulation.

In warmer temperatures, the goal is to prevent the body from overheating. Generally, in a warm or hot environment, less clothing should be worn and, if you are exercising outdoors, lighter colors should be chosen to diminish radiant heat transfer to the body. The clothing materials should allow for the transfer of moisture from the skin so that evaporation, which causes heat loss, can take place. Sweat that drips off or is wiped off the body does not produce any cooling.

In cooler temperatures, the goal is to prevent losing too much heat, which can result in hypothermia. A layered approach to dressing is recommended. When you exercise, even in the cold, you will produce body heat.

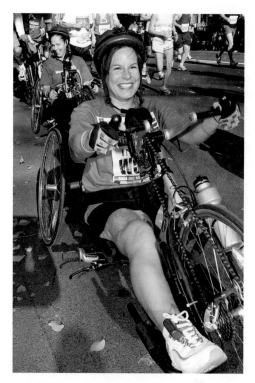

Wearing appropriate clothing and safety equipment and drinking adequate amounts of fluid are good strategies for any type of exercise.

Layering enables you to remove the outermost piece of clothing during exercise; you can put this layer back on during cooldown if you need to. The innermost layer should be made of a material that will transfer moisture away from your skin. Cotton is not recommended because it tends to absorb and retain moisture from sweat, which can increase the amount of heat loss in cold temperatures. The outermost layer should be of a material (such as Gore-Tex) that will shield your body from the wind but allow moisture to be transferred away from your body. Additionally, you should protect your extremities by wearing a hat that covers your ears and using gloves or mittens as dictated by the outdoor temperature.

In any environment, appropriate footwear is critical for safe and comfortable exercise; see the box "Choosing an Athletic Shoe" for specific guidelines for choosing shoes.

What Are Low-Impact Aerobic Activities?

Because long-term participation in some aerobic activities (for example, jogging, running, aerobic dancing, and rope skipping) may lead to injury of the hip, knee, and ankle joints, many fitness experts promote low-impact aerobic activities. Low-impact aerobic dancing, water aerobics, bench aerobics, and brisk walking are examples of this kind of fitness activity. Participants still conform to the principle components of a cardiorespiratory fitness program. THR levels are the same as in high-impact aerobic activities.

Choosing an Athletic Shoe

Proper-fitting sports shoes can enhance performance and prevent injuries. When shopping for new athletic shoes, use these tips to find a good shoe that fits well.

- Do the "wet test" to see what type of foot you have. Wet the bottoms of your feet and step onto a piece of paper or another surface where you'll be able to see the footprint you leave. A "blob" footprint with little arch indicates flat feet. Two "islands" with a lot of space between the heel and ball indicates high arches. A normal arch will look like the classic cartoon footprint.

- Choose a shoe for your foot type. If you have normal arches, get a shoe with good stability and a moderate amount of motion control. If you have high arches, get shoes with extra cushioning and flexibility. If you have flat arches, get shoes with a harder rubber or plastic area on the inner (arch support) side of the heel to control excess movement and provide support.

- Don't use running shoes for other sports, as they are not made for lateral movements, making ankle sprains more likely. Use only good quality court shoes or cross-trainers for other conditioning activities.

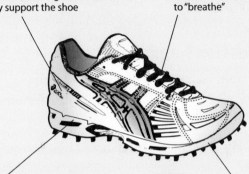

Heel counter (a cup shaped piece to stabilize the entire shoe): It should be made from a rigid material to firmly support the shoe

Upper (the entire top of the shoe): It should be made of material to allow the shoe to "breathe"

Midsole (the thick portion of the sole): It should be made of a shock-absorbing, yet lightweight material to provide cushioning

Outsole (the bottom portion of the shoe that contacts the ground): It should be made of a durable rubber and have a pattern to provide good traction

- Try on athletic shoes with the socks you plan to wear them in, and toward the end of the day when feet are larger.

- You should have about one thumb's width of room between your longest toe and the end of the shoe. Shoes should be wide enough that the foot does not feel pinched on the sides, but not a sloppy fit or one that slips at the heel.

It can be hard to choose from the many different types of athletic shoes available. Basic characteristics of a good athletic shoe are shown in the illustration. For additional advice on choosing shoes for physical activity, visit the websites listed in the InfoLinks section.

Source: Rogers M, Starting a running program, www.cpb.gov, February 2009.

InfoLinks

www.aofas.org

http://orthoinfo.aaos.org

www.runnersworld.com

The main difference between low-impact and high-impact aerobic activities is the use of the legs. Low-impact aerobics requires having one foot on the ground at all times. Thus, weight transfer does not occur with the forcefulness seen in traditional high-impact aerobic activities. In addition, low-impact activities may include exaggerated arm movements and the use of hand or wrist weights. All of these variations are designed to increase the heart rate to the THR without undo strain on the joints of the lower extremities. Low-impact aerobics are excellent for people of all ages, and they may be especially beneficial to older adults.

What Is Cross-Training?

Cross-training is the use of more than one aerobic activity to achieve cardiorespiratory fitness. For example, runners may use swimming, cycling, or rowing periodically to replace running in their training routines. Cross-training

allows certain muscle groups to rest and injuries to heal. Also, cross-training provides a refreshing change of pace for the participant. You will probably enjoy your fitness program more if you vary the activities.

What Is the Most Effective Way to Replace Fluids During Exercise?

Despite all the advertising hype associated with commercial fluid-replacement products, for an average person involved in typical fitness activities, water is still the best fluid replacement. The availability and cost are unbeatable. However, when activity is prolonged and intense, commercial sports drinks may be preferable to water because they contain electrolytes (which replace lost sodium and potassium) and carbohydrates (which replace depleted energy stores). However, the carbohydrates in sports drinks are actually simple forms of sugar. Thus, sports drinks tend to be high in calories, just like regular soft drinks. Regardless of the

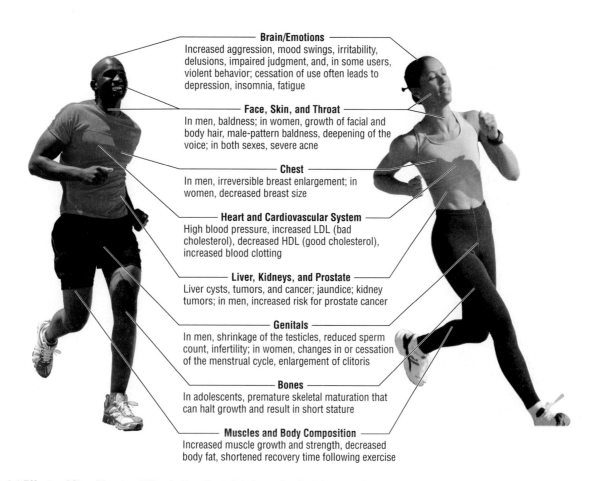

Brain/Emotions
Increased aggression, mood swings, irritability, delusions, impaired judgment, and, in some users, violent behavior; cessation of use often leads to depression, insomnia, fatigue

Face, Skin, and Throat
In men, baldness; in women, growth of facial and body hair, male-pattern baldness, deepening of the voice; in both sexes, severe acne

Chest
In men, irreversible breast enlargement; in women, decreased breast size

Heart and Cardiovascular System
High blood pressure, increased LDL (bad cholesterol), decreased HDL (good cholesterol), increased blood clotting

Liver, Kidneys, and Prostate
Liver cysts, tumors, and cancer; jaundice; kidney tumors; in men, increased risk for prostate cancer

Genitals
In men, shrinkage of the testicles, reduced sperm count, infertility; in women, changes in or cessation of the menstrual cycle, enlargement of clitoris

Bones
In adolescents, premature skeletal maturation that can halt growth and result in short stature

Muscles and Body Composition
Increased muscle growth and strength, decreased body fat, shortened recovery time following exercise

Figure 4-1 Effects of Steroids   In addition to the effects listed, people who inject steroids run the added risk of contracting or transmitting HIV infection or hepatitis.

Sources: *NIDA InfoFacts,* National Institute on Drug Abuse, March 2007; "Anabolic Steroids," *NIDA Community Drug Alert Bulletin,* National Institute on Drug Abuse, April 2000.

drink you choose, exercise physiologists recommend that you drink fluids before and at frequent intervals throughout the activity particularly in warm, humid environments. For more detailed information about this and other nutrition issues as they relate to athletic performance, see the report of the American College of Sports Medicine, Dieticians of Canada, and the American Dietetic Association.[10]

What Are Steroids, and Why Do Some Athletes Use Them?

Steroids are drugs that can be legally prescribed by physicians for a variety of health conditions, including certain forms of anemia, inadequate growth patterns, and chronic debilitating diseases. Steroids can also be prescribed to aid recovery from surgery or burns. **Anabolic steroids** are drugs that function like the male sex hormone testosterone. They can be taken orally or by injection.

Anabolic steroids are used by athletes who hope to gain weight, muscular size and strength, power, endurance, and aggressiveness. Over the last few decades, many bodybuilders, weight lifters, track athletes, and

football players have chosen to ignore the serious health risks posed by illegal steroid use.

The use of steroids is highly dangerous because of serious, life-threatening side effects and adverse reactions. These effects include heart problems, certain forms of cancer, liver complications, and even psychological disturbances. The side effects on female steroid users are as dangerous as those on men. Figure 4-1 shows the adverse effects of steroid use.

Steroid users have developed a terminology of their own. Anabolic steroids are called "roids" or "juice." "Roid rage" is an aggressive, psychotic response to chronic steroid use. "Stacking" means using multiple steroids, and possibly other drugs like stimulants, at the same time.

> **Key Terms**
>
> **anabolic steroids** Drugs that function like testosterone to produce increases in muscle mass, strength, endurance, and aggressiveness.

Most organizations that control athletic competition (for example, the National Collegiate Athletic Association, the Athletics Congress, the National Football League, and the International Olympic Committee) have banned steroids and are testing athletes for illegal use. Although athletes finally seem to be getting the message about the health risks associated with steroids, the temptation for improved performance via all possible means is still there.

 TALKING POINTS If you suspected that a young person you know was using steroids, what strategies would you use to encourage the person to change his or her behavior?

St. Louis Cardinal baseball player Mark McGwire's admitted use of androstenedione put this supplement in the national spotlight in the summer of 1998. That was the season when McGwire rocked the baseball world by surpassing Roger Maris's home run record, hitting 70 home runs. It is interesting, though, that during the 1999 baseball season McGwire opted to stop using andro, but still managed to hit nearly 70 home runs.

What Are the Risks and Benefits of Creatine?

Creatine is an amino acid found in meat, poultry, and fish. In a person's body, creatine is produced naturally in the liver, pancreas, and kidneys. Typically, people get one to two grams of creatine each day from their food intake. Creatine has recently received much attention for its use as a possible ergogenic aid.[10] **Ergogenic aids** are supplements taken to improve athletic performance. As an ergogenic aid, creatine performs its work in the muscles, where it helps restore the compound adenosine triphosphate (ATP). ATP provides quick energy for muscle contractions. It also helps to reduce the lactic acid buildup that occurs during physical exertion. This buildup causes a burning sensation that limits the amount of intense activity one can perform.

Early studies suggest that creatine can help athletes in anaerobic sports, which require short, explosive bursts of energy. However, the increase in performance has been small, the long-term health effects are unknown, studies have been restricted to highly trained subjects (not recreational athletes), and damage to kidneys is possible with high dosages. Users are cautioned to consume ample amounts of water to prevent cramping and dehydration.

All in all, creatine is unlikely to prove as potentially dangerous as androstenedione. If additional studies should indicate that creatine can consistently improve performance, this substance might be banned by many sports federations. For now, the safest, most prudent recommendation is for athletes to spend their time and energy improving their training programs rather than looking for a solution in a bottle.

How Worthwhile Are Commercial Health and Fitness Clubs?

The health and fitness club business is booming. Fitness clubs offer activities ranging from free weights to weight machines to step walking to general aerobics. Some clubs have saunas and whirlpools and lots of frills. Others have course offerings that include wellness, smoking cessation, stress management, time management, dance, and yoga. The atmosphere is friendly, and people are encouraged to have a good time while working out.

If your purpose in joining a fitness club is to improve your cardiorespiratory fitness, measure the program offered by the club against the ACSM standards. If your primary purpose is to meet people and have fun, request a trial membership for a month or so to see whether you like the environment.

Before signing a contract at a health club or spa, do some careful questioning. Find out when the business was established, ask about the qualifications of the employees, contact some members for their observations, and request a thorough tour of the facilities. You might even consult your local Better Business Bureau for additional information. Finally, make certain that you read and understand every word of the contract.

Similar consumer strategies should be used in evaluating fitness equipment. See the box "Infomercials and Advertisements for Fitness Equipment" for some specific suggestions.

Are Today's Children Physically Fit?

Major research studies published during the last 10 years have indicated that U.S. children and teenagers lead very sedentary lives. Children ages 6–17 score extremely poorly in the areas of strength, flexibility, and cardiorespiratory endurance. In many cases, parents are in better shape than their children are. A major consequence of these sedentary habits in children is obesity. The 2010 report from the National Center for Health Statistics indicates that 16.9 percent of children and adolescents ages 2–19 years are obese. Indeed, from the National Health and Nutrition Examination Surveys (NHANES) in 1976–80 to 2007–2008, the prevalence of obesity in adolescents has increased from 5.0 to 18.1 percent. The seriousness of these data is revealed by the fact that most obese children become obese adults.

This situation presents a challenge to educators and parents to emphasize the need for strenuous play activity. Television watching and parental inactivity were implicated as major factors in these studies.

How Do I Handle Common Injuries That May Be Caused by My Fitness Activities?

For the most part, emergency care for injuries that pertain to the bones or muscles should follow the RICE acronym.[11] Depending on the type and severity of the injury, the importance of rest (R), ice (I) or cold application, compression (C), and elevation (E) cannot be overstated. Each type of injury identified in Table 4.4 has a particular RICE protocol to follow. Any significant injury should be reported to your college student health center, an athletic trainer, a physical therapist, or a physician.

The major signs and symptoms of exercise injury include these:

- A delay of over one hour in your body's return to a fully relaxed, comfortable state after exercise
- A change in sleep patterns
- Any noticeable breathing difficulties or chest pains
- Persistent joint or muscle pain
- Unusual changes in urine composition or output (marked color change)
- Anything unusual (for example, headaches, nosebleeds, fainting, numbness in an extremity, and hemorrhoids)

If any of these signs or symptoms appear, stop exercise and contact your physician.

What Is the Female Athlete Triad?

In 2007, the American College of Sports Medicine updated their report that identified a three-part syndrome of disordered eating, **amenorrhea** (lack of menstruation), and osteoporosis as the female athlete triad.[12] The conditions of this syndrome appear independently in many women, but among female athletes they appear together. The female athlete triad is most likely to be found in athletes whose sport activities emphasize appearance (for example, diving, ice skating, or gymnastics).

Parents, coaches, trainers, and teammates should be watchful for signs of the female athlete triad. This syndrome has associated medical risks, including inadequate fuel supply for activities, inadequate iron intake, reduced cognitive function, altered hormone levels, reduced mental health, early onset of menopause, increased likelihood of skeletal trauma, altered blood fat profiles, and increased vulnerability to heart disease.[12] Vitally important is an early referral to a physician who is knowledgeable about the female athlete triad. The physician will likely coordinate efforts with a psychologist, a nutritionist, and an athletic trainer to improve the health of the athlete and prevent recurrences. More information about this syndrome can be found at www.femaleathletetriad.org.

Key Terms

ergogenic aids Supplements that are taken to improve athletic performance.

amenorrhea The absence of menstruation.

Table 4.4 Common Injuries Associated with Physical Activity

Injury	Condition
Achilles tendinitis	A chronic tendinitis of the "heel cord," or muscle tendon, located on the back of the lower leg just above the heel. It may result from any activity that involves forcefully pushing off with the foot and ankle, such as in running and jumping. This inflammation involves swelling, warmth, tenderness to touch, and pain during walking and especially running.
Ankle sprain	Stretching or tearing of one or several ligaments that provide stability to the ankle joint. Ligaments on the outside or lateral side of the ankle are more commonly injured by rolling the sole of the foot downward and toward the inside. Pain is intense immediately after injury, followed by considerable swelling, tenderness, loss of joint motion, and some discoloration over a 24- to 48-hour period.
Groin pull	A muscle strain that occurs in the muscles located on the inside of the upper thigh just below the pubic area and that results either from an overstretch of the muscle or from a contraction of the muscle that meets excessive resistance. Pain will be produced by flexing the hip and leg across the body or by stretching the muscles in a groin-stretch position.
Hamstring pull	A strain of the muscles on the back of the upper thigh that most often occurs while sprinting. In most cases, severe pain is caused simply by walking or in any movement that involves knee flexion or stretch of the hamstring muscle. Some swelling, tenderness to touch, and possibly some discoloration extending down the back of the leg may occur in severe strains.
Patellofemoral knee pain	Nonspecific pain occurring around the knee, particularly the front part of the knee, or in the kneecap (patella). Pain can result from many causes, including improper movement of the kneecap in knee flexion and extension; tendinitis of the tendon just below the kneecap, which is caused by repetitive jumping; bursitis (swelling) either above or below the kneecap; and osteoarthritis (joint surface degeneration) between the kneecap and thigh bone. It may involve inflammation with swelling, tenderness, warmth, and pain associated with movement.
Quadriceps contusion "charley horse"	A deep bruise of the muscles in the front part of the thigh caused by a forceful impact or by some object that results in severe pain, swelling, discoloration, and difficulty flexing the knee or extending the hip. Without adequate rest and protection from additional trauma, small calcium deposits may develop in the muscle.
Shin splints	A catch-all term used to refer to any pain that occurs in the front part of the lower leg or shin, most often caused by excessive running on hard surfaces. Pain is usually caused by strain of the muscles that move the ankle and foot at their attachment points in the shin. It is usually worse during activity. In more severe cases it may be caused by stress fractures of the long bones in the lower leg, with the pain being worse after activity is stopped.
Shoulder impingement	Chronic irritation and inflammation of muscle tendons and a bursa underneath the tip of the shoulder, which results from repeated forceful overhead motions of the shoulder, such as in swimming, throwing, spiking a volleyball, or serving a tennis ball. Pain is felt when the arm is extended across the body above shoulder level.
Tennis elbow	Chronic irritation and inflammation of the lateral or outside surface of the arm just above the elbow at the attachment of the muscles that extend the wrist and fingers. It results from any activity that requires forceful extension of the wrist. Typically occurs in tennis players who are using faulty techniques hitting backhand ground strokes. Pain is felt above the elbow after forcefully extending the wrist against resistance or applying pressure over the muscle attachment above the elbow.

Source: Prentice WE, *Get Fit, Stay Fit*, 5th ed. McGraw-Hill, 2009. Reproduced with permission of The McGraw-Hill Companies.

Taking Charge of Your Health

- Assess your level of fitness by completing the National Fitness Test on pages 92–93.
- Implement or maintain a cardiorespiratory fitness program that uses the most recent American College of Sports Medicine recommendations.
- Start a daily stretching program based on the guidelines in this chapter.

- Recognize that a comprehensive physical fitness program includes performing muscular fitness exercises at least twice a week.
- Make sure that you always include a warm-up and a cooldown with each exercise session.
- If you are currently sedentary, make a list of five benefits you would obtain by

becoming more active, and then develop three strategies for incorporating more physical activity into your daily routine.

SUMMARY

- Physical fitness allows one to engage in life's activities without unreasonable fatigue.
- The health benefits of exercise can be achieved through regular moderate exercise.
- Fitness comprises five components: cardiorespiratory endurance, muscular strength, muscular endurance, flexibility, and body composition.
- The American College of Sports Medicine's program for cardiorespiratory fitness has four components: mode of activity, frequency of training, intensity of training, and duration of training.
- ACSM now recommends that everyone also include resistance training and flexibility training.

- The target heart rate (THR) refers to the number of times per minute the heart must contract to produce a cardiorespiratory training effect.
- Training sessions should take place in three phases: warm-up, conditioning, and cooldown.
- Fitness experts are concerned about the lack of fitness in today's youths.
- Static stretching is usually recommended for stretching.
- Low-impact aerobic activities have a lower risk of muscle and joint injuries than do high-impact activities.
- College students who are interested in fitness should understand the important topics of steroid use, cross-training, fluid replacement, and the female athlete triad.

REVIEW QUESTIONS

1. Identify the five components of fitness described in this chapter. How does each component relate to health?
2. What is the difference between anaerobic and aerobic energy production? What types of activities are associated with anaerobic energy production? With aerobic energy production?
3. List some of the benefits of aerobic fitness.
4. Describe the various methods used to promote muscular strength.

5. What does the principle of overload mean in regard to fitness training programs?
6. Identify the ACSM's components of an effective cardiorespiratory conditioning program. Explain the important aspects of each component.
7. Under what circumstances should you see a physician before starting a physical fitness program?
8. Identify and describe the three parts of a training session.
9. Describe some of the negative consequences of anabolic steroid use. How do "andro" and creatine differ?

ANSWERS TO THE "WHAT DO YOU KNOW?" QUIZ

1. False   2. True   3. False   4. True   5. True   6. False   7. False

Visit the Online Learning Center (**www.mhhe.com/hahn11e**), where you will find tools to help you improve your grade including practice quizzes, key terms flashcards, audio chapter summaries for your MP3 player, and many other study aids.

SOURCE NOTES

1. U.S. Department of Health and Human Services. *Physical Activity and Health: A Report of the Surgeon General.* Centers for Disease Control and Prevention, National Center for Chronic Disease Prevention and Health Promotion, 1996.
2. American College of Sports Medicine. *Guidelines for Exercise Testing and Prescription* (8th ed.). Baltimore: Wolters Kluwer, 2009.
3. Pate RR, et al. Physical activity and public health: a recommendation from the Centers for Disease Control and Prevention and the American College of Sports Medicine. *Journal of the American Medical Association, 273,* 402–407, 1995.
4. Haskell WL, et al. Physical activity and public health: updated recommendations for adults from the American College of Sports Medicine and the American Heart Association. *Circulation, 116,* 1081–1093, 2007.
5. U.S. Department of Health and Human Services. *2008 Physical Activity Guidelines for Americans.* www.health.gov/PAguideline.

6. Casperson C, et al. *Public Health Reports,* 100, 126, 1985.
7. Brubaker PH, Kaminsky LA, Whaley MH. *Coronary Artery Disease.* Champaign, IL: Human Kinetics, 2002.
8. National Osteoporosis Foundation. *Physician's Guide to Prevention and Treatment of Osteoporosis.* Washington, DC, 2005.
9. Arthritis Foundation. Osteoarthritis treatment. www.arthritis.org/conditions/diseasecenter/OA/oa_treatment1.asp.
10. American College of Sports Medicine, American Dietetic Association, Dietitians of Canada. Nutrition and athletic performance. *Medicine and Science in Sports and Exercise, 41(3),* 709–731, 2009.
11. Arnheim DD, Prentice WE. *Essentials of Athletic Training.* New York: McGraw-Hill, 1999.
12. American College of Sports Medicine. The female athlete triad. *Medicine and Science in Sports and Medicine, 39(10),* 1867–1882, 2007.

Personal Assessment

What Is Your Level of Fitness?

You can determine your level of fitness in 30 minutes or less by completing this short group of tests based on the National Fitness Test developed by the President's Council on Physical Fitness and Sports. If you are over 40 years old or have chronic medical disorders such as diabetes or obesity, check with your physician before taking this or any other fitness test. You will need another person to monitor your test and keep time.

3-Minute Step Test

Aerobic capacity. Equipment: 12-inch bench, crate, block, or stepladder; stopwatch. Procedure: face bench. Complete 24 full steps (both feet on the bench, both feet on the ground) per minute for 3 minutes. After finishing, sit down, have your partner find your pulse within 5 seconds, and take your pulse for 1 minute. Your score is your pulse rate for 1 full minute.

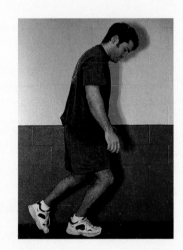

Scoring standards (heart rate for 1 minute)									
Age	18–29		30–39		40–49		50–59		60+	
Gender	F	M	F	M	F	M	F	M	F	M
Excellent	<80	<75	<84	<78	<88	<80	<92	<85	<95	<90
Good	80–110	75–100	84–115	78–109	88–118	80–112	92–123	85–115	95–127	90–118
Average	>110	>100	>115	>109	>118	>112	>123	>115	>127	>118

Sit and Reach

Hamstring flexibility. Equipment: yardstick, tape. Positioned parallel to your legs and between them, tape a yardstick to the floor. Sit with legs straight and heels about 5 inches apart, heels even with the 15-inch mark on the yardstick. While in a sitting position, slowly stretch forward as far as possible. Your score is the number of inches reached.

Scoring standards (inches)									
Age	18–29		30–39		40–49		50–59		60+	
Gender	F	M	F	M	F	M	F	M	F	M
Excellent	>22	>21	>22	>21	>21	>20	>20	>19	>20	>19
Good	17–22	13–21	17–22	13–21	15–21	13–20	14–20	12–19	14–20	12–19
Average	<17	<13	<17	<13	<15	<13	<14	<12	<14	<12

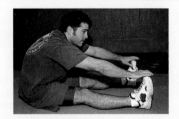

Arm Hang

Upper-body strength. Equipment: horizontal bar (high enough to prevent feet from touching the floor), stopwatch. Procedure: hang with straight arms, palms facing forward. Start watch when subject is in position. Stop when subject lets go. Your score is the number of minutes and seconds spent hanging.

Scoring standards (minutes:seconds)									
Age	**18–29**		**30–39**		**40–49**		**50–59**		**60+**
Gender	F	M	F	M	F	M	F	M	F	M
Excellent	>1:30	>2:00	>1:20	>1:50	>1:10	>1:35	>1:00	>1:20	>:50	>1:10
Good	:46–1:30	1:00–2:00	:40–1:20	:50–1:50	:30–1:10	:45–1:35	:30–1:00	:35–1:20	:21–:50	:30–1:10
Average	<:46	<1:00	<:40	<:50	<:30	<:45	<:30	<:35	<:21	<:30

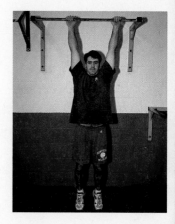

Curl-Ups

Abdominal and low back strength. Equipment: stopwatch. Procedure: Lie flat on upper back, knees bent, shoulders touching the floor, arms extended above thighs or by sides, palms down. Bend knees so that the feet are flat and 12 inches from buttocks. Curl up by lifting head and shoulders off the floor, sliding hands forward above thighs or the floor. Curl down and repeat. Your score is the number of curl-ups in 1 minute, without breaking a beat.

Scoring standards (number in 1 minute)									
Age	**18–29**		**30–39**		**40–49**		**50–59**		**60+**
Gender	F	M	F	M	F	M	F	M	F	M
Excellent	>45	>50	>40	>45	>35	>40	>30	>35	>25	>30
Good	25–45	30–50	20–40	22–45	16–35	21–40	12–30	18–35	11–25	15–30
Average	<25	<30	<20	<22	<16	<21	<12	<18	<11	<15

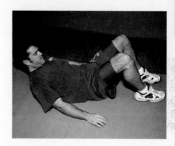

Push-Ups (Men)

Upper-body strength. Equipment: stopwatch. Assume a front-leaning position. Lower body until chest touches the floor. Raise and repeat for 1 minute. Your score is the number of push-ups completed in 1 minute, without breaking a beat.

Scoring standards (number in 1 minute)				
Age	**18–29**	**30–39**	**40–49**	**50–59**	**60+**
Excellent	>50	>45	>40	>35	>30
Good	25–50	22–45	19–40	15–35	10–30
Average	<25	<22	<19	<15	<10

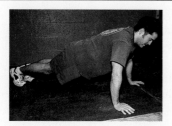

Modified Push-Ups (Women)

Upper-body strength. Equipment: stopwatch. Assume a front-leaning position with knees bent up, hands under shoulders. Lower chest to the floor, raise, and repeat. Your score is the number of push-ups completed in 1 minute, without breaking a beat.

Scoring standards (number in 1 minute)				
Age	**18–29**	**30–39**	**40–49**	**50–59**	**60+**
Excellent	>45	>40	>35	>30	>25
Good	17–45	12–40	8–35	6–30	5–25
Average	<17	<12	<8	<6	<5

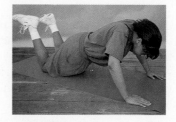

TO CARRY THIS FURTHER . . .

Note your areas of strengths and weaknesses. To improve your fitness, become involved in a fitness program that reflects the concepts discussed in this chapter. Talking with fitness experts on your campus might be a good first step.

Source: Data from the National Fitness Foundation.

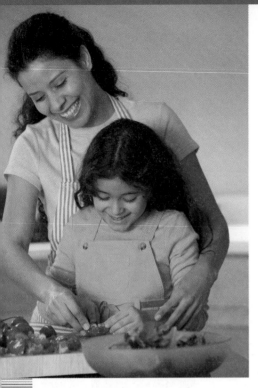

5

Understanding Nutrition and Your Diet

What Do You Know About Nutrition?

1. The USDA dietary guidelines recommend exercising for 60–90 minutes most days of the week for weight management. True or False?

2. Whole-grain bread does not have the same nutritional benefits as wheat bread. True or False?

3. Most people get enough vitamin D from sun exposure. True or False?

4. Saturated fats are the same thing as trans fats. True or False?

5. Most Americans eat enough fruits and vegetables. True or False?

6. Food allergies can be fatal. True or False?

7. Fruit juice is a good way to meet the dietary recommendations for the fruit group. True or False?

Check your answers at the end of the chapter.

Healthy eating is important throughout life, in order to maintain a high level of wellness. Food provides the body with the **nutrients** required to produce energy, repair damaged tissue, promote tissue growth, and regulate physiological processes.

Physiologically, these nutrients—carbohydrates, fat, protein, vitamins, minerals, dietary fiber, and water—are essential in adequate quantity. In addition, the production, preparation, serving, and sharing of food enrich our lives in other ways (see the box "Mealtime—A Chance to Share and Bond").

Types and Sources of Nutrients

Let's discuss the familiar nutrients first: carbohydrates, fats, and proteins. These three nutrients provide our bodies with **calories.** Calories are used quickly by our bodies in energy metabolism, or they are stored in the form of glycogen or adipose (fatty) tissue. The other nutrient groups, which are not sources of energy for the body, will be discussed later.

Carbohydrates

Carbohydrates are various combinations of sugar units, or saccharides, and are the major energy source for the body.[1]

Types and Sources of Carbohydrates Carbohydrates occur in three forms, depending on the number of saccharide (sugar) units that make up the molecule. Carbohydrates are divided into two categories: simple (monosaccharides and disaccharides) and complex carbohydrates (polysaccharides). Monosaccharides are carbohydrates with one saccharide unit. Disaccharides are carbohydrates with two saccharide units, one of which is always a glucose unit. Polysaccharides, or starches, are carbohydrates with more than two saccharide units. Polysaccharides include starches and dietary fiber. Examples are vegetables, breads, cereals, legumes, and pasta.

Both simple and complex carbohydrates contain 4 calories per gram, and both are digested into glucose. Simple carbohydrates are digested more quickly because they are composed of fewer saccharide units than complex carbohydrates. Complex carbohydrates also take longer to digest because they have more fiber, vitamins, and minerals.

How Much Carbohydrate Is Recommended? Each gram of carbohydrate contains 4 calories. Since the average person requires approximately 2,000 calories per day and about 45–65 percent of our calories come from carbohydrates, approximately 1,200 calories per day come from carbohydrates.[2] However, age, gender, and activity level affect the number of calories an individual requires each day.

Simple Sugars: The American Sweet Tooth According to the U.S. Department of Agriculture (USDA), the average adult American consumes about 22.2 teaspoons of sugar per day while the USDA recommendations are no more than 8 teaspoons per day, a difference of 335 calories. These sugars are usually found in sodas, candy, and bakery items, which have little nutritional value. Corn sweetener consumption has decreased since 2003

Key Terms

nutrients Elements in foods that are required for the growth, repair, and regulation of body processes.

calories Units of heat (energy); specifically, 1 calorie is the amount of heat required to raise the temperature of 1 gram of water by 1°C. In common usage, on food labels, and in this chapter, the term *calorie* is used to refer to a larger energy unit, *kilocalorie* (1,000 calories).

carbohydrates The body's primary source of energy for all body functioning; chemical compounds including sugar, starches, and dietary fibers.

from 79 pounds to 37.8 pounds per year. However, sugar consumption has increased to 47.2 pounds per year.

Much of the sugar we consume is hidden. For example, it is an ingredient in ketchup, salad dressings, cured meat products, and canned vegetables and fruits. High-fructose corn syrup, often found in these items, is a highly concentrated sugar solution. Whether the sugar is overt or hidden, the USDA has suggested a limit of 8 teaspoons of sugar per day for a 2,000-calorie diet.

Starches are complex carbohydrates composed of long chains of sugar units. However, these starches should not be confused with the adjective "starchy." When people talk about starchy foods, they usually mean complex carbohydrates, or "heavy" foods. True starches are among the most important sources of dietary carbohydrates. Starches are found primarily in vegetables, fruits, and grains. Eating true starches is overall nutritionally beneficial because most starch sources also contain much-needed vitamins, minerals, plant protein, and water.

Fats

Fats (lipids) have been given a bad name but are an important nutrient in our diets because they provide a concentrated form of energy (9 calories per gram). Fats provide a feeling of satiety and keep us from feeling hungry. Because fats take longer to leave the stomach than either carbohydrates or proteins do, our stomachs feel full for a longer period of time, decreasing our appetite. Fats also help give food its pleasing taste, and they carry the fat-soluble vitamins A, D, E, and K. Without fat, these vitamins would quickly pass through the body. Fat also insulates our bodies to help us retain heat.

Dietary sources of fat are often difficult to identify. The visible fats in our diet, such as butter, salad oils, and the layer of fat on some cuts of meat, represent only about 40 percent of the fat we consume. Most of the fat we eat is hidden in food.

Types of Fats   All dietary fat is made up of a combination of three forms of fat: saturated, monounsaturated, and polyunsaturated, based on chemical composition (see Figure 5-1). Paying attention to the amount of each type of fat in our diet is important because of the known link to heart disease (see Chapter 9). Not all fats are created equal.

Monounsaturated and Polyunsaturated Fats   Though monounsaturated fats can reduce the harmful low-density lipoproteins (LDLs), polyunsaturated fats reduce both LDLs and total cholesterol. However, polyunsaturated fats also lower the healthful high-density lipoproteins (HDLs), which is not a desirable outcome. Omega-3 fatty acids, found in most varieties of fish, are a type of polyunsaturated fat and have been associated with decreased risk of heart disease. Our bodies require omega-3 fatty acids, but we can't produce them on our own, and therefore we must get them from the foods

we eat. Flax seed, walnuts, and olive oil are other good sources for omega-3 fatty acids. You can also consume omega-3 fish oil as a dietary supplement.

Saturated and Trans Fats   Saturated fats, including those found in animal sources and vegetable oils to which hydrogen has been added (hydrogenated), becoming *trans-fatty acids,* need to be carefully limited in a healthy diet. Concern over the presence of trans-fatty acids (an altered form of a normal vegetable oil molecule) is associated with changes detrimental to the cell membrane, including those cells lining the artery wall. Among the changes being suggested is an increase in calcium deposits.[3] This could result in a rough surface, leading to plaque formation (see Chapter 9).

Processing can change the structure of fat, making it more saturated. As a result, the oils become semisolid and more stable at room temperature. The term *trans* describes the chemical makeup of a fatty acid. Most trans-fatty acids come from hydrogenated oil, which is found in foods such as stick margarine, peanut butter, and crackers. Trans-fatty acids are popular in food manufacturing because they can extend the shelf life of the food: The oil stays mixed in the food and doesn't rise to the top, and the food doesn't become too soft at room temperature. Many foods are fried with these fats in the fast-food industry.[4]

There has been a big push for restaurants and food manufacturers to discontinue using trans fats in their products, which has resulted in a 70 percent decrease in the use of trans fats over the past three years. Trans fat has been called a "dangerous and unnecessary ingredient" and has been banned for use in restaurants in New York City. The FDA now requires food manufacturers to list trans fat on any product that contains more than 0.5 gram of trans fat per serving. However, that means products that boast they contain "no trans fat" can have less than half a gram of trans fat per serving, and if you eat multiple servings you can easily consume more than the 2 grams of trans fat a day that is the USDA's suggested daily limit. Many food producers are jumping on the no-trans-fat bandwagon, and you will see more cereals, chips, crackers, and other foods labeled "No trans fat."

Trans fats can act like saturated fat, potentially raising LDL blood cholesterol levels and decreasing HDL cholesterol. This is the reason nutritionists encourage us to use butter rather than stick margarine. To reduce your intake of trans fat, make sure you check the labels on foods to see if they list "partially hydrogenated vegetable oil" as one of the ingredients. Foods such as cakes, cookies, crackers, snack foods, stick margarine, vegetable shortening, and fried foods are most likely to have hydrogenated vegetable oil as one of the ingredients. Trans fat should be limited to 2 grams or less daily.

Tropical Oils   Although all cooking oils (and fats such as butter, lard, margarine, and shortening) have the same

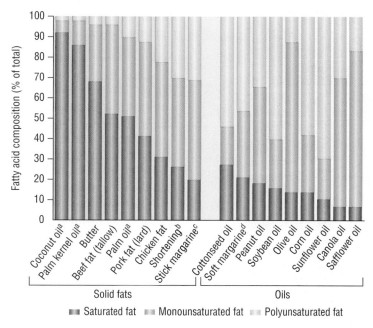

Figure 5-1 Fatty Acid Profiles of Common Fats and Oils

a Coconut oil, palm kernel oil, and palm oil are called oils because they come from plants. However, they are semi-solid at room temperature due to their high content of short-chain saturated fatty acids. They are considered solid fats for nutritional purposes.

b Partially hydrogenated vegetable oil shortening, which contains *trans* fats.

c Most stick margarines contain partially hydrogenated vegetable oil, a source of *trans* fats.

d The primary ingredient in soft margarine with no *trans* fats is liquid vegetable oil.

Source: U.S. Department of Agriculture, Agricultural Research Service, Nutrient Data Laboratory, USDA National Nutrient Database for Standard Reference, release 22, 2009. Available at http://www.ars.usda.gov/ba/bhnrc/ndl. Accessed July 19, 2010.

number of calories by weight (9 calories per gram), some oils contain high percentages of saturated fats. All oils and fats contain varying percentages of saturated, monounsaturated, and polyunsaturated fats. However, the tropical oils—coconut, palm, and palm kernel—contain much higher percentages of saturated fats than do other cooking oils. Coconut oil, for example, is 92 percent saturated fat. Tropical oils can still be found in some brands of snack foods, crackers, cookies, nondairy creamers, and breakfast cereals, although they have been removed from most national brands.

How Much Fat, and What Type, Is Recommended? The dietary guidelines recommend that no more than 20–35 percent of our calories come from fat. In addition it is suggested that people do the following:

- Consume less than 10 percent of calories from saturated fatty acids and less than 300 mg per day of cholesterol, and keep trans-fatty acid consumption as low as possible, no more than 2 grams per day.

- Get most fats from sources of polyunsaturated and monounsaturated fatty acids, such as fish, nuts, and vegetable oils.

- Make choices that are lean, low-fat, or fat-free when selecting and preparing meat, poultry, dry beans, and milk or milk products.

Children 2 to 3 years of age, however, need 30–35 percent fat in their diets for growth.[5]

Cholesterol **Cholesterol** is a white, fatlike substance found in cells of animal origin. It is not found in any vegetable product, so products such as peanut butter and margarine that claim they are cholesterol-free never had it in the first place. Cholesterol is used to synthesize cell membranes and also serves as the starting material for the synthesis of bile acids and sex hormones. Although we consume cholesterol in our diet—in such foods as shrimp and other shellfish, animal fat, and milk—we don't need to obtain cholesterol from external sources.

> **Key Terms**
>
> **satiety** (suh **tie** uh tee) The feeling of no longer being hungry; a diminished desire to eat.
>
> **saturated fats** Fats that promote cholesterol formation; they are in solid form at room temperature; primarily animal fats.
>
> **cholesterol** A primary form of fat found in the blood; lipid material manufactured within the body and derived from dietary sources.

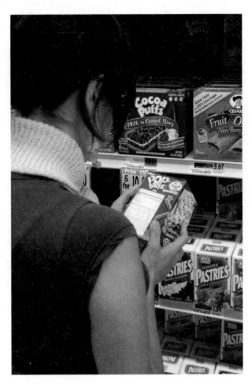

Food labels are an important source of information about the type and amount of fats, carbohydrates, and other nutrients contained in a food.

The human liver can synthesize enough of the substance to meet the body's needs.

Cholesterol is essential for many of the body's functions. However, if you have too much cholesterol, it builds up in your bloodstream and clogs arteries, putting you at risk for heart disease, heart attack, and stroke. There are different kinds of cholesterol. LDL is often referred to as "bad" cholesterol. LDL cholesterol builds up on the walls of arteries to form artery-clogging "plaques" that contribute to the development of heart disease and stroke. HDL, or "good" cholesterol, helps remove excess cholesterol from the blood and transports it back to the liver, where it can be eliminated from the body. You want to have lower LDL (under 130) and higher HDL (over 40), with total cholesterol under 200 (see Chapter 9). Almonds, oatmeal, fish, soy, and red wine (a limit of one glass daily) help lower overall cholesterol levels. Whole milk, processed meats, and foods with trans fats and tropical oils, such as fast food and baked goods, can increase overall cholesterol levels and should be avoided.

A number of medical conditions can give rise to high blood cholesterol, such as liver disease, kidney failure, hypothyroidism, and diabetes. Certain medications (some diuretics, for example) can also raise blood cholesterol, irrespective of diet. The USDA dietary guidelines recommend that people restrict their dietary intake of cholesterol to 300 mg or less per day. In addition, no more than 20–35 percent of your total caloric intake should come from fat, with most fats being monounsaturated and polyunsaturated.

Low-Fat Foods   *Low-fat* and *low-calorie* do not mean the same thing, but often people confuse the two. Fat-free, low-fat, and reduced-fat foods have been popular for many years with people thinking they can eat as much as they want of these foods. This is far from true; a fat-free or reduced-fat product may have as many if not more calories per serving than do regular products. For example, 2 tablespoons of fat-free caramel topping have 103 calories, the same number of calories as in the homemade-with-butter caramel topping.[6]

Fatty foods make people feel fuller longer than do fat-free foods; thus, people tend to eat more of the fat-free foods and so consume *more* calories. In general, the lower the fat, the higher the price tag because the food industry recognizes that Americans are willing to pay more for reduced-fat and fat-free brands. This situation may be changing since people have realized that lower fat with potentially higher calories doesn't equal weight loss or healthy weight management. However, foods such as low-fat sour cream, yogurt, or salad dressing are healthier choices because they have less saturated fat.

Proteins

Proteins are found in every living cell. Protein primarily promotes growth and maintenance of body tissue. However, when caloric intake falls, protein is broken down and converted into glucose. This loss of protein can impede the growth and repair of tissue. Protein also is a primary component of enzyme and hormone structure. It helps maintain the *acid-base balance* of our bodies and is a source of energy (4 calories per gram).

Types and Sources of Protein   Proteins are composed of chains of **amino acids.** Of the 20 naturally occurring amino acids, the body can synthesize all but 9 *essential amino acids** from the foods we eat. A food that contains all 9 essential amino acids is called a *complete protein* food. Examples are animal products, including milk, meat, cheese, and eggs. A food source that does not contain all 9 essential amino acids is called an *incomplete protein* food. Vegetables, grains, and legumes (peas or beans—including chickpeas, butter beans, and peanuts)—are principal sources of incomplete protein. Vegan vegetarians (discussed later in the chapter), people with limited access to animal-based food sources, and those who have significantly limited their meat, egg, and dairy product consumption need to understand how essential amino acids can be obtained from incomplete protein sources.

When even one essential amino acid is missing from the diet, a deficiency can develop. Soybeans are a good

*Eight additional compounds are sometimes classified as amino acids, so some nutritionists believe that there are more than 20 amino acids.

source of protein for vegetarians. Soybeans provide the same high-quality protein as animal protein.[7] Furthermore, soybeans contain no cholesterol or saturated fat. There has been much debate surrounding whether consuming foods with soybeans can reduce the risk of heart disease.[8]

How Much Protein Is Recommended?   The latest recommendations for protein intake are part of a set of standards known as the **Dietary Reference Intakes,** or DRIs. The recommended intake of protein is based on body weight and activity level. The current DRI for protein is 0.36 gram per pound of body weight per day, based upon a sedentary lifestyle, and is higher for athletes and those who are more active. In terms of percent energy intake, nutritionists recommend that 10–35 percent of our total caloric intake come from protein.[9]

Vitamins

Vitamins are organic compounds that are required in small amounts for normal growth, reproduction, and maintenance of health. Vitamins differ from carbohydrates, fats, and proteins because they do not provide calories or serve as structural elements for our bodies. Vitamins are *coenzymes.* By facilitating the action of **enzymes,** vitamins help initiate a wide variety of body responses, including energy production, use of minerals, and growth of healthy tissue.

Types and Sources of Vitamins   Vitamins can be classified as *water-soluble* (capable of being dissolved in water) or *fat-soluble* (capable of being dissolved in fat or lipid tissue). Water-soluble vitamins include the B-complex vitamins and vitamin C. Most of the excess of these water-soluble vitamins is eliminated from the body in the urine. Because water-soluble vitamins dissolve quickly in water, it's important not to lose them during the preparation of fresh fruits and vegetables. One method is not to overcook fresh vegetables. The longer vegetables are steamed or boiled, the more water-soluble vitamins will be lost. Some people save the water in which vegetables were boiled or steamed and use it for drinking or cooking. More vitamins are retained with microwave cooking than with stove-top cooking.

The fat-soluble vitamins are vitamins A, D, E, and K. Excessive intake of these vitamins causes them to be stored in the body in the adipose (fat) tissue. It is therefore possible to consume and retain too many of these vitamins, particularly vitamins A and D. Because excess fat-soluble vitamins are stored in the body's fat, organs that contain fat, such as the liver, are primary storage sites.

Dietary Reference Intakes for Vitamins   To ensure adequate vitamin intake, a good approach is to eat a variety of foods. DRIs have been set for all vitamins and are available from the Food and Nutrition Board website (www.iom.edu/cms/3788.aspx). Some vitamins of concern are discussed in this section.

The DRI for folic acid for adults is 300–400 µg daily; however, for pregnant women it is 600 µg a day and for lactating women it is 500 µg daily. There has been some debate about whether folic acid can prevent cardiovascular disease, cancer, and Alzheimer's disease. There still isn't enough evidence to make these claims. Some research suggests that folic acid can accelerate the spread of cancer in people with precancerous or cancer cells. Vitamin B_{12} deficiency is a concern for vegetarians because this vitamin is primarily obtained from liver, fish, cheese, and eggs. Anemia, disturbances in walking and balance, a loss of vibration sensation, confusion, and dementia can be caused by vitamin B_{12} deficiencies. The body requires B_{12} to make the protective coating surrounding the nerves, and inadequate B_{12} can expose nerves to damage. B_{12} can sometimes be difficult for the body to absorb. The DRI for vitamin B_{12} is 2.4 µg daily and for B_6 is 1.3 to 1.7 mg per day. Vitamin B_6 deficiency can lead to anemia, fatigue, poor appetite, and diarrhea. Good sources of B_6 are meat, liver, cereal, grains, bananas, and nuts.

Should You Take a Vitamin Supplement?   Unless there are special circumstances, such as pregnancy, lactation, infancy, or an existing health problem, usually anyone who eats a reasonably well-rounded diet consumes enough vitamins to prevent deficiencies. People often think taking megadoses of vitamins such as vitamin C can be health-enhancing, but actually the reverse is true. Taking large doses of vitamin C from a dietary supplement can put a strain on your kidneys, causing kidney stones and diarrhea. Too much niacin, vitamin B_6, and folate can also be harmful.[4]

Some professionals recommend that supplements be taken with food since they're really components of food

---

Key Terms

proteins Compounds composed of chains of amino acids; primary components of muscle and connective tissue.

amino acids The building blocks of protein; can be manufactured by the body or obtained from dietary sources.

Dietary Reference Intakes (DRIs) Measures that refer to three types of reference values: Estimated Average Requirement, Recommended Dietary Allowance, and Tolerable Upper Intake Level.

vitamins Organic compounds that facilitate the action of enzymes.

enzymes Organic substances that control the rate of physiological reactions but are not themselves altered in the process.

and help the body metabolize other food components. The fat-soluble nutrients should be taken with a little oil or fat to enhance absorption. The water-soluble nutrients are easily absorbed without food but may work better when taken with meals. In addition, some people complain of stomach upset when they take vitamins on an empty stomach.

Unfortunately, not all people eat a balanced diet based on a variety of foods. Recent studies suggest that a somewhat higher intake of vitamins A, C, and E for adults might reduce the risk of developing cancer, atherosclerosis, and depressed levels of high-density lipoprotein (HDL) cholesterol; however, several unanswered questions remain, including the amounts needed for effectiveness (see Chapter 9).[9]

Consuming an adequate amount of folic acid before and during pregnancy has been shown to reduce the incidence of birth defects. To ensure adequate folic acid intake (400 μg/day), in 1997 the Food and Drug Administration (FDA) began to require that bread and cereal products be supplemented with folic acid. The goal of this requirement is for pregnant women and women of childbearing age to receive at least 140 μg per day through dietary intake. Taking a daily multivitamin before and during pregnancy would easily provide the remaining amount of folic acid necessary to promote fetal neural tube closure (thus preventing spina bifida). Manufacturers of folic acid supplements may make claims about the product's ability to prevent neural tube defects in infants. Folic acid is also considered important in the prevention of cardiovascular disease.[10]

Initial research suggested that vitamin E supplements help reduce the risk of chronic diseases, such as cardiovascular disease, cancer, and Alzheimer's, as well as strengthen immunity. However, more recent studies don't substantiate these findings and in fact have found that taking megadoses of vitamin E can be harmful. Because vitamin E is fat-soluble, there is a risk of toxicity because it is stored in the body's fatty tissues and can cause liver damage. It also works as a blood thinner, so there may be a risk of hemorrhaging. Vitamin E can be obtained in your diet from high-fat foods like nuts and oils and from leafy green vegetables such as spinach and broccoli. Most nutritionists agree that it is best to meet your vitamin E requirements through a balanced, healthy diet.[11]

If you take a vitamin D supplement, look for vitamin D$_3$ (also called cholecalciferol) instead of vitamin D$_2$, which is 25 percent less potent. The DRI for vitamin D has been increased to 600 international units (IU) (higher for individuals over 50 years of age) with 50 μg or 2,000 IU as the Tolerable Upper Intake Level (UL). The recommended amount of calcium intake is 1,000 mg per day (1,200 if you are over 50 years of age).[12] Too much calcium may cause kidney stones and may block absorption of other substances such as antibiotics.

At the same time that many health experts are recommending some vitamin supplementation, the FDA has prohibited manufacturers of food supplements, including vitamins, from making unsubstantiated claims for the cure, treatment, and prevention of disease.

Phytochemicals

Certain physiologically active components are believed to deactivate carcinogens or function as **antioxidants.** Antioxidants are substances that may protect cells from the damage caused by unstable molecules known as *free radicals,* which can lead to cancer. Antioxidants may prevent cancer by interacting with and stabilizing free radicals. Examples of antioxidants include beta-carotene, lycopene, and vitamins C, E, and A. However, Americans' number-one source of antioxidants is coffee. Chocolate, green tea, and nuts are other popular sources of antioxidants for Americans.[13] The different types of **phytochemicals** include the carotenoids (from green vegetables), polyphenols (from onions and garlic), indoles (from cruciferous vegetables), and allyl sulfides (from garlic, chives, and onions). These phytochemicals may play an important role in sparking the body to fight and slow the development of some diseases such as cancer. At this time, however, the exact mechanisms through which the various phytochemicals reduce the formation of cancer cells is not understood. Although it is generally agreed that these foods are important in planning food selections, no precise recommendations regarding the amounts of various phytochemical-rich plants to consume have been made.

Minerals

Nearly 5 percent of the body is composed of inorganic materials, the *minerals.* Minerals function primarily as structural elements (in teeth, muscles, hemoglobin, and hormones). They are also critical in the regulation of body processes, including muscle contraction, heart function, blood clotting, protein synthesis, and red blood cell formation. Approximately 21 minerals have been recognized as essential for good health. Unlike vitamins, minerals are inorganic and can't be destroyed by heat or food processing.

Major minerals are those that exist in relatively high amounts in our body tissues. Examples are calcium, phosphorus, sulfur, sodium, potassium, and magnesium. Examples of **trace elements,** minerals seen in relatively small amounts in body tissues, include zinc, iron, copper, selenium, and iodine. Trace elements are required only in small quantities, fewer than 20 mg daily of each, but they are essential for good health. As with vitamins, the safest, most appropriate way to prevent a mineral deficiency is to eat a balanced diet. Good food sources for minerals include fish, shellfish, red meat, grains, eggs, poultry, soy, broccoli, lentils, beans, raisins, bananas, citrus fruits, avocados, and leafy green vegetables. However, calcium, a major mineral, can be taken as a supplement to help prevent osteoporosis.

Water and Other Fluids

Water may well be our most essential nutrient, since without water most of us would die from the effects of **dehydration** in less than a week. We could survive for weeks or even years without some of the essential minerals and vitamins, but not without water. More than half our body weight comes from water. Water provides the medium for nutrient and waste transport, controls body temperature, and functions in nearly all of our body's biochemical reactions.

Most people seldom think about the importance of an adequate intake of water and fluids. The average adult loses about 10 cups of water daily through perspiration, urination, bowel movements, and breathing. Physical activity and heat exposure contribute to water loss and an increased need for fluids. The Institute of Medicine's general recommendation for an average woman is approximately 2.7 liters (91 ounces) of total water (from all food and beverages) each day, and for an average man approximately 3.7 liters (125 ounces) daily. Recommendations for fluid intake vary with age, gender, metabolism, weight, and diet. About 80 percent of people's total water intake comes from drinking water and beverages, including caffeinated beverages, while the other 20 percent is derived from food. It is recommended to avoid beverages that are high in sugar, such as fruit juice, regular sodas, and flavored coffee drinks. For example, a Starbucks white chocolate mocha has 400 calories.[14]

To see if you're drinking enough fluid, check your urine. A small amount of dark-colored urine can be an indication that you are not consuming enough fluid and need to drink more. Urine that is pale or almost colorless means you are most likely taking in enough fluids. Needed fluids are also obtained from fruits, vegetables, fruit and vegetable juices, milk, and noncaffeinated soft drinks, although these can be high in sugar and calories.[15]

Fiber

Although not considered a nutrient by definition, **fiber** is an important component of sound nutrition. Fiber consists of plant material that is not digested but moves through the digestive tract and out of the body. Beans, fruits, and vegetables all provide us with dietary fiber.

Fiber can be classified into two large groups on the basis of water solubility. *Insoluble* fibers are those that can absorb water from the intestinal tract. By absorbing water, the insoluble fibers give the stool bulk and decrease the time it takes the stool to move through the digestive tract. In contrast, *soluble* fiber turns to a "gel" in the intestinal tract and binds to liver bile, to which cholesterol is attached. Thus, the soluble fibers may be valuable in removing cholesterol, which lowers blood cholesterol levels. How much fiber do you need? Women should eat 25 grams and men require 38 grams of fiber each day; however, most American adults eat only 11 grams per day.

Fiber has many benefits, including helping to curb your appetite and prevent overeating because it is filling, requires more chewing, stays in the stomach longer, and absorbs water, adding to the feeling of fullness. Fiber also helps to slow the absorption of sugar from the intestines, thus steadying the blood sugar and slowing down the absorption of fat from the foods you eat. Consuming adequate amounts of fiber has an important effect of reducing serious medical problems because soluble fiber lowers LDL cholesterol and protects against cardiovascular disease while insoluble fiber protects against developing colon cancer.[15] A high-fiber diet has been associated with lower risk of death from infectious and respiratory diseases as well.[16]

In recent years, attention has been given to three forms of soluble fiber—oat bran, psyllium (from the weed plantain), and rice bran—because of their ability to lower blood cholesterol levels.[17]

Oat bran can lower cholesterol levels by five to six points in people whose initial cholesterol levels are moderately high. To accomplish this reduction, a daily consumption of oat bran equal to a large bowl of cold oat bran cereal or three or more packs of instant oatmeal would be necessary. Oatmeal can also be eaten as a cooked cereal or used in other foods, such as hamburgers, pancakes, or meatloaf.

Planning a Healthy Diet

Several tools, including the USDA's MyPlate and the Dietary Guidelines for Americans, are available to help you plan a diet that will provide adequate nutrients, as well as reducing your risk of developing heart disease, cancer, and other chronic diseases.[18]

> ### Key Terms
>
> **antioxidants** Substances that may prevent cancer by interacting with and stabilizing unstable molecules known as free radicals.
>
> **phytochemicals** Physiologically active components of foods believed to deactivate carcinogens and to function as antioxidants.
>
> **trace elements** Minerals whose presence in the body occurs in very small amounts; micronutrient elements.
>
> **dehydration** Abnormal depletion of fluids from the body; severe dehydration can be fatal.
>
> **fiber** Plant material that cannot be digested; found in cereal, fruits, and vegetables.

The USDA Food Guide: MyPlate

The most effective way to take in adequate amounts of nutrients is to eat a balanced diet as outlined by the USDA's most current guidelines.[19] The latest version of the USDA food group plan is called MyPlate (see Figure 5-2). The USDA replaced MyPyramid with MyPlate in June 2011, thinking that a plate is a better visual icon to prompt Americans to make healthier food choices. The plate is a familiar and simpler icon to decipher. MyPlate recommends that fruits and vegetables take up half the plate (a little more vegetables than fruits), with grains and proteins on the other half of the plate (more grains than proteins). See Table 5.1 for specific recommendations based upon gender and age. The new MyPlate also suggests decreasing portion sizes, consuming at least half your grains from whole grains, drinking fat-free or low-fat milk, choosing food lower in sodium, and drinking water instead of sugary drinks. Most Americans do not follow the MyPyramid recommendations in their daily food intake, and it is hoped that MyPlate will be a better way to encourage people to follow the dietary guidelines.

(Figure 5-3 on page 108 shows how typical American diets compare to the recommended intake levels.) To evaluate and track your food intake and physical activity, visit MyPlate.gov. The "Rate Your Plate" Personal Assessment at the end of this chapter will also help you evaluate your current eating habits.

Fifteen percent of Americans are not meeting their nutritional needs according to the dietary guidelines. We will look at the specific recommendations and how Americans are meeting them.

Fruits MyPlate recommends that almost a quarter of your plate be filled with fruit for each meal (half your plate contains fruits and vegetables). The specific amount depends upon gender and age. The dietary guidelines recommend eating 2 cups of fruits per day for a 2,000-calorie/day adult diet. However, only a third of adults eat the recommended number of fruits per day. This is far below the Healthy People 2010 objective from the U.S. Department of Health and Human Services of having 75 percent of Americans meeting the daily fruit

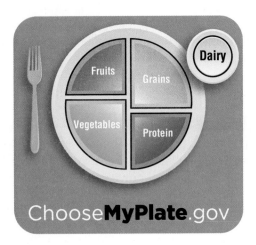

Balancing Calories
- Enjoy your food, but eat less.
- Avoid oversized portions.

Foods to Increase
- Make half your plate fruits and vegetables.
- Make at least half your grains whole grains.
- Switch to fat-free or low-fat (1%) milk.

Foods to Reduce
- Compare sodium in foods like soup, bread, and frozen meals – and choose the foods with lower numbers.
- Drink water instead of sugary drinks.

Figure 5-2 Choose MyPlate.gov The USDA changed the pyramid icon to a plate to prompt consumers to make healthier choices at meals.

Table 5.1 Find Your Calorie Count

			Activity Level	
	Age	Sedentary	Moderately Active	Active
Child	2–3	1,000	1,000–1,400	1,000–1,400
Female	4–8	1,200	1,400–1,600	1,400–1,800
	9–13	1,600	1,600–2,000	1,800–2,200
	14–18	1,800	2,000	2,400
	19–30	2,000	2,000–2,200	2,400
	31–50	1,800	2,000	2,200
	51+	1,600	1,800	2,000–2,200
Male	4–8	1,400	1,400–1,600	1,600–2,000
	9–13	1,800	1,800–2,200	2,000–2,600
	14–18	2,200	2,400–2,800	2,800–3,200
	19–30	2,400	2,600–2,800	3,000
	31–50	2,200	2,400–2,600	2,800–3,000
	51+	2,000	2,200–2,400	2,400–2,800

Sedentary means a lifestyle that includes only the light physical activity associated with typical day-to-day life.
Moderately active means a lifestyle that includes physical activity equivalent to walking about 1.5–3 miles per day at 3–4 miles per hour, in addition to the light physical activity associated with typical day-to-day life.
Active means a lifestyle that includes physical activity equivalent to walking more than 3 miles per day at 3–4 miles per hour, in addition to the light physical activity associated with typical day-to-day life.

Source: U.S. Department of Health and Human Services and U.S. Department of Agriculture. Dietary Guidelines for Americans, 2010, www.healthierus.gov/dietaryguidelines.

Table 5.2 USDA Food Guide at Six Different Calorie Levels

Daily Amount of Food from Each Group (vegetable subgroup amounts are per week)

Calorie Level	1,200	1,600	2,000	2,400	2,800	3,200
Food Group	Food group amounts are shown in cup (c) or ounce-equivalents (oz-eq), with number of servings (srv) in parentheses when it differs from the other units. Oils are shown in grams (g).					
Fruits	1 c (2 srv)	1.5 c (3 srv)	2 c (4 srv)	2 c (4 srv)	2.5 c (5 srv)	2.5 c (5 srv)
Vegetables	1.5 c (3 srv)	2 c (4 srv)	2.5 c (5 srv)	3 c (6 srv)	3.5 c (7 srv)	4 c (8 srv)
Dark green	1.5 c/wk	2 c/wk	3 c/wk	3 c/wk	3 c/wk	3 c/wk
Red and orange	1 c/wk	1.5 c/wk	2 c/wk	2 c/wk	2.5 c/wk	2.5 c/wk
Beans and peas	1 c/wk	2.5 c/wk	3 c/wk	3 c/wk	3.5 c/wk	3.5 c/wk
Starchy	2.5 c/wk	2.5 c/wk	3 c/wk	6 c/wk	7 c/wk	9 c/wk
Other	4.5 c/wk	5.5 c/wk	6.5 c/wk	7 c/wk	8.5 c/wk	10 c/wk
Grains	4 oz-eq	5 oz-eq	6 oz-eq	8 oz-eq	10 oz-eq	10 oz-eq
Whole	2	3	3	4	5	5
Other	2	2.5	3	4	5	5
Protein	3 oz-eq	5 oz-eq	5.5 oz-eq	6.5 oz-eq	7 oz-eq	7 oz-eq
Milk	2 c	3 c	3 c	3 c	3 c	3 c
Oils	17 g	22 g	27 g	31 g	36 g	51 g
Discretionary calorie allowance	171	182	267	362	426	648

Source: U.S. Department of Health and Human Services and U.S. Department of Agriculture, Dietary Guidelines for Americans, 2010, www.healthierus.gov/dietaryguidelines.

recommendations. One medium-sized fruit, ½ cup dried fruit, or 1 cup of fresh, frozen, or canned fruit is equivalent to 1 cup. Orange fruits such as mango, cantaloupe, apricots, and red or pink grapefruit are sources of vitamin A. Kiwi, strawberries, guava, papaya, cantaloupe, and citrus fruits are good sources of vitamin C. Oranges and orange juice also provide folate. Some good sources for potassium are bananas, plantains, dried fruits, oranges and orange juice, cantaloupe and honeydew melons, and tomato products. For the majority of your fruit intake, it is generally recommended that you consume whole fruits and avoid fruit juices to ensure adequate fiber and to avoid the high sugar content associated with fruit juices. The American Cancer Society indicates that this food group may play an important role in the prevention of certain forms of cancer.[20]

Vegetables MyPlate recommends that over a quarter of your plate contain vegetables at each meal, with half the plate being filled with fruits and vegetables. The specific amounts of vegetables depend on gender and age. Also, MyPlate includes red vegetables such as red peppers and tomatoes, making a "red and orange vegetable" subcategory of recommended intake. Two and one-half cups of vegetables per day is the recommendation for adults following a 2,000-calorie diet. Americans fall short in

this category as well, with only 27 percent meeting this recommendation. The Healthy People 2010 objective was for 50 percent of Americans to meet this recommendation. As with the fruit group, the important function of this group is to provide vitamins A and C, complex carbohydrates, and fiber. Because Americans tend to eat only a few vegetables, such as potatoes, corn, and carrots, the new guidelines give specific recommendations about the types of vegetable. One general rule is to "eat your colors," meaning you should consume a variety of vegetables over the course of a week. For a 2,000-calorie diet, the USDA recommends:

- Dark green vegetables (such as broccoli and spinach)—3 cups/week
- Red and orange vegetables (such as tomatoes, carrots, and sweet potatoes)—2 cups/week
- Beans and peas (such as soy, kidney, lentil, and pinto beans)—3 cups/week
- Starchy vegetables (such as corn, potatoes, and green peas)—3 cups/week
- Other vegetables (such as cauliflower, asparagus, and celery)—6½ cups/week

Again, avoid drinking vegetable juices as a way of meeting these requirements because they can be high in salt and sugar and don't provide the fiber intake that whole vegetables do. **Cruciferous vegetables,** such as broccoli, cabbage, brussels sprouts, and cauliflower, may be particularly helpful in the prevention of certain forms of cancer.[20]

Dairy MyPlate has changed the "milk and milk products" category to the "dairy" category to include foods such as yogurt and cheese. The dietary guidelines recommend consuming 3 cups of fat-free or low-fat milk each day, or its equivalent in another dairy product. The good news is that the consumption of whole milk is decreasing; however, chocolate milk is rising in popularity. Consumption rates for fat-free and 1 percent and 2 percent reduced-fat milk are holding steady, but it was hoped that more people would opt for either the low-fat or fat-free options, as 2 percent milk contains almost as much fat as whole milk. Overall, Americans are not getting 3 cups of milk per day as recommended by the dietary guidelines.

Dairy consumption has been associated with higher bone density and can help fight osteoporosis.[21] Calcium and high-quality protein, required for bone and tooth development, are two primary nutritional benefits provided by this food group. The guidelines further suggest that children 2–3 years old should consume 2 cups per day of fat-free or low-fat milk, or equivalent dairy products, whereas children 4–8 years of age should consume 2½ cups per day of fat-free or low-fat milk, or equivalent dairy products. Milk, cheese, yogurt, pudding, and ice cream are included in this food group. For individuals who are lactose-intolerant (lactose upsets their intestines) or are vegan (vegetarians who don't consume any animal products, including dairy products), soybeans, tofu, spinach, kale, okra, beet greens, and oatmeal are good alternative sources of calcium.

Protein MyPlate changed the "meat, poultry, fish, eggs, dry bean, and nuts" category to simply the "protein" category to encapsulate all of these foods. Our need for selections from this protein-rich group is based on our daily need for protein, iron, and the B vitamins. Meats include all red meat (beef, pork, and game), fish, and poultry. It is strongly recommended that we choose lean meats and low-fat or fat-free foods in this group. It is further recommended that we increase the amount and variety of seafood consumed and eat seafood instead of meat and poultry. Meat substitutes include dry beans, eggs, tofu, peanut butter, nuts, and seeds. The USDA guidelines recommend that adults eat 5–6 ounces of meat or protein foods each day. One ounce is equivalent to

- 1 ounce cooked lean meat, poultry, or fish
- 1 egg
- ¼ cup cooked dry beans
- ¼ cup tofu
- 1 tablespoon peanut butter
- ½ ounce nuts or seeds

The fat content of meat varies considerably. Some forms of meat are only 1 percent fat, whereas others may be as high as 40 percent fat. Poultry and fish are generally significantly lower in overall fat than are red meats. Interestingly, the higher the grade of red meat, the more fat is marbled throughout the muscle fiber. People may find that higher-grade steak usually tastes better, but that is because of its higher fat content.

Meats are generally excellent sources of iron. Iron is present in much greater amounts in red meats and organ meats (liver, kidney, and heart) than in poultry and fish. Iron plays a critical role in hemoglobin synthesis in red blood cells and thus is an important contributor to physical fitness (see Chapter 4) and overall cardiovascular health (see Chapter 9). However, meat and fish should be fresh, stored appropriately, and cooked adequately to reduce the likelihood of serious foodborne illnesses. This will be discussed later in this chapter.

Grains Bread, cereal, rice, and pasta are referred to as the "grain group" by the USDA. Rates of consumption in this food group are on the rise, as we now eat 25 percent more grains than Americans did in 1970. Corn flour, starch, and grits are the main grains for which consumption has increased, while the numbers have remained steady for oats.[21] There is a particular emphasis on consuming at least 3 of the 6 ounces of this group from whole grains. Whole grains can reduce the risk of chronic disease and help with weight maintenance.

Whole grains consist of the entire grain seed, or the kernel, and can't be identified by the color of the food. The FDA requires that food contain 51 percent or more whole-grain ingredients by weight and be low-fat in order to be called "whole grain." On food labels, "whole grain" should be the first ingredient listed. It is further advised that you avoid refined grains because the grain-refining process typically removes most of the bran and some of the germ, resulting in the loss of dietary fiber, minerals, vitamins, and other important nutrients. Wheat flour, enriched flour, and degerminated cornmeal are *not* whole grains.

Reading and understanding what food labels mean is important when you are trying to meet your whole-grain requirements. Optimally, you want the label to say "100% whole grain," meaning there is no refined flour in the food. However, if it says "Made with whole grain," then it has some whole grain but you don't know how much. "A good source of whole grain" indicates that the food may have as little as 8 grams of whole grains per serving, and "An excellent source of whole grain" means as little as 16 grams per serving. "Multigrain" means a mixture of grains that is mostly refined grain with some whole grains sprinkled in.

The food industry has risen to the challenge of providing nutritious whole-grain foods with improved taste and texture. For example, ConAgra spent millions of dollars to develop "white wheat" made from a naturally occurring albino variety of flour. It has 3½ times more dietary fiber, 11 times more vitamin E, 5 times more magnesium, and 4 times more niacin than does refined, unenriched wheat flour. It also tastes milder and sweeter than most whole grains do. It combines the best of both worlds—the nutrition of whole wheat and the taste of white flour.[21]

Some products are labeled **enriched,** meaning that some of the nutritional elements that were removed during processing are returned to the food; however, only three B vitamins (thiamine, niacin, riboflavin) and iron are replaced.

The nutritional benefit from the breads, cereals, rice, and pasta group lies in its contribution of B-complex vitamins and energy from complex carbohydrates. Some nutritionists believe that foods from this group promote protein intake, since many of them are prepared as complete-protein foods—for example, macaroni and cheese, cereal and milk, and bread and meat sandwiches.

The USDA recommends 6 ounces of grains daily, with at least 3 ounces coming from whole grains. One ounce is equivalent to

- 1 slice of bread
- 1 cup dry cereal
- ½ cup cooked rice, pasta, cereal

Oils   The USDA defines oils as fats that are liquid at room temperature, such as vegetable oils used in cooking. Oils come from many different plants and from fish. Some common oils are canola oil, corn oil, cottonseed oil, olive oil, safflower oil, soybean oil, and sunflower oil. Canola and olive oil are preferred over other types of oils. Some foods, such as nuts, olives, fish and avocados, are naturally high in oils. Foods that are mainly oil include mayonnaise, salad dressings, and soft margarine with no trans fats. A limit of 24 grams or 6 teaspoons of oils is the daily recommendation, although this can vary by age and gender. One teaspoon is equal to

- 1 teaspoon margarine
- 1 tablespoon low-fat mayonnaise
- 2 tablespoons light salad dressing
- 1 teaspoon vegetable oil

Empty Calories   Where do such items as beer, butter, candy, sodas, cookies, corn chips, and pastries fit into your diet? Most of these items contribute relatively little to healthful nutrition; they provide additional calories, generally from sucrose and significant amounts of salt and fat. Fats, salt, sugar, and alcohol are referred to as "empty calories" and are limited to 120–330 calories a day by the MyPlate food guide. As described earlier in this chapter, the recommended total daily fat intake

should be 20–35 percent of your total calories, with most fats coming from sources of polyunsaturated and mono-unsaturated fatty acids. Less than 10 percent of total calories should be from saturated fats, and less than 300 mg per day should come from cholesterol. Trans-fatty acid consumption should be kept to 2 grams or less daily.

The USDA also suggests that we choose and prepare foods and beverages with little added sugars or caloric sweeteners. The new food guide recommends no more than 8 teaspoons of added sugars per day, which is equivalent to ½ ounce of jelly beans or an 8-ounce glass of lemonade. Eating too much sugar is thought to be a major contributor to the increase in obesity in Americans.

Dietary Guidelines for Americans 2010

The Dietary Guidelines for Americans are science-based and summarize the most current scientific information regarding nutrition, health, physical activity, and food safety. The goal of these guidelines is to lower the risk of chronic disease and promote health through diet and physical activity. Together, these guidelines encourage Americans to take in fewer calories, make wiser food choices, and be more physically active. The key recommendations focus on increasing consumption of nutrient-dense food and fruits and vegetables, exercising regularly, decreasing portion sizes, and decreasing consumption of sodium, trans fat, saturated fatty acids, dietary cholesterol, sugar, refined grains, and alcohol. We will discuss these recommendations in the next section along with guidelines for food safety and special populations.

Focus on Nutrient Density   Many Americans consume too many calories and too much saturated and trans fat, cholesterol, added sugar, and sodium. At the same time, many people do not meet the recommended intake for fiber and a number of vitamins and minerals. Therefore, people should choose mostly **nutrient-dense foods,** which provide substantial amounts of vitamins and minerals and comparatively few calories. Junk foods typically are not nutrient-dense, because they are high in sugar and saturated and trans fats, high in calories, and low in vitamins

---

Key Terms

cruciferous vegetables   Vegetables, such as broccoli, whose plants have flowers with four leaves in the pattern of a cross.

enriched   Foods that have been resupplied with some of the nutritional elements (B vitamins and iron) removed during processing.

nutrient-dense foods   Foods that provide substantial amounts of vitamins and minerals and comparatively few calories.

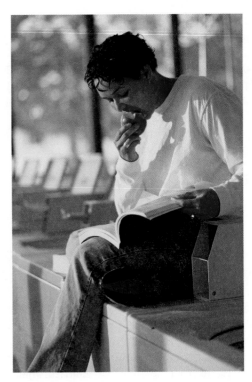

The Dietary Guidelines for Americans recommend that we increase our intake of fruits, vegetables, whole grains, and fat-free or low-fat dairy products. Fruit can be easily incorporated into the daily diet as part of a meal or as a snack.

and minerals. Choosing nutrient-dense foods can be especially challenging when eating out.

Following the recommendations in the MyPlate plan can help you choose nutrient-dense foods. In general, Americans are advised to consume more dark green and orange vegetables, legumes, fruits, whole grains, and low-fat milk and milk products.

Physical Activity Of course, part of managing your weight in a healthy manner includes physical activity. The Dietary Guidelines for Americans emphasize the important role that physical activity plays in our lives. It is proposed that adult Americans engage in 2 hours and 30 minutes of moderate-intensity aerobic physical activity spread over three days a week. This is in addition to the usual activities of daily life, at work or home on most days of the week to reduce the risk of chronic disease. It is further recommended that adults engage in strength training activities such as situps, push-ups, and weight lifting two times a week. Children and adolescents should engage in one hour or more of moderate- to vigorous-intensity physical activity every day, including strengthening activities such as climbing and jumping at least three times a week. Children younger than 5 are recommended to be active each day. Seventy-seven percent of Americans don't meet the USDA's recommendations for physical activity.

Weight Management The Dietary Guidelines for Americans define weight management as meaning "to maintain body weight in a healthy range, balance calories from foods and beverages with calories expended, and to prevent gradual weight gain over time, make small decreases in food and beverage calories and increase physical activity." The dietary guidelines were designed with the goal of weight management in mind, and the recommendations for the different food groups were developed to reach this goal. However, most Americans don't know how many calories they should consume each day to maintain their weight, making it difficult to achieve this goal. Chapter 6 will go into further detail on how to identify a healthy weight and manage your weight effectively.

Food Groups to Encourage: Fruits, Vegetables, Dairy, and Seafood Americans are advised to consume more fiber-rich whole grains, fruits and vegetables, seafood, and dairy products. Specifically, it is suggested that we consume 3–6 ounce-equivalents of whole-grain products per day, with the rest of the recommended grains coming from enriched or whole-grain products. In general, at least half the grains should come from whole grains. Americans are also encouraged to choose a variety of fruits and vegetables, selecting from all four vegetable subgroups: dark green, orange, and starchy vegetables and legumes. Drinking 3 cups of fat-free or low-fat milk or the equivalent per day is also encouraged, especially because milk consumption has been decreasing over the past 30 years. Americans are further encouraged to drink water instead of sugary drinks. There is also a push to eat seafood in place of meat and poultry.

Foods to Limit: Fats, Sugars, Sodium, and Alcohol

Choose Your Fats Wisely According to the USDA, we should limit our total fat intake to 20–35 percent of calories, with most fat calories coming from polyunsaturated and monounsaturated fatty acids. However, 34 percent of calories Americans consume come from fat intake. Less than 10 percent of our calories should come from saturated fatty acids, keeping our consumption of trans-fatty acids as low as possible. Also, we need to limit our cholesterol intake to less than 300 mg per day, getting our protein from low-fat, fat-free, or lean meat, poultry, dairy, and bean products.

Sugar Consumption This follows the upward trend in soda consumption, as well as the increased consumption of flavored coffees. The Dietary Guidelines for Americans suggest that we choose and prepare foods and beverages with little added sugar or noncaloric sweeteners. Most added sugar comes from soft drinks; energy, fruit, and sports drinks; desserts; and candy. For example, a regular 12-ounce soft drink contains 8 teaspoons of

Does seeing a television advertisement for a juicy, mouth-watering Steak and Shake burger make you hungry? Does a Dove chocolate waterfall cascading down the television screen make you salivate? Advertisers hope so and spend over $10 billion on food and beverage television ads each year, with the lowest amount of money being spent on advertising fruits, vegetables, and milk. Most of these ads are targeted toward children and adolescents, who view one food ad every five minutes of television screen time. Eighty-nine percent of these ads are for products that are high in sugar, fat, and/or sodium. Children as young as 2 years of age begin asking their parents to buy certain food items seen on television; this is known in the advertising industry as "pestering power" or "nag power." Most of these requests are for cereal, soft drinks, cookies, and candy, and parents comply with their children's request 50 percent of the time. The least nutritious, high-sugar cereals are the most heavily marketed to children.

Studies have shown that people do eat more after watching television food ads, regardless of how hungry they reported they were at the time. One study found that children ate 45 percent more after seeing a television food ad, compared to those who didn't view one, potentially contributing to a weight gain of 10 pounds per year. The

ads don't show viewers the whole picture such as caloric count or the fat, sodium, and sugar content of these foods. Nor do they tell viewers that the more people see these ads, the more they eat and the more they weigh.

So what is the answer? It is very difficult if not impossible to avoid these ads as they bombard us constantly. Do you think there should be regulation for food ads, such as requiring them to list the nutritional information for these foods? Should there be an equal number of ads for fruits, vegetables, and dairy products? One thing that we as consumers can do is educate ourselves about the nutritional information of these foods—that is, be more informed viewers and look at the ads with a more realistic and knowledgeable perspective.

Sources: Approximately how much money is spent each year marketing food products to children? *Purdue Extension*, March 16, 2010; Story M, French S, Food advertising and marketing directed at children and adolescents in the US. *International Journal of Behavior, Nutrition, and Physical Activity*, 5, 1, 2004; Taylor J, Are fast-food advertisers playing you? *WebMD*, March 20, 2011; Kids' cereals pour on the sugar and sodium, *USA Today*, October 26, 2009.

sugar. The dietary guidelines specifically focus on reducing Americans' consumption of sugary beverages for this reason. There is a further recommendation to decrease the amount of added sugars in foods. It is estimated that Americans consume 400 calories worth of added sugars daily. Added sugars have been associated with higher risk of obesity, heart disease, diabetes, and gout.[22] Shopping for foods that limit sugar can be a challenge, however; see the box "Does Watching Television Influence Your Eating?"

Sodium Intake The USDA guidelines recommend limiting sodium intake to less than 2,300 mg daily, and for Americans over 51, to less than 1,500 mg daily; however, the average American consumes 3,400 mg daily (see Figure 5-3). Most of our salt intake comes from processed or prepared foods. Many people are unaware of the high sodium content in prepared foods, sauces, soups, and canned foods, and so reading the labels for ingredients is extremely important. You might be surprised by some of the foods that contain salt—cookies, bread, salad dressings, soft drinks, and cereal. Too much sodium is linked to hypertension, and about 30 percent of Americans have sodium-sensitive high blood pressure, which can lead to heart attack or stroke. One study showed that a low-sodium diet reduced the risk of cardiovascular disease by 25–30 percent.[23] It is estimated that about 150,000 deaths each year are caused by consumption of too much salt.

For this reason, salt has been referred to as the "silent killer," and the USDA labeled salt as "public enemy No. 1." The Institute of Medicine issued a report in 2010 urging the government to reduce the maximum amount of sodium that manufacturers and restaurants can add to foods and beverages.[24] For example, the sodium content in McDonald's Big Mac is 1,040 mg, Panera's broccoli cheddar soup is 1,020 mg, and Olive Garden's spaghetti and meatballs is 2,180 mg.[24] Some companies are already acting in anticipation of this possible FDA regulation. Subway decreased its sodium content by 28 percent in its "fresh fit" sandwich line, following the lead of others who have already cut sodium in their products, such as PepsiCo, ConAgra, Del Monte, General Mills, Kraft, Heinz, Mars, Starbucks, and Campbell. Perhaps sodium will go the way of trans fat in being severely reduced in Americans' diet if the food and beverage industry continues the trend of decreasing the sodium in its products.

Alcohol Consumption The USDA states that "if alcohol is consumed, it should be consumed in moderation—up to one drink per day for women and two drinks per day for men—and only by adults of legal drinking age." One drink is defined as either 12 fluid ounces of regular beer, 5 fluid ounces of wine, or 1½ fluid ounces of 80-proof distilled spirits. Because alcoholic beverages tend to contribute calories but little nutrition, they are counterproductive to taking in sufficient nutrients while not going

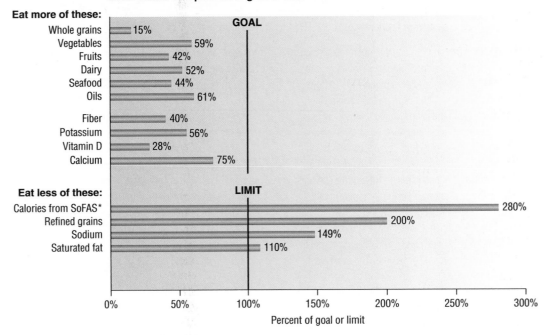

Usual intake as a percent of goal or limit

Figure 5-3 How Do Typical American Diets Compare to Recommended Intake Levels or Limits?

* SoFAS = Solid fats and added sugars.

Based on data from: U.S. Department of Agriculture, Agricultural Research Service, and U.S. Department of Health and Human Services, Centers for Disease Control and Prevention, What We Eat in America, NHANES 2001–2004 or 2005–2006.

over the daily caloric allotment. However, there are some indications that moderate alcohol consumption, such as having a glass of red wine each day, assists in decreasing the risk of coronary heart disease.

Food Safety Food safety has become an increasing concern with the numerous foodborne pathogens showing up in peanuts, seafood, meat, eggs, vegetables, and even dog food. The dietary guidelines suggest common-sense safety measures, such as making sure your hands and work surfaces are clean before you prepare food. Food should be cooked or chilled at appropriate temperatures (see the section "Food Safety" on page 116). It is further suggested that you *not* wash meat or poultry prior to preparing them, which is the opposite of what has been advised in the past. Avoid unpasteurized juices, milk, and milk products; raw or partially cooked eggs or foods containing raw eggs; undercooked meat and poultry; and raw sprouts. This will be discussed in more detail in the food safety section later in this chapter.

Recommendations for Special Populations There are also some special recommendations for specific population groups. For people over 50, consuming vitamin B$_{12}$ in its crystalline form (such as fortified foods or supplements) is recommended. Women of childbearing age need to eat iron-rich plant food or iron-fortified food with an enhancer for iron absorption, such as vitamin-C-rich foods. Taking in adequate amounts of folic acid

daily from fortified foods or supplements is important for pregnant women and women who may become pregnant. Pregnant or breast-feeding women are further recommended to consume 8–12 ounces of seafood per week, limiting tuna and abstaining from tilefish, shark, swordfish, and mackerel due to high mercury content. Older adults, people with dark skin, and those not exposed to enough sunlight need to consume extra vitamin D from vitamin-D-fortified foods and/or supplements.

Additional Eating Plans and Recommendations

Other eating plans are consistent with the Dietary Guidelines for Americans and appropriate for different groups. This section describes the DASH diet, introduces different types of vegetarian diets, and provides nutritional guidelines for older adults. The box "Diverse Food Pyramids" on page 110 describes food group plans based on different ethnic dietary patterns.

Dietary Approaches to Stop Hypertension (DASH) The DASH diet is not a weight loss program but an example of how to eat in accordance with the Dietary Guidelines for Americans. The DASH diet is constructed across a range of calorie levels to meet the needs of various age and gender groups. Originally developed to study the effects of an eating pattern on the prevention and treatment of hypertension, DASH is a balanced eating plan

Table 5.3 DASH Eating Plan

Food Groups	Servings/Day			
	1,600 Calories/Day	2,000 Calories/Day	2,600 Calories/Day	3,100 Calories/Day
Grains*	6	6–8	10–11	12–13
Vegetables	3–4	4–5	5–6	6
Fruits	4	4–5	5–6	6
Fat-free or low-fat milk and milk products	2–3	2–3	3	3–4
Lean meats, poultry, and fish	3–6	6	6	6–9
Nuts, seeds, and legumes	3/week	4–5/wk	1	1
Fats and oils	2	2–3	3	4
Sweets and added sugars	Less than 3	Less than 5	Less than 2	Less than 2

*Whole grains are recommended for most grain servings as a good source of fiber and nutrients.
Source: National Heart, Lung, and Blood Institute, Your Guide to Lowering Your Blood Pressure with DASH, 2010, www.nhlbi.nih.gov/health/public/heart/hbp/dash/how-make-dash.html.

consistent with the USDA'S dietary guidelines and similar to the Mediterranean diet. You can view examples of the DASH program on the National Institutes of Health website at www.nhlbi.nih.gov/health/public/heart/hbp/dash. Table 5.3 also shows the DASH diet varying by caloric intake requirements. A 25-year study of 88,000 women showed those who followed the DASH diet were 24 percent less likely to have a stroke than those women who didn't follow it.

Vegetarian Diets A *vegetarian diet* relies on plant sources for all or most of the nutrients needed by the body. This approach includes a range of diets, from those that allow some animal sources of nutrients to those that exclude all animal sources. Studies show that vegetarians who eat a balanced diet don't seem to have any more iron-deficiency problems than do meat eaters. Although the iron in plant food is not as well absorbed as the iron in animal food is, vegetarians tend to eat more iron-containing foods and more vitamin C foods, which help with the absorption of the iron.[15] In addition, vegetarians tend to get enough calcium from dairy foods, tofu, beans, soybeans, calcium-fortified cereals, and vegetables such as broccoli. There has been some concern about a vitamin B_{12} deficiency because animal foods are the best source for B_{12} and plant foods don't naturally contain the vitamin. However, soy foods may contain vitamin B_{12}, although it is not as biologically active as in animal foods. Many soy products are fortified with vitamin B_{12} as well. It is important also to note that the liver stores so much B_{12} that it would take years to become deficient in this vitamin.[15] Vegetarians tend to eat healthier diets; have lower rates of cardiovascular disease, lower blood pressure, lower levels of LDL cholesterol, and less incidence of diabetes; and weigh 15 percent less than do those who eat meat. Three types of vegetarian diets, beginning with the least restrictive, are summarized in

the following sections. The MyPlate food guide described earlier in the chapter can be used as a guide for all types of vegetarian diets.

Ovolactovegetarian Diet Depending on the particular pattern of consuming eggs (*ovo*) and milk (*lacto*) or using one but not the other, an **ovolactovegetarian diet** can be a very sound approach to healthful eating for adults. Most vegetarians in the United States fit into this category. Ovolactovegetarian diets provide the body with the essential amino acids and limit the high intake of fats involved in more conventional diets. The exclusion of meat as a protein source lowers the total fat intake, and the consumption of milk or eggs allows an adequate amount of saturated fat to remain in the diet. The use of vegetable products as the primary source of nutrients is consistent with the current dietary recommendations for an increase in fruits, vegetables, and fiber. Vegetarians who do consume dairy products face challenges when making food choices if they wish to avoid other animal products in their food. Because most cheese is made with rennet, a coagulating agent that usually comes from stomachs of slaughtered newborn calves, many vegetarians eliminate cheese from their diet or opt for rennet-less cheese. Vegetarian cheeses are manufactured using rennet from either fungal or bacterial sources. Similarly, yogurt is often made with gelatin derived from animal ligaments, skins, tendon, and bones (gelatin is also found in marshmallows, candies such as jelly beans and candy corn, some poptarts, and a variety of other foods).

> **Key Terms**
>
> **ovolactovegetarian diet** (oh voe **lack** toe veg a **ter** ee in)
> A diet that excludes all meat but does include the consumption of eggs and dairy products.

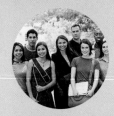

Learning from Our Diversity

Diverse Food Pyramids

Besides MyPlate, discussed earlier in this chapter, other food pyramids exist. The Mediterranean food pyramid emphasizes fruits, beans, legumes, nuts, vegetables, whole grains, and small amounts of meat. In fact, the latest version of the USDA pyramid and dietary guidelines are in keeping with what had already been suggested by the Mediterranean food pyramid—for example, using more olive oil; limiting consumption of alcohol; eating more whole grains, fruits, and vegetables; choosing lean meat; eating fish and shellfish; and exercising daily.

The Asian food pyramid limits meat consumption even more by recommending consumption of meat on a monthly basis and daily consumption of fish, shellfish, and dairy products. The Asian diet,

like the Mediterranean diet, encourages daily intake of fruit, legumes, vegetables, and whole grains. In addition, the Asian diet includes rice and noodles and suggests eating poultry, eggs, and sweets only once a week.

The Latin American food pyramid also advises consumption of meat, sweets, and eggs only once a week. Like the Asian diet, it encourages eating fish and shellfish on a daily basis, and unlike the Mediterranean and Asian diets, it advises consumption of poultry on a daily basis. As in the other food pyramids, fruit, vegetables, beans, and whole grains are to be consumed every day. Physical exercise and water consumption are emphasized by all three food pyramids.

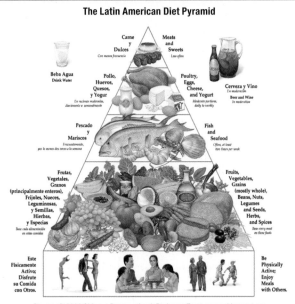

The Mediterranean Diet Pyramid

Meats and Sweets
Less often

Wine
In moderation

Poultry, Eggs, Cheese, and Yogurt
Moderate portions, daily to weekly

Fish and Seafood
Often, at least two times per week

Drink Water

Fruits, Vegetables, Grains (mostly whole), Olive oil, Beans, Nuts, Legumes and Seeds, Herbs and Spices
Base every meal on these foods

Be Physically Active; Enjoy Meals with Others

Source: © 2009 Oldways Preservation & Exchange Trust. www.oldwayspt.org

The Latin American Diet Pyramid

Carne y Dulces
Con menos frecuencia

Meats and Sweets
Less often

Beba Agua
Drink Water

Pollo, Huevos, Quesos, y Yogur
En raciones moderadas, diariamente a semanalmente

Poultry, Eggs, Cheese, and Yogurt
Moderate portions, daily to weekly

Cerveza y Vino
En moderación
Beer and Wine
In moderation

Pescado y Mariscos
Frecuentemente, por lo menos dos veces a la semana

Fish and Seafood
Often, at least two times per week

Frutas, Vegetales, Granos (principalmente enteros), Frijoles, Nueces, Leguminosas, y Semillas, Hierbas, y Especias
Base cada alimentación en estas comidas

Fruits, Vegetables, Grains (mostly whole), Beans, Nuts, Legumes and Seeds, Herbs, and Spices
Base every meal on these foods

Este Físicamente Activo; Disfrute su Comida con Otros.

Be Physically Active; Enjoy Meals with Others.

Source: © 2009 Oldways Preservation & Exchange Trust. www.oldwayspt.org

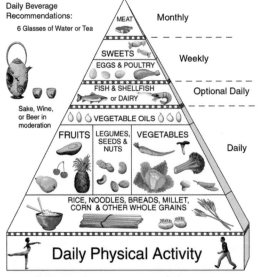

The Asian Diet Pyramid

Daily Beverage Recommendations:
6 Glasses of Water or Tea

MEAT — Monthly

SWEETS
EGGS & POULTRY — Weekly

FISH & SHELLFISH or DAIRY — Optional Daily

Sake, Wine, or Beer in moderation

VEGETABLE OILS

FRUITS — LEGUMES, SEEDS & NUTS — VEGETABLES — Daily

RICE, NOODLES, BREADS, MILLET, CORN & OTHER WHOLE GRAINS

Daily Physical Activity

Source: © 2000 Oldways Preservation & Exchange Trust. www.oldwayspt.org

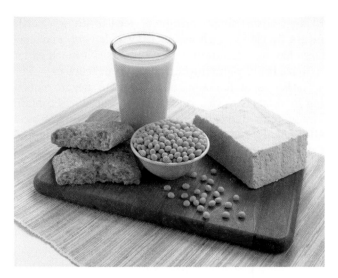

Soy foods are an important source of protein and other nutrients for vegetarians.

It has become easier to follow a vegetarian diet since stores have begun offering organic vegetarian items that do not contain these animal products. However, it can be difficult to avoid all animal products without being an avid and knowledgeable label reader.

Lactovegetarian and Ovovegetarian Diets People who include dairy products in their diet but no other animal products, including eggs, are *lactovegetarians*. In contrast, people who exclude dairy products such as milk and cheese, yet consume eggs, are ovovegetarians. Both diets carry the advantages of ovolactovegetarianism.

Vegan Vegetarian Diet A **vegan vegetarian diet** is one in which not only meat but also other animal products, including milk, cheese, and eggs, are excluded. When compared with the ovolactovegetarian diet, the vegan diet requires a higher level of nutritional understanding to avoid nutritional inadequacies.

One potential difficulty is that of obtaining all the essential amino acids. Since a single plant source does not contain all the essential amino acids, the vegan must learn to consistently employ a complementary diet. By carefully combining various grains, seeds, and legumes, amino acid deficiency can be prevented.

In addition to the potential amino acid deficiency, the vegan could have some difficulty in maintaining the necessary intake of vitamin B_{12}. Possible ramifications of inadequate B_{12} intake include depression, anemia, back pain, and menstrual irregularity. Vegans often have difficulty maintaining adequate intakes of iron, zinc, and calcium.[1] Calcium intake must be monitored closely by the vegan. In addition, vitamin D deficiencies can occur. Supplements and daily exposure to sunshine will aid in maintaining adequate levels of this vitamin.

Semivegetarian Diets People become vegetarians for many reasons. Some avoid meat and animal products for ethical or spiritual reasons. Others choose vegetarianism for health or environmental reasons. In recent years, some people have found a middle-ground style of eating that includes some meat consumption but an increase in vegetable consumption, referred to as *semivegetarianism*, or *flexitarian*. Semivegetarians occasionally add fish and poultry to the ovolactovegetarian diet, and some eat red meat infrequently as well. **Pesco-vegetarians** eat fish, dairy products, and eggs along with vegetables.

Nutrition and the Older Adult Nutritional needs change as adults age. Age-related changes to the structure and function of the body are primarily responsible for such altered nutritional requirements. These changes can involve the teeth, salivary glands, taste buds, oral muscles, gastric acid production, and peristaltic action. In addition, chronic constipation resulting from changes in gastrointestinal tract function can decrease the older adult's interest in eating.

The progressive lowering of the body's basal metabolism is another factor that will eventually influence the dietary patterns of older adults. As energy requirements fall, the body gradually senses the need for less food. In addition, a tendency to decrease activity levels also occurs with aging. Because of this decreased need for calories, nutrient density—the nutritional value of food relative to calories supplied—is an important consideration for older adults. The USDA dietary guidelines make some specific suggestions for people over 50. These include consuming more vitamin B_{12}, because older people tend to have difficulty absorbing this vitamin. Older adults are also encouraged to consume extra vitamin-D-fortified foods, since this vitamin may be lacking in this group.

Psychosocial factors also alter the role of food in the lives of many older adults. Social isolation, depression, chronic alcohol consumption, loss of income, transportation limitations, and housing restrictions are lifestyle factors that can lessen the ease and enjoyment associated with the preparation and consumption of food. Consequently, a person's food intake might decrease.

> **Key Terms**
>
> **vegan vegetarian diet** (**vee** gun *or* **vay** gun) A vegetarian diet that excludes all animal products, including eggs and dairy products.
>
> **pesco-vegetarian diet** A vegetarian diet that includes fish, dairy products, and eggs along with plant foods.

Special Nutrition Concerns: Challenges and Tools for Consumers

Food Labels

Since 1973, the FDA has required food manufacturers to provide nutritional information (labels) on products to which one or more nutrients have been added or for which some nutritional claim has been made. Originally, there was concern about whether the public could understand the labels and whether additional information would be required. So the FDA, in consultation with individual states and public interest groups, developed new labeling regulations. Revised labels began appearing on food packages in May 1993. The currently used label is shown in Figure 5-4. Specific types of information contained on this label are highlighted.

Foods that were not initially covered by the 1993 food-labeling guidelines are gradually being assigned labels. In 2008, the "Country of Origin" legislation took effect, requiring all fresh or frozen meats, fish, fruits, and vegetables to be identified by their country of origin. This identification may be made by using a sticker, sign, placard, or label to indicate the country of the product's origin. However, cooked and processed foods, such as frozen or cooked shrimp and smoked ham or fish, are exempt. Also exempt are foods packaged together, such as frozen peas and carrots. Fresh fruits and vegetables are not required to be labeled, but many stores do so voluntarily.

Recent additions to the 1993 requirements include the labeling of fruit juices for pasteurization (unpasteurized juice can be a source of *Escherichia coli [E. coli]* contamination), the identification of milk from cows whose food has been enhanced with bovine growth hormone, and the issuing of specific criteria for legal use of the term *organic*. Some supermarkets also label fresh and frozen poultry and seafood with information about how it was prepared and stored. This point-of-purchase labeling is voluntary.

As of January 2006, food makers are required by the FDA to put the amount of trans fat on food labels. The FDA has further recommended that food labels list calories in larger type print, list the percentage of the consumer's daily allotment of calories, and list the total amount of calories in the container, not just the calories per serving. For example, pretzels might be listed as having 100 calories per serving and approximately 15 servings per bag, and so it is up to you to compute how many servings and calories you have consumed. The FDA prohibits any nutrient claim that it has not defined. For example, the FDA recently defined *low-fat* as containing 3 grams or less of fat per serving. The FDA has not yet defined what can be considered to be *low-carb* even though many food makers and restaurants use this term in their advertising. Consumers need to know what is meant by claims such as *low-calorie, low-fat,* and *low-carb;* having a standard definition makes it much easier to make healthy and informed nutritional choices.

Also as of January 2006, the FDA began requiring food labels to clearly state if food products contain any proteins derived from any of the eight major food allergens. In addition, the Food Allergen Labeling and Consumer Protection Act of 2004 (FALCPA) requires manufacturers to clearly identify the presence of ingredients that contain protein derived from milk, eggs,

Nutrition Facts

Serving Size 1 Bar (40g)

	Amount Per Serving	
Check Calories	**Calories** 170	Calories from Fat 60
		% Daily Value*
Limit These Nutrients	**Total Fat** 7g	11%
	Saturated Fat 7g	15%
	Trans Fat 0g	
	Cholesterol 0mg	0%
	Sodium 160mg	7%
	Total Carbohydrate 24g	8%
	Dietary Fiber 3g	12%
	Sugars 10g	
	Protein 5g	
Get Enough of These Nutrients	Vitamin A 2%	Vitamin C 2%
	Calcium 20%	Iron 8%

Footnote

* Percent Daily Values are based on a 2,000 calorie diet. Your daily values may be higher or lower depending on your calorie needs:

	Calories:	2,000	2,500
Total Fat	Less than	65g	80g
Sat Fat	Less than	20g	25g
Cholesterol	Less than	300mg	300mg
Sodium	Less than	2,400mg	2,400mg
Total Carbohydrate		300g	375g
Dietary Fiber		25g	25g

Calories per gram:
Fat 9 • Carbohydrate 4 • Protein 4

Ingredients
Granola Bar (Brown Rice Syrup, Granola [rolled oats, honey, canola oil], Dry Roasted Peanuts, Soy Crisps [soy protein isolate, rice flour, malt extract, calcium carbonate], Crisp Brown Rice [organic brown rice flour, evaporated cane juice, molasses, rice bran extract, sea salt], Glycerine, Peanut Butter [ground dry roasted peanuts], Inulin, Whey Protein Isolate, Gold Flax Seeds, Quinoa Flakes, Calcium Carbonate, Salt, Natural Flavors, Water, Soy Lecithin [an emulsifier]), Dark Compound Coating (evaporated cane juice, palm kernel oil, cocoa [processed with alkali], palm oil, soy lecithin [an emulsifier]).

Figure 5-4 The Nutrition Facts Label and Ingredients List of a Granola Bar

Source: Dietary Guidelines for Americans, 2010.

Should You Take a Dietary Supplement?

Half of Americans take a dietary supplement for health, weight management, and athletic performance enhancement, spending $23 billion on them in 2009. But what are the risks? Dietary supplements do not have to have clinical trials to prove their safety or effectiveness and are not subject to regulation by the FDA. Due to the lack of quality control, supplements have been routinely found to contain metals, pesticides, high amounts of selenium and chromium, and prescription drugs. People have reported problems with breathing, liver failure, kidney failure, stroke, high blood pressure, heart attacks, joint pain, diarrhea, hair loss, finger- and toenails falling off, skin turning blue, whites of eyes turning yellow, and fatigue. Fatalities have been associated with taking dietary supplements as well.

Consumer Reports, along with the Natural Medicines Comprehensive Database, developed a list of the most dangerous supplements, ones they say should be avoided due to lack of safety and to adverse side effects. They are aconite, bitter orange, chaparral, colloidal silver, coltsfoot, comfrey, country mallow, germanium, greater celadine, kava, lobelia, and yohimbe. They have been associated with liver damage, kidney damage, heart failure, cancer, respiratory problems, and death.

If you do take a dietary supplement, be a cautious and informed consumer. Look for the "USP Verified" mark on the product indicating that the manufacturer has voluntarily undergone quality control testing by U.S. Pharmacopeia. USP is a nonprofit, private standard-setting authority that verifies the quality, purity, and potency of the product.

You can check out a list of verified products at www.uspverified.org. If the promises seem too good to be true, they probably are. It is illegal for dietary supplement companies to claim that their product can prevent, treat, or cure any disease other than ones caused by nutrient deficiencies. Be sure to tell your doctor or pharmacist if you are taking any dietary supplements to avoid negative interactions with prescription medications. If you experience any problems, consult your doctor immediately.

Source: Dangerous supplements, *Consumer Reports,* September 2010.

---

fish, crustacean shellfish, tree nuts, peanuts, wheat, or soybeans in the list of ingredients or to say "contains" followed by name of the food allergen after or adjacent to the list of ingredients. This is very important for those who suffer from food allergies, and there is a discussion of this topic later in this chapter. Additionally, some restaurant menus now state the nutritional content of some selections and provide cautionary notes about their safe cooking.

Anticipating that the FDA would eventually develop a system to indicate healthy food choices on packaging, some companies, such as PepsiCo, General Mills and Kellogg, implemented voluntary food labeling using a green check mark on the front of the item to indicate a "smart choice." However, this type of labeling came under fire as high-sugar foods such as Froot Loops and Cracker Jacks had these green "smart choice" check marks on their packages. Critics claimed that this labeling practice was more misleading than helpful, as it resulted in people not reading the nutritional information, assuming that the food was a healthy choice. Consumers may have believed that these food labels were regulated by the FDA when in reality they were not. The "smart choice" check marks are now being replaced by "nutrition keys" on the front of packages, listing calories, saturated fat, sodium, and sugars per serving. Again, this is a voluntary nutrition labeling system created by the Grocery Manufacturers' Association and the Food Marketing Institute, not the FDA.

A new law, part of the U.S. health care bill, mandates that nutrition information must be posted on the menu or menu board next to the menu item in any restaurant that has 20 or more locations. This law also applies to vending machine food. New York City, California, and Seattle already have this calorie-posting law. The hope is that Americans will make better-informed choices when eating out. As of 2012, the FDA requires nutrition labels on beef, poultry, lamb, and pork; previously, this was not required. The labels list calories, calories from fat, saturated fat, cholesterol, sodium, protein, and vitamins.[25]

Fast Foods

Fast foods deliver a high percentage of their calories from fat, often associated with their method of preparation (for example, frying in saturated fat). **Fat density** is a serious limitation of fast foods. In comparison with the recommended standard (20–35 percent of total calories from fat), 40–50 percent of the calories in fast foods come from fats. Although many fast-food restaurants are now using vegetable oil instead of animal fat for frying (to reduce cholesterol levels), this change has not lowered the fat density of these foods. The average fast-food meal supplies over one-half the amount of fat needed in a day.

> **Key Terms**
>
> **fat density** The percentage of a food's total calories that are derived from fat; above 30 percent is considered a high fat density.

I am always in a hurry and don't have time to cook, and so a lot of my meals end up being fast food. Are there better choices I can make when eating on the run?

The typical American eats about three hamburgers and four orders of French fries each week, so you aren't alone. With over 300,000 fast-food restaurants in the United States, fast food is definitely part of the American lifestyle. Here are some things to consider when eating at fast-food restaurants:

- Don't supersize! Go for the "small" or "regular" size.
- Don't wait until you are starving because that leads to overeating and supersizing!
- Decide what you want to order ahead of time, and don't be swayed by "value meal" or what "looks good."
- Ask for a nutritional guide for the menu. Look at the calories, fat grams, and sodium when making your selection.

- Order grilled instead of fried chicken or fish.
- Look for the "light" choices.
- Limit your condiments. Mustard, ketchup, salsa, and low-fat or fat-free condiments and dressings are preferable to regular mayonnaise or high-fat dressings.
- Bring fast food from home! Buy portable foods at the grocery store to take with you that can be eaten quickly and easily, such as portable yogurt, a banana or apple, low-fat granola bar, or breakfast bar.
- Order low-fat or skim milk or water instead of soda.
- Go to a variety of different kinds of fast-food restaurants so you aren't eating hamburgers every day, and set a limit on how many meals you are going to eat out each week.

In addition, fast foods are often high in sugar and salt. The restaurant and fast-food industry has received strong criticism lately for its contribution to creating overweight Americans. In response, Olive Garden, Wendy's, Applebee's, Chili's, and some other national restaurant chains are going trans-fat-free.

Despite these efforts, a recent study showed that those who said they ate out at fast-food restaurants at least twice a week gained 10 pounds more than those who did not. Another study showed that most people underestimate how many calories they have eaten when they eat fast food, often by as much as 681 calories. This makes some sense given that a study of restaurants found that menu items were 18 percent higher in calories than was listed in the nutritional information. Nutritional information for restaurants and fast-food chains can be found on websites such as www.chowbaby.com.

While fast-food restaurants are offering some healthy choices, they still have high-fat, high-calories options such as Hardee's Western Bacon Thickburger, weighing in at 900 calories, 470 from fat; Burger King's XT Steakburger at 970 calories, 549 from fat; and McDonald's Double Quarter Pounder with Cheese at 730 calories, 360 from fat, as well as supersize fries at 610 calories, 261 from fat, and 32-ounce chocolate shake at 770 calories, 160 from fat, for a grand total of 2,110 calories.

Who are these restaurants appealing to with these menu items? Research shows that men ages 18–24 make fast-food choices based on getting the most for the least amount of money, not on nutritional value. And don't be fooled by thinking that if it's salad it's healthy, because that can be far from the truth. Wendy's Baja Salad has 740 calories, 420 from fat and 1,990 mg of sodium. McDonald's Southwest Salad with Chicken without salad dressing has 430 calories, 20 grams of fat, and 920 mg of sodium.

On the other side of the coin, some healthy fast-food choices are Taco Bell's Chicken Soft taco with 150 calories, Wendy's Grilled Chicken Go Wrap with 127 calories, McDonald's Hamburger with 250 calories, and McDonald's Fruit and Yogurt Parfait with 160 calories.

See the box "Eating on the Run" for more suggestions on healthier fast-food choices.

TALKING POINTS Which fast-food restaurants are your favorites? Are you surprised at any of the information in this chapter regarding your favorite meals? Will you change your order next time you visit a fast-food restaurant?

Functional Foods

At the forefront of healthful nutrition is the identification and development of foods intended to affect a particular health problem or to improve the functional capability of the body. **Functional foods** contain not only recognized nutrients but also enhanced elements that impart medicine-like properties to the food. Alternative labels also exist for various subclasses of functional foods, such as *nutraceuticals,* or food elements that may be packaged in forms appearing more like medications (for example, pills or capsules), and *probiotics.*[26] **Probiotics** ("for life") are living bacteria ("good bugs") that are thought to help prevent disease and boost the immune system. Probiotic bacteria have been associated with alleviating allergies, irritable bowel, respiratory and urinary tract infections, and with cancer prevention. They make the environment in the digestive system inhospitable for harmful bacteria ("bad bugs"). More than 400 types of bacteria reside in and on our bodies and outnumber human cells 10 to 1. Yogurt is one example of a food that gives you a dose of these good bugs—*Lactobacillus bulgaricus.*

Examples of functional foods include garlic (believed to lower cholesterol), olive oil (thought to prevent heart disease), foods high in dietary fiber (which prevent constipation and lower cholesterol), and foods rich in calcium (which prevent osteoporosis). In addition, foods that contain high levels of vitamins A, C, and E—primarily fruits and vegetables—and provide the body with natural sources of antioxidants are functional foods.

Other functional foods are those that contain or are enriched with folic acid. These vitamin-B-family foods aid in the prevention of spina bifida and other neural tube defects and the prevention of heart disease. Foods that are rich in selenium are sometimes categorized as functional foods because of selenium's potential as an agent in cancer prevention. The FDA has approved a "heart healthy" label for foods that are rich in soy protein.[27] All of the functional foods discussed here are approved to carry **health claims** on the basis of current FDA criteria.[28] Phytosterols are another example of

a functional food. Phytosterols are found in plants and help lower cholesterol levels.[29] They can be found in oils, nuts, vegetables, fruits, and legumes.

One category of functional foods being researched is vegetables that are genetically engineered to produce a specific biological element that is important to human health. An example is tomatoes that are high in lycopene. Food technologists are interested in expanding the functional food family to include a greater array of health-enhancing food items.

Dietary Supplements

Americans spend $23 billion annually on a wide array of over-the-counter (OTC) products known collectively as *dietary supplements*. These unregulated, nonprescription products are legally described as[30]

- Products (other than tobacco) that are intended to supplement the diet, including vitamins, amino acids, minerals, glandular extracts, herbs, and other plant products such as fungi

- Products that are intended for use by people to supplement the total daily intake of nutrients in the diet

- Products that are intended to be ingested in tablet, capsule, soft gel, gelcap, and liquid form

- Products that are not in themselves to be used as conventional foods or as the only items of a meal or diet

Unlike prescription medications (see Chapter 12), dietary supplements have been available in the marketplace for years almost without restriction. However, dietary supplements now must be deemed safe for human use on the basis of information supplied to the FDA by the manufacturers. In addition, the labels on these products cannot make a direct claim, with the exception of calcium and folic acid supplements, that they can cure, treat, or prevent illnesses. However, other materials with such claims may be displayed close to the dietary supplements themselves. Further, the labels

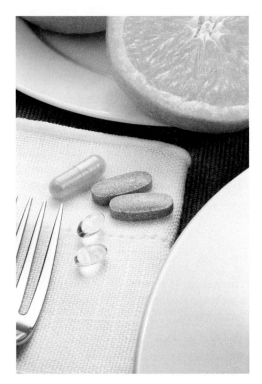

Consumers must decide for themselves whether to use dietary supplements.

Key Terms

functional foods Foods capable of contributing to the improvement/prevention of specific health problems.

probiotics Living bacteria ("good bugs") that help prevent disease and strengthen the immune system.

health claims Statements authorized by the FDA as having scientific proof of claims that a food, nutrient, or dietary supplement has an effect on a health-related condition.

---

on dietary supplements must remind consumers that the FDA doesn't have the authority to do the rigorous research required of prescription medications, and so the FDA cannot attest to their purity, quality, safety, or effectiveness. Beyond this, consumers are left to themselves to decide whether to purchase and use dietary supplements (see the box "Should You Take a Dietary Supplement?").

As was mentioned earlier, probiotic products, dietary supplements with live bacteria, are gaining in popularity, with sales of over $1.1 billion to date. Actimel is one of the biggest sellers, claiming to "help to strengthen your body's natural defenses" and enhance your immune system.[31]

Easily accessible to anyone, over 15,000 different dietary supplements can be purchased in grocery stores, drugstores, and discount stores; through mail-order catalogs; and over the Internet. Because of the great demand for these products, major pharmaceutical companies are now entering the dietary supplement field. Whether this trend leads to the development of more effective products, or to a greater effort on the part of the FDA to demand proof of effectiveness, remains to be seen. By definition, supplements are not foods but simply "supplements." Therefore, they remain free from requirements to substantiate their claims of effectiveness (as is now required for functional foods).

 TALKING POINTS A friend asks you about the advantages and disadvantages of taking a dietary supplement. What would you point out to your friend?

Food Allergies

Being intolerant to certain foods is not the same as being allergic to particular foods. **Food intolerance** means that a food upsets your intestines, usually because of an enzyme deficiency. A lactase deficiency, for example, causes lactose intolerance. Lactose intolerance affects 20 percent of Caucasian Americans, 75 percent of African Americans and Native Americans, 50 percent of Hispanic Americans, and 90 percent of Asian Americans. Intolerance to gluten (found in wheat, rye, barley, and perhaps oats) affects 1 of every 150 Americans and can cause malnutrition, premature osteoporosis, colon cancer, thyroid disease, diabetes, arthritis, miscarriage, and birth defects. The incidence of celiac disease has quadrupled in numbers; when someone with this autoimmune disease consumes gluten, an allergic reaction results.

A **food allergy** mistakenly calls the body's disease-fighting immune system into action, creating unpleasant and sometimes life-threatening symptoms. Peanuts, milk, eggs, shellfish, tree nuts, fish, soy, and wheat account for 90 percent of food allergies. Food allergies in American children have increased 18 percent over the past few years, with African American and Caucasian children having more food allergies than Hispanic children have. Eight percent of children and 2 percent of adults have food allergies. For some members of this group, food-based allergies may be serious or even life threatening.

Because food allergies generally develop slowly, initial symptoms may not be fully recognized or even associated with the food. It takes three exposures to the allergic food to obtain a significant food allergy reaction. The first time a person eats a food she is allergic to, she may have little or no reaction. The second time she eats this food, she will most likely have a more observable reaction, such as breaking out in hives, itching, having a runny nose, feeling a burning sensation in the mouth, and wheezing. The third exposure can bring on a full-blown reaction, which for peanut allergies, among others, can result in death within minutes. Also, food allergies can develop later in life. There is no cure for food allergies, and the treatment is to avoid these foods and to carry an EpiPen (epinephrine) at all times.

Food Safety

Technological advances in food manufacturing and processing have done much to ensure that the food we eat is fresh and safe. Yet concern is growing that certain recent developments may also produce harmful effects on humans. For example, the preparation, handling, and storage of food; irradiation of foods; and genetic engineering of foods all contribute to the safety of our food in terms of food contamination.

Preventing Foodborne Illness

Foodborne illness or food poisoning is the result of eating contaminated food. The symptoms of food poisoning can be easily mistaken for the flu—fatigue, chills, mild fever, dizziness, headaches, upset stomach, diarrhea, and cramps. Illness develops within one to six hours

Key Terms
food intolerance An adverse reaction to a specific food that does not involve the immune system; usually caused by an enzyme deficiency.
food allergy A reaction in which the immune system attacks an otherwise harmless food or ingredient; allergic reactions can range from mildly unpleasant to life threatening.

following ingestion of the contaminated food, and recovery is fairly rapid.[32] However, new research suggests that 10 percent of people who contract food poisoning from ingesting food with *Escherichia coli (E. coli)* develop a life-threatening illness, hemolytic uremic syndrome, which can cause kidneys and other major organs to eventually fail. Bacteria are the culprits in most cases of food poisoning, which can be the result of food not being cooked thoroughly to destroy bacteria or not being kept cool enough to slow their growth. In addition, nearly half of all cases of food poisoning can be prevented with proper hand washing so as to not contaminate food with viruses, parasites, or toxic chemicals. Food safety is such an important issue that the USDA incorporated it into the current dietary guidelines. Food should be refrigerated below 40° or kept warm above 140°. Between 40° and 140°, bacteria can double in number in as little as 20 minutes, so it is important to keep food at safe temperatures. (See Figure 5-5 on temperature rules for safe cooking and handling of foods.)

It is estimated that 1 of every 4 Americans is the victim of food poisoning each year, and about 5,000 of these people die.

Salmonella bacteria are the most common cause of foodborne illness and are found mostly in raw or undercooked poultry, meat, eggs, fish, peanut butter, fruits,

vegetables, unpasteurized milk, and even pet food. *Clostridium perfringens,* also called the "buffet germ," grows where there is little to no oxygen and grows fastest in large portions held at low or room temperatures. For this reason, buffet table servings should be replaced often and leftovers should be refrigerated quickly. Refrigerated leftovers may become harmful to eat after three days. The old adage "If in doubt, throw it out" applies to any questionable leftovers (see Table 5.4). A third type of food poisoning is botulism, which is rare but often fatal. It is caused by home-canned or commercially canned

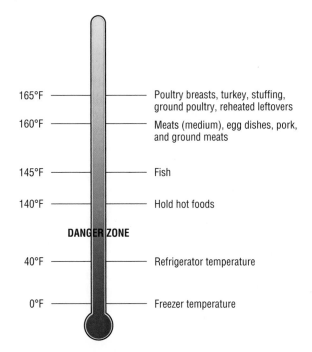

Figure 5-5 Temperature Rules for Cooking and Safe Handling of Food Keep food out of the danger zone between 40°F and 140°F, in which bacteria can multiply rapidly.

Source: U.S. Department of Health and Human Services and U.S. Department of Agriculture, Dietary Guidelines for Americans, 2010, www.healthierus.gov/dietaryguidelines.

Table 5.4 Cold Storage Limits	
Apples	3 weeks
Apricots, peaches, nectarines, pears	3–4 days
Bacon	1 week
Beans, green	3–4 days
Berries, cherries	1–2 days
Butter	1–3 months
Carrots	2 weeks
Cheese, hard	3–4 weeks
Cheese, soft	1 week
Chicken or turkey (fresh)	1–2 days
Chicken or turkey (cooked)	3–4 days
Citrus fruit	1–2 weeks
Deli and vacuum-packed products	3–5 days
Eggs (fresh, in shell)	3–5 weeks
Eggs (hard cooked)	1 week
Fish or seafood (fresh)	1–2 days
Fish (cooked)	3–4 days
Fish (canned, after opening)	3–4 days
Gravy and meat broth	1–2 days
Hot dogs (after opening)	1 week
Lettuce, leaf	3–7 days
Luncheon meat (after opening)	3–5 days
Margarine	4–5 months
Mayonnaise (after opening)	2 months
Milk (after opening)	5 days
Meat (fresh, ground)	1–2 days
Meat (fresh; steak, chops, roasts)	3–5 days
Meat (cooked)	3–4 days
Pizza (cooked)	3–4 days
Soups and stews	3–4 days
Spinach	1–2 days
Yogurt	7–14 days

Sources: Food Safety and Inspection Service, U.S. Department of Agriculture. Basics for Handling Food Safely, September 2006; Food Marketing Institute, *A Consumer Guide to Food Quality and Safe Handling.*

food that hasn't been processed or stored properly. Some warning signs are swollen or dented cans or lids, cracked jars, loose lids, and clear liquids turned milky. Can you tell if meat is spoiled by looking at it? Not necessarily. Some supermarkets package their meat with carbon monoxide, which reacts with the pigment in the meat to make it redder.

The Center for Science in the Public Interest found that fruits and vegetables account for the majority of foodborne illnesses. Salads are by far the biggest culprit. The reason for this seems to be that some of the water used to irrigate and wash produce is contaminated with human and animal feces. *E. coli* has historically been a harmless bacterium that resides in the guts of animals, including humans. A new and pathogenic strain called *E. coli* O157:H7 was identified in 1982 and now causes an estimated 73,000 cases of infection and 60 deaths in the United States each year. *E. coli* can be found in uncooked produce, raw milk, unpasteurized juice, contaminated water, and meat. Dozens of people contracted food poisoning from the green onions in food from Taco Bell restaurants in 2006. This same strain of *E. coli* was linked to the spinach that sickened 200 people in 2006. In 2009, over 600 people in 43 states were sickened by tainted peanut butter produced by the Peanut Corp of America (PCA). Twenty-three percent of these people were hospitalized and at least nine died as a result of salmonella poisoning. In its report on the PCA, the FDA found that poor sanitation in the form of bird feces, tainted water, and cockroaches accounted for the salmonella. In addition, the FDA contended that there were substandard food inspections so that the problem was not discovered and corrected quickly. In fact, the FDA issued a recall of the company's products from the previous two years, involving over 432 different products such as crackers, cookies, and ice cream.

A salmonella outbreak from eggs from infected hens occurred in 2010. Over 1,500 people became ill, and 550 million eggs from two facilities were recalled. Salmonella was found in chicken feed. A new FDA egg safety rule took effect later that year requiring new procedures for salmonella enteritidis testing and pasteurization. Another new food safety bill passed requiring that manufacturers alert government officials within 24 hours of knowledge of contaminated products, calling for more frequent inspections of food production facilities, giving regulators more power to recall products and suspend or shut down plants with poor safety records, and strengthening surveillance to track foodborne illnesses.[33]

Because produce comes from all over the world, this bacteria problem can be difficult to regulate or correct. Even the ready-to-eat bags of produce that boast they have been "thoroughly" or "triple" washed cannot be guaranteed to be bacteria-free. Washing the produce yourself may not solve the problem, either. Produce washes such as veggie wash don't claim to kill *E. coli,* but only to clean off wax, pesticides, and dirt. The best way to avoid getting sick from produce is to cook it so that you kill any remaining bacteria.

It is important to handle food properly to avoid food poisoning. Frequent hand washing is at the top of the list of food safety tips. Bacteria live and multiply on warm, moist hands, and hands can inadvertently transport germs from one surface to another. It is also important to clean work surfaces with hot, soapy water and keep nonfood items such as the mail, newspapers, and purses off the countertops. Some people advocate the use of antibacterial products; others maintain that if they are overused, these products can lose their effectiveness, and bacteria then become resistant to them. Utensils, dishes, cutting boards, cookware, and towels and sponges need to be washed in hot, soapy water and rinsed well.[34]

Food Irradiation

Because of the increasing concern about contaminated meat and meat products, the first irradiated meat, ground beef, arrived in American supermarkets in early 2000. Irradiated frozen chicken was introduced more recently. Irradiation is a process that causes damage to the DNA of disease-causing bacteria such as salmonella and *E. coli,* as well as of insects, parasites, and other organisms so that they can't reproduce. While irradiated meat has much lower bacteria levels than regular meat does, irradiation doesn't destroy all bacteria in meat. In fact, irradiation actually destroys fewer bacteria than does proper cooking.[35] The FDA also approved irradiation of spinach and lettuce to kill *E. coli* and other germs. There is some concern that irradiation will lull consumers into a false sense of security so that they erroneously believe that they don't have to take the usual precautions in food handling and preparation. For example, undercooking, unclean work surfaces, unwashed cooking utensils, and improper storage can still contaminate meat. Some also claim that irradiated meat has a distinct off-taste and a smell, like "singed hair."

Safe Farming Techniques

It has been suggested that there is an increase in the quality of meat when animals are treated humanely, with less bruising, more tenderness, lower incidence of dark-cutting beef, and lessened occurrence of pale, soft, and dry pork.

One important component in these reforms—some of which have been government mandated and others voluntarily adopted by the agricultural industry—relates to the feed given to beef cattle. The spread of bovine spongiform encephalopathy, more commonly known as mad cow disease, has largely been attributed to the use of animal feed containing the protein-rich by-products of slaughtered cows, including nerve tissue, the tissue most likely to harbor the disease. Such feed—which is believed to be the primary, if not the only, way the disease can be transmitted—was banned in the United States and Canada in August 1997.[32] However, from August 1997 to March 2004, 52 companies recalled 410 feed products because of suspected infectious prions, the proteins thought to spread mad cow disease. While the disease had been restricted to European cows, three cases of mad cow disease detected in American cattle from 2003 to 2006 encouraged the U.S. government to impose even stricter rules to protect the nation's beef supply from the disease, including banning the butchering of sick or injured cows, banning certain animal parts from the food supply, and increasing testing on suspect animals.[36]

Eliminating animal products from feed has also proven beneficial for hens. Many consumers choose to eat only poultry and eggs from free-range, vegetarian-fed chickens, for health and safety reasons. Several companies (such as Eggland's Best) claim that their vegetarian-fed hens produce eggs that have seven times more vitamin E, are lower in cholesterol, have a higher unsaturated/saturated fat ratio, and contain more omega-3 fatty acids than do factory-farmed eggs.[37]

There has also been increasing concern about giving chickens Roxarsone (3-Nitro) because it contains arsenic. It is given to chickens to fatten the birds faster and to kill microbes. Human antibiotics are also fed to chickens to increase their growth, but the bacteria in the chickens' intestines can develop resistance to the antibiotics. This can result in the antibiotic-resistant bacteria being passed along to people who consume this poultry, causing them to become ill and not respond to drugs typically prescribed to treat this illness.

In addition, recent studies have suggested that consumption of some types of fish may be hazardous to your health. Swordfish, halibut, albacore tuna, red snapper, flounder, freshwater bass, grouper, trout, marlin, king mackerel, tilefish, and shark all have been associated with toxic levels of mercury in people who consumed them regularly, some of whom had mercury levels more than double the amount the EPA deemed safe. Memory lapses, hair loss, stomach cramps, headaches, muscle and joint aches, nausea, and dizziness are the symptoms reported by people who had toxic levels of mercury from eating these fish. Mercury is also suspected to increase the risk of heart attack and has been linked with Alzheimer's disease and autism.[38]

Organic Foods

The USDA organic food labels went into effect in October 2002 to standardize regulations for food grown without

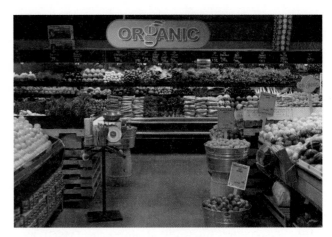

Organic products have grown in popularity in recent years and are now available in many major grocery stores.

synthetic pesticides or other chemicals. Under the new USDA rules, *organic* means the following:

- Meat, poultry, and eggs are from animals that have not been given growth hormones or antibiotics. Vitamin and mineral supplements are allowed. Livestock are given organic feed and live in conditions that allow for "exercise, freedom of movement, and reduction of stress."

- Products are not genetically engineered or irradiated to kill germs.

- Crops are grown on land that has not been fertilized with sewage sludge or chemical fertilizers.

- Pests and plant diseases are treated primarily with insect predators, traps, natural repellents, and other nonchemical methods.

- Weeds are controlled by mulching, mowing, hand weeding, or mechanical cultivation, not chemical herbicides.

There are different types of organic foods: "100 percent organic," which means the food contains all organic ingredients; "organic," which means at least 95 percent of the product is organic; and "made with organic ingredients," which means at least 70 percent of the food is organic as defined here.[39]

In recent years, the $24-billion organic food industry has enjoyed a 20 percent annual growth rate, much higher than that of the rest of the food industry. Almost 70 percent of people said they bought organic food at least once in the past three months. While organic foods have been found to have fewer pesticides, to do less damage to the environment, and possibly to have more nutrients, they can still contain some pesticide residue and chemical contaminants from the environment and have risk of *E. coli* contamination. See Chapter 16 for more information on the benefit of organic foods for health.

Food Additives

Today many people believe that the food they consume is unhealthy because of the 2,800 generally recognized as safe (GRAS) **food additives** that can be put into food during production, processing, and preparation. But should these additives be banned?

Food additives are substances added to food to preserve and improve its taste and appearance. Some additives are thickening agents, and some add color and prevent food from spoiling. Food additives are found in all types of foods and beverages, such as meat, soup, salad dressings, peanut butter, chips, cakes, cookies, and soda. Vinegar, food coloring, artificial sweeteners, white sugar, salt, monosodium glutamate (MSG), and antioxidants are some common examples of additives. For example, emulsifiers help give peanut butter a more consistent texture and prevent separation, while stabilizers and thickeners give ice cream a smoother, more uniform texture. The three most common additives are sugar, salt, and corn syrup.[40] Food additives must undergo FDA testing and approval to ensure that the benefits outweigh any risks associated with them. There has been some debate about how safe some additives are despite their FDA approval. Some of the ones in question are aspartame (NutraSweet); red, blue, yellow, and green food coloring; saccharin; propyl gallate; potassium bromate; sodium nitrate; and stevia. Many of these additives have been linked with an increased risk of cancer.

Genetically Modified Foods

Genetically modified foods are crops that are bred with genes engineered in labs so that they are more resistant to pests, disease, drought, and cold; produce higher yields; and have a higher nutritional content. Ten percent of farm acreage worldwide is planted with genetically engineered or biotech crops, an increase from 1 percent 15 years ago. Soybeans, corn, cotton, canola, sugar beets, alfalfa, papaya, summer squash, and potato are the most commonly grown genetically engineered crops.[41] The success of American agriculture, in terms of food quality and marketability, has been based on the ability to genetically alter food sources to improve yield, reduce production costs, and introduce new food characteristics. Today, however, genetic technology is so sophisticated that changes are being introduced faster than scientists can fully evaluate their effects. Concerned individuals and agencies in the United States and abroad called for more extensive longitudinal research into safety issues and stricter labeling requirements for genetically modified foods. In January 2001, the FDA determined that food companies did not need to label foods as having genetically modified components, although they could inform consumers the foods are "derived through biotechnology." They had argued that without these measures consumers would have been at risk for unrecognized problems.

In 2008, the FDA finally decided after seven years of discussion to allow the commercial use of genetically engineered animals. The FDA stated that it would allow animals to be genetically altered if such animals produce drugs, serve as models for human disease, produce industrial or consumer products, or have improved food-use qualities such as being more nutritious. Animals are considered genetically altered when either their genes are changed or genes from another animal are added for a specific purpose. This regulation is consistent with legislation concerning giving drugs to animals for similar reasons.[42]

Key Terms

food additives Chemical compounds intentionally added to the food supply to change some aspect of the food, such as its color or texture.

genetically modified foods Crops that are bred with genes engineered in labs so the crops are improved, such as being drought, pest, or cold resistant; producing a higher yield; and/or having a higher nutritional content.

Taking Charge of Your Health

- Take the Personal Assessment "Rate Your Plate" at the end of the chapter to rate your eating habits.

- Take the Personal Assessment "Are You Feeding Your Feelings?" at the end of the chapter to determine if you are an emotional eater.

- Look on MyPlate.gov to find your personal food plan.

- Keep track of your food intake for a week, using the pyramid tracker on MyPlate.gov, and see how well your intake reflects the new dietary guidelines.

- Make one change per week in your eating patterns, such as drinking skim milk or including a new fruit or vegetable.

- Assess your physical activity level using MyPlate.gov.

SUMMARY

- Carbohydrates are composed of sugar units and are the major source of energy for the body. About 45–65 percent of our calories should come from carbohydrates.
- Fats provide a concentrated source of energy for the body and keep us from feeling hungry. No more than 20–35 percent of our calories should come from fats, and most of these fats should be polyunsaturated or monounsaturated.
- Foods containing trans fats should be avoided as much as possible, and less than 10 percent of our calories should come from saturated fats, according to the current dietary guidelines.
- Protein primarily promotes growth and maintenance of body tissue, and is also a source of energy.
- The USDA Dietary Guidelines for Americans focus on the roles that trans fat, saturated fat, sugar, sodium, and alcohol play in weight management and health and disease.

These guidelines also address the importance of daily physical activity.
- Preventive strategies—such as hand washing and proper preparation, cooking, and storage of food—can help decrease foodborne illnesses.
- Vitamins serve as catalysts for body responses and are found in water-soluble and fat-soluble forms.
- Minerals are incorporated into various tissues of the body and participate in regulatory functions within the body.
- An adequate amount of water and other fluids is required by the body daily and is obtained from a variety of food sources, including beverages.
- Fast foods should play only a limited role in daily food intake because of their high fat density and their high levels of sugar and sodium.

REVIEW QUESTIONS

1. Which nutrients supply the body with calories?
2. What is the function of fat in nutritional health besides serving as the body's primary means of storage for excess calories? What is the basis of our current concern about saturated fats, cholesterol, and trans-fatty acids?
3. What is the principal role of protein in the body? How can complete protein be obtained by people who eat few or no animal products?
4. What role do vitamins play in the body? What is the current perception regarding the need for vitamin supplementation?
5. What functions do minerals have in the body? What is a trace element?
6. What do the Dietary Guidelines for Americans suggest in terms of physical activity, and what are the benefits of physical activity?
7. What is the recommendation for daily fluid intake?
8. What are the dietary recommendations regarding trans fat, saturated fat, and sodium intake?
9. Identify each of the food groups in MyPlate.
10. What information can be obtained from our current food labels?

ANSWERS TO THE "WHAT DO YOU KNOW?" QUIZ

1. True   2. True   3. False   4. False   5. False   6. True   7. False

Visit the Online Learning Center (**www.mhhe.com/hahn11e**), where you will find tools to help you improve your grade including practice quizzes, key terms flashcards, audio chapter summaries for your MP3 player, and many other study aids.

SOURCE NOTES

1. Wardlaw GM, Smith A. *Contemporary Nutrition: Issues and Insights.* New York: McGraw-Hill, 2010.
2. Wardlaw GM, Byrd-Bradbenner C, Moe G, Beshgetoor D, Berning J. *Perspectives in Nutrition* (8th ed.). New York: McGraw-Hill, 2002.
3. Kummerow FA, Zhou Q, Mahfouz MM. Effect of trans-fatty acids on calcium influx into human arterial endothelial cells. *American Journal of Clinical Nutrition,* 70(5), 832–838, 1999.
4. Duyff R. *American Dietetic Association Complete Food and Nutrition Guide* (3rd ed.). Hoboken, NJ: Wiley, 2006.
5. *Caring for Your School-Age Child: 5–12.* American Academy of Pediatrics, 2001.
6. National Institutes of Health. *Practical Guide to the Identification, Evaluation, and Treatment of Overweight and Obesity in Adults.* Bethesda, MD: Author, 2001.
7. Soyonara: tough times for the miracle bean. *Nutrition Action,* October 2006.
8. Soy what? *Nutrition Action,* November 2009.
9. National Academy of Sciences. *Dietary Reference Intakes.* Washington, DC: National Acadamies Press, 2004.
10. Jacques PF, et al. The effect of folic acid fortification on plasma folate and total homocysteine concentrations. *New England Journal of Medicine,* 340(19), 1449–1454, 1999.
11. Vitamin E. *Vegetarian Times,* October 2006.
12. Getting enough: what you don't eat can hurt you. *Nutrition Action,* September 2010.
13. Antioxidants: still hazy after all these years. *Nutrition Action,* November 2005.
14. www.starbucks.com/menu.
15. Sears W, Sears M. *The Family Nutrition Book.* New York: Little, Brown, 1999.
16. Study: eating more fiber could mean longer life. *USA Today,* February 15, 2011.

17. FDA allows whole oat foods to make health claims on reducing the risk of heart disease. *FDA Talk Paper,* January 1998.
18. The changing American diet. *Nutrition Action,* April 2006.
19. www.health.gov/dietary/guidelines/dga, 2010.
20. American Cancer Society. *Cancer Facts and Figures.* The Association, 2010.
21. Flour power: a slice of multigrain can taste like bread. *USA Today,* August 9, 2004.
22. Sugar overload. *Nutrition Action,* January/February 2010.
23. Cook N, Cutler J, Osborzanck E, Buring I, Rexrode K, Kummyika S., et al. Long-term effects of sodium reduction on cardiovascular disease outcomes: observational follow-up of trials of hypertension. Prevention (TOMP). *British Medical Journal,* 334, 885, April 2007.
24. Keeping a lid on salt: not so easy. *USA Today,* April 28, 2010.
25. Debuting in 2012: what's in the beef? *USA Today,* December 29, 2010.
26. Some bacteria for brunch? *U.S. News & World Report,* December 10, 2007.
27. FDA approves new health claim for soy protein and coronary heart disease [FDA talk paper]. U.S. Food and Drug Administration Center for Food Safety and Applied Nutrition, October 20, 1999. www.fda.gov/fdac/bbs/topics/ANSWERS/ANS00980.html.
28. Kurtzweil P. Staking a claim to good health, *FDA Consumer,* November–December 1998.
29. 10 mega-trends in the supermarket. *Nutrition Action,* May 2003.
30. Dietary Supplement Health and Education Act of 1994, U.S. Food and Drug Administration, Center for Food Safety and Applied Nutrition, December 1, 1995.
31. A bug for what's bugging you. *USA Today,* July 9, 2003.
32. Oppel RA, Jr. Infected cow old enough to have eaten now-banned feed. *New York Times,* December 30, 2003.
33. Egg crisis piques interest in bill. *USA Today,* August 25, 2010.
34. Rinzler C. *Nutrition for Dummies* (4th ed.). Hoboken, NJ: Wiley, 2006.
35. The truth about irradiated meat. *Consumer Reports,* 34–37, August 2003.
36. Grady D. U.S. imposes stricter safety rules for preventing mad cow disease. *New York Times,* December 31, 2003.
37. Corporate website, www.eggland.com.
38. Jetter, A. How safe is your food? *Reader's Digest,* August 2003.
39. USDA gives bite to organic label. *USA Today,* October 16, 2002.
40. Insel P, Turner E, Ross D. *Nutrition.* Sudbury, MA: Jones & Bartlett, 2007.
41. Farmers growing more genetically engineered crops. *USA Today,* February 23, 2011.
42. FDA moves on genetically altered animals. *USA Today,* September 19, 2008

Personal Assessment

Rate Your Plate

Take a closer look at yourself, your current food decisions, and your lifestyle. Think about your typical eating pattern and food decisions.

Do You . . .

	Usually	Sometimes	Never
Consider the MyPlate nutrition model when you make food choices?	❏	❏	❏
Try to eat regular meals (including breakfast), rather than skip or skimp on some?	❏	❏	❏
Choose nutritious snacks?	❏	❏	❏
Try to eat a variety of foods?	❏	❏	❏
Include new-to-you foods in meals and snacks?	❏	❏	❏
Try to balance your energy (calorie) intake with your physical activity?	❏	❏	❏

Now for the Details

Do You . . .

	Usually	Sometimes	Never
Consume half your grains as whole-grain products?	❏	❏	❏
Eat at least 2½ cups of vegetables daily?	❏	❏	❏
Eat at least 2 cups of fruits daily?	❏	❏	❏
Consume at least 3 cups of milk, yogurt, or cheese daily?	❏	❏	❏
Choose low-fat foods?	❏	❏	❏
Choose low-sodium foods?	❏	❏	❏
Drink 8 or more cups of fluids daily?	❏	❏	❏
Limit alcoholic beverages (no more than 1 daily for a woman or 2 for a man)?	❏	❏	❏

Score Yourself

Usually = 2 points
Sometimes = 1 point
Never = 0 points

If you scored . . .

24 or more points—Healthful eating seems to be your fitness habit already. Still, look for ways to stick to a healthful eating plan—and to make a "good thing" even better.

16 to 23 points—You're on track. A few easy changes could help you make your overall eating plan healthier.

9 to 15 points—Sometimes you eat smart—but not often enough to be your "fitness best."

0 to 8 points—For your good health, you're wise to rethink your overall eating style. Take it gradually—step by step!

TO CARRY THIS FURTHER . . .

Whatever your score, make moves for healthful eating. Gradually turn your "nevers" into "sometimes" and your "sometimes" into "usually." Try some of the suggestions from the discussion of MyPlate and the Dietary Guidelines for Americans.

Source: Adapted from *The American Dietetic Association's Monthly Nutrition Companion: 31 Days to a Healthier Lifestyle*, by R. Duyff, Chronimed Publishing, 1997. Copyright © 1997 American Dietetic Association. Reproduced with permission of John Wiley & Sons, Inc. and the Leap First Literary Agency.

Personal Assessment

Are You Feeding Your Feelings?

Sometimes people use food as a way of coping with their emotions and problems. To identify how you might be using food as a coping strategy and what feelings you tend to associate with eating, complete the following inventory.

0 = Never
1 = Rarely
2 = Occasionally
3 = Often
4 = Always

1. _____ Do you eat when you are angry?
2. _____ When you feel annoyed, do you turn to food?
3. _____ If someone lets you down, do you eat to comfort yourself?
4. _____ When you are having a bad day, do you notice that you eat more?
5. _____ Do you eat to cheer yourself up?
6. _____ Do you use food as a way of avoiding tasks you don't want to do?
7. _____ Do you view food as your friend when you are feeling lonely?
8. _____ Is food a way for you to comfort yourself when your life seems empty?
9. _____ When you are feeling upset, do you turn to food to calm yourself down?
10. _____ Do you eat more when you are anxious, worried, or stressed?
11. _____ Does eating help you to cope with feeling overwhelmed?
12. _____ Do you eat more when you are going through big changes or transitions in your life?
13. _____ Do you reward yourself with food?
14. _____ When you think you have done something wrong, do you punish yourself by eating?
15. _____ When you are feeling badly about yourself, do you eat more?
16. _____ When you feel discouraged about your efforts to improve yourself, do you eat more, thinking "What's the use of trying"?

_____ **TOTAL SCORE**

Interpretation

If you scored . . .
0 to 16—You don't eat to cope with your emotions. Your eating may not be related to your emotional state. However, you may avoid eating when you are upset or having trouble coping with your feelings. You may run away from food rather than running to food to cope.

17 to 47—Although you fall in the average range, you may use food to deal with specific situations or feelings such as anger, loneliness, or boredom. See the breakdown of scores below to identify how you may be using food to cope with particular feelings.

48 to 64—You run to food to cope with your emotions, and you may want to consider developing other ways of appropriately expressing your feelings.

Next, look more closely at your specific responses . . .
If you answered "3" or "4" to most of questions 1–4, this can be indicative of eating when you are angry.

If you answered "3" or "4" to most of questions 5–8, this can be indicative of eating when you are lonely or bored.

If you answered "3" or "4" to most of questions 9–12, this can be an indication that you are a stress eater.

If you answered "3" or "4" to most of questions 13–16, this can be an indication that you are using food to cope with feelings of low self-esteem and self-worth.

TO CARRY THIS FURTHER . . .

- Use the assessment scores to help you learn to recognize the triggers for your emotional eating.
- Make a list of things to do when you get the urge to eat and you're not hungry. Try going for a walk or calling a friend to distract yourself.
- Do something fun if you are tempted to eat to avoid work or a dreaded task.
- Reward yourself with things other than food.

Source: Adapted from *Nutrition for Healthy Living.* Courtesy of Marcy Leeds.

6

Maintaining a Healthy Weight

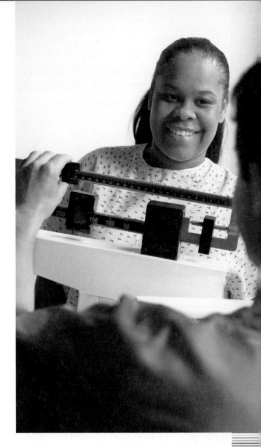

What Do You Know About Weight Management?

1. The number of Americans who are overweight or obese has been increasing over the past few years. True or False?

2. Body mass index (BMI) is a good way to assess body composition to determine if you are under- or overweight or in the normal weight range. True or False?

3. Socioeconomic status is not a contributing factor to developing obesity. True or False?

4. Most diets are effective for long-lasting weight management if you follow them correctly. True or False?

5. A goal of losing 5 pounds per week is a reasonable goal. True or False?

6. Diet pills and supplements are an effective method to manage your weight. True or False?

7. Bulimia nervosa is the most common eating disorder. True or False?

Check your answers at the end of the chapter.

Body Weight and Wellness

Weight management has become an obsession in American culture, as well as a significant health problem. In the United States, obesity has risen at an epidemic rate during the past 20 years. In fact, obesity is now equal to smoking as a threat to Americans' health. While smoking causes more deaths, obesity is related to more illnesses. One of the national health objectives for the year 2010 was to reduce the prevalence of obesity among adults to less than 15 percent.[1] Research indicates that the situation is worsening rather than improving. According to the National Center for Chronic Disease Prevention and Health Promotion, an estimated 66 percent of adult Americans are either overweight or obese (see Figure 6-1).[2] Currently, 34.3 percent, or 73 million, adult Americans are obese with more women (35 percent) than men (33 percent) meeting the criteria for obesity. The incidence of obesity was highest for people 40–59 years of age for both men and women. Rates were higher for African American women (50 percent) than for Mexican American women (45 percent) or Caucasian women (40 percent). Up 74 percent since 1991, the number of overweight children and adolescents has tripled in the past 20 years.[3]

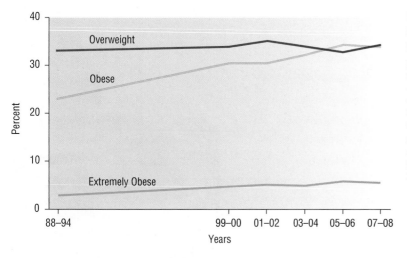

Figure 6-1 Trends in Overweight, Obesity, and Extreme Obesity Among Adults Aged 20 and Over, United States, 1988–2008

Notes: Age-adjusted by the direct method to the year 2000 U.S. Census Bureau estimates, using the age groups 20–39, 40–59, and 60 years and over. Pregnant females were excluded. Overweight is defined as a body mass index (BMI) of 25 or greater but less than 30; obesity is a BMI greater than or equal to 30; extreme obesity is a BMI greater than or equal to 40.

Source: Centers for Disease Control and Prevention, National Center for Health Statistics, National Health and Nutrition Examination Survey III 1988–1994, 1999–2000, 2001–2002, 2003–2004, 2005–2006, and 2007–2008.

People who are overweight are 40 percent more likely to die prematurely than people who are at a healthy weight. Obesity may account for as many as 400,000 deaths annually.[4]

Defining Overweight and Obesity

What's the difference between overweight and obesity? Doctors usually define **overweight** as a condition in which a person's weight is 1–19 percent higher than normal, as defined by a standard height/weight chart. **Obesity** is usually defined as a condition in which a person's weight is 20 percent or more above normal weight (see Figure 6-1). *Morbid obesity* refers to being 50–100 percent above normal weight, more than 100 pounds over normal weight, or sufficiently overweight to interfere with health or normal functioning.[4]

Some clinicians and laypersons continue to use standard height/weight tables to determine when weight is excessive. However, more precise techniques to determine body composition are currently available. Several of these techniques, including waist-to-hip ratio, body mass index, "Bod Pod" assessment, electrical impedance, skinfold measurements, and hydrostatic weighing, are described in the following sections.

Key Terms

overweight A condition in which a person's excess fat accumulation results in a body weight that exceeds desirable weight by 1–19 percent.

obesity A condition in which a person's body weight is 20 percent or more above desirable weight as determined by standard height/weight charts.

body image One's subjective perception of how one's body appears to oneself and others.

Obesity and Disease

Among the health problems caused by or complicated by obesity are increased surgical risk, hypertension, various forms of heart disease, stroke, type 2 diabetes, several forms of cancer, deterioration of joints, arthritis, complications during pregnancy, gallbladder disease, and an overall increased risk of mortality. Obesity is so closely associated with these chronic conditions that medical experts now recommend that obesity itself be defined and treated as a chronic disease.[5]

Research shows that women who have more fat concentrated around their waist, as opposed to their hips, have a greater risk of cardiovascular disease and diabetes. This has been referred to as the "apple versus pear shape" phenomenon. Whether you're an apple or a pear depends on where your body stores its excess fat. If fat tends to gather high around your abdomen, you're an apple. If it collects more around your hips and thighs, you're a pear.

 TALKING POINTS If a friend or close family member were dangerously overweight or obese, how would you express your concern?

Body Image and Sociocultural Standards for Weight

While the definition of overweight is clearly delineated as being above the norm in terms of the standards for height, weight, and gender, there still remains a great deal of confusion about who fits into this category. What is normal? Sociocultural ideals of body image, as discussed in the box "Mirror, Mirror on the Wall," vary significantly from the standards set in the height/weight charts. **Body image** refers to the subjective perception of how one's body appears to oneself and others. Current cultural standards suggest that women should be tall and very thin and men should be tall and muscular. People often compare themselves to actors and models and look to

Mirror, Mirror on the Wall

Television, magazines, billboards, movies, and a variety of other sources constantly bombard us with messages about how we should look. How realistic are these images? While the average woman's measurements are 37-29-40 (chest, waist, hips), store mannequins measure 38-18-28. The average American woman is 5 feet 4 inches tall, weighs 140 pounds, and wears a size 12–14. The average American female model is 5 feet 11 inches tall, weighs 117 pounds, and wears a size 2. Very early in our lives, we receive messages about how we should aspire to look with unrealistic models such as the Barbie doll, whose measurements at life-size would be equivalent to a person who is 5 feet 9 inches tall, weighs 110 pounds, and measures 39-18-33. G.I. Joe in life-size form would have a 55-inch chest and 27-inch biceps. Batman would be 7 feet tall with a 57-inch chest, a 30-inch waist, and 27-inch biceps. Fairy tales reinforce these messages as the thin, beautiful heroine becomes a princess and finds true love while the ugly, larger-bodied women are the villains, the evil stepmothers or stepsisters. Beauty is the most important quality for women, the evil queen tells us in *Snow White,* as she asks her magic mirror each day, "Who is the fairest of us all?" Men are not immune to these messages—the strong, handsome men are the princes who have the wealth and the beautiful women, while those who are not as attractive are seen as weak, pitiful, or evil.

Do we really buy into these messages? Researchers found that girls in middle school who read dieting articles were two to three times more likely to develop eating-disordered behaviors than those who didn't. While 44 percent of girls reported reading diet articles, only 14 percent of boys did, and this didn't seem to translate into these boys developing eating problems later in life. Another study showed that after women looked at a fashion magazine for three minutes, 70 percent of them became significantly more depressed and felt guilty and ashamed. A recent poll of 1,000 women showed that they would take extreme measures to attain their ideal weight, as 21 percent said they would give up 10 years of their lives, 23 percent said they would spend a week in jail, 23 percent said they would shave their head, and 22 percent said they would wear a bikini on television in order to do so. Eighty-five percent said they would rather have an extra toe than weigh 50 pounds more than they currently weigh. Certainly, it appears that these media messages have a strong negative influence on women's self-esteem, body image, and behavior.

Dove's "Real Beauty" ad campaign has broken out of this mold and takes a risk by featuring real women, not models, sizes 6–14, to advertise its beauty and soap products. Rather than claiming that its beauty products will morph you into a smaller, thinner, unrealistic image, Dove is suggesting in its ads that if you buy its products, you will feel more self-accepting and confident.

Bath & Body Works is focusing on preteens and teens in its line of shampoos and lotions under the American Girl brand, and their advertising addresses beauty "inside and out." Nike has also employed this type of advertising campaign with its use of a mixture of real women and pro athlete models showing their "big butts" and "thunder thighs." Wal-Mart's ads use real women to show that "fashion is reachable for everybody," and Wal-Mart has been using employees and their families in its ads since 1989. There was a great furor in Spain's top fashion show in 2006 when 30 percent of the models were ejected from the show for being too thin, having a body mass index under 18 when under 18.5 is considered underweight and unhealthy. This is quite a reverse from the trend of models being anorexic-looking and being rejected if they are not underweight.

What can you do as a consumer? Support companies such as Dove, Nike, and Wal-Mart that are moving in the right direction in terms of allowing for a broader definition of beauty. Don't read magazines that will quickly make you feel bad about yourself. Choose not to watch television programs such as *The Biggest Loser: Weight Loss Edition,* or *Extreme Makeover;* instead, watch programs such as *Glee,* which sends the message that being smart, genuine, and passionate about life is more important than appearance. Focus on body self-acceptance and attaining self-esteem and self-worth from all aspects of yourself, not just appearance.

What do you think about the message in this outdoor ad from the Dove "Real Beauty" campaign?

Sources: What's a girl to do? Hot and brainy brings mixed emotions, *USA Today,* July 25, 2006; Ad campaigns tell women to celebrate who they are, *The Star Press,* July 10, 2005; Unhealthy obsession: girls who read diet articles show later signs of eating disorders, *The Star Press,* January 2, 2007; Real curvy women betray media image of beauty, *The Star Press,* August 27, 2005; Dove ads enlist all shapes, styles and sizes, *USA Today,* August 29, 2005; Would you trade 10 years of life to be an ideal weight? *USA Today,* January 7, 2008.

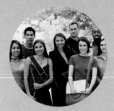

Learning from Our Diversity

Gender, Clothing Sizes, and Body Image Around the World

You are in London, England, and decide to buy some of the latest British fashions. You find a pair of pants you like and try them on. They don't fit. In fact, nothing in your size fits. Why not? Because not all sizes are the same for women.

As you can see from the table below, if you wear a size 12 in American stores, you will need to find a size 14 in British stores or an 11 in Japanese stores or a 42 in Parisian boutiques.* Is this true for men's clothing? No, you will find that a waist size of 38 is the same in American, British, and Japanese clothing. Why is this? Well, it is the same reason that you will find that not all women's size-12 clothing is the same even in the same country! What you will find is that the more expensive the clothing, the smaller the size compared to its true size. In other words, you can compare a pair of jeans from a discount store to the identical pair of pants in an expensive department store and find that the expensive pants are labeled one to two sizes smaller than the pants in the discount store. You will also discover that the smaller-size pants have

a much larger price tag. Again, does this hold true for men's clothing? No, it doesn't. The reason is that women will pay more for a smaller size, a lot more, while most men will not. There is not a market for smaller-size clothing for men the way there is for women. The fashion industry calls this "faith-based sizing" because consumers want to believe that they are the size the label tells them they are even if the scale says something different. This is also referred to as "vanity sizing."[†]

Men, however, are not immune to the trend of rising obesity around the world. In Cyprus, the Czech Republic, Finland, Germany, Greece, Malta, and Slovakia, proportionately more men are overweight or obese than in America. Although the Mediterranean diet has been touted as a healthy diet, the rate of obesity is also higher in the Mediterranean countries.[‡]

Eating disorders and distorted eating are more prevalent in cultures adopting Westernized values. One startling example of how quickly and significantly Western ideals of beauty can influence others was seen when television first came to the island of Fiji in 1995. Before the introduction of television, a common compliment given to someone was "you've gained weight," and dieting was almost nonexistent. Telling someone that he or she looked thin was a way of saying that the person didn't look well. Within three years of having television, the number of teenagers at risk for eating disorders more than doubled; 74 percent of teens said they felt too big or too fat, and 62 percent reported that they had been dieting in the past month.[§]

In the United States and other Westernized societies, the cultural ideal for beauty is becoming thinner and thinner. A generation ago, a model weighed 8 percent less than the average woman did, but she now weighs 23 percent less. With clothing available in sizes as low as 00, there is a message for women to aspire to nothingness. What can be done about this alarming trend? Women can refuse to buy more expensive clothes just because they are labeled with smaller sizes, as men have done for years. We can glorify all sizes and shapes of women. As Angel, a 17-year-old high school basketball player from West Los Angeles stated, "I'm 5 feet 8 inches and 165 pounds. I'm not a size 4. I'm tall. I'm muscular. I'm a thick girl. I accept that."[**]

Clothing Size Comparisons

Women's Clothing

USA	4	6	8	10	12	14	16	18	20
UK	6	8	10	12	14	16	18	20	22
Russia	40	42	44	46	48	50	52	54	56
Spain/France	34	36	38	40	42	44	46	48	50
Italy	38	40	42	44	46	48	50	52	54
Germany	32	34	36	38	40	42	44	46	48
Japan	3	5	7	9	11	13	15	17	19

Men's Clothing

Suits, Sweaters, Jackets, and Pants

USA	34	36	38	40	42	44	46	48
UK	34	36	38	40	42	44	46	48
Europe	44	46	48	50	52	54	56	58
Japan	S	–	M	–	–	L	–	–

Shirt Collars

USA	14	14½	15	15½	16	16½	17	17½
UK	14	14½	15	15½	16	16½	17	17½
Europe	36	37	38	39	40	41	42	43
Japan	36	37	38	39	40	41	42	43

Source: www.hostelscentral.com/hostels-article-34.html.

*International clothes sizes compared, www.hostelscentral.com.
[†]Faith-based sizing, *Newsweek*, October 18, 2006.
[‡]Some European countries more obese than in U.S., *USA Today*, March 28, 2005.
[§]Kilbourne, J, *Can't Buy My Love* (New York: Simon & Schuster, 1999).
[**]The new girls, *Oprah Magazine*, May 2004.

them for the standards for beauty. However, the average actress or model is thinner than 95 percent of the female population and weighs 23 percent less than the average woman.[6]

People may become dissatisfied and concerned about their inability to achieve these ideals. The scope of this dissatisfaction is evident as 75 percent of women think they need to lose weight and 60 percent are dissatisfied with their stomachs, hips, and thighs.[7] When

this type of dissatisfaction exists, people begin to question their attractiveness, and their self-esteem tends to decline.

Overall, men report feeling more comfortable with their weight and perceive less pressure to be thin than women do. A national survey showed that 41 percent of men were dissatisfied with their weight, with many of these men wanting to gain weight and increase muscle mass. While the average American woman wants to lose

11 pounds, the average American man wants to lose 1 pound or is happy with his weight.[8]

See the box "Gender, Clothing Sizes, and Body Image Around the World" for more on issues related to weight and self-concept.

Measuring and Assessing Weight and Body Fat Composition

Some of the techniques used to determine overweight and obesity are common and are routinely used by the general public. Others are expensive and of limited availability.

Body Mass Index

One method for assessing healthy body weight is the **body mass index (BMI).** BMI is calculated metrically as weight divided by height squared (kg/m²). The BMI does not reflect body composition (fat versus lean tissue) or consider the degree of fat accumulated in the central body cavity. It is, nevertheless, widely used in determining obesity. Overweight is defined as a BMI between 25 and 29.9. Individuals are considered obese with a BMI of 30 or above. Severe or morbid obesity is when the BMI is greater than 40.[9] See Table 6.1 on page 130 to determine the healthy BMI range for your height.

Once you have determined your BMI, you can find out whether it falls within a healthy range by using Table 6.1.

Height/Weight Tables

Height/weight tables were originally developed in 1983 to assist people in determining the relationship between their weight and desirable standards. Nearly every version of these tables has come under criticism for not considering variables such as gender, age, frame size, and body composition.[10] Some versions were thought to be too rigorous in establishing cutoff points for ideal or **desirable weight,** and others were deemed too generous. Although still available, these tables are being gradually replaced by other assessment techniques.

Waist and Hip Measurement

You can determine your **healthy body weight** by using the weight guidelines found in the Dietary Guidelines for Americans. This assessment involves two body measurements: BMI and waist circumference. Another method to determine if you are at a healthy body weight is using the waist-to-hip ratio (WHR). An acceptable WHR for women is near the lower end of each weight range, and for men it is at the higher end of each weight range.

To make a WHR determination, follow these steps:

1. Measure around your waist near your navel while you stand relaxed (not pulling in your stomach).
2. Measure around your hips, over the buttocks where the hips are largest.
3. Divide the waist measurement by the hip measurement.

Women with a WHR of less than 0.80 generally have a body weight that falls within the healthy range for their age and height; men with a WHR of less than 0.90 will also probably fall within the range considered healthy for their age and height.

This system was developed because of the growing concern over the relationship between the amount of fat located around the waist, the "spare tire," and the development of several serious health problems. As a point of interest, the Dietary Guidelines for Americans do not use WHR as a clinical marker for the treatment of obesity; instead, they use only waist circumference. The risk of health problems such as heart disease and diabetes increases at a waist measurement of 35 inches for women and 40 inches for men, regardless of height.[11]

Appearance

While it may seem as though the simplest method of determining one's body size is to look in the mirror, for most people this is not an accurate measure. In a study of college students, 42 percent underestimated their weight.[12]

There is also an important difference between one's internal concept of one's body and actual body perception, and this is particularly problematic for people with eating disorders.

Home Scale

Most people use scales at home or in a gym to determine their weight, but scales can be highly inaccurate, as evidenced by weighing yourself on a variety of scales and getting different readings. Also, you will probably weigh

---

Key Terms

body mass index (BMI) A mathematical calculation based on weight and height; used to determine desirable body weight.

desirable weight The weight range deemed appropriate for people, taking into consideration gender, age, and frame size.

healthy body weight Body weight within a weight range appropriate for a person with an acceptable waist-to-hip ratio.

Table 6.1 Body Mass Index (BMI)

BMI	Normal (18.5–24.9)						Overweight (25–29.9)					Obese (≥ 30)										Extreme Obesity
	19	20	21	22	23	24	25	26	27	28	29	30	31	32	33	34	35	36	37	38	39	40
Height (inches)											Body Weight (pounds)											
58	91	96	100	105	110	115	119	124	129	134	138	143	148	153	158	162	167	172	177	181	186	191
59	94	99	104	109	114	119	124	128	133	138	143	148	153	158	163	168	173	178	183	188	193	198
60	97	102	107	112	118	123	128	133	138	143	148	153	158	163	168	174	179	184	189	194	199	204
61	100	106	111	116	122	127	132	137	143	148	153	158	164	169	174	180	185	190	195	201	206	211
62	104	109	115	120	126	131	136	142	147	153	158	164	169	175	180	186	191	196	202	207	213	218
63	107	113	118	124	130	135	141	146	152	158	163	169	175	180	186	191	197	203	208	214	220	225
64	110	116	122	128	134	140	145	151	157	163	169	174	180	186	192	197	204	209	215	221	227	232
65	114	120	126	132	138	144	150	156	162	168	174	180	186	192	198	204	210	216	222	228	234	240
66	118	124	130	136	142	148	155	161	167	173	179	186	192	198	204	210	216	223	229	235	241	247
67	121	127	134	140	146	153	159	166	172	178	185	191	198	204	211	217	223	230	236	242	249	255
68	125	131	138	144	151	158	164	171	177	184	190	197	203	210	216	223	230	236	243	249	256	262
69	128	135	142	149	155	162	169	176	182	189	196	203	209	216	223	230	236	243	250	257	263	270
70	132	139	146	153	160	167	174	181	188	195	202	209	216	222	229	236	243	250	257	264	271	278
71	136	143	150	157	165	172	179	186	193	200	208	215	222	229	236	243	250	257	265	272	279	286
72	140	147	154	162	169	177	184	191	199	206	213	221	228	235	242	250	258	265	272	279	287	294
73	144	151	159	166	174	182	189	197	204	212	219	227	235	242	250	257	265	272	280	288	295	302
74	148	155	163	171	179	186	194	202	210	218	225	233	241	249	256	264	272	280	287	295	303	311
75	152	160	168	176	184	192	200	208	216	224	232	240	248	256	264	272	279	287	295	303	311	319
76	156	164	172	180	189	197	205	213	221	230	238	246	254	263	271	279	287	295	304	312	320	328

Note: At any BMI a waist circumference of more than 40 inches for men and 35 inches for women is associated with a significantly increased risk of chronic disease.

Source: Adapted from *Clinical Guidelines on the Identification, Evaluation, and Treatment of Overweight and Obesity in Adults: The Evidence Report,* National Institutes of Health, 2010.

---

less in the morning when you first wake up and more in the evening, after having eaten during the day. So, if you are using a scale to monitor your weight, you need to do so on the same scale, at the same time of day, and with approximately the same weight of clothing. Also, remember that muscle weighs more than fat, which explains why some toned and muscular athletes can weigh as much as someone who is sedentary and overweight. In general, risk of disease increases with a higher percentage of body fat, not weight.

Body Fat Measurement

Young adult men normally have a body fat percentage of 10–15 percent. The normal range for young adult women is 22–25 percent. The higher percentage of fat typically found in women is related to preparation for pregnancy and breast-feeding. When a man's body fat is higher than 20 percent and a woman's body fat is above 30 percent, these people are considered to be obese. There are many ways to assess body fat. The Bod Pod, skinfold measurements, and hydrostatic weighing are some of the most common methods for assessing body fat composition.

Bod Pod (Body Composition System) The **Bod Pod** is an egg-shaped chamber that uses computerized pressure sensors to determine the amount of air displaced by the person's body (larger people displace more air than smaller people). From this measure, you can then calculate the person's body density and percentage of body fat.[13]

Skinfold Measurements *Skinfold measurements* are another way to measure body composition. In this assessment procedure, constant-pressure **calipers** are used to measure the thickness of the layer of fat beneath the skin's surface, the *subcutaneous fat layer*. These measurements are taken at key places on the body. Through the use of specific formulas, skinfold measurements can be used to calculate the percentage of body fat. The percent body fat value can also be used in determining desirable weight.[14] There are several drawbacks to this type of measure: First, another person may be required to perform the test, because it is sometimes difficult to get an accurate measurement on yourself. Second, skinfolds are notoriously hard to locate precisely, and being just a few millimeters off can make a significant difference.[3]

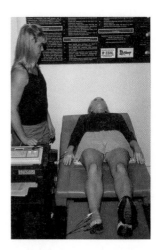

A woman undergoes bioelectric impedance analysis to determine body fat composition.

Hydrostatic Weighing   *Hydrostatic* (underwater) *weighing* determines a person's percentage of body fat by comparing the underwater weight with the body weight out of water and dry. The need for expensive facilities (a tank or pool) and experienced technicians limits of this procedure to small-scale applications, such as at a large research university or teaching hospital.[14]

Bioelectric impedance analysis, dual energy x-ray, absorpitometry, near infrared interactance, magnetic resonance imaging, total body electrical conductivity, and computed tomography are other ways of measuring body fat.

Causes of Obesity

Genetic, physiological, metabolic, environmental, psychological, and other factors may all play a part in obesity. In the past decade, the overall prevalence of obesity has increased so that currently one-third of all Americans are obese. Moreover, in the last 20 years, the number of overweight children in the United States has tripled to one in five children.[15] Genetics, dietary practice, and activity level all seem to play a role in this dramatic increase.

Four additional factors may play a significant role in the prevalence of obesity: gender, age, socioeconomic status, and race. Biology accounts for only 33 percent of the variation in body weight, so the environment can also exert an enormous influence. Among women, obesity is strongly associated with socioeconomic status, being twice as common among those with lower socioeconomic status as it is among those with higher status.[16] Although prevalence among Black and White men does not differ significantly, obesity is far more common among Black than among White women, affecting 50 percent of Black women compared with 42 percent of White women ages 40–59.

While the precise causes of obesity remain unclear, we do know that obesity is a complex condition caused by a variety of factors. Until we are sure what causes obesity, it will remain difficult to develop effective ways of managing overweight.

Calorie Balance: Energy Intake Versus Energy Output

What accounts for the high percentage of Americans defined as overweight or obese? Experts point to two salient factors: greater daily caloric consumption and a relatively low level of consistent physical activity. Women eat 335 more calories and men eat 168 more calories per day than they did 30 years ago. In addition, nearly two-thirds of Americans are not physically active on a regular basis and 25 percent are completely sedentary.[17] (See Chapter 4.) In fact, freshman college students spend 16.5 hours a week exercising while seniors exercise 6 hours per week. No wonder seniors tend to be 18 pounds heavier than freshmen.

The increase in weight occurs, of course, when the body is supplied with more energy than it can use and the excess energy is stored in the form of **adipose tissue,** or fat. This is called a **positive caloric balance.** Consuming about 3,500 calories a week more than is needed results in a weight gain of 1 pound of fat per week.[18] Weight remains constant when caloric input and caloric output are equal. This is called **caloric balance.** To maintain a specific weight, people must balance their energy intake with their energy expenditure. To lose weight, an individual must achieve a **negative caloric balance,** which involves expending more calories than are taken in. A negative caloric balance can be created

> ### Key Terms
>
> **Bod Pod** Body composition system used to measure body fat through air displacement.
>
> **calipers** A device used to measure the thickness of a skinfold from which percentage of body fat can be estimated.
>
> **adipose tissue** Tissue made up of fibrous strands around which specialized cells designed to store liquefied fat are arranged.
>
> **positive caloric balance** Caloric intake greater than caloric expenditure, resulting in weight gain.
>
> **caloric balance** Caloric intake and caloric expenditure are equal, and body weight remains constant.
>
> **negative caloric balance** Caloric intake is less than caloric expenditure, resulting in weight loss.

by reducing caloric intake, increasing physical activity, or both. The key to losing weight and keeping it off is regular aerobic exercise and a balanced diet that is consistent with the current dietary guidelines as described in Chapter 5.[19] In other words, eat healthfully and exercise regularly.

What are our energy needs? How many calories should we consume (or burn) to achieve a healthy weight? The USDA dietary guidelines are based on consuming 2,000 calories a day (see Chapter 5). We all vary in our specific energy needs, depending on our (1) basal metabolic rate (also referred to as resting energy expenditure, or REE), (2) activity requirements, and (3) the thermic effect of food. Gender also plays a role in caloric intake requirements; men tend to need more calories than women. We also need fewer calories as we age because our metabolism is slowing down, and we tend to become less active.

Basal Metabolic Rate Of the three factors that determine energy needs, basal metabolism uses the highest proportion (50–70 percent) of the total calories required by each person. **Basal metabolic rate (BMR)** is a measure of resting energy expenditure that is taken upon awakening, 10–12 hours after eating, or 12–18 hours after significant physical activity. A closely related construct, resting metabolic rate (RMR), is often used interchangeably with BMR. In comparison with the BMR, the RMR is measured at rest, without the stringent control on physical activity required in measuring BMR. RMR measures the calories needed for functioning such as blood circulation, respiration, brain activity, muscle function, body temperature, and heartbeat.[20]

Basal metabolism changes as people age. For both males and females, the BMR is relatively high at birth and continues to increase until the age of 2. Except for a slight rise at puberty, the BMR then gradually declines throughout life.[21] If people fail to recognize that their BMR decreases as they grow older (2 percent per decade), they might also fail to adjust their food intake and activity level accordingly. Thus, they may gradually put on unwanted pounds as they grow older.

Activity Requirements Each person's caloric *activity requirements* vary directly according to the amount of their daily physical activity. When weight-management experts are asked to identify the single most important reason that obesity rates are so high in today's society, they are most certain to point to inactivity. People of all ages tend to be less active and burn fewer calories than did their ancestors only a few generations ago. Both adults and children spend less time devoted to exercise as a result of longer work hours at sedentary jobs, a decline in physical education programs in school, and increased participation in sedentary recreational activities, such as browsing the Internet, playing video games, and watching television.

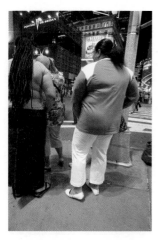

A variety of genetic, physiological, metabolic, social, environmental, and lifestyle factors contribute to the development of obesity.

In addition, many of the labor-saving devices and increased automation in the home and workplace have contributed to increased inactivity. According to some studies, it is not surprising that as inactivity becomes the norm, so does overweight.

Physical activity uses 20–40 percent of caloric intake. You can find more information on how many calories are burned depending upon type of exercise at www.bodybuilding.com.

Thermic Effect of Food **Thermic effect of food (TEF)** refers to the amount of energy our bodies require for the digestion, absorption, and transportation of food. This energy breaks down the bonds that hold complex food molecules together, resulting in smaller nutritional units that can be distributed throughout the body. The amount of TEF burned varies for different types of food, with some food, such as fat, requiring less energy to convert to energy stores and others, such as protein and carbohydrates, requiring more. The TEF peaks in about one hour after eating and accounts for approximately 10 percent of total energy expenditure.[20]

Genetic Factors

Through years of research, we do know that heredity plays a major role in the development of body size and obesity.[4] Based on studies comparing both identical and fraternal (nonidentical) twins raised together and separately, it's evident that both environment and genetics influence obesity. In fact, it is estimated that heredity accounts for 25–40 percent of the development of obesity.[3] Women have a higher percentage of body fat than do men, and this seems stable across cultures and dietary habits.[21]

The thrifty gene hypothesis, suggested by geneticist James Neel, theorizes that medical conditions such as diabetes and obesity were advantageous to humans in the past but now are detrimental. Neel speculates that heavier people would have had a better chance of survival when food was scarce because of their ability to store fat. Now that food is abundant in modern culture, this genotype is no longer beneficial but instead is problematic.[22]

A complex interplay of genetic factors very likely influence the development of obesity, since more than 250 genes may play a role in obesity. Promising research has explored how the leptin gene influences obesity. Discovered in the mid-1990s, the leptin gene, referred to as the "fat gene," is thought to influence satiety, or the feeling of fullness.[23] Experiments on mice revealed that when the leptin gene was faulty, it produced lower leptin levels, and the mice experienced excessive weight gain. However, when the leptin gene was normal, the leptin levels were higher, and the mice were able to maintain normal weight. It has been theorized that leptin resistance may be involved in weight gain and the maintenance of excessive weight, but much more research needs to be conducted in this area.[24]

Physiological and Hormonal Factors

Building on the new information about the genetic and neuropsychological basis of obesity, researchers have identified centers for the control of eating within the hypothalamus of the central nervous system (CNS). These centers—the feeding center for hunger and the satiety center for fullness—tell the body when it should begin consuming food and when food consumption should stop. It takes 20 minutes on average for these signals to go from the stomach to the brain to relay the message "stop eating."[25]

Hormonal factors also influence obesity. Obesity can be caused by a condition called **hypothyroidism,** in which the thyroid gland produces an insufficient amount of thyroxin, a hormone that regulates metabolism. Over 5 million Americans have this common medical condition, and as many as 10 percent of women may have some degree of thyroid hormone deficiency. In such individuals, the underactive thyroid makes burning up food difficult, and so weight gain is common. As we acquire greater understanding of the hormones and neurotransmitters that influence hunger and satiety, drugs designed to influence their actions will be developed. Some of these drugs already exist and will be described later in this chapter.

The effects of hormonal changes on eating can be seen each month just before a woman's menstrual cycle; many women say that they crave salty and sugary foods during this time. Pregnancy brings about another host of hormonal and metabolic changes. During a normal pregnancy, a woman requires an extra 300 calories a day to support the developing fetus and supportive tissues, and to fuel her elevated maternal metabolism. In addition, pregnant women will develop approximately 9 extra pounds of adipose tissue that will be used as an energy source during lactation. The average woman is expected to gain 25–35 pounds during pregnancy.[26] Many women express concern about their ability to lose this weight following the birth of the child, and some women do gain much more than the recommended amount of weight. However, the majority of women lose their pregnancy weight within six months to a year after having a baby. Nevertheless, obesity is one of the most frequent causes of complications in pregnancy. Women who are obese during pregnancy have a much higher risk of hypertension and gestational diabetes. Obesity has also been associated with infertility, poor pregnancy outcomes, and miscarriage.[27]

Typically, breast-feeding can help women to burn more calories and return to their prepregnancy weight, although extra fat may linger, since nature intended this to be a store of energy for breast-feeding. Breast-feeding requires an additional 500 calories a day.[26] Mothers who breast-feed tend to lose more weight when their babies are 3–6 months old than do formula-feeding mothers who consume fewer calories.[26]

Many researchers believe that the number of fat cells a person has is initially determined during the first two years of life. Babies are born with about 10 billion fat cells, and if they are overfed they develop a greater number of fat cells than do babies who receive a balanced diet of appropriate, infant-sized portions. When these children reach adulthood, they will have more fat cells. Individuals at a healthy weight have 10–20 billion fat cells, while an obese person can have up to 100 billion. An overweight person doesn't have an excess number of fat cells but, rather, increasingly larger fat cells. Dieting reduces only the size of fat cells, not the number of fat cells. People who have an abnormally high number of fat cells are biologically limited in their ability to lose weight.[28]

> **Key Terms**
>
> **basal metabolic rate (BMR)** The amount of energy, expressed in calories, that the body requires to maintain basic functions.
>
> **thermic effect of food (TEF)** The amount of energy our bodies require for the digestion, absorption, and transportation of food.
>
> **hypothyroidism** A condition in which the thyroid gland produces an insufficient amount of the hormone thyroxin.

Metabolic Factors

Traditional theory has suggested that the energy expenditure and energy storage centers of the body possess a genetically programmed awareness of the body's most physiologically desirable weight, called the **set point.** [29] However, the term *set point* is somewhat misleading in that it refers not to a certain number or point but to a weight range that the body is genetically programmed to maintain. When the body falls below its natural set point, one's metabolism reacts by slowing down the body's functioning in order to conserve energy. In other words, the body senses that it is not receiving enough calories to maintain healthy functioning, and so it sends calories to essential areas of the body and uses the energy as efficiently as possible. Alternatively, when someone consumes more calories than is needed, the body begins to increase the rate of metabolism in an effort not to gain weight above the set point. The process of storing or burning more energy to maintain the body's "best" weight is called **adaptive thermogenesis.** This process also explains why 90 percent of people who go on any diet gain all the weight back plus more within a year of going off the diet. When dieting, people reduce their caloric intake, which in turn lowers their metabolism. When they discontinue the diet, they typically eat more calories and foods with higher fat content on a lowered metabolism. This is a good formula for weight gain. In addition, dieters tend to lose muscle and regain their weight as fat.

There is a great deal of debate on how an individual's set point can be altered. The number of fat cells in the body, the blood level of insulin, and regions of the brain such as the hypothalamus all seem to play a role in determining set point. Certain drugs, such as amphetamines and other diet pills and herbal supplements, can act on the brain to temporarily lower the set point. However, once these drugs are discontinued, the set point returns to the previous level or perhaps an even higher level, and weight increases as a result. Healthier and more permanent methods of changing one's set point involve regular exercise and healthy eating patterns. In fact, a study of 8,000 successful dieters found that the majority of them used "my own diet and exercise regimen" and did not follow any formal weight reduction program. [30]

The body's requirement for energy to maintain basic physiological processes decreases progressively with age. This change reflects the loss of muscle tissue as both men and women age. This loss of muscle mass eventually alters the ratio of lean body tissue to fat. As the proportion of fat increases, the energy needs of the body are more strongly influenced by the lower metabolic needs of the fat cells. [17] This excess energy is then stored in the fat cells of the body. A gradual decrease in caloric intake and a conscious effort to expend more calories can effectively prevent this gradual increase in weight leading to obesity.

Family, Social, and Cultural Factors

Ethnic and cultural differences also relate to the incidence of obesity and what is considered to be a healthy weight. The statistics are startling: 50 percent of African American women and 37 percent of African American men are obese. For Mexican Americans, 43 percent of women and 34 percent of men are obese. Thirty-three percent of Caucasian women and 32 percent of Caucasian men are obese. [31] Until recently, Asian Americans had a lower rate of obesity than the general population; however, new figures show that 8 percent of Chinese children 10–12 years of age are obese and 15 percent are overweight, which is closer to the overall 19 percent of 6- to 11-year-old American children who are overweight.

Obesity disproportionately affects women of color and women of lower socioeconomic classes. Acculturation also has a significant effect on the rates of obesity—the more an ethnic group has adapted to and absorbed Western culture, the higher the rate of obesity within that group. [32]

Socioeconomic status is also an important influence on obesity. Women of higher socioeconomic status tend to be thinner than those of lower socioeconomic status, while among men there is not such a pattern. [33] Limited access to health care, lower education levels, lower income levels, and increased stress are some of the reasons cited for this disparity. [34] There are also regional differences among Americans related to obesity. The 10 states with the highest obesity rates in 2009, from highest to lowest, were Mississippi, Alabama/Tennessee (tie), West Virginia, Louisiana, Oklahoma, Kentucky, Arkansas, South Carolina, and Michigan/North Carolina (tie). Colorado had the lowest obesity rate, followed by Massachusetts, Utah, Hawaii, Connecticut, Rhode Island, California, New Mexico, Idaho, and Montana. [35]

Another way people can become obese is with a pattern of overeating over a long period of time. If an infant's cries for food are immediately responded to, that child will be more likely to learn what the sensation of hunger is and what the appropriate response is. If crying unrelated to hunger is responded to with the offer of a cookie or candy, the child will learn to soothe him- or

Key Terms

set point A genetically programmed range of body weight, beyond which a person finds it difficult to gain or lose additional weight.

adaptive thermogenesis The physiological response of the body to adjust its metabolic rate to the presence of food.

herself with food. Studies show that children become confused about what hunger is and how to satisfy it if their hunger needs are neglected or overindulged in infancy.[36]

Some of the first power struggles between parents and their children revolve around issues of food. A child who has little power in her life can exert some power and control through refusing to eat certain foods, and demanding other foods, and determining when she wants to eat. Parents who use food as a reward for good behavior ("If you get an A on your test, I will treat you to ice cream"), as punishment ("You weren't behaving so you can't have dessert"), or as a guilt trip ("Don't waste food. Clean your plate. Children are starving in the world") may inadvertently be creating negative dietary practices that will continue throughout the child's life. Interestingly, research has shown that children are extraordinarily adept at meeting their nutritional needs when left to their own devices. One study allowed children to eat whatever they wanted for a week. Did they always pick high-fat, high-sugar foods? No. Actually, when we look at each day's intake, they didn't eat a balanced diet. However, when one takes the full week into consideration, they met their nutritional needs perfectly.

What your parents *say* to you has a tremendous influence on your eating behavior; what they *do,* their own eating practices, can have an even greater impact. Children are exposed to different foods and model what their parents eat. If a parent makes comments such as "I shouldn't eat that because I will get fat" or doesn't eat fruits or vegetables, or sits down with a bag of chips in front of the television every night, the child will probably do the same. In the same vein, when parents exercise regularly, eat a balanced diet, and make positive comments about their weight, children tend to mimic this behavior.

 TALKING POINTS What were the messages you received in childhood regarding food? What positive and negative eating habits have you learned from your family?

Environmental Factors

Certainly, environmental factors such as the smell or sight of freshly made cookies, or an advertisement for a candy bar, can affect your eating habits. And the clock signaling it is "time to eat" can encourage us to eat even when we aren't hungry. While this may seem adaptive and helpful in regulating our food intake, Dr. Kelly D. Brownell, a professor of psychology at Yale and an expert on eating disorders, has gone so far as to label American society a "toxic environment" when it comes to food. Researchers contend that the local environment has a powerful effect on eating. Factors such as portion size, price, advertising, the availability of food, and the number of food choices

presented all can influence the amount the average person consumes. For example, moviegoers will eat 50 percent more popcorn if given an extra-large tub instead of a container one size smaller, even if the popcorn is stale. If a tabletop in the office is stocked with cookies and candy, coworkers tend to nibble their way through the workday, even if they are not hungry. One study found that moving a candy dish from on top of a secretary's desk to 6 feet away reduced the amount of candy eaten by over half, equal to 12 pounds of weight over a year's time.[37] Similarly, men eat 29 percent and women 10 percent more if they serve themselves at the table rather than having the plate filled for and served to them. Eating with someone who eats faster than you typically results in your consuming more calories, while eating with someone who eats slowly will result in your eating less food, called the "mimicry effect."[37] Women eat the same amount as other women around them, regardless of the other women's size or whether they know them. This was not found to be true for men, who tend to eat faster than women and to return for seconds without waiting for others to finish their first serving.

Packaging and price can also influence the amount people consume, a concept of which advertisers, restaurants, and grocery stores are well aware. Dropping the price of the low-fat snacks by even a nickel resulted in dramatically increased sales. In contrast, stickers signaling low-fat content or cartoons promoting the low-fat alternatives had a great deal of influence over which snacks were more popular. This is true not only of food but also of beverages: People tend to drink *more* from short, wide glasses than from thin, tall ones, thinking they are drinking less.[38] Our plate size has increased from 10 inches to 12 inches, and so has our portion sizes, by 22 percent. We eat less from smaller packages such as the 100-calorie packages. Even the names of food influence our eating. Changing the name from "Italian pasta" to "succulent Tuscany pasta" resulted in a 27 percent increase in sales according to one study.[37]

Having more choices also appears to make people eat more. In one study, people ate more when offered sandwiches with four different fillings than they did when they were given sandwiches with their single favorite filling. In another study, participants who were served a four-course meal with meat, fruit, bread, and pudding ate 60 percent more food than did those served an equivalent meal of only their favorite course. Note that these findings apply to people of all body sizes, not just people who are overweight or obese, as is often the misconception. This phenomenon is referred to as "unit bias," or the tendency to think that a single unit of food is the right amount to eat or drink no matter what size it is. We often don't make a conscious decision about how much to eat—the choice is made for us by the portion size that is offered to us. We mindlessly eat food without questioning the amount.[38] We also tend to eat or drink whatever is offered to us—whether a large cookie or a small one, we think of them as the same amount of calories because each is one cookie. In response to these and other findings, many public schools have begun offering only healthy foods in their cafeterias, replacing soft drinks, candy, and chips with juice, milk, fruit, and granola bars.

Psychological Factors

Psychological factors related to overeating concern the reasons people eat other than physiological hunger. Individuals with eating disorders often report that they don't know when they are hungry and often eat when they are not hungry and don't eat when they have a biological reason for doing so. Why do people eat if not in response to hunger? Frequently, people eat in response to their emotions—for example, to comfort themselves or when bored, tired, stressed, or depressed.[39] Some people say they use food as a way of coping with hurt, sadness, and anger, "swallowing" their feelings and putting food on top of them. Others eat out of habit and associate food with certain activities, such as eating popcorn at a movie, eating chips in front of the television, and having dessert after dinner. Certainly, many people think of chocolate when they want to cheer themselves up. Food is also part of celebrations, holidays, and family bonding, and a mainstay of socialization. It is difficult to think about social activities we engage in that don't involve food in some way.

Some people develop relationships with food that substitute for real human relationships or to fill other psychological or spiritual needs. Comments such as "Food is my best friend" and "A great meal is better than sex" are indicative of the degree to which many people rely on food to fill their needs. As we'll learn in our discussion of eating disorders later in the chapter, psychological issues with food can become serious, even life-threatening problems.

Weight-Management Strategies

Weight loss occurs when the calories consumed are fewer than required by the body for physiological maintenance and activity. This may sound overly simplified, and certainly the $50-billion-a-year weight loss industry would like us to think it is much more complicated than this.

Weight loss followed by weight gain may be less healthy and more frustrating than maintaining body weight, even at weight above the desirable levels. When a diet or weight loss strategy fails, the person, not the diet, is blamed. This causes people to jump to another weight loss method and then another, in a vicious cycle. However, committing to a lifestyle change of eating in healthy ways and engaging in regular exercise seem to be the most effective strategies for weight loss and weight maintenance.

Lifestyle Approaches for Lifetime Healthy Weight Management

To maintain a healthy weight, you need to eat a balanced diet supported by portion control, participate in regular physical activity, get consistent and sufficient sleep, and develop healthy ways of coping and problem solving. These key components to healthy weight management are discussed further in the next sections; see the box "Tips for Losing Weight Successfully" for some specific guidelines.

Balanced Diet Supported by Portion Control A diet that reduces caloric intake is the most common approach to weight loss. The choice of foods and the amount of food are the two factors that distinguish the wide range of diets currently available. Note, however, that dieting alone usually does not result in long-term weight loss. In a recent study, after one year, people who exercised regularly and followed a healthy diet lost 21 pounds, the healthy-eaters-but-no-exercise group lost 18 pounds, and the exercise-only group lost 5 pounds.[40] Effective and long-lasting weight management requires a lifestyle change, not just going on a diet for a specific time period only to return to your old patterns of eating. This is the problem many people face when they go on strict diets and overly restrict their calories. Because the diet is so restrictive and demanding, they are unable to continue to follow it for very long, and they return to their previous eating patterns. In addition, people tend to overeat the foods they denied themselves while dieting because they feel deprived and the forbidden food seems even more alluring. This can also lead to binge eating. Thus, diets tend not to work in the long run (see the box "Tips for Losing Weight Successfully").

A healthy and successful approach to weight loss and subsequent weight maintenance is to establish a nutritionally sound, balanced diet (see Chapter 5) that controls portions. Many people are confused about the difference between a portion size and a serving size. Food scales or food models can assist in gaining an understanding of portion sizes.

The USDA dietary guidelines outline the breakdown of daily caloric intake for each food group. You can get a personalized dietary guideline by inputting your gender, age, and activity level at MyPlate.gov. One study showed that people cut 256 calories a day just by trimming their portion sizes by 25 percent.

Maintaining a balanced diet and watching your portion sizes are especially important on the weekends. Many people throw their good eating habits out the window on the weekends, as evidenced by a recent study reporting that Americans eat an average of 115 extra calories per day from Friday to Sunday compared with the rest of the week. Most of these calories came from alcohol and increased fat consumption. The extra calories can result in a gain of 5 pounds over the course of a year.

Physical Activity Most Americans attempting to lose weight fail to include a physical activity component in their dietary approach. How much exercise is enough? The USDA dietary guidelines (Chapter 5) advise American adults to engage in at least 150 minutes of moderately intense aerobic exercise each week for weight maintenance and 300 minutes of this type of exercise for weight loss. Weight training has become a more important factor in weight management. (See Chapter 4 for further recommendations on physical fitness.) As a result, exercise boot-camp workouts are becoming more popular in gyms. These military-style exercise programs involve drills with running, jumping jacks, push-ups, squats, sit-ups, and weight lifting led by a trainer who looks, sounds, and acts more like a drill sergeant.

Like most things, too much or too little exercise is not beneficial and can be unhealthy. As will be discussed in a later section, some people with eating disorders tend to overexercise, which gives them diminishing returns.

Sleep Research has recently revealed that not getting enough sleep doesn't just make you grumpy and sluggish—it can make you gain weight as well! People who sleep 2–4 hours a night have been found to be 73 percent more likely to be obese than those who sleep 7–9 hours. Sleeping 5 hours a night results in a 50 percent chance of being obese compared to those consistently sleeping 7–9 hours. Twenty-three percent of people who sleep 6 hours tend to be obese. In other words, the higher the BMI, the less sleep the person got.[41]

Why does less sleep equal more weight? We used to think that sleeping too much made us gain weight and staying up meant we were more active and so burned calories, but this has been disproved. People tend to watch television, read, or be online late at night, and so they are not active. In addition, people tend to eat

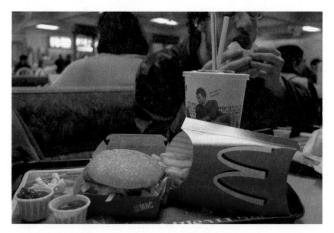

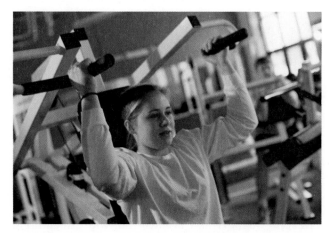

Lifestyle approaches to weight management address two key components of energy balance—energy in as food and energy out as physical activity. Strategies for creating a negative energy balance include reducing your intake of large portions of high-calorie foods (such as fast food) and increasing your level of physical activity.

high-fat, high-sugar foods while they are engaging in these activities. Some people say that they eat sugary foods in order to give themselves more energy to stay up late to study or to get work done. Two hormones, ghrelin and leptin, have been found to regulate both sleep and hunger. A sleep study at the University of Chicago found that leptin levels were 18 percent lower and ghrelin levels 28 percent higher after subjects slept 4 hours. Sleep-deprived subjects reported feeling the hungriest and craved carbohydrates, the energy food. Ghrelin has been referred to as the accelerator for eating. When ghrelin levels are up, people feel hungrier. Leptin is the brake for eating; higher levels are associated with feeling full and decreased appetite.

These sleep studies seem to indicate that a hormonal relationship exists between sleep and hunger. The ghrelin level in people who routinely slept 5 hours a night was 15 percent higher, compared to 15 percent lower leptin levels in people who slept 8 hours a night. The first group also had higher BMIs than did individuals sleeping 8 hours a night. Studies have also found that children are not getting the 10–11 hours of sleep a night they require, which may also help explain the increase in childhood obesity.[42]

So, one way for us to manage our weight is to manage our sleep better. This means managing our time better—prioritizing our commitments and activities and not overloading our schedules, so that we can get the rest we need.

Lifestyle Support and Problem Solving   In addition to committing yourself to a lifestyle that features regular physical activity and careful food choices, build a support system that nurtures your efforts. Successful dieters have consistently reported that having a coach, counselor, or someone else whom they can meet with on a regular basis to be accountable with has made a tremendous difference in their weight loss efforts and in maintaining a healthy weight.

It may be helpful for you to reevaluate your perception of food and eating. Do you use food as a way of coping with stress, boredom, or other feelings? Consider finding new ways to cope with stressors, using nonfood options such as talking with friends or family, exercising, or writing in a journal. You may want to take the Personal Assessment at the end of this chapter to see if you are eating mindlessly. (See also the box "Learning to Eat Mindfully.") Additionally, if you tend to use food as a way to reward yourself for hard work or completing something, you might want to generate other types of rewards, such as engaging in a hobby or another activity you enjoy.

The lifestyle choices suggested here will significantly lower your chances of developing a weight problem or a weight-related health problem in your lifetime. Again, genetics will exert its effects to some degree on weight and body composition, but you can counteract these effects by employing the methods just discussed.

Specific Dietary Approaches

There are many strategies for losing weight, and they vary in effectiveness, harmfulness, cost, and ease of use. The next section will cover the most popular weight loss methods: temporary caloric restriction, low-calorie foods and controlled serving sizes, controlled fasting, formal or commercial weight reduction programs, weight loss drugs, herbal supplements, and surgical interventions. The box "Health Halo Foods" considers yet another aspect of the weight-management conundrum.

Temporary Caloric Restriction   People use fad diets in an attempt to lose weight quickly. Currently, there are over 150 popular diets, often promoted by people who claim to be nutrition experts. With few exceptions, these approaches are both ineffective and potentially dangerous. In addition, some involve significant expense (see Table 6.2).

The main problem with dieting is that it is a temporary, quick fix. Most diets will result in temporary weight loss if followed correctly, and they usually promise rapid weight loss. Of course, much of this initial weight lost is water weight and not fat. Research shows that 90 percent of all people who diet gain back their weight, plus more, within a year. Oprah Winfrey is a good example of what happens to most dieters. She lost 67 pounds in four months consuming only Optifast. She kept this weight off for only one day. The first day she went off her diet and went back to her old eating patterns, she began gaining weight. She weighed 211 pounds prediet and she weighed 226 pounds postdiet. Look at Figure 6-2 to see why people struggle with losing weight.

Diets don't teach us how to eat; they teach us how not to eat! The restriction of calories is the basis of all diets. Some suggest limiting the consumption of fat or carbohydrates, or the caloric intake is dangerously low for all food groups. Many diet plans, such as the South Beach Diet and the Atkins Diet, advocate the restriction of carbohydrates, which can cause ketosis. Ketosis can cause the blood to become too acidic, and dehydration can occur. The body requires a minimum of 50–100 grams of carbohydrates per day to avoid ketosis.[21] Low-carbohydrate diets are characterized by initial rapid weight loss, which is appealing to most people, but this is primarily due to water loss, not fat loss. Complications associated with low-carbohydrate, high-protein diets include dehydration, hypertension, cancer, electrolyte loss, calcium depletion, weakness due to inadequate dietary carbohydrates, nausea due to ketosis, vitamin and mineral deficiencies, and possible kidney problems. The risk of coronary heart disease may be higher in those who stay on the diet a long time, due to the increased consumption of foods high in saturated fat and cholesterol.

Most diets are temporary in nature because they are medically unhealthy and potentially harmful. They are also too restrictive, and people end up craving the very foods they are being told to avoid. Dieters begin to feel deprived and resentful, and they respond by retaliating against the diet and bingeing on the "forbidden" foods.

A recent two-year study of whether low-fat or low-carbohydrate diets yielded better results found that they produced similar weight loss results and medical benefits. The key seemed to be a diet that you can stick with and that represents a lifestyle change. All of the participants who kept their weight off for two years also exercised regularly and kept track of what they ate.[43]

Table 6.2   Rating the Diets

	Overall Score	Nutritional Analysis	Short-Term Weight Loss	Long-Term Weight Loss
Volumetrics	Good	Excellent	Good	Good
Weight Watchers	Good	Excellent	Fair	Fair
Jenny Craig	Good	Excellent	Good	Good
Slim Fast	Good	Excellent	Good	Good
eDiets	Good	Excellent	Below avg	Below avg
Zone Diet	Good	Excellent	Fair	Below avg
Ornish Diet	Fair	Fair	Fair	Fair
Atkins Diet	Below avg	Poor	Good	Fair

Source: New diet winners, *Consumer Reports,* June 2007.

What's the major reason people want to lose weight?

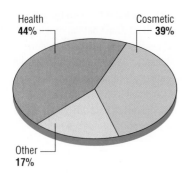

Health
44%

Cosmetic
39%

Other
17%

What's the main reason people resist changing their eating habits?

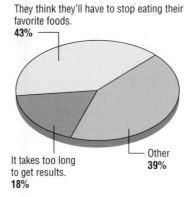

They think they'll have to stop eating their favorite foods.
43%

It takes too long to get results.
18%

Other
39%

Figure 6-2 Why Weight Loss Is Often Pie-in-the-Sky   *USA Today* surveyed 126 of the nation's top registered dietitians about trends in obesity and weight loss. Selected findings are shown here.

Source: From *USA Today*, July 11, 2006, p. 9A. Reprinted with permission.

What's the biggest mistake people make when trying to lose weight?

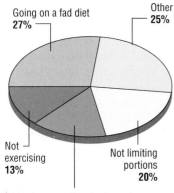

Going on a fad diet
27%

Other
25%

Not exercising
13%

Not limiting portions
20%

Setting inappropriate goals, such as wanting to lose quickly
15%

What's the main reason people don't exercise or increase physical activity to manage weight?

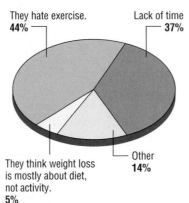

They hate exercise.
44%

Lack of time
37%

They think weight loss is mostly about diet, not activity.
5%

Other
14%

Controlled Fasting   In cases of extreme obesity, some patients are placed on a complete fast in a hospital setting. The patient consumes only water, electrolytes, and vitamins. Weight loss is substantial because the body is forced to begin **catabolism** of its fat and muscle tissues. Inadequate protein and sodium and potassium loss are particular health concerns.

Today, some people regularly practice unsupervised modified fasting for short periods. Solid foods are removed from the diet for a number of days. Fruit juice, water, protein supplements, and vitamins are used to minimize the risks associated with total fasting. However, unsupervised short-term fasting that is done too frequently can be dangerous and is not recommended.

Formal or Commercial Weight Reduction Programs   In virtually every area of the country, at least one version of the popular weight reduction programs, such as TOPS (Take Off Pounds Sensibly), Jenny Craig, NutriSystem, and Weight Watchers, can be found. These programs generally feature a format consisting of (1) a well-balanced diet emphasizing portion control and moderate-fat, low-saturated-fat, and high-complex-carbohydrate foods,

(2) specific weight loss goals to be attained over a set period of time, (3) encouragement from supportive leaders and fellow group members, (4) emphasis on regular physical activity, and (5) a maintenance program (follow-up program).

In theory, these programs offer an opportunity to lose weight for people who cannot or will not participate in a physical activity program. But their effectiveness is very limited. In fact, the limited success of these programs and the difficulty that working people have in attending meetings have resulted in falling enrollment and the development of online programs. All these programs are costly when compared with self-directed approaches, especially when the program markets its own food products (see Table 6.2).

Weight Loss Drugs

Another approach to weight loss involves over-the-counter weight loss drugs, herbal supplements, and prescription drugs. These are designed to either suppress hunger, increase metabolism, or block fat absorption in order to manage weight.

Over-the-Counter (OTC) Weight Loss Drugs and Herbal Supplements Most OTC and herbal supplements are designed to suppress hunger and increase metabolism. None of them are recommended for long-term use, as they can cause serious health problems and can be addictive. It is difficult to stop taking these pills, because weight loss occurs only while taking them and weight gain usually occurs once the drug or supplement is discontinued. Most of these contained ephedra or ephedrine until it was banned by the FDA in 2003[44] following the death of 23-year-old Baltimore Orioles pitcher Steve Bechler, whose death was linked to an ephedra supplement. Ephedra has been associated with heart attacks, strokes, high blood pressure, seizures, heart irregularities, insomnia, anxiety, tremors, and even death.

Herbal weight loss supplements are available as pills, bars, teas, and powders to mix in liquids. Some people see herbal supplements like Stackers, Mini Thins, Hoodia, and Fat Burner as safe because they are "natural," and yet they can be more dangerous and deadly than prescription medications because they are not inspected for the purity and accuracy of the contents or the potency of the ingredients. The Dietary Supplement Health and Education Act (DSHEA) of 1994 relegated herbal supplements to the category "dietary supplements," limiting the FDA's power to regulate these products to ensure that they meet certain standards or are safe and effective. In fact, it is difficult to stop the sale of dietary supplements that appear dangerous because there must be enough proof to substantiate the health risks.

However, some evidence links these diet supplements to heart attacks, strokes, hepatitis, headaches, tremors, anxiety, extreme irritability, and insomnia in consumers of all ages.[45] After the FDA banned ephedra, other supplements with questionable safety took its place. For example, a diet pill containing bitter orange called Slimming Beauty also contained dangerous amounts of sibutramine and has been associated with heart attacks and strokes, similar to ephedra. Hydroxycut supplements were recalled by the FDA after reports of serious liver damage and death associated with the supplement.[46,47]

Some diet supplements, such as cascara and aloe, act as strong stimulant laxatives; others, often derived from caffeine, act as diuretics. Juniper seeds, dandelion, equistine, horsetail, and shavegrass are examples of these and have been linked to renal damage, brain damage, and cancer. Acai berry, another herbal supplement promising weight loss, is really just a laxative. The Federal Trade Commission has received thousands of complaints from consumers who signed up for a free trial of this pill and were charged $45–$65 monthly, adding up to $100 million at last count. Other diet pills, such as glucomannan and guar gum, create a feeling of fullness because of their dietary fiber content and have been associated with gastrointestinal and esophageal obstructions.

There is also a danger in the potential interactions between prescription medications and herbal agents. Users are often unaware of this danger, and physicians may overlook them because 70 percent of patients do not disclose their use of herbal supplements to them. Chromium, pyruvate, 5-hydroxytryptophan (5-HTP), chitosan, and carnitine are some common herbal supplements used for weight loss; however, there are hundreds of herbal supplements, and it is impossible to list them all. It is important to look at the labels and read the ingredients in diet pills to see what you are really ingesting and know how these herbs affect your body. In addition, these dietary supplements have not been shown to be effective in helping users lose weight!

One particular OTC weight loss medication containing **phenylpropanolamine (PPA)** merits mentioning. In 2000, drug companies making these products were asked to stop manufacturing them because PPA had been associated with an increased risk for stroke. The FDA issued a public health advisory warning consumers not to use any products containing PPA for this reason. PPA was also found in OTC cough and cold medications.

Prescription Weight Loss Drugs Some prescription medications have been shown to produce serious side effects. Two such medications, phentermine and fenfluramine, have been prescribed for patients who wanted to lose weight. Both drugs affect levels of serotonin, the neurotransmitter associated with satiety. This popular combination, referred to as *phenfen*, gradually raised concern among health experts because of the side effects it produced in people with angina, glaucoma, and high blood pressure. In addition, reports began to surface that some patients had developed a rare but potentially lethal condition called *pulmonary hypertension*.

In September 1997, the FDA requested voluntary withdrawal of fenfluramine and dexfenfluramine from the market because of reports of heart valve damage in those using these drugs in combination.[48] Manufacturers responded by ceasing all distribution of the drugs. Phentermine remains on the market and is used in combination with various antidepressants, such as Prozac, Zoloft, and Paxil.

> **Key Terms**
>
> **catabolism** The metabolic process of breaking down tissue for the purpose of converting it into energy.
>
> **phenylpropanolamine (PPA)** (**fen** ill **pro** puh **nol** uh meen) An active chemical compound still found in some over-the-counter diet products and associated with increased risk of stroke.

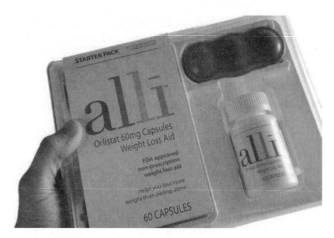

An over-the-counter version of the prescription drug orlistat (Xenical) was approved by the FDA in 2007.

Another serotonin-specific obesity drug, sibutramine (Meridia), was voluntarily removed from the U.S. market by its manufacturer in 2010 at the request of the FDA because it had been linked to heart attacks, high blood pressure, strokes, and death.

Manufacturers of three new prescription weight loss drugs—Qnexa, lorcaserin hydrochloride, and Contrave—recently requested approval by the FDA. Only Contrave was approved; the other two were deemed too dangerous as they were linked to heart problems and cancer. Contrave is a combination of the antidepressant bupropion and naltrexone, used for opioid and alcohol addictions. It helps to combat food cravings. Common side effects include nausea, constipation, and headaches.[49]

Fat-Blocking Drugs A non-serotonin-influencing drug, orlistat (Xenical), has also been used for weight loss. Unlike the serotonin-specific drugs, orlistat reduces fat absorption in the small intestine by about 30 percent. The drug is intended for use among people who are 20 percent or more above ideal weight. It could cause a 10 percent loss of body weight without significant dietary restrictions. Some concern exists about the lack of absorption of fat-soluble vitamins among people taking the drug. Additionally, anal leakage may accompany the drug's use, particularly following meals with high fat content.

For the first time, the FDA has approved a prescription diet pill, Xenical (orlistat), as an OTC medication, called Alli.[50] Costing about $50 for a two-month supply, Alli contains half the dosage of Xenical. Alli is not without its risks, as it has the same problematic side effects as Xenical including sudden diarrhea, commonly referred to as "alli-oops" because of the lack of warning and soiled pants Alli users have reported experiencing. Some have intense stomach pain when taking this pill, and it has also been linked with precancerous lesions in the colon.[50]

Surgical Interventions

It used to be that surgical measures were undertaken only if the person's weight was severely endangering his or her health and other less invasive methods had been unsuccessful. Now surgeries such as liposuction, tummy tucks, and gastric bypass, and gastric band surgeries are becoming increasingly popular and commonplace, especially among teenagers. Insurance companies are approving these expensive surgeries because the cost of obesity and its related medical problems is even more costly. Gastric bypass surgery, vertical banded gastroplasty, and laparoscopic adjustable gastric banding all involve major surgery.

These surgeries can also be very expensive, costing $20,000–50,000, and some insurance companies will not pay for them, claiming they are cosmetic even though there are significant medical risks associated with obesity. Even so, the number of obesity surgeries being performed has increased 600 percent over the past five years.[51] Although obesity surgeries are not recommended for use on patients under age 18 due to the risks, in 2007 surgeons performed almost 1,000 of them on children and teens. With the increase in obesity among children, along with improved surgical techniques, there has been a push for the FDA to approve these surgeries for those under 18 years of age.

All three operations limit the amount of food a person can eat at one time, because overeating results in vomiting or severe diarrhea. Because the stomach is made smaller, individuals who have undergone these procedures must limit their food intake to half a cup to a cup of food at each "meal." However, it is possible to regain weight by eating small portions of high-calorie foods on a consistent basis. Individuals lose weight because this type of surgery limits the amount of food that can be digested, therefore decreasing the amount of calories that you can eat at one time.

Gastric Bypass Surgery Gastric bypass is the most common type of weight loss surgery, and it has gained popularity since celebrities such as singer Carnie Wilson, *American Idol* judge Randy Jackson, and weatherman Al Roker have gone public about their experiences with this surgery. It is a major operation that involves dividing the stomach into two compartments to create a pouch, the size of a thumb, for food to enter. The small intestine is cut below the stomach and connected to a smaller portion of the stomach, bypassing the larger stomach and a section of the intestine, which are no longer used (see Figure 6-3A–D). An average of 205,000 people each year undergo gastric bypass surgeries (also referred to as *bariatric surgeries*), compared to 16,800 in 1993. The average cost per surgery is $26,000–$35,000, and the death rate is 1 in 200. Candidates for this surgery typically have a BMI above 40 or are 100 pounds or more

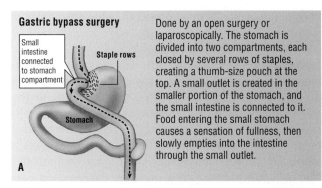

Gastric bypass surgery

Done by an open surgery or laparoscopically. The stomach is divided into two compartments, each closed by several rows of staples, creating a thumb-size pouch at the top. A small outlet is created in the smaller portion of the stomach, and the small intestine is connected to it. Food entering the small stomach causes a sensation of fullness, then slowly empties into the intestine through the small outlet.

A

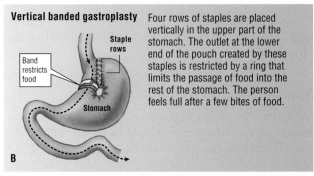

Vertical banded gastroplasty

Four rows of staples are placed vertically in the upper part of the stomach. The outlet at the lower end of the pouch created by these staples is restricted by a ring that limits the passage of food into the rest of the stomach. The person feels full after a few bites of food.

B

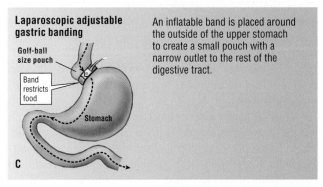

Laparoscopic adjustable gastric banding

An inflatable band is placed around the outside of the upper stomach to create a small pouch with a narrow outlet to the rest of the digestive tract.

C

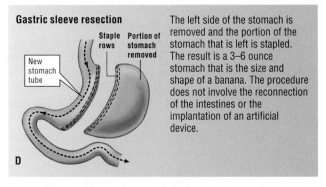

Gastric sleeve resection

The left side of the stomach is removed and the portion of the stomach that is left is stapled. The result is a 3–6 ounce stomach that is the size and shape of a banana. The procedure does not involve the reconnection of the intestines or the implantation of an artificial device.

D

Figure 6-3 Four Types of Obesity Surgery

Source: A–D from *USA Today*, May 5, 2004. Reprinted with permission.

(men) or at least 80 pounds (women) overweight. People with a BMI between 35 and 40 who suffer from type 2 diabetes or life-threatening cardiopulmonary problems may also be candidates for surgery.

Gastric sleeve resection is the newest option for weight loss surgery. It is typically used for individuals whose BMI is over 60 as part of a two-stage bypass surgical procedure. It involves removing two-thirds of the stomach by stapling, resulting in the stomach becoming tube shaped (see Figure 6-3D). It is not reversible.

Gastric bypass surgery tends to result in greater weight loss (93.3 pounds on average) than does gastroplasty (67 pounds on average) after one year. Over two years, gastric bypass surgery patients have been shown to lose two-thirds of excess weight. These surgeries are not without their risks—of hernias, ulcers, liver damage, infection, internal leaks, and even death. They are not a cure-all for weight management; individuals who have these operations must continue to exercise regularly, take nutritional supplements, eat small portions very slowly, and decrease intake of high-sugar foods in order to maintain their weight loss.[52]

Gastric Band Surgery There are two types of gastric band surgery (also known as lap band surgery): vertical banded gastroplasty and laparoscopic adjustable gastric banding. Vertical banded gastroplasty uses both a band and staples to create a small stomach pouch, limiting the passage of food into the rest of the stomach. This results in a feeling of fullness after only a few mouthfuls of food. This used to be the most common weight loss surgery, but it has decreased in popularity with the rise of gastric bypass surgery. Weight loss is not as rapid as with gastric bypass surgery. However, some insurance companies will pay for this surgery because it costs half as much as gastric bypass. Laparoscopic adjustable gastric banding, a less invasive procedure, involves placing an inflatable band around the upper end of the stomach, again creating a small pouch. A narrow passage is also made into the rest of the stomach. The band is inflated with a salt solution through a tube that connects the band to an access port positioned under the skin. In this way, the band can be tightened or loosened over time to change the size of the passageway into the stomach. This procedure is reversible. It too can involve postsurgical complications, such as band slippage, erosion and deflation, obstruction of the stomach, dilation of the esophagus, infection, nausea, stomach wall deterioration, ulcers, vomiting, heartburn, and difficulty swallowing.

In 2010, the FDA approved the use of lap band surgery for individuals with a BMI of 35 or higher and a BMI of 30–35 if the individual has at least one weight-related medical problem, such as diabetes, sleep apnea, or hypertension. Previously, individuals didn't qualify to undergo lap band surgery unless they had a BMI of 40 or higher (35 or higher with a related medical problem). This means that an additional 12 million people would qualify for lap band surgery.[52]

Cosmetic Surgeries and Procedures Cosmetic surgeries have increased 38 percent since 2000, with over 12 million Americans undergoing these surgeries, 219,000 them on teens. Some call it "addictive," because once they have one procedure, they notice other parts of their bodies that they want to change. In her book *Beauty Junkies: Inside Our $15 Billion Obsession with Cosmetic Surgery*, Alex Kuczynski talks about her pursuit of perfection through plastic surgery. Reality TV star Heidi Montag is a good example of this addictive behavior. She underwent 10 cosmetic procedures in one day: breast implants to increase her cup size to a triple D (she had one three years ago as well), brow lift, nose job revision (again, she had this three years ago), liposuction on her stomach and thighs, buttocks augmentation, Botox on her forehead, fat injections in her cheeks and lips, chin reduction, neck liposuction, and her ears pinned back. She said the reason she underwent these surgeries was because she was bullied about her appearance when she was younger and she felt insecure about her appearance. She called herself "an ugly duckling" prior to the surgeries.[53] Some believe that changing their bodies will improve their body image and their overall satisfaction with their lives. With the convenience and ease of being able to do some of the more minor procedures over the lunch hour, some people now view cosmetic surgery as being similar to getting a haircut. The most common cosmetic surgeries are liposuction, breast augmentation, eyelid surgery, abdominoplasty (tummy tuck), and breast reduction.

Liposuction and Abdominoplasty Liposuction is the most frequent cosmetic operation in the United States in which fat tissue is removed. Liposuction involves removing unwanted fat from specific areas, such as the abdomen, hips, buttocks, thighs, knees, upper arms, chin, cheeks, and neck. A small tube is inserted through the skin, and adipose tissue is vacuumed out. This is more of a sculpting or contouring operation than a weight loss surgery because little weight is lost. Potential risks and outcomes include infection; the formation of fat clots or blood clots, which may travel to the lungs and cause death; excessive fluid loss, which can lead to shock or fluid accumulation that must be drained; friction burns or other damage to the skin or nerves; numbness; skin discoloration; irregular body contours; and sagging skin. Approximately 400,000 people undergo liposuction each year. The cost of liposuction ranges from $3,000 to $8,500, depending upon the part of the body receiving the surgery and the size of the patient.[54]

Abdominoplasty, known more commonly as a "tummy tuck," is a major surgical procedure to remove excess skin and fat from the middle and lower abdomen and to tighten the muscles of the abdominal wall. It leaves a permanent scar, which can extend from hip to hip. Infection and blood clots are some of the potential risks. A balanced diet and regular exercise are required to maintain the results from this surgery. There have been reported 20 deaths for every 100,000 patients who underwent liposuction, a rate 20 times higher than for other types of surgeries.[55]

Lipodissolve Lipodissolve, also referred to as "fat melting shots," involves injecting soy lecithin and bile salt directly into problem areas such as the hips, waist, thighs, and buttocks, purportedly destroying the fat cells' walls and metabolizing and excreting the cells' contents. This process necessitates six to eight visits one every two weeks and costs approximately $2,000 for each area treated. The FDA has been cracking down on this procedure, as there is no clinical evidence proving its safety or effectiveness. Allergic reactions, skin ulcerations, scarring, and infections are some of the reported side effects of this procedure.

Approaches for Weight Gain

For some, the lack of adequate body weight is a serious concern. These people would likely fall into a BMI category of less than 18.5 and be 10–20 percent below normal on a standard height/weight table. One population that tends to struggle more with being too thin is the elderly. The CDC found that extreme thinness is associated with death in people over the age of 70. Also significant, unintentional weight loss has been associated with later development of Alzheimer's disease. A weight loss of 5 percent or more in a month is considered significant.

Nutritionists believe that the healthiest way to gain weight is to increase the intake of calorie-dense food. These foods are characterized by high fat density resulting from high levels of vegetable fats (polyunsaturated fats). Foods that meet this requirement include dried fruits, bananas, nuts, granola, and cheeses made from low-fat milk. These foods should be consumed later in a meal so that the onset of satiety that quickly follows eating fat-rich foods does not occur. The current recommendation is to eat three calorie-dense meals of moderate size per day, interspersed with two or three substantial snacks. Using MyPlate (see Chapter 5) as a guide, **underweight** people should increase intake from each group.[56]

A second component of weight gain for those who are underweight is an exercise program that uses weight-training activities intended to increase muscle mass. As detailed in Chapter 4, the use of anabolic drugs without highly competent medical supervision has no role in healthful weight gain. In addition, carefully monitored aerobic activity should be undertaken in sessions that adequately maintain heart-lung health. At the same time, unnecessary activity that expends calories should be restricted. See Chapter 4 to review the female athlete triad and its relationship to underweight.

For those who cannot gain weight, even by using these approaches, a medical evaluation may offer an explanation. If no medical reason can be found, the person may be among the 5 percent of the population who are naturally underweight.

When individuals fall below 80 percent of their desirable weight on standard height/weight tables and have BMIs below 16, it is highly probable that they are not only underweight but, more important, *undernourished* as well. This condition suggests clinically significant deficiencies in both the quantity of food being consumed and its nutritional value. Whether the undernourishment is associated with anorexia nervosa, other medical conditions characterized by weight loss (such as inflammatory bowel disease), or poverty or famine, affected people are in danger of death from starvation.

Eating Disorders

Given the pressure most people feel to maintain the cultural ideal of beauty, and being bombarded with images of very thin models and actresses such as Kate Bosworth, Mary-Kate Olsen, and Nicole Richie, it is no wonder that some develop serious medical and psychological disorders associated with body image, weight, and food. It is also not surprising that many of the very models we are trying to emulate also have eating disorders, as they succumb to the pressure to be even thinner. Anorexia nervosa, bulimia nervosa, binge eating, and disordered eating are frequently found in college populations. These topics are included in this chapter because most eating disorders begin with dieting. However, most eating disorders also involve inappropriate food choices and psychological issues (discussed in Chapters 2 and 5).

In the United States, conservative estimates indicate that after puberty 5–10 million females and 1 million males are struggling with eating disorders such as anorexia, bulimia, or binge eating. It is estimated that approximately 8 percent of college women will develop an eating disorder, and the population most at risk for developing bulimia is college freshman women. Ninety to 95 percent of people with eating disorders are women, although the prevalence of eating disorders in men is on the rise. Athletes such as dancers, gymnasts, swimmers, runners, and wrestlers are at risk for developing eating disorders because of the focus on weight and appearance for successful performance. In fact, any group in which success is influenced by weight or attractiveness is at risk for the development of an eating disorder, such as those involved in the performance arts, theater, television, and modeling.

Anorexia Nervosa

Anorexia nervosa is an eating disorder in which a person denies his or her own feelings of hunger and avoids food, with marked weight loss occurring. Anorexics tend to avoid food in the relentless pursuit of thinness,

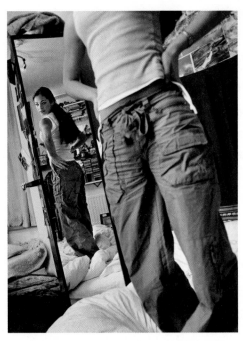

Preoccupation with weight and shape, inappropriate dieting, and perfectionism are factors associated with the development of eating disorders.

although they perceive themselves as never thin enough. To meet the diagnostic criteria for anorexia nervosa, the individual has to have an intense fear of gaining weight, even though he or she weighs less than 85 percent of the expected weight for his or her age, gender, and height, and, in females, menstruation ceases for at least three consecutive months.[57] In addition, people with anorexia perceive themselves as overweight, as much larger than they really are. Anorexics lose their ability to recognize when they are hungry and have difficulty eating even if they want to do so. Depression, irritability, withdrawal, perfectionism, and low self-esteem are some of the psychological problems associated with anorexia. In addition, anorexics tend to feel cold most of the time because they have very little body fat (2–10 percent) and also suffer from lightheadedness, dizziness, insomnia, hair

---

Key Terms

underweight A condition in which the body is below the desirable weight.

anorexia nervosa An eating disorder in which the individual weighs less than 85 percent of the expected weight for his or her age, gender, and height; has an intense fear of gaining weight; and, in females, ceases to menstruate for at least three consecutive months. People with anorexia perceive themselves as overweight, even though they are underweight.

Recognizing Anorexia Nervosa and Bulimia Nervosa

The American Psychological Association uses the following diagnostic criteria to identify anorexia nervosa and bulimia nervosa.

Anorexia	Bulimia
• Body weight 15 percent or more below desirable weight	• Binge eating two or more times a week for at least three months
• Fear of weight gain	• A lack of control over bingeing
• Distorted body image	• Inappropriate compensatory behavior, such as purging two or more times a week for at least three months to prevent weight gain
• In women, the absence of three or more menstrual periods (younger girls may not start menstruating at the appropriate age); in men, decrease in sex hormones	• Overly concerned about body image

Characteristic symptoms include the following. Note that it is unlikely that all the symptoms will be evident in any one individual.

Anorexia	Bulimia
• Looks thin and keeps getting thinner	• Uses bathroom immediately after eating
• Skips meals, cuts food into small pieces, moves food around plate to appear to have eaten	• Eats in secret
• Irregular or loss of menstrual periods and possible infertility	• Spends excessive time (and money) food shopping
• Wears baggy clothes in an attempt to disguise weight loss and to keep warm	• Shops for food at several stores instead of one store
• Experiences significant hair loss, develops lanugo (fine downy body hair)	• Has menstrual irregularities and possible fertility problems
• Has extreme sensitivity to cold	• Is excessively constipated
• Experiences dizziness, lightheadedness, headaches	• Has swollen and/or infected salivary glands, sore throat
• Is withdrawn, irritable, depressed	• Has bursting blood vessels in the eyes
• Suffers from insomnia, fatigue, loss of energy	• Experiences dental erosion in teeth and gums
• Has decreased sex drive	• Suffers dehydration and kidney dysfunction
• Is dehydrated, has kidney dysfunction	• Has significant hair loss, dry, brittle hair and nails
• Has decreased concentration	• Suffers from increased acne and skin problems
• Experiences heart irregularities, heart failure	• Experiences heart irregularities, heart failure

loss, muscle cramps, stress fractures, fatigue, decreased memory and concentration, and gastrointestinal problems. More serious complications include heart and kidney failure, hypothermia, osteoporosis, infertility, and, in 25 percent of cases, death. See the box "Recognizing Anorexia Nervosa and Bulimia Nervosa" for more information.

As with other eating disorders, anorexia nervosa also involves a sense of feeling out of control in one's life and attempting to find control through food and weight loss. It is not a coincidence that anorexia nervosa typically begins around puberty: Most individuals with anorexia have a fear of growing up and all that goes with being an adult, such as assuming financial responsibility, having sexual relationships, leaving one's family, and becoming more autonomous and independent.

Anorexia often begins with dieting but may also begin as a result of an illness, such as the stomach flu, or a relationship that breaks up, or after dental surgery, when it might be expected that one would temporarily eat less. However, anorexics will tell you that the disorder begins to take on a life of its own after what started as wanting to lose a few pounds turns into losing 15 percent or more of body weight and still not feeling satisfied with one's appearance. Friends and family might initially encourage the person on his or her weight loss and say complimentary things about his or her appearance but soon become concerned when the person's weight continues to dramatically decrease.

Anorexia has become more common as changing cultural ideals for beauty have changed. Our standards have gone from Marilyn Monroe, who was 5 feet 4 inches tall and 140 pounds, to Kate Moss, who has been reported to be 5 feet 7 inches tall and 105 pounds.[6] Now the "lollipop look" is considered the "in look" in Hollywood, with actresses and models having stick-thin bodies, making their heads seem huge. Many have admitted to having had anorexia—for example, the 2008 Miss America Kirsten Haglund, Spice Girl Victoria Beckham, singer Whitney Houston, and actresses Christina Ricci, Mary-Kate Olsen, Calista Flockhart, and Portia de Rossi. Because many of these stars are seen as the standard for the American body ideal, they may be contributing to the increasing number of women with eating disorders.

Denial of problems plays a major role in eating disorders in that the individual refuses to acknowledge that there is anything wrong, even though she is becoming thinner and wasting away, and family and friends are expressing great concern. Anorexia nervosa is considered a serious medical and psychological disorder; however, some anorexics argue that "anorexia is a lifestyle, not a disorder." Heated debates and discussions often take place on pro-anorexia websites. With names like "Thinspiration," "Stick Figures," and "Anorexic and Proud," these pro-anorexia forums have become very popular and deadly in the past few years. These websites show computer-enhanced pictures of models and actresses making them appear thinner and more skeletal than they really are.[58]

Messages on these websites include tips on how to starve, how to purge, and how to hide one's disorder, as well as encouragement to lose more weight. There has been a push among health providers, educators, and health organizations to eliminate these types of websites, and they have been somewhat successful. However, these sites still do exist, although somewhat disguised and underground.[59]

The three groups that have traditionally been overlooked in the incidence of anorexia are women of color, female athletes (see the discussion of the female athlete triad in Chapter 4), and men. The research shows a significant increase in the incidence of anorexia among these three groups. More focus has been given to anorexia among women of color, and it has been proposed that this group might be more vulnerable to developing eating disorders than Caucasian women are because of ethnocultural identity issues. It has been suggested that the more pressure women of color feel to fit into the dominant culture's standards of beauty and thinness, the more likely they are to develop eating disorders.

Often female athletes are not diagnosed with eating disorders because the symptoms of anorexia—absence of menses, low body fat and weight, and osteoporosis—are referred to as the female athlete triad and are not uncommon among athletes and don't necessarily signify the presence of an eating disorder.

The incidence of anorexia nervosa (as well as bulimia nervosa, which we'll cover next) has traditionally been much lower in men than in women. Today, however, the incidence of both conditions is increasing in men as they begin to feel some of the same pressures that women feel to conform to the weight and body composition standards imposed by others. The "lean look" of young male models serves as a standard for more and more young men, whereas the requirement to "make weight" for various sports drives others. Runners, jockeys, swimmers, wrestlers, and gymnasts frequently must lose weight quickly to meet particular standards for competition or the expectations of coaches and trainers. Researchers report that men are less inclined than women are to admit that they may have an eating disorder, thinking it is a "woman's illness." Thus, they are less likely to seek treatment. In addition, physicians tend not to suspect men of having eating disorders, and so they go untreated.

Fortunately, psychological treatment in combination with medical and dietary interventions can return the person with anorexia nervosa to a more life-sustaining pattern of eating. The person with anorexia needs to receive the care of professionals experienced in the treatment of this disorder. It is not uncommon for this treatment to take three to five years. If others, including friends, coworkers, roommates, and parents, observe this condition, they should consult a health care provider for assistance.

Bulimia Nervosa

Whereas anorexics are underweight, people with **bulimia nervosa** often are of a normal weight. These individuals use food and weight as a way of coping with stress, boredom, conflict in relationships, and low self-esteem. It is not uncommon in our society to comfort ourselves with food, to have social activities based on food, and to eat as a way of putting off a dreaded activity. However, people with bulimia take this to the extreme, engaging in recurrent bingeing—consuming unusually large amounts of food and feeling out of control with their eating.[57]

While anorexics run away from food, bulimics run to food to cope with their emotions, problems, and stress. Because they feel so guilty, ashamed, and anxious about the food they have consumed, people with bulimia **purge**

> ### Key Terms
>
> **bulimia nervosa** An eating disorder in which individuals engage in episodes of bingeing—consuming unusually large amounts of food, feeling out of control, and engaging in some compensatory purging behavior to eliminate the food.
>
> **purging** Using vomiting, laxatives, diuretics, enemas, or other medications, or means such as excessive exercise or fasting, to eliminate food.

by self-induced vomiting, taking an excessive number of laxatives and diuretics, or excessively exercising or fasting. There is a strong preoccupation with weight, calories, and food among sufferers of bulimia. Most people with bulimia constantly count calories, weigh themselves throughout the day, and frequently make negative statements concerning different parts of their bodies, primarily focusing on the thighs, stomach, and waist. As with anorexia, bulimia is associated with depression, isolation, anxiety, perfectionism, and low self-esteem. Dental erosion, hair loss, esophageal lesions, blood in vomit and stools, loss of voluntary gag reflex, kidney damage, heart failure, gastrointestinal problems, ketosis, edema, infertility, parotid gland swelling, depression, and insomnia are just some of the medical problems associated with bulimia nervosa.

Many celebrities have acknowledged struggling with this disorder, including Lady Gaga, Demi Lovato, Elton John, Jane Fonda, Paula Abdul and Katharine McPhee (*American Idol*), Felicity Huffman (*Desperate Housewives*), Joan Rivers, and the late Princess Diana. All these individuals have talked about the pressures to be thin in order to be successful in their careers and how they succumbed to this pressure by developing an eating disorder.

Bulimia often begins around 17 to 18 years of age when young adults are separating from their families and are forging lives of their own; some conflict arises around issues of independence, autonomy, and relationships with family. There is a higher incidence of bulimia than anorexia, although some bulimics may have had anorexia in the past. There is also a higher rate of bulimia among female college students as compared to their peers who are not attending college. Treatment for bulimia nervosa involves nutritional counseling, psychological counseling, and consultation with a physician. Often people with bulimia recover from this disorder within a year of beginning treatment.

Key Terms

binge eating disorder An eating disorder formerly referred to as compulsive overeating disorder; binge eaters use food to cope in the same way that bulimics do and also feel out of control, but do not engage in compensatory purging behavior.

body dysmorphic disorder (BDD) A secret preoccupation with an imagined or slight flaw in one's appearance.

bigorexia An obsession with getting bigger and more muscular, and thinking that your body is never muscular enough.

Binge Eating Disorder

Binge eating disorder is the newest term for what was previously referred to as compulsive overeating. It is the most common of all of the eating disorders, affecting 3.5 percent of women and 2 percent of men. It is also strongly linked to obesity. Binge eaters use food to cope in the same way that bulimics do and also feel out of control and unable to stop eating during binges. People with this disorder report eating rapidly and in secret or snacking all day. They tend to eat until they feel uncomfortably full, sometimes hoarding food and eating when they aren't physically hungry.[57] Like people with bulimia, they feel guilty about and ashamed of their eating habits and have a great deal of self-loathing and body hatred. People who have binge eating disorder do not engage in purging behavior, which differentiates them from people with bulimia nervosa. Typically, binge eaters have a long history of diet failures, feel anxious, are socially withdrawn from others, and are overweight. Heart problems, high blood pressure, joint problems, abnormal blood sugar levels, fatigue, depression, and anxiety are associated with binge eating. The treatment of this eating disorder involves interventions similar to those described for treating bulimia nervosa.

Chewing and Spitting Out Food Syndrome

Chewing and spitting out food without swallowing it has also been used as a method for weight loss or weight management. This is a common eating disorder and falls within the "eating disorder not otherwise specified" diagnosis. It differs from bulimia nervosa, and researchers contend that chewing and spitting out food without swallowing may indicate a more severe eating disorder.[60]

Night Eating Syndrome

Night eating syndrome has not yet been formally defined as an eating disorder. The signs and symptoms of this syndrome include eating more than half of one's daily food intake after dinner and before breakfast; feeling tense, anxious, and guilty while eating; having difficulty falling or staying asleep at night; and having little to no appetite in the morning. Unlike binge eating, night eating involves eating throughout the evening hours rather than in short episodes. Note that there is a strong preference for carbohydrates among night eaters. Some researchers speculate that night eating may be an unconscious attempt to self-medicate mood problems because eating carbohydrates can trigger the brain to produce so-called feel-good neurochemicals. About 60 percent of women and 40 percent of men suffer from night eating syndrome. It is also related to obesity. Research is underway to examine the underlying causes of this syndrome and develop subsequent treatment interventions. It seems likely that a combination of biological, genetic, and psychological factors contribute to this problem.

Body Dysmorphic Disorder

Body dysmorphic disorder (BDD) is a secret preoccupation with an imagined or slight flaw in one's appearance. Sometimes, people become almost completely fixated on concerns regarding body image, leading to repeatedly weighing themselves, checking mirrors throughout the day, compulsively dieting and exercising, and undergoing cosmetic surgery.[61] Perceptions of an imperfect body may lead to psychological dysfunction, such as not wanting to leave the house because of imagined defects. People with this disorder are 45 times more likely to commit suicide than the general population, demonstrating how their self-loathing can take a devastating toll on them.

Bigorexia

Bigorexia has been characterized as a "reverse anorexia nervosa" in which people want to be more muscular but see themselves as puny and scrawny.[62] Some say a better term for this would be *muscle dysmorphia,* because these people can never be muscular enough to satisfy their self-esteem. It has also been referred to as the *Adonis complex,* but women also suffer from this disorder, though not as frequently as men. Many people with bigorexia take anabolic steroids (see Chapter 4) or diet supplements to get bigger and more buff. People with this preoccupation obsessively lift weights for hours each day, sometimes sacrificing important social relationships, jobs, or physical

health. They can also become preoccupied with decreasing their fat as they increase their muscle, and they may develop eating disorders. Similar to people with anorexia, they tend to wear bigger clothes to hide their bodies, tend not to be seen in public, and avoid social situations because they have a negatively distorted view of themselves.

Treatment for Eating Disorders

The treatment for eating disorders is multimodal and multidimensional, involving nutritionists, psychologists, physicians, family, and friends. There are different treatment modalities, such as individual, group, and family counseling. Sometimes, treatment requires inpatient hospitalization to medically stabilize the individual. In extreme cases, a feeding tube may be inserted to treat starvation, especially if the person refuses to eat. Behavioral modification and cognitive therapy are utilized in counseling people with eating problems. Medications such as antidepressants are often used to decrease obsessive-compulsive behavior, reduce anxiety, alleviate depression, and improve mood. Some medications can stimulate or reduce appetite as well. There is some debate over the efficacy of using an addictions model, similar to the 12-step Alcoholics Anonymous philosophy, with eating disorders. Overeaters Anonymous utilizes this model in helping people with eating problems, and many hospital programs employ this model in their treatment programs. While there seems to be some overlap with substance abuse problems such as denying one's problems, feeling out of control of one's behavior, and using food or drugs or alcohol to cope with problems, this is where the similarities end—obviously, one needs food to live, which is not the case with drugs and alcohol.

Taking Charge of Your Health

- Investigate the resources available on your campus that you could use to determine your healthy weight and body composition profile.
- Evaluate your eating behaviors to find out if you are using food to cope with stress. If you are, develop a plan to use nonfood options, such as exercise or interaction with friends or family members, to deal with stress.

- Formulate a realistic set of goals for changing your weight and body composition in a time frame that allows you to do so in a healthful way.
- Establish a daily schedule that lets you make any necessary dietary and physical activity adjustments.
- Keep a daily journal of your weight-management efforts.

- Monitor your progress toward meeting your weight-management goals.
- Design a reward system for reaching each goal.
- Learn to accept your body, including the imperfections.
- Focus on other aspects of yourself besides your appearance.

SUMMARY

- Weight management has become an obsession in American culture, as well as a significant health problem; an estimated 66 percent of U.S. adults are either overweight or obese.
- Doctors usually define "overweight" as a condition in which a person's weight is 1–19 percent higher than "normal," as defined by a standard height/weight chart. Obesity is usually defined as a condition in which a person's weight is 20 percent or more above normal weight. "Morbid obesity" refers to being 50–100 percent over normal weight, more than 100 pounds over normal weight, or sufficiently overweight to interfere with health or normal functioning.
- Some of the methods for assessing one's weight are body mass index (BMI), current height/weight tables, waist-to-hip ratios, electrical impedance, Bod Pod, skinfold measurements, hydrostatic weighing, and home scales.
- Basal metabolic rate (BMR) is a measure of resting energy expenditure that is taken upon awakening, 10–12 hours after eating, or 12–18 hours after significant physical activity.
- Four factors seem to play a significant role in the prevalence of obesity: gender, age, socioeconomic status, and race.
- Psychological reasons for eating refer to eating not out of hunger but as a way of coping with feelings and socializing and celebrating with others, and by associating certain activities with eating.
- Weight loss occurs when the calories consumed are less than the energy the body needs for physiological maintenance and activity.
- The primary types of weight-management techniques include dietary alterations, surgical interventions, medications, weight loss programs, and physical activity.
- A commitment to a lifestyle change of eating in healthy ways and engaging in regular aerobic exercise seems to be the most effective strategy for weight loss and weight maintenance.
- Anorexia nervosa is a psychological condition in which the individual weighs less than 85 percent of his or her expected weight for his or her age, gender, and height.
- People with bulimia nervosa use food and weight as a way of coping with stress, boredom, conflict in relationships, and low self-esteem. They engage in recurrent bingeing and purging to eliminate the food from their bodies. Binge eaters use food to cope in the same way that bulimics do. They also feel out of control and unable to stop eating during binges but do not engage in purging behaviors.

REVIEW QUESTIONS

1. What percentage of U.S. adults are either overweight or obese?
2. How have the average caloric intake and physical activity levels for Americans changed over the past two decades?
3. Define *overweight, obesity,* and *morbid obesity.*
4. List at least four of the methods used for assessing weight.
5. Define basal metabolic rate (BMR).
6. What are four factors that seem to play a significant role in the prevalence of obesity?
7. Give four examples of how environmental factors can influence the amount the average person consumes.
8. Give examples of four different types of weight-management techniques.
9. What is the most effective strategy for weight loss and weight maintenance?
10. Describe the symptoms of anorexia nervosa, bulimia nervosa, and binge eating disorder.

ANSWERS TO THE "WHAT DO YOU KNOW?" QUIZ

1. True   2. True   3. False   4. False   5. False   6. False   7. True

Visit the Online Learning Center (**www.mhhe.com/hahn11e**), where you will find tools to help you improve your grade including practice quizzes, key terms flashcards, audio chapter summaries for your MP3 player, and many other study aids.

SOURCE NOTES

1. National Research Council. *Healthy People 2010.* www .healthypeople.com.
2. National Center for Chronic Disease Prevention and Health Promotion. *Defining Overweight and Obesity,* October 2008.
3. Centers for Disease Control and Prevention, Division of Nutrition, Physical Activity, and Obesity, National Center for Chronic Disease Prevention and Health Promotion, March 3, 2011.
4. Brownell KD, Fairburn CG. *Eating Disorders and Obesity: A Comprehensive Handbook.* New York: Guilford Press, 2005.
5. Field AE, et al. Impact of overweight on the risk of developing common chronic disease during a 10-year period. *Archives of Internal Medicine,* 161(13), 1581–86, 2001.
6. Poulton T. *No Fat Chicks.* Secaucus, NJ: Carol, 1997.
7. Dreisbach S. Exclusive body-image survey: 16,000 women tell their body confidence secrets. *Glamour,* March 23, 2009.
8. Kruger J, Lee C, Ainsworth B, Macera C. Body size satisfaction and physical activity levels among men and women. *Obesity,* 16(8), 1976–79, 2008.
9. National Institutes of Health Body Mass Index Table www.nhlbi.nih. gov/guidelines/obesity/bmi.tbl.htm.
10. Gaesser G. *Big Fat Lies.* Carlsbad, CA: Gurze Books, 2002.
11. Waist management: gauging your risk. *Consumer Reports,* 48, August 2003.
12. Binkley E, Fry M, Brown T. The relationship of college students' perceptions of their BMI and weight status to their physical self-concept. *American Journal of Health Education,* 40(3), 139–145, 2009.
13. International Health Racquet and Sportsclub Association. BOD POD body composition system to descend on San Francisco's IHRSA convention. As reported in the 29th Anniversary Exhibition in San Francisco's Moscone Convention Center, March 22–24, 2001.
14. Davis J. Experts rate the best and worst body fat measurements. *WebMD Health,* June 9, 2005.
15. America the fit. *Time Magazine,* June 23, 2008.
16. Ogden C, Carroll M, Curtin L, et al. Prevalence of overweight and obesity in the United States, 1999–2004. *Journal of the American Medical Association,* 295, 1549–55, 2006.
17. Harvard Women's Health Watch: Panel issues new guidelines for healthy eating. *Harvard Medical School,* 10(3), November 2002.
18. Kirby J. *Dieting for Dummies* (2nd ed). New York: Wiley, 2004.
19. *Dietary Guidelines for Americans,* www.health.gov/ dietaryguidelines. 2010.
20. Wardlaw GM, Byrd-Bredbenner C, Moe G, Beshgetoor D, Berning J. *Perspectives in Nutrition* (8th ed.). McGraw-Hill, 2008.
21. Wadden TA, Stunkard AJ. *Handbook of Obesity Treatment.* New York: Guilford Press, 2004.
22. Connor S. Scientists link obesity to "thrifty gene" of our ancestors. *The London Independent,* June 6, 2008.
23. Margetic S, Gazzola C, Pegg G, Hill R. Leptin: a review of its peripheral actions and interactions. *International Journal of Obesity and Related Metabolic Disorders,* 26(11), 1407–33, 2002.
24. Myers M, Cowley M, Münzberg H. Mechanisms of leptin action and leptin resistance. *Annual Review of Physiology,* 70, 537–556, 2008.
25. Cumming D, Overduin, J. Gastrointestinal regulation of food intake. *Journal of Clinical Investigation,* 117(1), 13–23, 2007.
26. La Leche-International. *The Womanly Art of Breastfeeding* (7th ed.). 2010.
27. Boyles S. Obesity linked to infertility in women. *WebMD Health,* December 11, 2007.
28. Gillman M, et al. Risk of overweight among adolescents who were breastfed as infants. *Journal of the American Medical Association,* 285(19), 2461–67, 2001.
29. Blackburn G. *Break Through Your Setpoint.* New York: HarperCollins, 2007.
30. The truth about dieting. *Consumer Reports,* 26–31 June 2002.
31. Flegal K, Carroll M, Ogden C, Curtin L. Prevalence and trends in obesity among U.S. adults, 1999–2008. *Journal of the American Medical Association,* 235–241, 2010.
32. Fitzgerald N, Himmelgreen D, Damio G, Segura-Pérez S, Peng Y-K, Pérez-Escamilla R. Acculturation, socioeconomic status, obesity and lifestyle factors among low-income Puerto Rican women in Connecticut, U.S., 1998–1999. *Rev Panam Salud Publica,* 19(5), 306–313, 2006.
33. Stunkard AJ, Wadden TA. *Obesity: Theory and Therapy.* New York: Raven Press, 2004.
34. Statistics related to overweight and obesity. National Institute of Health, August 2005.
35. Centers for Disease Control and Prevention. Behavioral risk factor surveillance system survey data. U.S. Department of Health and Human Services, 2011.
36. Craighead L. *The Appetite Awareness Workbook.* Oakland, CA: New Harbinger, 2006.
37. Under the influence: how external cues make us overeat. *Nutrition Action,* May 2011.
38. Goode E. Obesity in America. *New York Times,* August 19, 2003.
39. Overweight people gain when stressed. *USA Today,* July 9, 2009.
40. Middle age isn't too late to lose. *USA Today,* October 28, 2009.
41. Sleep loss may equal weight gain. *USA Today,* December 7, 2004.
42. One more reason to get enough sleep. *Harvard Women's Health Watch,* May 2005.
43. Foster G, Wyatt H, Hill J, Rosenbaum D, et al. Weight and metabolic outcomes after 2 years on a low-carbohydrate versus low-fat diet: a randomized trial. *Annals of Internal Medicine,* 153(3), 147–157.
44. Ephedra ban puts herb industry on notice. *New York Times,* December 31, 2003.
45. Ephedra-free doesn't mean risk-free. *WebMD Health,* September 9, 2005.
46. FDA recalls hydroxycut supplements after reports of liver damage. *Consumer Reports,* November 2, 2009.
47. FDA warns against some diet pills sold on the web. *USA Today,* December 22, 2008.
48. Center for Drug Evaluation and Research, U.S. Food and Drug Administration. FDA announces withdrawal of fenfluramine and dexfenfluramine. News release 97–32, September 15, 1997.
49. Diet pills in the pipeline. *USA Today,* October 22, 2009.
50. Taking the diet pill . . . alli. *People,* July 9, 2007.
51. Obesity surgery increases 600 percent. ABC News, May 31, 2006.
52. Panel back expanding use of stomach bands. *Star Press,* December 4, 2010.
53. Addicted to plastic surgery. *People Magazine,* January 13, 2010.
54. Grazer FM, de Jong RH. Fatal outcomes from liposuction: census survey of cosmetic surgeons. *Plastic Reconstructive Surgery,* 105(1), 436–446, 2000.
55. Center for Drug Evaluation and Research, FDA. FDA announces withdrawal of fenfluramine and dexfenfluramine. News Release no. 97–32, September 15, 1997.
56. American Dietetic Association. Gaining weight: a healthy plan for adding pounds. *Hot Topics.* www.eatright.org/nfs10html. 2009.
57. *Diagnostic and Statistical Manual of Mental Disorders IV-TR.* Washington, DC: American Psychiatric Association, 2000.
58. Gotthelf M. The new anorexia outrage. *Self Magazine,* 82–84, August 2001.
59. Lilenfeld L. Academy members debate over pro-anorexia websites. *Academy of Eating Disorders Newsletter,* June 2001.
60. Update: chewing and spitting out food. *Eating Disorders Review,* July/ August, 2002.
61. A dangerous duo: body dysmorphic disorder with anorexia nervosa. *Eating Disorders Review,* 4–5, November/December 2002.
62. Pope H, Phillips K, Olivardia R. *The Adonis Complex.* New York: Simon & Schuster, 2000.

Personal Assessment

Do You Eat Mindfully or Mindlessly?

Below is a collection of statements about your everyday experiences. Using the 1–6 scale, indicate how frequently or infrequently you currently have each experience. Answer according to what really reflects your experience rather than what you think your experience should be. Treat each item separately from every other item.

1 = Almost always	2 = Very frequently	3 = Somewhat frequently	4 = Somewhat infrequently	5 = Very infrequently	6 = Almost never

1. I could be experiencing some emotion and not be conscious of it until sometime later. 1 2 3 4 5 6
2. I break or spill things because of carelessness, not paying attention, or thinking of something else. 1 2 3 4 5 6
3. I find it difficult to stay focused on what's happening in the present. 1 2 3 4 5 6
4. I tend to walk quickly to get where I'm going without paying attention to what I experience along the way. 1 2 3 4 5 6
5. I tend not to notice feelings of physical tension or discomfort until they really grab my attention. 1 2 3 4 5 6
6. I forget a person's name almost as soon as I've been told it for the first time. 1 2 3 4 5 6
7. It seems I am "running on automatic," without much awareness of what I'm doing. 1 2 3 4 5 6
8. I rush through activities without being really attentive to them. 1 2 3 4 5 6
9. I get so focused on the goal I want to achieve that I lose touch with what I'm doing right now to get there 1 2 3 4 5 6
10. I do jobs or tasks automatically, without being aware of what I'm doing. 1 2 3 4 5 6
11. I find myself listening to someone with one ear, doing something else at the same time. 1 2 3 4 5 6
12. I drive places on "automatic pilot" and then wonder why I went there. 1 2 3 4 5 6
13. I find myself preoccupied with the future or the past. 1 2 3 4 5 6
14. I find myself doing things without paying attention. 1 2 3 4 5 6
15. I snack without being aware that I'm eating. 1 2 3 4 5 6

Interpretation

To find your score, add up your scores for all 15 items and then divide by 15. (This will give you your mean score.) The higher your mean score, the higher your level of mindfulness.

TO CARRY THIS FURTHER . . .

If you scored low on this assessment, try some of the suggestions in the box "Learning to Eat Mindfully" to become a more mindful eater.

Personal Assessment

Body Love or Body Hate?

When you catch a glimpse of yourself in a mirror, do you smile or grimace at what you see? The following quiz will help you to assess your body self-esteem associated with your appearance. Please answer using the following rating scale:

1 = Rarely or never
2 = Sometimes
3 = Almost always or always

Add up your scores to determine your total score, and look at the interpretation of your scores.

_____ 1. I worry about my weight and weighing "too much."

_____ 2. I prefer to eat by myself and not with other people.

_____ 3. My mood is determined by the scale and how I feel about my appearance.

_____ 4. I make negative comments about my appearance to myself and others.

_____ 5. I think I look less attractive on days that I haven't exercised.

_____ 6. I have a difficult time accepting compliments about my appearance from others.

_____ 7. I compare myself to other people and find myself lacking.

_____ 8. I ask other people how I look.

_____ 9. I avoid social situations, activities, and events involving food.

_____ 10. I feel more anxious about my body in the summertime because of the need to wear bathing suits and clothing suitable for warmer temperatures.

_____ **TOTAL POINTS**

Interpretation

10 to 15—You have positive body self-esteem and are accepting of yourself and your appearance.

16 to 23—You scored in the average range.

24 to 30—You have poor or low body self-esteem.

TO CARRY THIS FURTHER . . .

If you scored in the average range: While you are in good company, feeling about your body the way most people do, you may want to reframe your body image and develop more of an appreciation for your body and appearance.

If you have poor body self-esteem: Your self-esteem in general is probably driven by how you see yourself, and you may be putting too much emphasis on your appearance and are too self-critical. You may feel as though you never are thin enough or look good enough and can always find a flaw when looking in the mirror. To improve your body self-esteem, focus on other aspects of yourself, focus on the positive aspects of your body, and be more accepting of yourself and less perfectionistic.

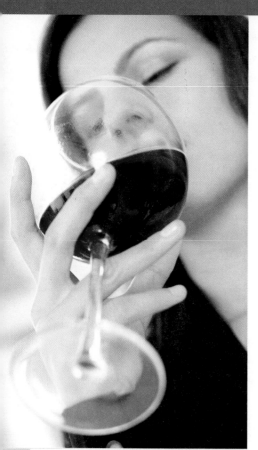

7

Making Decisions About Drug and Alcohol Use

What Do You Know About Drug and Alcohol Use?

1. Intravenous drug injection is the most efficient and fastest way to administer a drug. True or False?

2. Women absorb alcohol into their bloodstream faster than men do. True or False?

3. The vomiting reflex prevents an individual from becoming poisoned by alcohol. True or False?

4. Drug use is highest for 18- to 25-year-olds, compared to any other age group. True or False?

5. The use of all drugs has been increasing over the years. True or False?

6. Energy drinks such as Red Bull can have dangerous effects on the heart. True or False?

7. Putting someone in a cold shower, giving them coffee, or walking them around are good ways to sober them up. True or False?

Check your answers at the end of the chapter.

Each of us may have different ideas about what qualifies as a **drug.** The most accepted definition is "any substance, natural or artificial, other than food, that by its chemical or physical nature alters structure or function in the living organism."[1] Included in this broad definition is a variety of psychoactive drugs, medicines, and substances that many people do not usually consider to be drugs.

Psychoactive drugs alter the user's feelings, behavior, perceptions, or moods; they include stimulants, depressants, hallucinogens, opiates, and inhalants. Prescription medications function to heal unhealthy tissue, as well as to ease pain, prevent illness, and diagnose health conditions. Although some psychoactive drugs are used for medical reasons, as in the case of tranquilizers and some narcotics, the most commonly prescribed medicines are antibiotics, hormone replacement drugs, sulfa drugs, diuretics, oral contraceptives, and cardiovascular drugs. Legal substances are also considered to be drugs, such as caffeine, tobacco, alcohol, aspirin, and other over-the-counter (OTC) preparations. These substances are used so commonly in our society that they are rarely perceived as drugs.

For organizational reasons, this chapter primarily deals with psychoactive drugs including alcohol. The effects of tobacco are discussed in Chapter 8. Prescription and OTC drugs and medicines are explored further in Chapter 14. Anabolic steroids, drugs used primarily for increasing muscle growth, are discussed in Chapter 4.

Drug Misuse and Abuse

What is the difference between use, misuse, and abuse? The term *use* is all-encompassing and describes drug taking in the most general way. For example, Americans use drugs of many types. The term *use* can also refer more narrowly to misuse and abuse. **Misuse** is defined as the inappropriate use of legal drugs intended to be medications. **Abuse** is any use of drugs in a way that is detrimental to one's physical, psychological, social, or occupational functioning. Misuse or abuse of drugs can lead to **intoxication,** which literally means poisoning by a drug or toxic substance. Drug intoxication usually involves dysfunctional and disruptive changes in physiological and psychological functioning, mood, and cognitive processes, resulting from the consumption of a psychoactive substance. Over time, misuse and abuse of drugs can result in **psychological dependence.**

Dependence

Psychoactive drugs and alcohol have a strong potential for the development of **dependence.** When users take a psychoactive drug or use alcohol, the patterns of nervous system functions are altered. If these altered functions provide perceived benefits for the user, the substance use

---

Key Terms

drug Any substance, natural or artificial, other than food, that by its chemical or physical nature alters structure or function in the living organism.

psychoactive drug Any substance capable of altering feelings, moods, or perceptions.

misuse Inappropriate use of drugs intended to be medications.

abuse Any use of a drug in a way that is detrimental to health.

intoxication Dysfunctional and disruptive changes in physiological and psychological functioning, mood, and cognitive processes resulting from the consumption of a psychoactive substance.

psychological dependence Craving a drug for emotional reasons and to maintain a sense of well-being; also called *habituation*.

dependence A physical or psychological need to continue using a drug.

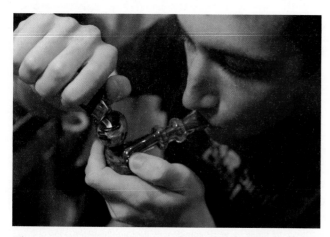

The way a drug enters the body influences the speed of its effects, and more rapid effects are associated with a higher risk of dependence. A drug reaches the brain quickly when administered by inhalation.

may continue, perhaps at increasingly larger dosages. If persistent use continues, the user can develop a dependence on the drug. Pharmacologists have identified two types of dependences: physical and psychological.

A person can be said to have developed a *physical dependence* when the body cells have become reliant on a drug. Continued use of the drug is then required because body tissues have adapted to its presence.[2] The person's body needs the drug to maintain homeostasis, or dynamic balance. If the drug is not taken or is suddenly withdrawn, the user experiences **withdrawal.** The symptoms of withdrawal reflect the attempt by the body's cells to regain normality without the drug. Common withdrawal symptoms include anxiety, sweating, tremors, vomiting, insomnia, irritability, and depression. Abrupt withdrawal from some drugs, such as alcohol or barbiturates, can be life threatening. In this chapter, the term *addiction* is used interchangeably with *physical dependence.*

Continued use of most drugs can lead to **tolerance.** Tolerance is an acquired reaction to a drug in which continued intake of the same dose has diminishing effects.[2] The user needs larger doses of the drug to receive the same effect. The continued use of depressants, including alcohol, and opiates can cause users to quickly develop a tolerance to the drug.

Tolerance developed for one drug may carry over to another drug within the same general category. This phenomenon is known as **cross-tolerance.** The heavy abuser of alcohol, for example, might require a larger dose of a preoperative sedative to become relaxed before surgery than the average person would. The tolerance to alcohol "crosses over" to the other depressant drugs.

A person who possesses a strong desire to continue using a particular drug is said to have developed a *psychological dependence.* People who are psychologically dependent on a drug believe that they need to consume the

drug to maintain a sense of well-being. They crave the drug for emotional reasons despite having persistent or recurrent physical, social, psychological, or occupational problems caused or worsened by the drug use. Abrupt withdrawal from a drug by such a person would not trigger the fully expressed withdrawal, although some unpleasant symptoms of withdrawal might be felt. The term **habituation** is often used interchangeably with *psychological dependence.*

Drugs whose continued use can quickly lead to both physical and psychological dependence are depressants (barbiturates, tranquilizers, and alcohol), narcotics (the opiates, which are derivatives of the Oriental poppy: heroin, morphine, and codeine), and synthetic narcotics (Demerol and methadone). Drugs whose continued use can lead to various degrees of psychological dependence and occasionally to significant (but not life-threatening) physical dependence in some users are the stimulants (amphetamines, caffeine, and cocaine), hallucinogens (LSD, peyote, mescaline, and marijuana), and inhalants (glues, gases, and petroleum products).

Addictive Behavior

Drug and alcohol use are two of the many forms of addictive behavior. People can also be addicted to behaviors that are detrimental to their lives and relationships, such as gambling, shopping, gaming, and sexual activity. These are referred to as **process addictions.** Similar to the dependence upon drugs, process addictions can cause serious financial, emotional, social, and health problems. People believe that they have control over their shopping, gambling, and gaming activities, but it becomes apparent after a while to others around them that they are out of control and their behavior is excessive and unhealthy. People with process addictions feel a compulsion to engage in this behavior and use the behavior as a stress reliever and coping strategy. Addiction may or may not include physical dependence on a drug and focuses on the person's behavior while dependence involves physiological functioning.

The Process of Addiction The process of developing an addiction has been a much-studied topic. Three common aspects of addictive behavior are exposure, compulsion, and loss of control.

Exposure An addiction can begin after a person is exposed to a drug (such as alcohol) or a behavior (such as gambling) that he or she finds enjoyable (see the box "Improving Your Mood Without Drugs or Alcohol"). This initial pleasure gradually, reinforces the addictive behavior, which can then lead to compulsive behavior.

Compulsion Increasingly, the person spends more energy, time, and money pursuing the drug use or behavior. At this point in the addictive process, the person can be said to have a compulsion for the drug or behavior. Frequently, repeated exposure to the drug or behavior continues despite negative consequences.

During the compulsion phase, a person's life often degenerates as the person feels a strong urge to experience the effects of the drug or the behavior. An addicted person's family, friends, work, or school become less important than does the search for more and better "highs." The development of tolerance and withdrawal may develop at this point. (These terms are discussed later in the chapter.)

Why some people develop compulsions and others do not is difficult to pinpoint, but addiction might be influenced by genetic makeup, family dynamics, physiological processes, personality type, peer groups, and available resources for help.

Loss of Control   Over time, the person experiences both an increased need for the drug or behavior and a desire to avoid the effects of withdrawal. Addicted people lose the ability to control their behavior. Despite overwhelming negative consequences (for example, deterioration of health, alienation of family and friends, or loss of all financial resources), addicted people continue to behave in ways that make their lives worse. The person addicted to alcohol continues to drink heavily, the person addicted to shopping continues to run up large debts, and the person addicted to sex continues to have sex indiscriminately. Frequently, a person has addictions to more than one drug or behavior or may switch from one addiction to another.

 TALKING POINTS How would you tell a friend that her video game playing is becoming an addiction that needs to be controlled?

Codependence   In some cases, people close to a person with an addiction develop a codependent relationship, in which they deny the addiction and enable the addicted person. Enabling behaviors include things like making excuses and providing assistance to keep the individual's work, academic, and/or family life intact. These actions help the addicted person continue with his or her behavior without experiencing all the negative consequences, possibly delaying treatment. People in codependent relationships are at increased risk for developing addictive behaviors themselves and for facing a variety of psychological consequences related to guilt, loss of identity and self-esteem, depression, and anxiety. Both private and public programs are available to help codependent people learn new behaviors and new ways of interacting.

Basic Terminology and Concepts

Before we move on to discussing specific types of drugs, it is important to review general principles of addictive behavior, how psychoactive drugs affect the body, and how different methods and patterns of use influence drug effects and health.

Actions of Drugs on the Central Nervous System

To better understand the disruption caused by the actions of psychoactive drugs, a general knowledge of the normal functioning of the nervous system's basic unit, the **neuron,** is required.

First, stimuli from the internal or external environment are received by the appropriate sensory receptor, perhaps an organ such as an eye or an ear. Once sensed, these stimuli are converted into electrical impulses. These impulses are then directed along the neuron's **dendrite,** through the cell body, and along the **axon** toward the *synaptic junction* near an adjacent neuron. On arrival at the **synapse,** the electrical impulses stimulate the production and release of chemical messengers called neurotransmitters.[3] These neurotransmitters transmit the electrical impulses from one neuron to the dendrites of adjoining neurons. Thus, neurons function in a coordinated fashion to send information to the brain for interpretation and to

Key Terms

withdrawal Uncomfortable, perhaps toxic response of the body as it attempts to maintain homeostasis in the absence of a drug; also called *abstinence syndrome.*

tolerance An acquired reaction to a drug; continued intake of the same dose has diminished effects.

cross-tolerance Transfer of tolerance from one drug to another within the same general category.

habituation The development of psychological dependence on a drug after a period of use.

process addictions Addictions in which people compulsively engage in behaviors such as gambling, shopping, gaming, or sexual activity to such an extreme degree that these addictions cause serious financial, emotional, social, and health problems similar to those resulting from drug and alcohol addictions.

neuron (**noor** on) A nerve cell.

dendrite (**den** drite) The portion of a neuron that receives electrical stimuli from adjacent neurons; neurons typically have several such branches or extensions.

axon The portion of a neuron that conducts electrical impulses to the dendrites of adjacent neurons; neurons typically have one axon.

synapse (**sinn** aps) The location at which an electrical impulse from one neuron is transmitted to an adjacent neuron; also referred to as a *synaptic junction.*

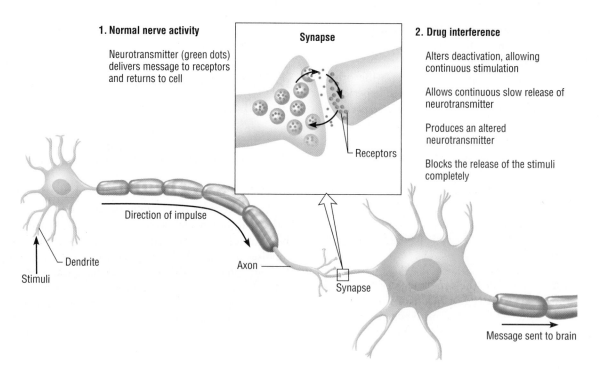

1. Normal nerve activity

Neurotransmitter (green dots) delivers message to receptors and returns to cell

Synapse

Receptors

2. Drug interference

Alters deactivation, allowing continuous stimulation

Allows continuous slow release of neurotransmitter

Produces an altered neurotransmitter

Blocks the release of the stimuli completely

Direction of impulse

Dendrite

Stimuli

Axon

Synapse

Message sent to brain

Figure 7-1 The Action of Psychoactive Drugs on the Central Nervous System   Neurotransmitters are chemical messengers that transfer electrical impulses across the synapses between nerve cells. Psychoactive drugs interrupt this process, thus disrupting the normal functioning of the nervous system.

relay appropriate response commands back to the tissues of the body.

The role of neurotransmitters is critical to the relay of information within the system. A substance that has the ability to alter some aspect of transmitter function also has the potential to seriously disrupt the otherwise normally functioning system. Psychoactive drugs (including alcohol) are capable of exerting these disruptive influences on the neurotransmitters. Drugs change the way neurotransmitters work, often by blocking the production of a neurotransmitter or forcing the continued release of a neurotransmitter (see Figure 7-1).

With some drugs, the higher the dose, the stronger the effect on the body. For other drugs, there is an all-or-none response, so when the body responds it is at the maximum level and further additions of the drug have no effect. This is called the **dose-response curve,** in which the size of the response is related to the amount of the drug administered. The smallest amount of a drug that produces a response is referred to as the **threshold dose,** meaning that any amount less than that would not have an observable effect on the body. For example, a very low dose of a sedative may have no observable effect, while a moderate dose might cause drowsiness and feelings of relaxation; a high dose of a sedative would result in loss of consciousness.

Routes of Drug Administration

Drugs generally enter the body through one of four methods: ingestion, injection, inhalation, or absorption.

Ingestion, or oral administration, is the entry of drugs through the mouth and into the digestive tract. *Injection* refers to the use of a needle to insert a drug into the body. With *inhalation,* the drug enters the body through the lungs. *Absorption* refers to the administration of a drug through the skin or mucous membranes.

Different routes of administration can have different effects. In inhalation and injection, the drug reaches the brain quickly, and these methods of use are associated with a greater risk of dependence. Injection use carries a higher risk of overdose, because large amounts of the drug can be administered at one time, as well as a risk for infection such as HIV and hepatitis.

Major Drug Classifications

Drugs can be categorized according to the nature of their physiological effects. Most psychoactive drugs fall into one of six general categories: stimulants, depressants, hallucinogens, cannabis, narcotics, and inhalants (see Table 7.1).

> **Key Terms**
>
> **dose-response curve** The size of the effect of a drug on the body related to the amount of the drug administered.
>
> **threshold dose** The least amount of a drug to have an observable effect on the body.

Table 7.1 Drugs of Abuse: Uses and Effects

Drugs	Trade or Other Names	Medical Uses	Dependence Physical	Dependence Psycho-logical	Tolerance	Duration (hours)	Usual Method	Possible Effects	Effects of Overdose	Withdrawal Syndrome
Narcotics										
Heroin	Diamorphine, horse, smack, black tar, *chiva, negra*	None in U.S., analgesic, antitussive	High	High	Yes	3–4	Injected, snorted, smoked	Euphoria, drowsi-ness, respiratory depression, constricted pupils, nausea	Slow and shallow breathing, clammy skin, convulsions, coma, possible death	Water eyes, runny nose, yawning, loss of appetite, irritability, tremors, panic, cramps, nausea, chills and sweating
Morphine	MS-Contin, Rox-anol, Oramorph SR, MSIR	Analgesic	High	High	Yes	3–12	Oral, injected			
Hydro-codone	Hydrocodone w/ acetaminophen, Vicodin, Vicoprofen, Tus-sionex, Lortab	Analgesic, antitussive	High	High	Yes	3–6	Oral			
Hydro-morphone	Dilaudid	Analgesic	High	High	Yes	3–4	Oral, injected			
Oxyco-done	Roxicet, Oxycodone w/ acetaminophen, OxyContin, Endo-cet, Percocet, Percodan	Analgesic	High	High	Yes	3–12	Oral			
Codeine	Acetaminophen, Guaifenesin or Promethazine w/ codeine, Fiori-nal, Fioricet or Tylenol w/codeine	Analgesic, antitussive	Moderate	Moderate	Yes	3–4	Oral, injected			
Other narcotics	Fentanyl, Demerol, Methadone, Darvon, Stadol, Talwin, Paregoric, Buprenex	Analgesic, antidiarrheal, antitussive	High-Low	High-Low	Yes	Variable	Oral, injected, snorted, smoked			
Depressants										
Gamma hydroxybu-tyric acid	GHB, Liquid Ecstasy, Liquid X, Sodium Oxybate, Xyrem®	None in U.S., anesthetic	Moderate	Moderate	Yes	3–6	Oral	Slurred speech, disori-entation, drunken behavior without odor of alcohol, impaired memory of events, interacts with alcohol	Shallow respiration, clammy skin, dilated pupils, weak and rapid pulse, coma, possible death	Anxiety, insomnia, tremors, delirium, convulsions, possible death
Benzodiaz-epines	Valium, Xanax, Halcion, Ativan, Restoril, Rohypnol (Roofies, R-2), Klonopin	Antianxiety, sedative, anti-convulsant, hypnotic, muscle relaxant	Moderate	Moderate	Yes	1–8	Oral, injected			
Other depressants	Ambien, Sonata, Meprobamate, Chloral Hydrate, barbiturates, Methaqualone (Quaalude)	Antianxiety, sedative, hypnotic	Moderate	Moderate	Yes	2–6	Oral			

(continued)

Table 7.1 Drugs of Abuse: Uses and Effects *(continued)*

Drugs	Trade or Other Names	Medical Uses	Dependence — Physical	Dependence — Psychological	Tolerance	Duration (hours)	Usual Method	Possible Effects	Effects of Overdose	Withdrawal Syndrome
Stimulants										
Cocaine	Coke, flake, snow, crack, *coca, blanca, perico, nieve,* soda	Local anesthetic	Possible	High	Yes	1–2	Snorted, smoked, injected	Increased alertness, excitation, euphoria, increased pulse rate and blood pressure, insomnia, loss of appetite	Agitation, increased body temperature, hallucinations, convulsions, possible death	Apathy, long periods of sleep, irritability, depression, disorientation
Amphetamine/ methamphetamine	Crank, ice, crystal, glass meth, speed, Adderall, Dexedrine, Desoxyn	Attention deficit hyperactivity disorder, narcolepsy, weight control	Possible	High	Yes	2–4	Oral, injected, smoked			
Methylphenidate	Ritalin (Illy's), Concerta, Focalin, Metadate	Attention deficit hyperactivity disorder	Possible	High	Yes	2–4	Oral, injected, snorted, smoked			
Hallucinogens										
MDMA and analogs	(Ecstasy, XTC, Adam), MDA (love drug), MDEA (Eve), MBDB	None	None	Moderate	Yes	4–6	Oral, snorted, smoked	Heightened senses, teeth grinding, dehydration	Increased body temperature, electrolyte imbalance, cardiac arrest	Muscle aches, drowsiness, depression, acne
LSD	Acid, microdot, sunshine, boomers	None	None	Unknown	Yes	8–12	Oral	Illusions and hallucinations, altered perception of time and distance	(LSD) Longer, more intense "trip" episodes	None
Phencyclidine and analogs	PCP, angel dust, hog, loveboat, Ketamine (Special K), PCE, PCPY, TCP	Anesthetic (Ketamine)	Possible	High	Yes	1–12	Smoked, oral, injected, snorted		Inability to direct movement, feel pain, or remember	Drug-seeking behavior
Other hallucinogens	Psilocybin mushrooms, mescaline, peyote cactus, Ayahausca, DMT, Dextromethorphan (DXM)	None	None	None	Possible	4–8	Oral			
Cannabis										
Marijuana	Pot, grass, sinsemilla, blunts, *mota, yerba, grifa*	None	Unknown	Moderate	Yes	2–4	Smoked, oral	Euphoria, relaxed inhibitions, increased appetite, disorientation	Fatigue, paranoia, possible psychosis	Occasional reports of insomnia, hyperactivity, decreased appetite
Hashish and hash oil	Hash, hash oil	None	Unknown	Moderate	Yes	2–4	Smoked, oral			

(continued)

Table 7.1 Drugs of Abuse: Uses and Effects *(continued)*

								Inhalants			
Nitrous oxide	Laughing gas, balloons, whippets	Anesthetic	Unknown	Low	No	0.5	Inhaled	Impaired memory, slurred speech, drunken behavior, slow-onset vitamin deficiency	Vomiting, respiratory depression, loss of consciousness, possible death	Trembling, anxiety, insomnia, vitamin deficiency, confusion, hallucinations, convulsions

Source: Hart C, Ksir C, Ray O, *Drugs, Society, and Human Behavior*. New York: McGraw-Hill, 2009.

Marijuana is the only drug that shows a significant increase in use over the past few years (see Figure 7-2). According to the 2009 NSDUH National Findings for Alcohol and Drug Information, American Indians had the highest rate of substance abuse and dependence (18.3 percent) while Asians had the lowest rate (3.7 percent); 7.9 percent of Hispanics and 9.6 percent of African Americans reported substance abuse or dependence in 2009.

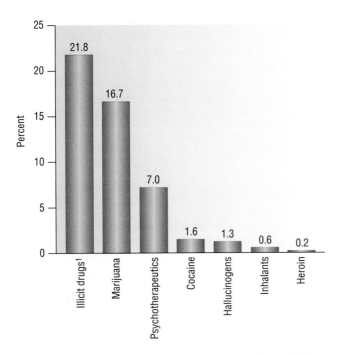

[1]Illicit Drugs include marijuana/hashish, cocaine (including crack), heroin, hallucinogens, inhalants, or prescription-type psychotherapeutics used nonmedically.

Figure 7-2 Past-Month Use of Selected Illicit Drugs Among Americans Ages 12 and Older   Marijuana is the most commonly used illicit drug, followed by nonmedical use of prescription drugs (psychotherapeutics).

Source: Substance Abuse and Mental Health Services Administration, Office of Applied Studies. *Results from the 2009 National Survey on Drug Use and Health: National Findings* (NSDUH Series H-34, DHHS Publication No. SMA 08-4343). Rockville, MD, 2010.

Stimulants

In general, **stimulants** excite or increase the activity of the central nervous system (CNS). Also called "uppers," stimulants alert the CNS by increasing heart rate, blood pressure, and the rate of brain function. Users feel uplifted and less fatigued. Examples of stimulant drugs include caffeine, amphetamines, and cocaine. Most stimulants produce psychological dependence and tolerance relatively quickly, but they are unlikely to produce significant physical dependence when judged by life-threatening withdrawal symptoms. The important exception is cocaine, which seems to be capable of producing psychological dependence and withdrawal so powerful that continued use of the drug is inevitable for some users.

Caffeine   Caffeine is a CNS stimulant found in chocolate, some soft drinks, energy drinks, coffee, tea, some aspirin products, and OTC "stay-awake" pills. It is a relatively harmless stimulant when consumed in moderate amounts.[4] Approximately 72 percent of Americans drink coffee daily, consuming an average of 3.4 cups per day per person, earning the United States the name "Caffeine Nation."[5]

For the average healthy adult, moderate consumption of caffeine is unlikely to pose any serious health threat. However, excessive consumption, also called caffeine intoxication, can occur when a person takes in more than 500 mg/day of caffeine. Consuming more than this amount of caffeine can lead to anxiety, diarrhea, restlessness, insomnia, headache, and heart palpitations. Most experts agree that 400 mg/day of caffeine, which is equivalent to 4 cups of coffee, is a moderate amount of caffeine consumption. Energy drinks, an increasingly

> **Key Terms**
>
> **stimulants** Psychoactive drugs that stimulate the function of the central nervous system.

Chapter Seven Making Decisions About Drug and Alcohol Use   **161**

popular source of caffeine, can range in caffeine content; an 8-ounce can of Red Bull contains 80 mg of caffeine, and a 16-ounce can of Monster Energy contains 160 mg of caffeine (see the box "The Buzz on Energy Drinks"). Pregnant women are advised to avoid caffeine consumption.[6]

Amphetamines   Amphetamines produce increased activity and mood elevation in almost all users. The amphetamines include several closely related compounds: amphetamine, dextroamphetamine, and methamphetamine. These compounds do not have any natural sources and are completely manufactured in the laboratory. Medical use of amphetamines is limited primarily to the treatment of obesity, **narcolepsy,** and **attention deficit hyperactivity disorder (ADHD).**

Amphetamines can be ingested, injected, or inhaled (shorted). At low-to-moderate doses, amphetamines elevate mood and increase alertness and feelings of energy by stimulating receptor sites for two naturally occurring neurotransmitters. They also slow the activity of the stomach and intestines and decrease hunger. In the 1960s and 1970s, in fact, amphetamines were commonly prescribed for dieters. Later, when it was discovered that the appetite suppression effect of amphetamines lasted only a few weeks, most physicians stopped prescribing them. At high doses, amphetamines can elevate heart rate and blood pressure to dangerous levels. As amphetamines are eliminated from the body, the user becomes tired.

When chronically abused, amphetamines produce rapid tolerance and strong psychological dependence. Other effects of chronic use include impotence and episodes of psychosis. When use is discontinued, periods of depression may develop.

Methamphetamine   Today the abuse of amphetamines is a more pressing concern than it has been in the recent past because of the sharp increase in abuse of methamphetamine. Known by a variety of names and forms, including "crank," "ice," "crystal," "meth," "speed," "crystal meth," and "zip," methamphetamine is produced in illegal home laboratories.[7]

Crystal meth, or ice, is among the most dangerous forms of methamphetamine. Ice is a very pure form of methamphetamine that looks like rock candy.[8] When ice is smoked or injected, its effects are felt in about seven seconds as a wave of intense physical and psychological exhilaration. This is due to the drug "telling" the brain to release large amounts of dopamine.[9] This effect lasts for several hours (much longer than the effects of *crack*), until the user becomes physically exhausted. When ingested orally or snorted, methamphetamine induces euphoria that may result in a quick addiction. Abuse can lead to memory loss, violence, and cardiac and neurological damage. Chronic use can result in Parkinson-like symptoms, rotten teeth ("meth mouth"), stroke, anorexia, increased heart rate and blood pressure,

The Buzz on Energy Drinks

The sales of energy drinks have skyrocketed in recent years, making it the $3.4-billion-per-year industry it is today. Consumers of energy drinks say that they have increased energy, alertness, and stamina. The energy in these drinks comes primarily from caffeine and sugar, as they have 80–350 mg per can or bottle. Dizziness, light-headedness, rapid heartbeat, dehydration, and numbness and tingling in the hands and feet are some of the side effects of these drinks. When consuming numerous cans or the ones with higher levels of caffeine, people have experienced seizures, stroke, and even death, as was the case of the 18-year-old athlete in France who died after consuming four cans of Red Bull. Redline Power Rush, a 74-milliliter bottle with 350 mg of caffeine, comes with a warning to drink it in multiple servings, not all at one time; it also states that it is not meant for people under age 18. However, 65 percent of energy drinkers are teenagers. Another concern related to energy drinks is their use with alcohol. This combination has been associated with higher blood alcohol levels than drinking alcohol alone, with more drunk driving as people do not feel as impaired when drinking energy drinks with alcohol, and with binge drinking. An estimated 50 percent of college students drink alcohol and energy drinks.

Withdrawal symptoms from energy drinks include irritability, tremors, fatigue, and headaches. Because of the problems associated with these drinks, you are advised not to combine energy drinks with alcohol and to limit your consumption of these drinks. Further, it is important to drink plenty of water if consuming energy drinks to prevent dehydration.

Sources: Thombs DL, O'Mara RJ, Tsukamoto M, Rossheim ME, Weiler RM, Merves ML, Goldberger BA, Event-level analyses of energy drink consumption and alcohol intoxication in bar patrons, *Addictive Behaviors,* 35, 325–330, 2010; Energy drinks are hot, but medical concerns growing, *USA Today,* March 17, 2011; Doctors say: Energy drinks can harm kids, *USA Today,* February 14, 2011.

nutritional difficulties, weight loss, reduced resistance to infection, damage to the liver, lungs, and kidneys, and death.[7] Psychological dependence is quickly established. Withdrawal causes acute depression and fatigue but not significant physical discomfort.

Key Terms

narcolepsy (nar co **lep** see) A sleep disorder in which a person has a recurrent, overwhelming, and uncontrollable desire to sleep.

attention deficit hyperactivity disorder (ADHD) Above-normal rate of physical movement; often accompanied by an inability to concentrate on a specified task; also called *hyperactivity.*

Ritalin and Adderall Abuse on College Campuses

Ritalin and Adderall abuse on college campuses continues to rise. Studies have shown that one in every five college students has used Ritalin or Adderall illegally. Students who take Ritalin or Adderall without a prescription are using these drugs to help enhance concentration during late-night study sessions, to obtain a cocainelike high, or to suppress their appetites. However, students may not realize the serious side effects they can experience from misusing these drugs.

Side effects of Adderall and Ritalin can include nervousness, insomnia, loss of appetite, headaches, increased heart and respiratory rates, dilated pupils, dry mouth, perspiration, and feelings of superiority. Higher doses can result in tremors, convulsions, paranoia, and/or a sensation of bugs crawling under the skin. These health risks are considerably higher if Ritalin or Adderall are snorted. Death can occur from abusing Ritalin and Adderall.

Adderall has been used as a weight loss drug and can decrease appetite; however, addiction and dependence can develop, meaning more and more of the medication is needed to produce the same effect. Chronic misuse of Adderall can lead to liver damage, cardiovascular problems, anxiety, irritability, insomnia, and sometimes psychotic behavior.

Abrupt withdrawal from chronic use of Adderall can cause weight gain, decreased energy, and lack of concentration.

Sources: The Johns Hopkins News-Letter, *Ritalin Abuse Is Increasing,* www.jhunewsletter.com/vnews/display.v/ART/2002/11/22/3ddd766faebeb, February 21, 2005; The Johns Hopkins News-Letter, *Hopkins Students Turning to Drugs to Keep Grades Up,* www.jhunewsletter.com/vnews/display.v/ART/2004/04/02/406cd1793dfb2?in_archive=1, February 21, 2005; Attention Deficit Disorder Help Center, *Adderall Side Effects,* www.add-adhd-help-center.com/adderall_side_effects.htm, February 21, 2005.

Methamphetamine can be made using common household ingredients including pseudoephedrine, which is found in cold medications. For this reason, many meth labs are found in houses and apartments, creating a toxic environment for those living in and around these areas. Toxic fumes, fires and explosions, and absorption of methamphetamine through one's skin from residue on countertops and other surfaces are some of the dangers associated with meth labs. In addition, normal cleaning doesn't remove methamphetamine, which may remain on floors, furniture, and countertops. In an effort to obstruct methamphetamine production, some states (Missouri, California, Kentucky, and Oklahoma) are considering further limiting access to decongestants. Oregon is the only state to require a prescription for decongestants, and it had only 10 meth lab seizures in the year after passing this law.[10]

Ritalin and Adderall There is increasing concern about the misuse and abuse of psychostimulants such as methylphenidate (Ritalin) and dextroamphetamine (Adderall), as the number of children and teens taking these medications increased 311 percent over the past 15 years. Adderall, Ritalin, Strattera (atomoxetine), Concerta (methylphenidate), and Vyvanse (lisdexamfetamine) are typically prescribed to help focus attention in those who have attention deficit disorder (ADD) or ADHD. However, many people misuse these medications, using them to stay awake longer, control weight, and increase concentration (see the box "Ritalin and Adderall Abuse on College Campuses"). Strattera and Vyvanse don't have the tendency for abuse because they don't have the same stimulating effects as other medications for ADD and ADHD.

Cocaine Cocaine, perhaps the strongest of the stimulant drugs, has received much media attention. It is the primary psychoactive substance found in the leaves of the South American coca plant.[11] The effects of cocaine are brief, lasting 5–30 minutes. Regardless of the way in which it is consumed, cocaine produces an immediate, near-orgasmic "rush," or feeling of exhilaration. This euphoria is quickly followed by a period of marked depression. Used only occasionally as a topical anesthetic, cocaine is usually inhaled (snorted), injected, or smoked (as *freebase* or crack). There is overwhelming scientific evidence that users quickly develop a strong psychological dependence. There is considerable evidence that physical dependence also rapidly develops. Cocaine users risk a weakened immune system, making them "more susceptible to infections, including HIV."[12] However, physical dependence on cocaine does not lead to death upon withdrawal.

Freebasing Freebasing and the use of crack cocaine are the most recent techniques for maximizing the psychoactive effects of the drug. Freebasing first requires that the common form of powdered cocaine (cocaine hydrochloride) be chemically altered (alkalized). This altered form is then dissolved in a solvent, such as ether or benzene. This liquid solution is heated to evaporate the solvent. The heating process leaves the freebase cocaine in a powder form that can then be smoked, often through a water pipe. Because of the large surface area of the lungs, smoking cocaine facilitates fast absorption into the bloodstream.

One danger of freebasing cocaine is the risk related to the solvents used. Ether is a highly volatile solvent capable of exploding and causing serious burns. Benzene is a known carcinogen associated with the development of leukemia. Clearly, neither solvent can be used without increasing the level of risk typically associated with cocaine use. This method of making smokable cocaine led to a new epidemic of cocaine use, smoking crack.

Crack Cocaine　In contrast to freebase cocaine, crack is made by combining cocaine hydrochloride with common baking soda. When this pastelike mixture is allowed to dry, a small, rocklike crystalline material remains. This crack is heated in the bowl of a small pipe, and the vapors are inhaled.[13] Some crack users spend hundreds of dollars a day to maintain their habit.

The effect of crack is almost instantaneous. Within 10 seconds after inhalation, cocaine reaches the CNS and influences the action of several neurotransmitters at specific sites in the brain. As with the use of other forms of cocaine, convulsions, seizures, respiratory distress, and cardiac failure have been associated with this sudden, extensive stimulation of the nervous system.

Within about six minutes, the stimulating effect of crack is completely expended, and users frequently become depressed. Dependence develops within a few weeks, since users consume more crack in response to the short duration of stimulation and rapid onset of depression.

Intravenous administration has been the preferred route for cocaine users who are also regular users of heroin and other injectable drugs. Intravenous injection results in an almost immediate high, which lasts about 10 minutes. A "smoother ride" is said to be obtained from a "speedball," the injectable mixture of heroin and cocaine (or methamphetamine). This type of mixture can be volatile and even fatal.

Bath Salts

Many states have placed an emergency ban on the sale of a synthetic drug known as bath salts, which act similarly to cocaine or methamphetamine. Both salts are usually snorted, injected, smoked, or eaten and are highly addictive. Also referred to as "cloud nine," "ivory way," and "blue silk," bath salts contain methylenedioxy-pyrovalerone (MDV), which is not approved for medical use in the United States but is sold as an insect repellent or plant food. Users have reported psychotic experiences, anxiety, hypertension, and agitation. Deaths have also been associated with this drug.

Depressants

Depressants (or sedatives) sedate the user, slowing down CNS function. Drugs included in this category are alcohol, barbiturates, and tranquilizers. We will discuss alcohol in more detail later in this chapter. Depressants produce tolerance in abusers, as well as strong psychological and physical dependence.

Barbiturates　Barbiturates are the so-called sleeping compounds that function by enhancing the effect of inhibitory neurotransmitters. They depress the CNS to the point where the user drops off to sleep or, as is the case with surgical anesthetics, the patient becomes anesthetized. Medically, barbiturates are used in widely varied dosages as anesthetics and for treatment of anxiety,

insomnia, and epilepsy.[1] Regular use of a barbiturate quickly produces tolerance—eventually, such a high dose is required that the user still feels the effects of the drug the next morning. Some abusers then begin to alternate barbiturates with stimulants, producing a vicious cycle of dependence. Other misusers combine alcohol and barbiturates or tranquilizers, inadvertently producing toxic or even lethal results. Abrupt withdrawal from barbiturate use frequently produces a withdrawal syndrome that can involve seizures, delusions, hallucinations, and even death.

Methaqualone (Quaalude, "ludes," Sopor) was developed as a sedative that would not have the dependence properties of other barbiturates.[1] Quaaludes were occasionally prescribed for anxious patients. Today, compounds resembling Quaaludes are manufactured in home laboratories and sold illegally so that they can be combined with small amounts of alcohol for an inexpensive, drunklike effect.

Tranquilizers　Tranquilizers are depressants that are intended to reduce anxiety and to relax people who are having problems managing stress. Because of their sedating effects, they have also been prescribed to treat insomnia. Lorazepam (Ativan), alprazolam (Xanax), diazepam (Valium), and chlordiazepoxide (Librium) are some of the most commonly prescribed. Unfortunately, some people become addicted to these and other prescription drugs.[13]

All tranquilizers can produce physical and psychological dependence and tolerance.

"Date Rape" Drugs　"Date rape" drugs or club drugs are commonly used on college campuses. These drugs are usually slipped into the drink of an unsuspecting person and can result in a coma, seizures, or even death.

Common date rape drugs include GHB (gammahydroxybutyrate), also known as G, Liquid Ecstasy, Easy-Lay, Georgia Home Boy, and Rohypnol ("roofies"). They are odorless, colorless, and tasteless. When these drugs are consumed, they cause a drunklike or sedative state that can last for hours. It is during this time that unsuspecting individuals are taken advantage of, against their will and sometimes without their knowledge. GHB acts quickly, within 10–20 minutes of ingestion, and lasts about 4 hours.[14]

For this reason, it is wise not to accept drinks from people you don't know and not to leave your drink unattended. This recommendation extends to all parties where drinkers do not know what has been added to the punch or other drinks.

In 1996, Congress passed the Drug-Induced Rape Prevention and Punishment Act, and it is now a federal crime to give someone a drug, without the user's knowledge, to aid in sexual assault. The maximum penalty for this crime is 20 years in prison and a $250,000 fine.[15] GHB (G, Liquid Ecstasy) and ketamine (K, Special K, Cat) are additional depressants that are being used as date rape drugs.[15] These drugs should serve as a reminder to all partygoers to keep an extremely careful watch over their drinks.

Hallucinogens

As the name suggests, hallucinogenic drugs produce hallucinations—perceived distortions of reality. Also known as *psychedelic drugs* or *phantasticants,* **hallucinogens** reached their height of popularity during the 1960s. At that time, young people were encouraged to use hallucinogenic drugs to "expand the mind," "reach an altered state," or "discover reality." Not all the reality distortions, or "trips," were pleasant. Many users reported "bad trips," or trips during which they perceived negative, frightening distortions.

Hallucinogenic drugs include laboratory-produced lysergic acid diethylamide (LSD), mescaline (from the peyote cactus plant), and psilocybin (from a particular genus of mushroom). Consumption of hallucinogens seems to produce not physical dependence but mild levels of psychological dependence. The development of tolerance is questionable. *Synesthesia,* a sensation in which users report hearing a color, smelling music, or touching a taste, is sometimes produced with hallucinogen use.

The long-term effects of hallucinogenic drug use are not fully understood. Questions about genetic abnormalities in offspring, fertility, sex drive and performance, and the development of personality disorders have not been fully answered. One phenomenon that has been identified and documented is the development of *flashbacks*—the unpredictable return to a psychedelic trip that occurred months or even years earlier. Flashbacks are thought to result from the accumulation of a drug within body cells.

LSD   The most well-known and powerful hallucinogen is lysergic acid diethylamide. LSD ("acid") is a drug that helped define the counterculture movement of the 1960s. During the 1970s and the 1980s, this drug lost considerable popularity. LSD use peaked in 1996, with an annual prevalence of 8.8 percent of high school seniors experimenting with the drug.[16] There was a sharp decline in the use of LSD between 2002 and 2003, which was attributed to the increase in Ecstasy use. The rates have continued to decrease since that time. Part of the appeal of LSD is its low cost and ready availability.

LSD is manufactured in home laboratories and frequently distributed in absorbent blotter paper or gelatin squares. It is odorless, colorless, and tasteless.[17] Users place the paper on their tongues or chew the paper to ingest the drug. LSD can produce a psychedelic (mindviewing) effect that includes altered perception of shapes, images, time, sound, and body form. Synesthesia is common to LSD users. Ingested in doses known as "hits," LSD produces a 6- to 9-hour experience.

Although the typical doses today are about half as powerful as those in the 1960s, users still tend to rapidly develop a high tolerance to LSD. The effects of LSD depend on the dose. Physical dependence does not occur. Not all LSD trips are pleasant, as hallucinations produced from LSD can be frightening and dangerous. Users can injure or kill themselves accidentally during a bad trip. Dangerous side effects include panic attacks, flashbacks, and occasional prolonged psychosis.

Ecstasy and Designer Drugs   In recent years, chemists who produce many of the illicit drugs in home laboratories have designed versions of drugs listed on **FDA Schedule 1.** Under the Controlled Substances Act, substances regulated by the Food and Drug Administration are placed in one of five schedules. Schedule 1 contains the most dangerous drugs that have no medical use.[18] These *designer drugs* are similar to the controlled drugs on the FDA Schedule 1 but are sufficiently different that they escape governmental control. Either designer drugs are newly synthesized products that are similar to already outlawed drugs but against which no law yet exists, or they are reconstituted or renamed illegal substances. Designer drugs are said to produce effects similar to those of their controlled drug counterparts.

People who use designer drugs do so at great risk because the manufacturing of these drugs is unregulated.

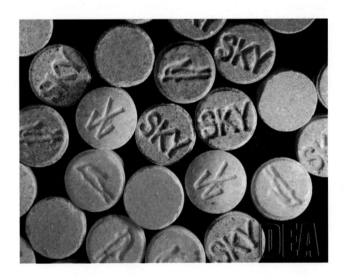

MDMA (Ecstasy) is a designer drug that has both stimulant and hallucinogenic effects. Heavy or long-term use has a number of negative effects, including memory impairment, possibly caused by depletion of the neurotransmitter serotonin.

Key Terms

hallucinogens   Psychoactive drugs capable of producing hallucinations (distortions of reality).

FDA Schedule 1   A list of drugs that have a high potential for abuse but no medical use.

The neurophysiological effects of these homemade drugs can be quite dangerous. So far, a synthetic heroin product (MPPP) and several amphetamine derivatives with hallucinogenic properties have been designed for the unwary drug consumer.

DOM (STP), MDA (the "love drug"), and MDMA (Ecstasy or "XTC") are examples of amphetamine-derivative, hallucinogenic designer drugs. These drugs produce mild, LSD-like hallucinogenic experiences, positive feelings, and enhanced alertness. They also have a number of potentially adverse effects. Experts are particularly concerned that Ecstasy can produce strong psychological dependence and can deplete serotonin, an important excitatory neurotransmitter associated with a state of alertness and mood. Heavy or long-term users can experience depression, anxiety, paranoia, hallucinations, panic attacks, and hostility. Heavy MDMA users commonly have memory loss and are sometimes called "E-tards."[19] Permanent brain damage is possible.[1]

Phencyclidine Phencyclidine (PCP, or "angel dust") has been classified variously as a hallucinogen, a stimulant, a depressant, and an anesthetic. PCP was studied extensively in the 1950s and 1960s and was found to be an unsuitable animal and human anesthetic.[20] PCP is an extremely unpredictable and dangerous drug. Easily manufactured in home laboratories in tablet or powder form, PCP can be injected, inhaled, taken orally, or smoked. The effects vary. Some users report mild euphoria, although most report bizarre perceptions, paranoid feelings, and aggressive behavior. PCP can increase blood pressure and body temperature and decrease coordination. People also report feeling an increased state of drowsiness, a decreased sensitivity to pain, and a sense of disconnection from reality. PCP overdose may cause convulsions, cardiovascular collapse, and damage to the brain's respiratory center.

In a number of cases, the aggressive behavior caused by PCP has led users to commit brutal crimes against both friends and innocent strangers. PCP accumulates in cells and may stimulate bizarre behavior months after initial use.

Salvia Divinorum Salvia divinorum (salvia), a plant from the mint family, has been used by Mazatec people for centuries in religious ceremonies. Referred to as "magic mint," it has a hallucinatory effect that lasts about an hour. Salvia leaves can be smoked, chewed, or drunk in tea. Some people use it as a substitute for marijuana. People using salvia may experience dizziness, lack of coordination, and slurred speech, and there is a risk of injury or death as a result of impaired sensory and cognitive functioning. Salvia is not controlled by any federal law; however, many states have passed laws to restrict its use, and the Drug Enforcement Administration (DEA) is studying whether it should be banned on the federal level.

Cannabis

Cannabis (marijuana) was labeled a mild hallucinogen for a number of years. However, most experts now consider it to be a drug category in itself. Marijuana produces mild effects like those of stimulants and depressants. Marijuana has been implicated in a large number of traffic fatalities. Marijuana is actually a wild plant (*Cannabis sativa*) whose fibers were once used in the manufacture of hemp rope. When the leafy material and small stems are dried and crushed, users can smoke the mixture in rolled cigarettes ("joints"), cigars ("blunts"), or pipes. The resins collected from scraping the flowering tops of the plant yield a marijuana product called *hashish*, or *hash*, commonly smoked in a pipe.[21]

The potency of marijuana's hallucinogenic effect is determined by the percentage of the active ingredient tetrahydrocannabinol (THC) present in the product. The concentration of THC averages about 3.5 percent for marijuana, 7–9 percent for sinsemilla (a higher-quality marijuana), 8–14 percent for hashish, and as high as 50 percent for hash oil.[1] Today's marijuana has THC levels that are higher than in past decades.

Short-Term Effects THC is a fat-soluble substance and thus is absorbed and retained in fat tissues within the body. Before being excreted, THC can remain in the body for up to a month. With the sophistication of today's drug tests, trace **metabolites** of THC can be detected for up to 30 days after consumption.[1]

Once marijuana is consumed, its effects vary from person to person (see Table 7.2). Being "high" or "stoned" or "wrecked" means different things to different people. Many people report heightened sensitivity to music, cravings for particular foods, and a relaxed mood. There is a consensus that marijuana's behavioral effects include four probabilities: (1) Users must learn to recognize what a marijuana high is like, (2) marijuana impairs short-term memory, (3) users overestimate the passage of time, and (4) users lose the ability to maintain attention to a task.[1]

Long-Term Effects The long-term effects of marijuana use are still being studied. Chronic abuse may lead to an **amotivational syndrome** in some people. The irritating effects of marijuana smoke on lung tissue are more pronounced than those of cigarette smoke, and some of the over 400 chemicals in marijuana are now linked to lung cancer development. In fact, one of the most potent carcinogens, benzopyrene, is found in higher levels in marijuana smoke than in tobacco smoke. Marijuana smokers tend to inhale deeply and hold the smoke in the lungs for long periods. It is likely that at some point the lungs of chronic marijuana smokers will be damaged.

Long-term marijuana use is also associated with damage to the immune system and to the male and female reproductive systems, and with an increase in birth defects in babies born to mothers who smoke marijuana.

Table 7.2 Effects of Marijuana

Short-Term Effects	Long-Term Effects
• Increased heart rate and blood pressure • Feeling of elation • Drowsiness and sedation • Increased appetite • Red eyes • Food cravings • Slow reaction time • Feelings of depression, excitement, paranoia, panic, and euphoria • Problems with attention span, memory, learning, problem solving, and coordination • Sleeplessness	• Lung damage • Increased risk of bronchitis • Emphysema • Lung cancer • Heart attack • Loss of motivation and short-term memory • Increased panic or anxiety • possible tolerance • Damage to lungs, immune system, and reproductive organs • Present in the body for up to a month • Birth defects in offspring • Five times more damaging to the lungs than tobacco products

Source: National Institute on Drug Abuse, National Institutes of Health, *NIDA Research Report–Marijuana Abuse*, www.nida.nih.gov/ResearchReports/Marijuana/default.html, February 15, 2005.

Chronic marijuana use lowers testosterone levels in men, sometimes resulting in enlarged breast size and decreased sperm count. For women who are chronic marijuana users, their testosterone level increases, which can cause irregular menstrual cycles and infertility.

There are no legally sanctioned medical uses for marijuana, as the U.S. Supreme Court ruled that the federal government can ban the use of medicinal marijuana. Individuals who use marijuana for medicinal purposes risk federal legal action, with state laws providing no defense.

K2 or Spice K2 or Spice is a packet of herbs coated with a synthetic chemical and is marketed as an herbal incense. However, people are smoking it and using it as a substitute for marijuana. Smoking K2 can produce a rapid heart rate, dangerously high blood pressure, hallucinations, paranoia, vomiting, convulsions, anxiety, disorientation, and aggressive behavior. Currently, many states have banned the sale of K2, and the DEA placed an emergency ban for a year on the chemical needed to make K2.

Narcotics

The **narcotics,** or opiates, are among the most dependence-producing drugs. Medically, narcotics are used to relieve pain and induce sleep. On the basis of origin, narcotics can be subgrouped into the natural, quasisynthetic, and synthetic narcotics.

Natural Narcotics Naturally occurring substances derived from the Oriental poppy plant include opium (the primary psychoactive substance extracted from the Oriental poppy), morphine (the primary active ingredient in opium), and thebaine (an opium alkaloid). Morphine

and related compounds have medical use as analgesics in the treatment of mild-to-severe pain.

Overdose can be lethal and can occur the first time a person takes the drug. People using narcotics experience a rush of pleasure followed by a dreamy, drowsy state in which they feel little pain. Breathing slows, sometimes to the point of respiratory failure. Users also report that their skin flushes and their pupils become pinpointed, and they feel nauseous and may vomit. Depending upon how quickly the drug is metabolized in the liver, the effects of most narcotics are experienced for 4–6 hours. The effects from taking methadone can last 12–24 hours.[19]

Quasisynthetic Narcotics Quasisynthetic narcotics are compounds created by chemically altering morphine. These laboratory-produced drugs are intended to be used as analgesics, but their benefits are largely outweighed by a high dependence rate and a great risk of toxicity. The best known of the quasisynthetic narcotics is heroin. Although heroin is a fast-acting and very effective analgesic, it is extremely addictive. Once injected into a

> **Key Terms**
>
> **metabolite** A breakdown product of a drug.
>
> **amotivational syndrome** Behavioral pattern characterized by lack of interest in productive activities.
>
> **narcotics** Opiates; psychoactive drugs derived from the Oriental poppy plant. Narcotics relieve pain and induce sleep.

vein or "skin-popped" (injected beneath the skin surface), heroin produces dreamlike euphoria and, like all narcotics, strong physical and psychological dependence and tolerance.

As with the use of all other injectable illegal drugs, the practice of sharing needles increases the likelihood of transmission of various communicable diseases, including hepatitis C and HIV (see Chapter 11). Abrupt withdrawal from heroin use is rarely fatal, but the discomfort during cold turkey withdrawal is reported to be overwhelming. The use of heroin has increased during the last decade. The purity of heroin has improved while the price has dropped. Cocaine abusers may use heroin to "come down" from the high associated with cocaine.

Synthetic Narcotics Meperidine (Demerol) and propoxyphene (Darvon), common postsurgical painkillers, and methadone, the drug prescribed during the rehabilitation of heroin addicts, are *synthetic narcotics*. These opiatelike drugs are manufactured in medical laboratories. They are not natural narcotics or quasisynthetic narcotics because they do not originate from the Oriental poppy plant. Like true narcotics, however, these drugs can rapidly induce physical dependence. One important criticism of methadone rehabilitation programs is that in some cases, they merely shift the addiction from heroin to methadone.

OxyContin OxyContin, also known by such names as "hillybilly heroin," "Oxy," and "Oxycotton," is a time-released legal prescription drug used to treat individuals with moderate-to-severe pain.[22] Illegal use of OxyContin gained national attention when individuals in rural areas of the country were found abusing this drug. Now abuse of OxyContin is continuing to spread across the country.[23] Classified as a narcotic, OxyContin is an addictive controlled substance with an addiction potential similar to morphine. This prescription drug is considered extremely dangerous as an illicit drug. Some methods of usage that increase the likelihood of dangerous effects, including death, are chewing the tablets, snorting crushed tablets, and dissolving the tablets in water and then injecting the drug. When OxyContin is not taken in tablet form, the controlled-release dosage is defeated and the user has a strong possibility of receiving a lethal dose due to the drug being released immediately into one's system.[23] Other long-term consequences of OxyContin abuse are physical dependence and severe respiratory depression that may lead to death. Common withdrawal symptoms include restlessness, muscle and bone pain, insomnia, diarrhea, vomiting, cold flashes with goose bumps, and involuntary leg movements.[23] The FDA continues to monitor the abuse of OxyContin and has approved the strongest warning labels for this drug with the intent of changing prescription practices as well as increasing the physician's focus on the potential for abuse.[24]

Painkillers are the second most abused drug (marijuana is the first). Painkillers represent the fastest-growing drug problem, one the Centers for Disease Control and Prevention have termed an "epidemic." The number of people over 12 years of age receiving treatment for dependence on painkillers has grown 400 percent (from 2.2 percent to 9.8 percent) and has doubled for those over 50 years of age.

Inhalants

Inhalants constitute a class of drugs that includes a variety of volatile (quickly evaporating) compounds that generally produce unpredictable, drunklike effects and feelings of euphoria in users.[25] Users of inhalants may also have some delusions and hallucinations. Some users may become quite aggressive. Drugs in this category include anesthetic gases (chloroform, nitrous oxide, and ether), vasodilators (amyl nitrite and butyl nitrite), petroleum products and commercial solvents (gasoline, kerosene, plastic cement, glue, typewriter correction fluid, paint, and paint thinner), and certain aerosols (found in some propelled spray products, fertilizers, and insecticides).

Most of the danger in using inhalants lies in the damaging, sometimes fatal effects on the respiratory and cardiovascular systems. Furthermore, users may unknowingly place themselves in dangerous situations because of the drunklike hallucinogenic effects. Aggressive behavior might also make users a threat to themselves and others.

Combination Drug Effects

Drugs taken in various combinations and dosages can alter and perhaps intensify effects.

A **synergistic drug effect** is a dangerous consequence of taking different drugs in the same general category at the same time. The combination exaggerates each individual drug's effects. For example, the combined use of alcohol and tranquilizers produces a synergistic effect greater than the total effect of each of the two drugs taken separately. In this instance, a much-amplified, perhaps fatal sedation will occur. In a simplistic sense, "one plus one equals four or five."

When taken at or near the same time, drug combinations produce a variety of effects. Drug combinations have additive, potentiating, or antagonistic effects. When two or more drugs are taken and the result is merely a combined total effect of each drug, the result is an **additive effect.** The sum of the effects is not exaggerated. In a sense, "one plus one plus one equals three."

When one drug intensifies the action of a second drug, the first drug is said to have a **potentiated effect** on the second drug. One popular drug-taking practice during the 1970s was the consumption of Quaaludes and beer. Quaaludes potentiated the inhibition-releasing, sedative effects of alcohol. This particular drug combination

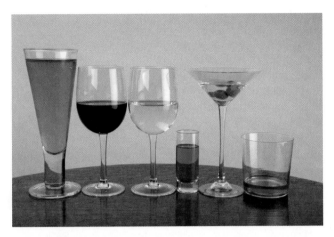

Different types of alcoholic beverages have differing concentrations of pure alcohol—different proof values. A 12-ounce beer, a 5-ounce glass of wine, and 1.5 ounces of liquor in a mixed drink or as a shot all contain equivalent amounts of pure alcohol and are counted as "one drink." Moderate drinking is defined as no more than two drinks per day for men and no more than one drink per day for women.

produced an inexpensive but potentially fatal drunklike euphoria in the user.

An **antagonistic effect** is an opposite effect one drug has on another drug. One drug may be able to reduce another drug's influence on the body. Knowledge of this principle has been useful in the medical treatment of certain drug overdoses, as in the use of tranquilizers to relieve the effects of LSD or other hallucinogenic drugs.

Alcohol: America's Number-One Drug Problem

Alcohol remains the preferred drug for most American adults, including college students, but as a society, we are increasingly uncomfortable with the ease with which alcohol can be misused. Like other drugs, alcohol has immediate intoxication effects that can be dangerous both to the user and to others. Over the long term, chronic overuse of alcohol can lead to many medical, social, and family problems.

The Nature of Alcoholic Beverages

Alcohol (also known as *ethyl alcohol* or *ethanol*) is the principal product of **fermentation.** In this process, yeast cells act on the sugar content of fruits and grains to produce alcohol and carbon dioxide.[26]

The alcohol concentration in beverages such as whiskey, gin, rum, and vodka is determined through a process called **distillation.** Distillation values are expressed by the term *proof,* a number that is twice the

percentage of alcohol by volume in a beverage. Thus, 70 percent of the fluid in a bottle of 140-proof gin is pure alcohol. Most proofs in distilled beverages range from 80 to 160. The familiar pure *grain alcohol* that is often added to fruit punches and similar beverages has a proof of almost 200. Some states are allowing beer to have an alcohol content as high as 13.9 percent.

"Lite" beers and low-calorie wines have been introduced in response to concerns about the number of calories that alcoholic beverages provide. They are not low-alcohol beverages but merely low-calorie beverages. Only beverages marked "low alcohol" contain a lower concentration of alcohol than the usual beverages of that type. And ice beers actually contain a higher percentage of alcohol than other types of beer.

Alcoholic beverages produced through modern processing methods contain nothing but empty calories—about 100 calories per fluid ounce of 100-proof distilled spirits and about 150 calories for each 12-ounce bottle or can of beer.[27] Pure alcohol contains only simple carbohydrates; it has no vitamins or minerals, and no fats or protein.

The Physiological Effects of Alcohol

First and foremost, alcohol is classified as a drug—a very strong CNS depressant. The primary depressant effect of alcohol occurs in the brain and spinal cord. Any temporary sensations of elation, confidence, or friendliness are

> ### Key Terms
>
> **cold turkey** Immediate, total discontinuation of use of a drug; associated with withdrawal discomfort.
>
> **inhalants** Psychoactive drugs that enter the body through inhalation.
>
> **synergistic drug effect** (sin er **jist** ick) Heightened, exaggerated effect produced by the concurrent use of two or more drugs.
>
> **additive effect** The combined (but not exaggerated) effect produced by the concurrent use of two or more drugs.
>
> **potentiated effect** (poe **ten** she ay ted) Phenomenon whereby the use of one drug intensifies the effect of a second drug.
>
> **antagonistic effect** Effect produced when one drug reduces or offsets the effects of a second drug.
>
> **fermentation** A chemical process whereby plant products are converted into alcohol by the action of yeast cells on carbohydrate materials.
>
> **distillation** The process of heating an alcohol solution and collecting its vapors into a more concentrated form.

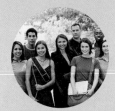

Learning from Our Diversity

Women and Alcohol

Do women drink for the same reasons as men? The research says no. There are some important differences in alcohol use for men and women. Women with low self-esteem are twice as likely to drink alcohol, whereas no such relationship exists for men. This is true for teenage girls and for college women. Women who were sexually or physically abused in childhood are much more likely than men to have alcohol-related problems. Peer pressure, a family history of alcohol abuse, and maternal drinking during pregnancy are more predictive of a likelihood to have alcohol problems for women than for men. Genetics plays a role to some degree in the variation between the genders; however, this does not account for all of these differences.

There are critical periods in women's lives when they are more likely to develop alcohol-related problems. For instance, the freshman year in college shows an increase in binge drinking for women, as compared to the rate of female high school seniors who reported binge drinking. Compared to men, women have more late-onset alcoholism (developing alcoholism after age 59). Life transitions, stressful life events, crises or losses, loneliness, and boredom are triggers for women to develop problems with alcohol.

Because women have different triggers for their alcohol-related problems, they require different approaches for treatment. We are beginning to see specialized groups and treatment facilities that focus on women's issues related to alcohol abuse and dependence.

One such group, Women for Sobriety, is a mutual aid organization for women with alcohol problems that was founded in 1975 by Dr. Jean Kirkpatrick. The WFS program focuses on improving self-esteem; members achieve sobriety by taking responsibility for their actions and by learning not to dwell on negative thoughts. Another alternative, Rational Recovery, is open to both men and women. RR, which is based on psychologist Albert Ellis's rational emotive therapy, also uses a cognitive, nonspiritual approach that fosters cohesiveness and provides the emotional support sought by people to gain and maintain sobriety.

Particularly for "marginalized" alcoholic women such as lesbians, racial and ethnic minorities, and those of non-Christian religious backgrounds, alcoholism treatment professionals increasingly are being encouraged to present the full range of support group options, including but not emphasizing the approach of Alcoholics Anonymous.

If you were seeking help to achieve and maintain sobriety, would you be more inclined to attend a program based on spirituality, or one that offers a rational, cognitive approach? Why?

Sources: Galanter M, et al., Rational recovery: alternative to AA for addiction? *American Journal of Drug and Alcohol Abuse,* 19, 499, 1993; Hall J, Lesbians' participation in Alcoholics Anonymous: experience of social, personal, and political tensions, *Contemporary Drug Problems,* 23(1), 113, 1996; Kaskutas L, A road less traveled: choosing the "Women for Sobriety" program, *Journal of Drug Issues,* 26(1), 77, 1996; Women for Sobriety, Inc., www.womenforsobriety .org/, March 10, 2005; The National Center on Addiction and Substance Abuse at Columbia University, *Women Under the Influence* (Baltimore: Johns Hopkins University Press, 2006).

attributable to alcohol's ability as a depressant drug to reduce personal inhibitions and provide temporary relief from tension.

How Is Alcohol Absorbed in the Body?

Eighty percent of alcohol is absorbed by the small intestine, and the stomach absorbs the other 20 percent. Then the alcohol enters the bloodstream, where it is carried throughout the body to all the organs. More than 90 percent of the alcohol is **metabolized** in the liver. Less than 2 percent of alcohol is excreted unchanged through the skin, breath, and urine.

Factors That Influence the Absorption of Alcohol

The rate of **absorption** of alcohol is influenced by several factors, most of which can be controlled by the individual. These factors include the following:

- *Alcohol concentration.* The stronger the concentration of alcohol in the beverage, the more alcohol is absorbed. Also, carbonated liquids such as sodas or champagne speed up absorption, whereas water will dilute the concentration and slow the rate of absorption.[1]
- *Number of drinks consumed.* As more drinks are consumed, more alcohol is absorbed.
- *Speed of consumption.* If consumed rapidly, even relatively few drinks will result in a large concentration gradient that leads to high blood alcohol concentration.
- *Presence of food.* Food can compete with alcohol for absorption into the bloodstream, slowing the absorption of alcohol. When alcohol absorption is slowed, the alcohol already in the bloodstream can be removed. Slow absorption favors better control of blood alcohol concentration. Your peak blood alcohol level can be three times higher when your stomach is empty than when you consume alcohol after eating something.
- *Degree of hydration.* Having more body water will help to dilute alcohol.
- *Genetics.* Genetics accounts for 50 percent of the risk for alcoholism, for both men and women; however, that means that environment accounts for the other half. Researchers have been trying to locate the specific genes linked to the risk for developing alcoholism, as this would help in predicting who may be at risk and developing better treatment for alcoholism

- *Race/ethnicity.* Research suggests that alcohol tolerance levels may range from weak to strong based on an individual's race/ethnic origin. Genetics may also help protect some Asians from developing alcoholism. About half of all Far East Asians produce low levels of an important enzyme that helps metabolize alcohol. These people cannot tolerate even small amounts of alcohol. Genetic factors pertaining to the absorption rates of alcohol in the intestinal tract have been hypothesized to predispose some Native Americans to alcoholism. It is likely that more research will be undertaken concerning the role of genetic factors in all forms of chemical dependence.

- *Gender.* Women absorb about 30 percent more alcohol into the bloodstream than men do, even if they have an identical number of drinks and equal body weight. The reason for this is that women produce much less alcohol dehydrogenase than men do.[28] This enzyme is responsible for breaking down alcohol in the stomach.

There are other reasons that help explain why women tend to absorb alcohol more quickly than men of the same body weight. First, women have proportionately more body fat than men. Since alcohol is not stored easily in fat, it enters the bloodstream relatively quickly. Second, women's bodies have proportionately less water (52 percent) than do men's bodies of equal weight (66 percent). Thus, alcohol consumed does not become as diluted as in men. Third, alcohol absorption is influenced by a woman's menstrual cycle. Alcohol is more quickly absorbed during the premenstrual phase of a woman's cycle. Also, there is evidence that women using birth control pills absorb alcohol faster than usual.[28]

For more on issues related to gender, see the box "Women and Alcohol."

Blood Alcohol Concentration   A person's **blood alcohol concentration (BAC)** rises when alcohol is consumed faster than it can be removed (oxidized) by the liver. A fairly predictable sequence of events takes place when a person drinks alcohol at a rate faster than one drink every hour. Table 7.3 shows changes in mood, motor functioning, vision, hearing, and physiological effects at different BAC levels. When the BAC reaches 0.05 percent, initial measurable changes in mood and behavior take place. Inhibitions and everyday tensions appear to be released, while judgment and critical thinking are somewhat impaired (see Table 7.3).

At a level of 0.08 percent, the drinker typically loses significant motor coordination and experiences impairment in motor functioning, speech, vision, and hearing. At this BAC, most states consider a drinker legally intoxicated and thus incapable of safely operating a vehicle.

As the BAC rises from 0.20 to 0.50 percent, the health risk of acute alcohol intoxication increases rapidly.

A person with a BAC of 0.20 tends to feel disoriented, and a blackout is likely to occur. A 0.30 percent BAC produces further depression and stuporous behavior, and the drinker becomes so confused that he or she may not be capable of understanding anything. Often people pass out at this point and are difficult to wake up. The 0.40–0.50 percent BAC produces a coma. At this level, a person can die, since the brain centers that control body temperature, heartbeat, and breathing may shut down.

An important factor influencing the BAC is the individual's blood volume. The larger the person, the greater the amount of blood into which alcohol can be distributed. Conversely, the smaller person has less blood into which alcohol can be distributed, and as a result, a higher BAC will develop (see Table 7.4).

The amount of alcohol that can be metabolized is the same no matter how much alcohol is in the blood. This rate is about ¼–⅓ ounce per hour. As previously mentioned, the activity of the enzyme alcohol dehydrogenase is the major factor in determining the rate of alcohol metabolism.[1] So, doing things like drinking coffee or exercising has no effect on alcohol metabolism. To find out what a BAC level would be for your age and gender and the type and number of alcoholic drinks, go to www.healthstatus.com/calculate/bac.

Alcohol Oxidation: Sobering Up   Alcohol is removed from the bloodstream principally through the process of **oxidation.** Oxidation occurs at a constant rate (about ¼–⅓ ounce of pure alcohol per hour) that cannot be appreciably altered. Since each typical drink of beer, wine, or distilled spirits contains about ½ ounce of pure alcohol, it takes about two hours for the body to fully oxidize one typical alcoholic drink.[1]

Although people may try to sober up by drinking hot coffee, taking cold showers, or walking around, the oxidation rate of alcohol is unaffected by these measures.

Key Terms

metabolism   The chemical process by which substances are broken down or synthesized in a living organism to provide energy for life.

absorption   The passage of nutrients or alcohol through the walls of the stomach or the intestinal tract into the bloodstream.

blood alcohol concentration (BAC)   The percentage of alcohol in a measured quantity of blood; BACs can be determined directly through the analysis of a blood sample or indirectly through the analysis of exhaled air.

oxidation   The process that removes alcohol from the bloodstream.

Table 7.3 Blood Alcohol Concentration and Levels of Impairment

Blood Alcohol Concentration	Level of Impairment
0.02–0 .03	No loss of coordination, slight euphoria, loss of shyness. Depressant effects not apparent. Mildly relaxed, maybe a little lightheaded.
0.04–0.06	Feeling of well-being and relaxation, lower inhibitions, sensation of warmth. Euphoria. Some minor impairment of reasoning and memory, lowering of caution. Behavior may become exaggerated and emotions intensified.
0.07–0.09	Slight impairment of balance, speech, vision, reaction time, hearing. Euphoria. Judgment and self-control reduced; caution, reason, and memory impaired. 0.08 legally impaired, illegal to drive at this level. You will probably believe you are functioning better than you really are.
0.10–0.125	Significant impairment of motor coordination, loss of good judgment. Speech slurred; balance, vision, reaction time, hearing impaired. Euphoria.
0.13–0.15	Gross motor impairment, lack of physical control. Blurred vision, major loss of balance. Euphoria reduced, dysphoria (anxiety, restlessness) beginning to appear. Judgment and perception severely impaired.
0.16–0.19	Dysphoria predominates, nausea possible. Appearance of a "sloppy drunk."
0.20	Feeling dazed, confused, otherwise disoriented. May need help to stand or walk. If you injure yourself, you may not feel the pain. Nausea, vomiting possible. Gag reflex impaired, choking possible if you do vomit. Blackouts likely, so you may not remember what has happened.
0.25	All mental, physical, sensory functions severely impaired. Increased risk of asphyxiation from choking on vomit and of seriously injuring yourself from falls or other accidents.
0.30	Stupor—little comprehension of where you are. You may pass out suddenly and be difficult to awaken.
0.35	Coma possible—the level of surgical anesthesia.
0.40 and up	Onset of coma, possible death due to respiratory arrest.

Thus far, the FDA has not approved any commercial product that can help people achieve sobriety. Since alcohol causes dehydration, rehydration and the passage of time remain the only effective remedies for diminishing alcohol's effects.

Alcohol Poisoning People who drink heavily over a short period of time may develop alcohol poisoning, also called **acute alcohol intoxication.** The first real danger signs of alcohol poisoning are the typical signs of **shock.** The drinker will already be unconscious and will not be able to be aroused from a deep stupor. A person's BAC level can continue to rise even when she or he has stopped drinking, is sleeping, or is unconscious. The person will probably have a weak, rapid pulse (over 100 beats per minute). The skin will be cool and damp, and breathing will be increased to once every 3 or 4 seconds. These breaths may be shallow or deep but will certainly occur in an irregular pattern. Skin will be pale or bluish. (In the case of a person

with dark skin, these color changes will be more evident in the fingernail beds or in the mucous membranes inside the mouth or under the eyelids.) Whenever any of these signs are present, seek emergency medical help immediately.

Involuntary regurgitation (vomiting) can be another potentially life-threatening condition for a person who has drunk too much alcohol. When a drinker has consumed more alcohol than the liver can oxidize, the pyloric valve at the base of the stomach tends to close. Additional alcohol remains in the stomach. This alcohol irritates the lining of the stomach so much that involuntary muscle contractions force the stomach contents to flow back through the esophagus. By removing alcohol from the stomach, vomiting may be a life-saving mechanism for conscious drinkers.

An unconscious drinker who vomits may be lying in such a position that the airway becomes obstructed by the vomitus. This person is at great risk of dying from **asphyxiation.** Unconscious drinkers should always be rolled onto their sides to minimize the chance of airway

Table 7.4 Blood Alcohol Concentration Effects for Women and Men

BAC Table for Women									
	Body Weight in Pounds								**Condition**
Drinks	90	100	120	140	160	180	200	220	240	
0	.00	.00	.00	.00	.00	.00	.00	.00	.00	Only Safe Driving Limit
1	.05	.05	.04	.03	.03	.03	.02	.02	.02	Driving Skills Significantly Affected
2	.10	.09	.08	.07	.06	.05	.05	.04	.04	
3	.15	.14	.11	.10	.09	.08	.07	.06	.06	Possible Criminal Penalties
4	.20	.18	.15	.13	.11	.10	.09	.08	.08	
5	.25	.23	.19	.16	.14	.13	.11	.10	.09	
6	.30	.27	.23	.19	.17	.15	.14	.12	.11	Legally Intoxicated
7	.35	.32	.27	.23	.20	.18	.16	.14	.13	
8	.40	.36	.30	.26	.23	.20	.18	.17	.15	Criminal Penalties
9	.45	.41	.34	.29	.26	.23	.20	.19	.17	
10	.51	.45	.38	.32	.28	.25	.23	.21	.19	Death Possible

Subtract .01% for each 40 minutes of drinking.
1 drink = 1.5 oz. 72 proof liquor, 12 oz. beer, or 5 oz. wine.

BAC Table for Men									
	Body Weight in Pounds								**Condition**
Drinks	100	120	140	160	180	200	220	240	
0	.00	.00	.00	.00	.00	.00	.00	.00	Only Safe Driving Limit
1	.04	.03	.03	.02	.02	.02	.02	.02	Driving Skills Significantly Affected
2	.08	.06	.05	.05	.04	.04	.03	.03	
3	.11	.09	.08	.07	.06	.06	.05	.05	Possible Criminal Penalties
4	.15	.12	.11	.09	.08	.08	.07	.06	
5	.19	.16	.13	.12	.11	.09	.09	.08	
6	.23	.19	.16	.14	.13	.11	.10	.09	Legally Intoxicated
7	.26	.22	.19	.16	.15	.13	.12	.11	
8	.30	.25	.21	.19	.17	.15	.14	.13	Criminal Penalties
9	.34	.28	.24	.21	.19	.17	.15	.14	
10	.38	.31	.27	.23	.21	.19	.17	.16	Death Possible

Subtract .01% for each 40 minutes of drinking.
1 drink = 1.5 oz. 72 proof liquor, 12 oz. beer, or 5 oz. wine.

Source: Virginia Tech Alcohol Abuse Prevention Center. © 2006.

obstruction. If you are with someone who is vomiting, make certain that his or her head is positioned lower than the rest of the body. This position minimizes the chance that vomitus will obstruct the air passages. People who are unconscious from alcohol intoxication may also "swallow their tongue." While it is physically impossible to swallow your tongue, when someone is unconscious the muscles relax and the tongue can fall backward into the throat, obstructing the airway. Again, rolling the person on his or her side can help prevent this from happening. Monitoring the physical condition of anyone who becomes unconscious from heavy drinking is crucial because of the risk of death. This is the reason you don't want to let a drunk friend "sleep it off," as the BAC can rise during sleep or unconsciousness, resulting in death. Instead, you need to constantly monitor the physical condition of anyone who becomes unconscious from drinking or take the person to the emergency room if you are unable to monitor him or her or are uncertain about his or her physical condition.

Patterns of Alcohol Use

Although alcohol is a widely used drug, many people choose not to drink. Among drinkers, there is a great deal of variation in the amount and circumstances of their alcohol consumption. It is important to distinguish between light, responsible drinking and patterns of alcohol use that are potentially harmful in the short or long term.

Why Do People Drink? People drink alcoholic beverages for many different reasons. Most people drink alcohol because it is an effective, affordable, and legal substance for altering the brain's chemistry. As **inhibitions**

Key Terms

acute alcohol intoxication A potentially fatal elevation of the BAC, often resulting from heavy, rapid consumption of alcohol.

shock Profound collapse of many vital body functions; evident during acute alcohol intoxication and other health emergencies.

asphyxiation Death resulting from lack of oxygen to the brain.

inhibitions Inner controls that prevent a person from engaging in certain types of behavior.

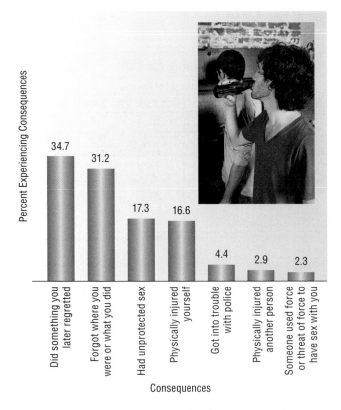

34.7 — Did something you later regretted
31.2 — Forgot where you were or what you did
17.3 — Had unprotected sex
16.6 — Physically injured yourself
4.4 — Got into trouble with police
2.9 — Physically injured another person
2.3 — Someone used force or threat of force to have sex with you

Percent Experiencing Consequences

Consequences

Figure 7-3 Negative Consequences of Alcohol and Drug Use
Reported consequences experienced by college students after drinking alcohol in the past school year.

Source: Spring 2009 Survey, *Journal of American College Health,* 55, January/February 2010.

are removed by the influence of alcohol, behavior that is generally held in check is expressed (see Figure 7-3). At least temporarily, drinkers become a different version of themselves—more outgoing, relaxed, and uninhibited.

From magazines to billboards to television, alcohol is one of the most heavily advertised consumer products in the country.[29] You cannot watch television, listen to the radio, or read a newspaper without being encouraged to buy a particular brand of beer, wine, or liquor. The advertisements create a warm aura around alcohol use. The implications are clear: Alcohol use will bring you good times, handsome men or beautiful women, exotic settings, and a chance to forget the hassles of work and study.

How Much Do People Drink?   Before we discuss how much alcohol people drink, we need to define some terms. What counts as "one drink"? The National Survey on Drug Use and Health (NSDUH) defines "one drink" as "a can or bottle of beer, a glass of wine or a wine cooler, a shot of liquor, or a mixed drink with liquor in it."[29] (More precisely, this means 12 ounces of beer, 5 ounces of wine, or 1.5 ounces of liquor.) Over half of Americans ages 12 and over (over 130 million people) reported being current

drinkers in the 2009 survey. **Current use** is defined as "at least one drink in the past 30 days." Twenty-three percent of people 12 and older (59.6 million Americans) reported having engaged in binge drinking at least once in the past month. **Binge drinking** is defined as "five or more drinks on the same occasion (at the same time or within a couple of hours of one another) on at least 1 day in the last 2-week period." In 2009, 6.8 percent of Americans 12 and older (17 million) reported heavy drinking, "five or more drinks on the same occasion on each of 5 or more days in the past 30 days."

People who plan to drive, women who are pregnant, people recovering from alcohol addiction, people under age 21, people taking medications, and those with existing medical concerns should not consume alcohol. Elderly people are limited to no more than one drink each day, again because of a higher percentage of body fat. Additionally, although some studies have shown that low levels of alcohol consumption may have minor psychological and cardiovascular benefits, nondrinkers are not advised to start drinking.

Who Drinks?   As Figure 7-4 shows, current use, binge use, and heavy use were highest for the 21–25 age group and then decreased with increasing age. On average, more men than women drink; however, for the 12- to 17-year-old age range, drinking was the same for males and females. Caucasians had the highest drinking rate (56.7), followed by African Americans (42.8), Hispanics (41.7), Asians (37.7), and American Indians (37.1). Asian youths had the lowest rates of alcohol use, and the binge drinking rate was lowest for Asians of any age group. One increasing concern is the alcoholism rate of U.S. military personnel, which has doubled since 2003 to 11.4 percent.[30] In the United States, drinking rates are lowest in the South (47.6 percent) and highest in the Northeast (56.7 percent).

College Drinking   The National College Health Assessment 2009 reported that 72.5 percent of college students drank at the last party they attended. However, students thought that 97 percent of college students drank when actually 21 percent reported never drinking. The NSDUH study actually found that college students were more likely to drink than their same-age peers who weren't in college, and drinking increased with level of education. Rates of binge and heavy drinking were also higher among college students than among same-age peers who were not in college.[31]

Binge Drinking   Binge drinking refers to the consumption of five drinks in one sitting, at least once during the previous two-week period. Pregaming and drinking games are a form of binge drinking in which individuals consume large amounts of alcohol in a small period of time. A long-term study by the University of Michigan found that about 37 percent of college students engage in

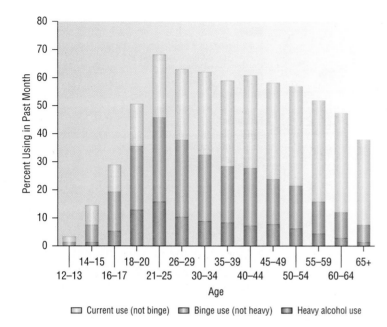

Figure 7-4 Current, Binge, and Heavy Alcohol Use Among Persons Ages 12 and Older Alcohol use is highest among Americans 21–25 years old. Binge use is having five or more drinks on the same occasion in the past month. Heavy use is having five drinks on the same occasion on five or more days during the past month.

Source: Substance Abuse and Mental Health Services Administration, *Results from the 2009 National Survey on Drug Use and Health: National Findings* (Office of Applied Studies, NSDUH Series H-34, DH HS Publication No. SMA 08-4343). Rockville, MD: 2010.

binge drinking.[32] The strongest predictors for bingeing for college students were living in a fraternity or sorority house, adopting a party-centered lifestyle, and engaging in other risky behavior.

Binge drinking can be dangerous. Drunk driving, physical violence, property destruction, date rape, police arrest, and lowered academic performance are all closely associated with binge drinking. There is a direct correlation between the amount of alcohol consumed and lowered academic performance; consequences include impaired memory, verbal skill deficiencies, and altered perceptions.[33]

For some students, the college years are a time when they drink more heavily than at any other time in their life. These years will also mark the entry into a lifetime of problem drinking for some.

Alcohol-Related Medical Problems

Heavy alcohol use causes a variety of changes to the body that lead to an increase in morbidity and mortality. Figure 7-5 describes these changes.

Effects of Chronic Alcohol Use on the Body Because alcohol goes to every organ in the body, with chronic use it can negatively affect every organ in your body. Chronic malnutrition can result from consuming alcohol instead of calories with nutritional value. This in turn can result in brain damage, such as **Wernicke-Korsakoff syndrome,** which results from vitamin B_1 deficiency. This syndrome is characterized by symptoms such as impaired short-term memory, psychosis, impaired coordination, and abnormal eye movements, and is often irreversible. Liver disorders such as cirrhosis of the liver are related to chronic drinking and are the seventh-leading cause of death in the United States.[1] Heart disease, hypertension,

stroke, and cancer are also commonly associated with chronic alcohol use. Infectious diseases such as tuberculosis, pneumonia, yellow fever, cholera, and hepatitis B have also been linked with chronic alcohol use.

Fetal Alcohol Syndrome and Fetal Alcohol Effects A growing body of scientific evidence indicates that alcohol use by pregnant women can result in birth defects in unborn children.

Alcohol exposure has disastrous consequences for the developing fetus. Low birth weight, mental retardation, facial abnormalities (for example, small head or widely spaced eyes), and heart problems are often seen in such children (see Figure 7-6 on page 177). This combination of effects is called **fetal alcohol syndrome.** Recent estimates indicate that the full expression of this

Key Terms

current use At least one drink in the past 30 days.

binge drinking Five or more drinks on the same occasion (at the same time or within a span of a couple of hours) on at least one day in the last two-week period.

Wernicke-Korsakoff syndrome A syndrome that results from vitamin B_1 deficiency, often the result of alcoholism. Symptoms include impaired short-term memory, psychosis, impaired coordination, and abnormal eye movements.

fetal alcohol syndrome Characteristic birth defects noted in the children of some women who consume alcohol during their pregnancies.

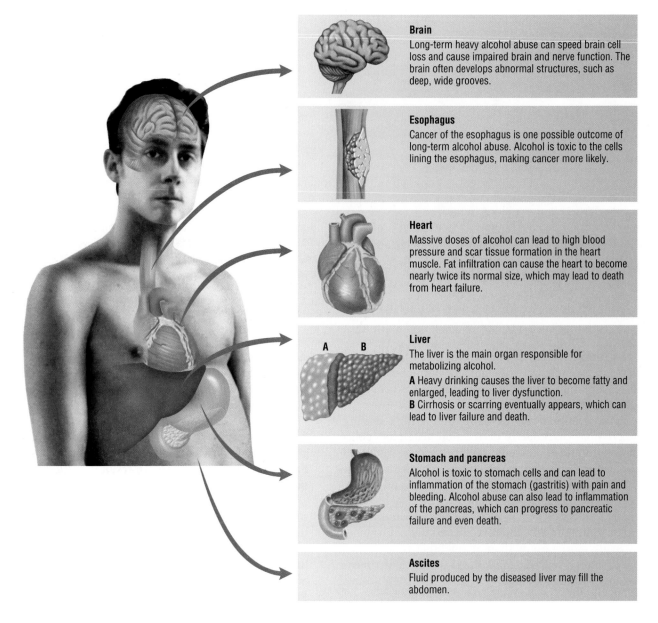

Brain
Long-term heavy alcohol abuse can speed brain cell loss and cause impaired brain and nerve function. The brain often develops abnormal structures, such as deep, wide grooves.

Esophagus
Cancer of the esophagus is one possible outcome of long-term alcohol abuse. Alcohol is toxic to the cells lining the esophagus, making cancer more likely.

Heart
Massive doses of alcohol can lead to high blood pressure and scar tissue formation in the heart muscle. Fat infiltration can cause the heart to become nearly twice its normal size, which may lead to death from heart failure.

Liver
The liver is the main organ responsible for metabolizing alcohol.
A Heavy drinking causes the liver to become fatty and enlarged, leading to liver dysfunction.
B Cirrhosis or scarring eventually appears, which can lead to liver failure and death.

Stomach and pancreas
Alcohol is toxic to stomach cells and can lead to inflammation of the stomach (gastritis) with pain and bleeding. Alcohol abuse can also lead to inflammation of the pancreas, which can progress to pancreatic failure and even death.

Ascites
Fluid produced by the diseased liver may fill the abdomen.

Figure 7-5 Effects of Alcohol Use on the Body

Source: Wardlaw G, Hampl J, *Perspectives in Nutrition,* 7th ed. Copyright © 2007 The McGraw-Hill Companies, Inc. Reproduced by permission of The McGraw-Hill Companies.

syndrome occurs at a rate of 1–3 per 1,000 births. Partial expression (fetal alcohol effects [FAE]) can be seen in 3–9 per 1,000 live births. In addition, it is likely that many cases of FAE go undetected.[33]

Since no one can accurately predict the effect of drinking even small amounts of alcohol during pregnancy, the wisest plan is to avoid alcohol altogether.

Alcohol-Related Psychological Problems

Depending on the amount and pattern of alcohol use, inappropriate or chronic drinking may be classified as alcohol dependence (alcoholism) or alcohol abuse (problem drinking).

Alcohol Dependence (Alcoholism)   **Alcohol dependence,** or alcoholism, is a primary, chronic disease with genetic, psychosocial, and environmental factors influencing its development and manifestations. The disease is often progressive and fatal. It is characterized by lack of control over drinking, preoccupation with alcohol, use of alcohol despite adverse consequences (such as endangering one's job, relationships, financial situation, and health), and distortions in thinking, most notably denial. Tolerance to alcohol develops so that the alcoholic needs to drink more alcohol to gain the same effect. Each of these symptoms may be continuous or periodic.[34]

Unlike problem drinking, alcoholism involves a physical addiction to alcohol. For the true alcoholic,

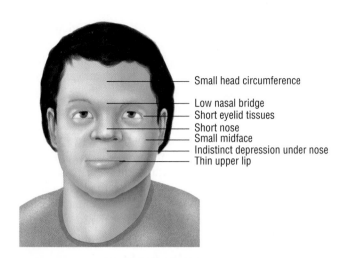

- Small head circumference
- Low nasal bridge
- Short eyelid tissues
- Short nose
- Small midface
- Indistinct depression under nose
- Thin upper lip

Figure 7-6 Fetal Alcohol Syndrome The facial features shown are characteristic of affected children. Additional abnormalities in the brain and other internal organs accompany fetal alcohol syndrome but are not obvious in the child's appearance.

when the body is deprived of alcohol, physical and mental withdrawal symptoms become evident. These withdrawal symptoms can be life threatening. Uncontrollable shaking can progress to nausea, vomiting, hallucinations, shock, and cardiac and pulmonary arrest. Uncontrollable shaking combined with irrational hallucinations is called *delirium tremens (DTs),* an occasional manifestation of alcohol withdrawal.[35]

We do know that individuals with a family history of alcoholism are five times more likely to develop alcoholism due to this predisposition, and sons of alcoholic fathers are nine times more likely to have a drinking problem. Two forms of alcoholism are thought to be inherited: type 1 and type 2. Type 1 is thought to take years to develop and may not surface until midlife. Type 2 is a more severe form and appears to be passed primarily from fathers to sons. This form of alcoholism frequently begins earlier in a person's life and may even start in adolescence.

Factors ranging from unusually low self-esteem to an antisocial personality have been implicated in contributing to the development of alcoholism. Additional factors making people susceptible to alcoholism may include depression, anxiety, impulsivity, low stress tolerance, loneliness, hypersensitivity, and compulsiveness.

Alcohol Abuse (Problem Drinking) **Alcohol abuse,** also referred to as problem drinking, is considered less severe than alcohol dependence. School and job performance suffers, responsibilities are neglected, and interpersonal conflicts arise when individuals abuse alcohol. They may drive while intoxicated, have legal problems, experience **blackouts,** and know that their drinking is causing them problems, but they persist in their drinking. Instead of helping them to cope with their stress, alcohol is now creating problems in their lives. One

major difference between dependence and abuse is that the definition of dependence includes tolerance, withdrawal, or a pattern of compulsive use, but the definition of abuse does not. Abuse refers to experiencing harmful consequences from repeated use of alcohol.[36]

For college students, two clear indications of alcohol abuse, or **problem drinking,** are missed classes and lowered academic performance. Problem drinkers are not always heavy drinkers; they might not be daily or even weekly drinkers. Unlike alcoholics, problem drinkers do not need to drink to maintain "normal" body functions. Problem drinkers are more likely than other drinkers to eventually develop alcoholism.

 TALKING POINTS How would you know if your family or friends show signs of problem drinking? What might you do to help them?

Alcohol-Related Social Problems

Alcohol abuse is related to a variety of social problems. These problems affect the quality of interpersonal relationships, employment stability, and the financial security of both the individual and the family.

Accidents The four leading causes of accidental deaths in the United States (motor vehicle collisions, falls, drownings, and fires and burns) have significant statistical connections to alcohol use.

Motor Vehicle Collisions Data from the National Highway Traffic Safety Administration (NHTSA) indicate that in 2007 over 13,000 alcohol-related vehicular crash deaths occurred.[37]

> **Key Terms**
>
> **alcohol dependence** Tolerance, withdrawal, and a pattern of compulsive use of alcohol. A primary, chronic disease with genetic, psychosocial, and environmental factors influencing its development. Also called *alcoholism.*
>
> **alcohol abuse** Patterns of alcohol use that create problems for the drinker's school and job performance, other responsibilities, and interpersonal relationships. Also called *problem drinking.*
>
> **blackout** A temporary state of amnesia experienced by a drinker; an inability to remember events that occurred during a period of alcohol use, including things that person said or did during that time.
>
> **problem drinking** An alcohol use pattern in which a drinker's behavior creates personal difficulties or difficulties for other people. Also called *alcohol abuse.*

Presently in the United States, an alcohol-related car crash fatality occurs every 31 minutes. Every 2 minutes, an alcohol-related car crash injury happens. In 2007, an estimated 275,000 people were injured in such crashes. The NHTSA reported that approximately 1.5 million drivers were arrested for drunk driving, reflecting an arrest rate of 1 for every 130 licensed drivers in the United States.[37] One out of every 12 drivers reported drinking and driving drunk at least once a year.

One response to drunk driving has been for all states to raise the minimum legal drinking age to 21 years. Another response is that all states have lowered the driving standard to 0.08 percent BAC. You can search the MADD (Mothers Against Drink Driving) website at www.madd.org to find out current 0.08 percent BAC law information.[38]

Many states have enacted **zero-tolerance laws** to help prevent underage drinking and driving. Also included have been efforts to educate bartenders to recognize intoxicated customers, to use off-duty police officers as observers in bars, to place police roadblocks, to develop mechanical devices that prevent intoxicated drivers from starting their cars, and to encourage people to use designated drivers.

Falls   Many people are surprised to learn that falls are the second leading cause of accidental death in the United States. Alcohol use increases the risk for falls. Various studies suggest that alcohol is involved in 21–77 percent of deadly falls and 18–53 percent of nonfatal falls.[39]

Drownings   Drownings are the third leading cause of accidental death in the United States. Studies have shown that alcohol use is implicated in 21–47 percent of these deaths.[39] High percentages of recreational boaters have been found to drink alcohol while boating.[39] Alcohol can impair judgment and swimming ability and reduce body temperature.[40]

Fires and Burns   Fires and burns are responsible for an estimated 5,000 deaths each year in the United States, the fourth leading cause of accidental death. This cause is also connected to alcohol use: Studies indicate that half of burn victims have BACs above the legal limit.

Crime and Violence   The connection of alcohol to crime has a long history. Prison populations have large percentages of alcohol abusers and alcoholics; people who commit crimes are more likely to have alcohol problems than are people in the general population. This is especially true for young criminals. Furthermore, alcohol use has been reported in 53–66 percent of all homicides, with the victim, the perpetrator, or both found to have been drinking. In rape situations, rapists

are intoxicated 50 percent of the time, and victims 36 percent of the time.[27]

It seems clear that in a large number of families, alcohol is associated with violence and other harmful behavior, including physical abuse, child abuse, psychological abuse, and abandonment.[41]

Suicide   Alcohol use has been related to large percentages of suicides. Alcoholism plays a role in 30 percent of completed suicides.[42] Also, alcohol use is associated with impulsive suicides rather than premeditated ones. Drinking is also connected with more violent and lethal means of suicide, such as the use of firearms.[42]

Alcohol-Related Family Problems

Considerable disruption occurs in the families of alcoholics, not only from the consequences of the drinking behavior (such as violence, illness, and unemployment) but also because of the uncertainty of the family's role in causing and prolonging the situation. Family members often begin to adopt a variety of dysfunctional roles that allow them to cope with the presence of the alcoholic in the family. Unless family members receive appropriate counseling, these unhealthy roles may remain intact for a lifetime.[43]

Once an alcoholic's therapy has begun, family members are encouraged to participate in many aspects of the recovery. This participation will also help them understand how they are affected by alcoholism. Family members are encouraged to become affiliated with support groups.[44]

Responses to Drug and Alcohol Use

During the last 25 years, society has responded to illegal drug and alcohol use with growing concern (see the box "Do Public Service Announcements Make a Difference?"). Most adults see drug abuse as a clear danger to society. This position has been supported by the development of community, school, state, and national organizations directed toward the reduction of drug and alcohol abuse. These organizations have included such diverse groups as Parents Against Drugs, Partnership for a Drug-Free America, Mothers Against Drunk Driving (MADD), Narcotics Anonymous, and the U.S. Drug Enforcement Administration. Certain groups have concentrated their efforts on education, others on enforcement, and still others on the development of laws and public policy.[45]

The personal and social issues related to drug abuse are complex. Innovative solutions continue to be devised. Some believe that only through early childhood education will people learn alternatives to drug use. Starting drug education in the preschool years may have a more positive effect than waiting until the upper elementary or junior high school years. Recently, the focus on reducing young people's exposure to **gateway drugs** (especially tobacco, alcohol, and marijuana) may help slow down the move to other addictive drugs.

Some people advocate harsher penalties for drug use and drug trafficking, including heavier fines and longer prison terms. Others support legalizing all drugs and making governmental agencies responsible for drug regulation and control, as is the case with alcohol. Advocates of this position believe that drug-related crime and violence would virtually cease once the demand for illegal products was reduced. The United States now spends nearly $18 billion annually to fight the drug war. About $11 billion is spent on law enforcement (supply reduction) and $6 billion on education, prevention, and treatment (demand reduction).[46]

Action is also taking place on college campuses. Among college fraternity organizations, the attitudes toward the indiscriminate use of alcohol are changing. Many rush functions are now conducted without the use of alcohol, and growing numbers of fraternities are alcohol-free.

Another encouraging sign on college campuses is the increasing number of alcohol-use task forces. Although each of these groups has its own focus and title, many are meeting to discuss alcohol-related concerns on their particular campus. These task forces often try to formulate detailed, comprehensive policies for alcohol use across the entire campus community.

> **Key Terms**
>
> **zero-tolerance laws** Laws that severely restrict the right to operate motor vehicles for underage drinkers who have been convicted of driving under any influence.
>
> **gateway drug** An easily obtainable legal or illegal drug that represents a user's first experience with a mind-altering drug.

Responsible Drinking

Drinking alcohol in a responsible way means reducing the potential negative consequences of drinking and increasing your safety and the safety of others around you. It involves some practical strategies, such as the following:

- Don't make getting drunk the goal or drinking the focus of your activity.
- Eat food before drinking.
- Set a limit on the number of drinks you will consume.
- Limit alcoholic drinks to one an hour, and drink water or soda in between.
- Don't use alcohol to manage feelings such as stress, boredom, anger, or loneliness.
- When going to a party or bar, have a designated driver.
- Don't leave your drinks unattended.

Drinking responsibly helps you avoid the negative legal, social, and medical consequences that can be associated with alcohol use.

Drug Testing

Society's response to concern over drug use includes the development and growing use of drug tests. Most of the testing is done by corporations that screen employees for commonly abused drugs. Among these are amphetamines, barbiturates, benzodiazepines (the chemical bases for prescription tranquilizers such as Valium and Librium), cannabinoids (THC, hashish, and marijuana), methaqualone, opiates (heroin, codeine, and morphine), and PCP. With the exception of marijuana, most traces of these drugs are eliminated by the body within a few days after use. Marijuana can remain detectable up to 30 days after use. Drug tests will likely identify 90 percent of recent drug users. Most Fortune 500 companies, the armed forces, various government agencies, and nearly all athletic organizations have already implemented mandatory drug testing.

Treatment

The good news for people with drug and alcohol problems is that help is available through inpatient hospitalization, intensive outpatient care, self-help groups such as Narcotics Anonymous, and medical and mental health professions. The bad news is that treatment can be costly. Inpatient hospital treatment can cost thousands per day. Figure 7-7 shows the barriers people report in not getting substance abuse treatment. Most said that cost was the number-one obstacle. Additionally, addicts typically make numerous attempts at drug treatment before they find lasting recovery. Most people reported going to a self-help group such as Alcoholics Anonymous or Narcotics Anonymous for treatment, followed by outpatient rehabilitation (see the box "The Spiritual Component in Alcoholics Anonymous"). Cost most likely played heavily into these treatment decisions.

Medical treatment for the management of drug problems may be obtained through a local community mental health center, private clinic, or local hospital. Treatment may be on an inpatient or outpatient basis.

Medical management might include detoxification, treatment of secondary health complications and nutritional deficiencies, and therapeutic counseling for chemical dependence. Disulfiram (antabuse) is a prescription drug frequently used to prevent alcoholics from drinking, because drinking alcohol within two weeks of taking disulfiram will cause extreme nausea. Naltrexone and Campral have also been prescribed to reduce craving for alcohol, as well as to diminish the pleasurable effects of alcohol.

Drug and alcohol treatment is also available in college or university counseling centers. The emphasis of treatment is on the behavioral dimensions of substance abuse. Trained counselors and psychologists who specialize in chemical dependence counseling will work with students to (1) analyze their particular concerns, (2) establish constructive ways to cope with stress, and (3) search for alternative ways to achieve new "highs" (see the Personal Assessment at the end of this chapter).

Intervention

Another obstacle to receiving treatment is users' denial that they have a problem. As Figure 7-7 shows, "Not ready to stop using" is a major reason people do not enter

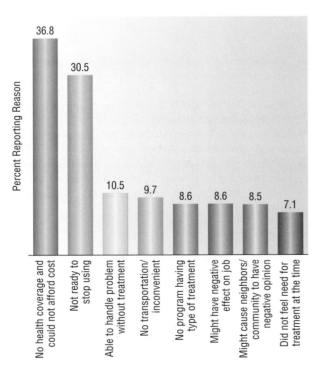

(A) Reasons for not receiving substance abuse treatment

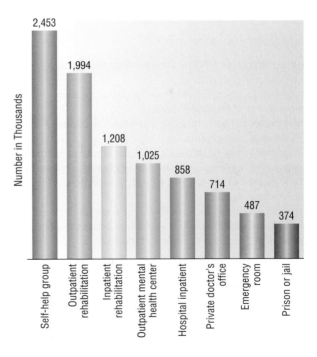

(B) Location of substance abuse treatment

Figure 7-7 Facts About Substance Abuse Treatment   (a) Among people who tried and failed to obtain drug abuse treatment, lack of insurance and cost were cited as the top barrier. (b) Among people who did obtain treatment, self-help groups and outpatient programs were the most commonly reported treatment locations.

Source: Substance Abuse and Mental Health Services Administration, Office of Applied Studies, *Results from the 2009 National Survey on Drug Use and Health: National Findings* (NSDUH Series H-34, DHHS Publication No. SMA 08-4343). Rockville, MD: 2009.

drug treatment. A treatment approach called **intervention** has shown promise in convincing people with drug problems to enter treatment programs. An intervention is usually coordinated by family and friends, with the assistance of a mental health professional. People who live or work with chemically dependent people are encouraged to confront them directly about how their addiction has personally affected them and the negative behaviors they have witnessed from this individual. The focus is on the person's behavior, such as not meeting financial or work obligations, withdrawing from the family, creating tension in relationships, and not keeping promises. The goal of the intervention is to motivate the person with the drug problem to seek professional help.

> **Key Terms**
>
> **intervention** An organized process that involves encouraging a chemically addicted individual to enter into drug treatment; usually coordinated by family and friends along with a mental health professional.

Taking Charge of Your Health

- Calculate the amount of caffeine you consume daily. If you're drinking more than three cups of caffeinated beverages per day, develop a plan to reduce your overall intake.

- Prepare a plan of action to use if someone you know needs professional assistance with a drug or alcohol problem.

- Identify five activities that can provide you with a drug-free high.

- Analyze your drug and alcohol use patterns (if any), and assess the likelihood that you might fail a pre-employment drug test.

- If you think you have a drug or alcohol problem, join a support group or see a mental health professional.

SUMMARY

- A drug affects the CNS by altering neurotransmitter activity on the neuron.
- *Drug misuse, abuse tolerance,* and *dependence* are important terms to understand.
- Drugs enter the body through ingestion, injection, inhalation, or absorption.
- Drugs can be placed into six categories: stimulants, depressants, hallucinogens, cannabis, narcotics, and inhalants.
- Many factors affect the rate of absorption of alcohol into the bloodstream.
- Problem drinking, also called alcohol abuse, reflects an alcohol use pattern in which a drinker's behavior creates personal difficulties or problems for others.

- Alcoholism, or alcohol dependence, is a primary, chronic disease with a variety of possible causes and characteristics.
- Recovery and rehabilitation programs can be effective in helping substance abusers to recover.
- Federal legislation has pushed all states to lower the legal driving BAC standard to 0.08 percent.
- Society's response to drug abuse has been widely varied and has included education, law enforcement, treatment, testing, and the search for drug-free ways to achieve highs.

REVIEW QUESTIONS

1. Describe how neurotransmitters work.
2. Identify and explain the three steps in the process of addiction.
3. How is the term *drug* defined in this chapter? What are psychoactive drugs? How do medicines differ from drugs?
4. Define the four routes of administration. Select a drug that reflects each of the ways drugs enter the body.
5. Explain what dependence means. Identify and explain the two types of dependence.
6. Define the word *tolerance*. What does cross-tolerance mean? Give an example of cross-tolerance.

7. Differentiate among drug misuse, drug abuse, and drug dependence.
8. List the six general categories of drugs. For each category, give several examples of drugs, and explain the effects they would have on the user. What are designer drugs?
9. Identify and explain the various factors that influence the absorption of alcohol. Why is it important to be aware of these factors?
10. What is BAC? Describe the general sequence of physiological events that takes place when a person drinks alcohol at a rate faster than the liver can oxidize it.

ANSWERS TO THE "WHAT DO YOU KNOW?" QUIZ

1. False   2. True   3. True   4. True   5. False   6. True   7. False

Visit the Online Learning Center (**www.mhhe.com/hahn11e**), where you will find tools to help you improve your grade including practice quizzes, key terms flashcards, audio chapter summaries for your MP3 player, and many other study aids.

SOURCE NOTES

1. Hart O, Ksir C, Ray O. *Drugs, Society and Human Behavior* (13th ed.). New York: McGraw-Hill, 2009.
2. Pinger R, Wayne R, Hahn D, Hahn E. *Drug Issues for Today* (3rd ed.). New York: McGraw-Hill, 2001.
3. Shier D, Butler J, Lewis R. *Hole's Essentials of Human Anatomy and Physiology* (10th ed.). New York: McGraw-Hill, 2008.
4. The Coffee Science Information Centre. *Caffeine.* www.cosic.org/. March 7, 2005.
5. Caffeine nation, CBS News, September 7, 2003.
6. *Caffeine.* Johns Hopkins online newsletter, September 2002. www.intelihealth.com. March 7, 2005.
7. National Institute on Drug Abuse, National Institutes of Health. NIDA InfoFacts, *Methamphetamine.* www.nida.nih.gov/Infofax/methamphetamine.html. March 7, 2007.
8. U.S. Department of Justice, Drug Enforcement Administration. *Methamphetamine.* www.usdoj.gov/dea/concern/meth.htm. December 31, 2001.
9. Frackelmann K. Breaking bonds of addiction: compulsion traced to part of the brain. *USA Today,* April 18, 2002.
10. States mull Rx rule for meth ingredients. *USA Today,* February 1, 2010.
11. U.S. Department of Justice, Drug Enforcement Administration. *Drugs of Abuse.* www.dea.gov/pubs/abuse/5-stim.htm. 2005 edition.
12. Cocaine weakens immune system. *Boston Herald,* March 7, 2003.
13. National Institute on Drug Abuse, National Institutes of Health. NIDA Research Report, *Prescription Drugs Abuse and Addiction.* www.drugabuse.gov/ResearchReports/prescription/prescription.html, NIH publication No. 01-4881. July 2001.
14. National Institute on Drug Abuse. NIDA InfoFacts, *Rohypnol and GHB.* www.nida.nih.gov/Infofax/RohypnolGHB.html. February 14, 2004.
15. National Institute on Drug Abuse, National Institutes of Health NIDA InfoFacts, *Club Drugs.* www.drugabuse.gov/Infofax-/Clubdrugs.html. March 7, 2005.
16. Johnston LD, O'Malley PM, Bachman JG, Schulenberg JE. *Monitoring the Future: National Survey Results on Drug Use: 1975–2003. Volume I: Secondary School Students.* www.monitoringthefuture.org/pubs/monographs/vol1_2003.pdf. NIH Publication No. 04-5507. Bethesda, MD: 2004.
17. National Institute on Drug Abuse. NIDA InfoFacts, *LSD.* www.nida.nih.gov/Infofax/lsd.html. 2007.
18. U.S. Drug Enforcement Administration. Controlled Substances Act. www.usdoj.gov/dea/agency/csa.htm. 2007.
19. Kuhh C, Swartzwelder S, Wilson W. *Buzzed: The Straight Facts About the Most Used and Abused Drugs from Alcohol to Ecstasy* (3rd ed.). New York: Norton, 2008.
20. National Institute on Drug Abuse, National Institutes of Health. NIDA InfoFacts, *PCP (Phencyclidine).* www.nida.hih.gov/Infofax/pcp.html. 2009.
21. National Institute on Drug Abuse, National Institutes of Health. NIDA InfoFacts, *Marijuana.* www.nida.nih.gov/Infofax/marijuana.html. 2010.
22. OxyContin questions and answers. Drug Information, U.S. Food and Drug Administration, Center for Drug Evaluation and Research. www.fda.gov/cder/drug/infopage/oxycontin/oxycontin-qa.htm. March 7, 2008.
23. *OxyContin Addiction and Treatment and Rapid Detox Services.* www.oxycontin-detox.com/index-overture-kw-oxycontin.html. March 7, 2009.
24. U.S. Food and Drug Administration. *FDA Strengthens Warnings for OxyContin.* www.fda.gov/bbs/topics/answer/2001/ans01091.html. March 7, 2009.
25. Frackelmann K. Inhalants' hidden treat: Access makes huffing popular but kids can recover with help. *USA Today,* June 25, 2002.
26. Zest for Life. Alcohol and ethanol information page. www.anyvitamins.com/alcohol-ethanol-info.htm. March 9, 2005.
27. Kinney J. *Loosening the Grip: A Handbook of Alcohol Information* (8th ed.). New York: McGraw-Hill, 2005.
28. Be Responsible About Drinking. Women and alcohol. www.brad21.org/alcohol_and_women.html. March 9, 2005.
29. Substance Use and Mental Health Services Administration. Results from the 2009 National Survey on Drug Use and Health: National Findings (Office of Applied Studies, NSDUH Series H-30 DHHS Publication No. SMA 06-4194). Rockville, MD: 2009.
30. Alcohol abuse weighs on Army. *USA Today,* February 2, 2010.
31. American College Health Association. Spring 2006, Survey *Journal of American College Health,* 55, January–February 2007.
32. College parties, minus the beer binges. *The Wall Street Journal,* February 16, 2011.
33. ADA: Division of Drug and Alcohol Abuse. *As a Matter of Fact . . . Fetal Alcohol Syndrome.* www.well.com/user/woa/fsfas.htm. March 9, 2009.
34. Morse R M, et al. The definition of alcoholism. *Journal of the American Medical Association,* 268(8), 1012–14, 1992.
35. Burns M. *Delirium Tremens.* emedicine.com. November 8, 2004.
36. *Diagnostic and Statistical Manual of Mental Disorders* (4th ed.). Washington, DC: American Psychiatric Association, 2000.
37. *Traffic Safety Facts 2009: Alcohol.* U.S. Department of Transportation, National Highway Traffic Safety Administration.
38. Mothers Against Drunk Driving. *About Us.* www.madd.org. March 9, 2005.
39. The Trauma Foundation. *Alcohol and Unintentional Injury: A Brief Review of the Literature.* The Trauma Foundation. www.tf.org/tf/alcohol/ariv/reviews/injurev5.html. June 16, 2003.
40. Training Guide for USLA Safety Tips: General Information on Drowning. USLA Lifeguards for Life. www.usla.org/PublicInfo/safety.asp. June 16, 2003.
41. Vaughn C. *Children of Alcoholics: At Risk for Family Violence.* U.S. Department of Health and Human Services and SAMHSA's National Clearinghouse for Alcohol and Drug Information, February 10, 2003.
42. *Facts About Suicide.* Centers for Disease Control and Prevention, National Center for Health Statistics, 2009.
43. Woititz J. *The Complete ACOA Sourcebook.* Deerfield Beach, FL: Health Communications, 2002.
44. Website information, Al-Anon/Alateen. www.al-anon.alateen.org/. May 2001.
45. SADD History. Students Against Drunk Driving. www.saddonline.com. March 1, 2005. www.bacchusgamma.org/. March 1, 2005.
46. www.whitehousedrugpolicy.gov/publications/policy/04budget/exec_sum.pdf. May 21, 2003.

Personal Assessment

Risk Assessment for Marijuana Dependence or Abuse

You may wonder if your use or a friend's use of marijuana fits the criteria for being at risk for developing marijuana dependence or abuse. The following questions may help you decide whether you have cause for concern. Answer each question with a yes or no.

1. Have you tried to cut down or stop smoking marijuana and not been able to do so?
2. Do you use daily?
3. Is it hard for you to imagine life without marijuana?
4. Does your social life revolve around your marijuana use?
5. Do you use marijuana to avoid dealing with your problems?
6. Do you use marijuana to cope with your feelings?
7. Has your marijuana use created conflict in your relationships?
8. Has your marijuana use created problems for you at work?
9. Has your marijuana use negatively affected your academic performance?
10. Has your marijuana use caused problems with memory or concentration?
11. When you don't have access to marijuana, do you feel anxious or worried about how to get more?
12. Do you plan your life around your marijuana use, thinking about the next time you will use?
13. Have friends or family members ever complained that your marijuana use is damaging your relationship with them?
14. Have you or others noticed a decrease in your overall motivation level?
15. Do you find that your marijuana use has increased over time?
16. Are you more apathetic about things such as personal hygiene, exercise, and going out with nonusing friends?

Interpretation

Any yes answer could indicate problematic use of marijuana.

TO CARRY THIS FURTHER . . .

If you answered yes to many of these questions, you may want to reevaluate your marijuana use and talk to a medical or mental health care provider about a further assessment for drug abuse or dependence. If you are concerned about a friend's use, you might point to these specific behavioral criteria in sharing your concerns and encourage your friend to seek professional assistance.

Source: Adapted from Ball State University Health Questionnaire, 2010.

Personal Assessment

Do You Have a Drinking Problem?

The **CAGE** questionnaire (the acronym refers to the survey's four questions) is a widely used method of screening for alcoholism. Please answer yes or no to the following questions:

1. Have you ever felt you needed to **C**ut down on your drinking?
2. Have people **A**nnoyed you by criticizing your drinking?
3. Have you ever felt **G**uilty about drinking?
4. Have you ever felt you needed a drink first thing in the morning (**E**ye-opener) to steady your nerves or to get rid of a hangover?

Interpretation

If you answered yes to two out of four of these questions, it is an indicator that you may have a problem with alcohol.

TO CARRY THIS FURTHER . . .

If you are concerned about whether you may have a drinking problem and answered yes to at least half of the CAGE questions, it is recommended that you consult with a physician or mental health provider for further evaluation.

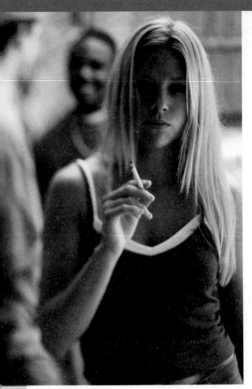

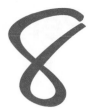

Rejecting Tobacco Use

What Do You Know About Tobacco Use?

1. Of all educational levels, those with a college degree have the highest rate of cigarette smoking. True or False?

2. Internal documents of the tobacco industry demonstrate that the tobacco industry neither knew of the health risks associated with its products nor intentionally marketed its products to young adolescents. True or False?

3. Nicotine dependence is easily (and quickly) established in the majority of people who begin cigarette use. True or False?

4. Carbon dioxide, produced during the combustion of tobacco, is the gaseous element in tobacco smoke that reduces the oxygen-carrying capacity of the blood. True or False?

5. When homicide and suicide are removed from death-related statistics, the life expectancy of smokers is virtually the same as that of their nonsmoking peers. True or False?

6. When assessed at the end of one year, well over half of the people who successfully completed a 10- to 12-week smoking cessation program will still be tobacco-free. True or False?

7. In public places, today's smokers are more likely to be asking "Where can I smoke?" rather than "Where can't I smoke?" True or False?

Check your answers at the end of the chapter.

Tobacco Use in American Society

If you were to visit certain businesses, entertainment spots, or sporting events in your community, you might leave convinced that virtually every adult is a tobacco user. Certainly, for some segments of society, tobacco use is the rule rather than the exception. You may be quite surprised to find out that the great majority of adults do not use tobacco products.

Table 8.1 indicates that only three states have a percentage of smokers above 25 percent, with Kentucky and West Virginia having the highest percentage at 25.6 percent,[1] whereas Utah, a state in which nearly three-fourths of the residents are Mormons and thus refrain from tobacco and alcohol use, reports the lowest percentage of tobacco users (9.8 percent).[2] When 14 states were asked what percentage of their households were "totally smoke-free," findings ranged from 63.6 percent in Kentucky to 82.9 percent in Arizona; "totally smoke-free workplaces" ranged from a low of 54.8 percent in Kentucky to a high of 85.5 percent in West Virginia.[3] Why do citizens in some states appear to care more about "freedom from tobacco smoke" than do those in other states?

Following the surgeon general's 1964 report (the first official statement of concern by the federal government regarding the dangers of smoking), the prevalence of smoking began a decline that lasted until 1991, when a leveling off was noted that lasted for the next three years. Since 1994, the percentage of the population who smoke has declined slowly but progressively. Current statistics reveal that 20.6 percent of American adults smoke cigarettes on a daily or near-daily basis.

Table 8.2 provides specific information on the percentage of Americans based on age who smoke regularly. The percentage of Americans over 18 who smoke (20.6 percent) is lower than in previous years, but it is still well above the 12 percent goal stated in *Healthy People 2010: Understanding and Improving Health,* described in Chapter 1.

Cigarette Smoking Among College Students

Until very recently, the rate of cigarette smoking among college graduates was lower than that reported for the population as a whole, and it was significantly lower than the rate for persons with very little formal education. In fact, the prevalence of smoking among college students decreased progressively from 21 percent in 1964 to 14 percent in 1995. However, it was noted that in the late 1990s and early 2000s, 30.6 percent of full-time enrolled students reported that they had smoked, and 42.7 percent of part-time students had smoked within the preceding months.[4] In contrast, smoking among twelfth-graders during 2007 reached its lowest level in several years with only 6 percent smoking daily.[5] Based on current data, a range of 21.7–24.9 percent suggests continuing movement downward in the number of college students who self-report cigarette smoking. The rate for men is higher (23.4–28.8 percent) and lower (19.0–22.9 percent) for women.[1] However, factors that more likely reflect college life, in comparison to high school, may well intervene in a negative direction.

When a college community is viewed as a whole regarding which segments of the student body are most likely to smoke, there appears to be a direct relationship between the level of alcohol consumption and cigarette smoking. Additional direct relationships appear between smoking and other drug use and in housing where smoking is permitted. Similar, although perhaps less influential, relationships are seen among tobacco use and coping style, depression, and perceptions of life satisfaction.[6]

The historically predictable relationship between higher levels of completed education and the lessened likelihood of smoking remains evident even today, particularly for those who have graduated from college, and even more so for persons holding a graduate degree.

The most disturbing aspect of the reported smoking among college students, beyond the eventual influence it will have on health and life expectancy, is its negation of the traditional belief that the college and university experience "protects" this segment of society from making some ill-informed choices. As recently as the mid-1990s, it was still possible to believe that the college population was "too well informed" and "too future oriented" to engage widely in an addictive behavior that fosters dependence, compromises health, and shortens life. Today that proposition seems to lack some of its former validity, but one hopes that the corner is being turned.

Table 8.1 Prevalence of Current Cigarette Smoking Among Adults (top 10 and bottom 10 states/areas)

State/Area	Percentage
Top 10	
Nevada	22.0
Tennessee	22.0
Louisiana	22.1
Alabama	22.5
Indiana	23.1
Missouri	23.1
Mississippi	23.3
Oklahoma	25.5
Kentucky	25.6
West Virginia	25.6
Bottom 10	
Utah	9.8
California	12.9
Washington	14.9
Massachusetts	15.0
Rhode Island	15.1
Maryland	15.2
District of Columbia	15.3
Connecticut	15.4
Hawaii	15.4
New Hampshire	15.8

Source: Centers for Disease Control and Prevention (CDC), Vital signs: current cigarette smoking among adults aged ≥ 18 years—United States, 2009, *Morbidity and Mortality Weekly Report,* 59 (43) September 10, 2010.

Table 8.2 Percentage of Persons Aged ≥ 18 Years Who Smoke* (by characteristic)

Characteristic	Percentage
Age group (yrs)	
18–24	21.8
25–44	24.0
45–64	21.9
≥ 65	9.5
Race/Ethnicity	
White, non-Hispanic	22.1
Black, non-Hispanic	21.3
Hispanic	14.5
American Indian/Alaska Native	23.2
Asian, non-Hispanic	12.0
Multiple race, non-Hispanic	29.5
Education	
0–12 yrs (no diploma)	26.4
≤ 8 yrs	17.1
9–11 yrs	33.6
12 yrs (no diploma)	28.5
GED	49.1
High school graduate	25.1
Some college (no degree)	23.3
Associate degree	19.7
Undergraduate degree	11.1
Graduate degree	5.6
Poverty Status	
At or above poverty level	19.4
Below poverty level	31.1
Unspecified	17.3
Region	
Northeast	20.0
New England	19.4
Mid-Atlantic	20.2
Midwest	23.1
East north central	23.8
West north central	21.8
South	21.8
South Atlantic	20.1
East south central	25.8
West south central	22.5
West	16.4
Mountain	18.8
Pacific	15.3
Total	20.6

*Persons who reported smoking at least 100 cigarettes during their lifetimes and who, at the time of the interview, reported smoking every day or some days.

Sources: Centers for Disease Control and Prevention, Cigarette smoking among adults—United States, 2007, *Morbidity and Mortality Weekly,* 57(42), November 14, 2008; U.S. Substance Abuse and Mental Health Services Administration, *Results from the 2007 National Survey on Drug Use and Health: National Findings* (NSDUH Series H-34, DHHS Publication No. SMA 08-4343). Rockville, MD: U.S. Department of Health and Human Services, Office of Applied Statistics, 2008.

Other Demographic Factors Influencing Tobacco Use

In addition to gender, race, ethnicity, and education level, other demographic factors appear to influence the extent to which smoking occurs. Included among these factors are the age groups into which persons fall, the region of the country in which they live, the size of their communities, and their employment status. Table 8.2 provides specific information on many of these demographic categories. Further, careful study of the information provides the basis for several interesting questions.[6]

Given the age-related information in Table 8.2, why do you think the percentage of smokers declines as age increases? What most likely accounts for the significant drop in smokers in the 45–64 age range and for persons who are 65 years of age and older? Also speculate on the differences that exist in terms of regions of the country.

An additional set of demographic categories, not presented in Table 8.2, further depicts the increased likelihood of heavy smoking among the unemployed. Specifically, for those persons who have spent more than 24 hours on the street, have lived in a shelter, or have been in a jail or prison, 56.2 percent are smokers. In 2004 this population included 9.5 million adults.[7]

For information on tobacco use in other countries, see the box "Smoking Around the World."

Marketing of Tobacco Products

Shredded plant material, wrapped in paper or leaf, ignited with a flame, and then placed on or near the delicate tissues of the mouth . . . what other human behavior does this resemble? If you answered "None!" to this question, then you appreciate that smoking is unique and, therefore, that it must be learned. How it is learned is currently a less than fully understood process that most likely requires a variety of stimuli ranging from modeling to actual experimentation. The role of advertising as a source of models has long been suspected and intensely debated. Today, as in the past, controversy surrounds the intent of the tobacco industry's advertising. Are the familiar logos seen in a variety of media intended to challenge the brand loyalty of those who have already decided to smoke, as the industry claims? Or are the ads intended to entice new smokers—older children and young adolescents—in sufficient numbers to replace the 3,000 smokers who die each day from the consequences of tobacco use? This latter objective is now known, by admission of the tobacco industry, to have been pursued for decades.

Master Tobacco Settlement Agreement A significant roadblock to the tobacco industry's success in addicting another generation of cigarette smokers emerged in

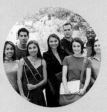

Learning from Our Diversity

Smoking Around the World

People in less-developed areas of the world are becoming increasingly exposed to the cultural influences of the postindustrial world, including behavioral patterns and access to products. Among the most harmful of these behavioral patterns is cigarette smoking, which is supported by access to imported cigarettes and the technology to manufacture cigarettes locally. Tragically today, as the postindustrial countries of the world turn way from cigarette smoking and move toward improved health, in less-developed countries the exact opposite is occurring. Already in these countries, the level of cigarette smoking is double or even triple the levels in the United States and Western Europe.

According to the American Cancer Society, the following levels of adult smoking were reported for 2005. In the United States, the rates of cigarette smoking are only slightly above 20 percent—so we can imagine the level of smoking-related illnesses being experienced in and projected for the future in less-developed areas of the world.

Given the astronomical levels of smoking in some countries, and worldwide levels in excess of the approximately 20 percent level in the United States, it is heartening to know that various types of regulation and cessation programs are now being seen on the world stage. Recent examples, reported by the Associated Press in 2011, include "harsh" smoking bans in Spain virtually eliminating locations in which smoking once was permitted; Honduras's consideration of a restriction on smoking in homes of nonsmokers, with arrest resulting, should a person attempt to smoke and the police are notified by the home owner; and China's restriction on smoking in films and on television shows (China's cigarette consumption surpasses one-third of the world total).

Countries Reporting Heavy Levels of Smoking, 2005

Males		Females	
Russian Federation	70.1%	Nauru	52.4%
Ukraine	63.8	Serbia and Montenegro	43.8
Belarus	63.7	Austria	40.1
Greece	63.6	Greece	39.8
Indonesia	62.1	Bosnia and Herzegovina	35.1
Tonga	61.8	Hungary	33.9
Lao People's Democratic Republic	61.1	Portugal	31.0
China	59.5	Chile	30.5
Korea, Democratic People's Republic of Korea	58.6	Nive	30.4
Georgia	57.1	Netherlands	30.3

Source: Shafey O, Eriksen M, Ross H, Mackay J, *The Tobacco Atlas* (3rd ed.). American Cancer Society, 2009.

the early 1990s when previously secret documents from the five largest cigarette manufacturers were leaked to the public. The fortuitous availability of these documents gave rise to a massive suit by the attorneys general of all 50 states. Using information regarding the tobacco industry's decades-old knowledge of the health risks of their products, the states brought suit against the industry to recoup Medicaid money paid by the states in treating illness due to smoking. This huge class-action suit was brought in 1998, leading to a Master Tobacco Settlement Agreement in 1999.

Although the settlement is far too complex to detail in this text, two significant components of the settlement are the monetary award to the states of $246 billion, to be paid over 25 years, and the implementation of restrictions on the tobacco industry regarding multiple aspects of its marketing of cigarettes and other tobacco products.

Since the Master Settlement In the decade and a half since the 1999 master settlement was reached, the $246 billion won by the 50 states has largely been depleted. The money, initially intended to pay for tobacco use prevention education and smoking cessation programs, was misappropriated by most of the states to help cover financial shortfalls due largely to the poor business practices of state-level governments and the recession that began in 2008. Relatively little was used for its intended purpose.

On a more positive note, lawsuits brought by chronically debilitated smokers and the families of deceased smokers (often filed as class action suits) are frequently won, with settlements against the tobacco industry approaching $100 billion.

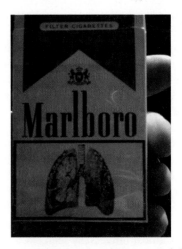

The FDA has proposed 36 new graphic warning labels for cigarette packages, including one showing a toe tag on a corpse. Cigarette manufacturers have vowed to fight the labels in federal court, saying they violate the right to property and free speech.

Smoking in Film

It is well established that most smokers begin using cigarettes in early adolescence and that adolescent smoking is influenced by an interplay of factors including parental smoking and parental supervision of media exposure, as well as the adolescent's personality and group affiliations. Particularly influential is the extent to which preadolescents and adolescents see movies in which cigarette use is portrayed and the attractiveness of the film characters who are seen smoking.

In a series of studies in which hundreds of G-, PG-13-, and R-rated films were assessed, researchers identified literally thousands of scenes depicting smoking by one or more characters. The percentage of characters who smoked closely approximated the percentage of adult smokers in the general population (approximately 22 percent), with men smoking a bit more often than women (approximately 25 percent versus 20 percent). Further, of the film characters who smoke in comparison to those who do not, white male antagonists (often favored by young adolescents) from lower socioeconomic classes and with little apparent education were the most likely to smoke. Interestingly, largely independent of the socioeconomic status of the youthful movie attendees, characters in today's films meeting the "smoker profile" described seem to hold a near-universal attractiveness to pre- and early-adolescent viewers.

Adding to the tobacco-positive message portrayed by the highly attractive smokers is the cumulative power of characters' presence.

Consider, for example, that in a single financially successful film, the number of scenes in which smoking occurs multiplied by the number of preteens and younger adolescents seeing the films easily equals billions of worldwide "hits" beneficial to the tobacco industry. This amazing reality fuels the tobacco industry's willingness to spend tens of thousands of dollars per film on product placement.

Parents and others who worry about the continued trend of early-onset smoking among today's younger adolescents would do well to pay attention to the role movies play in the lives of their children. Certainly, parents must discuss the intentions of the tobacco industry and the reasons film production companies purposely let some of a film's characters be depicted engaging in a practice that is so dangerous to real people.

On a positive note, in July 2011, the CDC announced that between 2005 and 2010 the percentage of characters seen smoking in G-, PG-, and PG-13-rated films declined by 72 percent.

Sources: Sargent JD, Tanski SE, Gibson J, Exposure to movie smoking among U.S. adolescents aged 10 to 14 years: a population estimate, *Pediatrics*, 119(5), e1167–e1176, May 2007; Hanewinkel R, Sargent JD, Exposure to smoking in internationally distributed American movies and youth smoking in Germany, *Pediatrics*, 121(1), e108–e117, January 2008.

Tobacco Use and the Development of Dependence

Although not true for every tobacco user (see the discussion of "chippers" later in this section), the vast majority of users, particularly cigarette smokers, will develop a dependency relationship with the nicotine contained in tobacco. This state of **dependence** causes users to consume greater quantities of nicotine over extended periods of time, further endangering their health.

Dependence can imply both a physical and a psychological relationship. Particularly with cigarettes, physical dependence or addiction, with its associated tolerance, withdrawal, and **titration,** is strongly developed by 40 percent of all smokers. The development of addiction reflects a strong genetic predisposition to physical dependence. Most of the remaining population of smokers will experience lesser degrees of physical dependence. Psychological dependence, or habituation, with its accompanying psychological components of compulsion and indulgence, is almost universally seen.

Compulsion reflects a strong emotional desire to continue tobacco use despite restrictions on smoking and the awareness of health risks. Very likely, users are "compelled" to engage in continual tobacco use in fear of the unpleasant physical, emotional, and social effects that result from discontinuing use. In comparison to compulsion, indulgence is seen as "rewarding" oneself for aligning with a particular behavior pattern—in this case, smoking. Indulgence is made possible by the existence of various reward systems built around the use of tobacco, including a perceived image, group affiliation, and even appetite suppression intended to foster weight control.

Much to the benefit of the tobacco industry, dependence on tobacco is easily established. Many experts believe that physical dependence on tobacco is far more easily established than is physical dependence on alcohol, cocaine (other than crack), or heroin. Of all people who experiment with cigarettes, 85 percent develop various aspects of a dependence relationship.

Key Terms

dependence A physical or psychological need to continue the use of a drug.

titration (tie **tray** shun) The particular level of a drug within the body; adjusting the level of nicotine by adjusting the rate of smoking.

bolus theory A theory of nicotine addiction based on the body's response to the bolus (ball) of nicotine delivered to the brain with each inhalation of cigarette smoke.

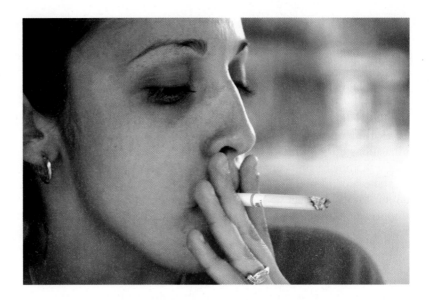

Laboratory tests, using newer technology, have indicated that nicotine content in cigarettes has increased by approximately 11 percent since 2000—a finding that the tobacco industry rejects.

A small percentage of smokers, known as "chippers," can smoke on occasion without becoming dependent. Most likely, chippers respond differently to environmental cues than do more dependent smokers, thus smoking less frequently. Chippers, once described as "social smokers," smoke in a wide variety of settings, including when alone, when socializing or indulging in activities, and when eating and consuming alcohol, just as heavy smokers do. The primary difference is that chippers have a highly developed level of control over their smoking. In contrast, heavy smokers do not have such control, smoke in a wider array of settings, and when smoking, cannot easily limit the number of cigarettes they smoke.[8] Unfortunately, many inexperienced smokers feel that they too are only "social smokers"; however, a few months, or even a few days, of this type of occasional smoking can be a transitional period into a dependence pattern of tobacco use.

Sandwiched between regular smokers and chippers is a newly emerging group of smokers—part-time smokers. Today these smokers constitute about 20 percent of all smokers. Also called *nondaily smokers,* these part-time smokers show many of the same types of negative health effects as seen in daily smokers, although in part-time smokers they are not as well established or as debilitating. That said, nondaily smokers can show classic signs of withdrawal, such as irritability, restlessness, and disrupted concentration, if nonsmoking intervals approach one week. Further, among nondaily smokers who tried to quit, one-fourth were unsuccessful.[9]

As to why nondaily smokers exist, perhaps it reflects the high cost of cigarettes and restrictions in the workplace and other public spaces.

Theories of Nicotine Addiction

The establishment and maintenance of physical dependence or addiction is less than fully understood. Most experts, however, believe that for a specific individual, addiction has a multifaceted etiology, or cause, with increasing attention being directed toward a genetic basis for addiction. Accordingly, several theories have been proposed to explain the development of dependence. We present a brief account of some of these theories. Readers are reminded that many of these theories are technically sophisticated and only a most basic description can be provided in a personal health textbook. The more emotional aspects of dependence formation are discussed later in the chapter.

Genetic Influences Although the specific genetic pathways that influence both the initiation and maintenance of smoking (or other forms of tobacco use) are less than fully understood, a role for genetic influence is evident. Applying new statistical techniques to earlier studies of smoking patterns in families and by identical twins, it is now believed that initiation and maintenance of initial smoking is somewhat more heavily driven by genetic and genetic/environmental interplay than by only environmental factors.[10]

Once the relatively brief period of initial exposure (initiation) and early maintenance is passed, the role of genetic influences may be even more powerful—providing a majority portion (nearly 70 percent) of the maintenance stimulus required over decades of smoking. Environmental and personality factors subside accordingly.[11]

On the basis of the growing evidence pointing to the powerful role of genetics in cigarette dependence, the risk of early experimentation is akin to "walking on very thin ice." First-time smokers have little or no indication of their genetic susceptibility to a dependence on nicotine, and they might end up "choosing" a lifetime of addiction and habituation.

Bolus Theory In the **bolus theory** of nicotine addiction, one of the oldest and most general theories of addiction, each inhalation of smoke releases into the blood a concentrated quantity of nicotine (a ball or bolus) that reaches the brain and results in a period of neurohormonal (neurochemical) excitement. The smoker perceives this period of stimulation as pleasurable but, unfortunately, short-lived. Accordingly, the smoker attempts to reestablish this pleasurable feeling by again inhaling and sending another bolus of nicotine on its way to the brain. The 70,000 or more inhalations during the first year of smoking serve to condition the novice smoker, resulting in a lifelong pattern of cigarette dependence. The level needed for arousal is different for each individual smoker, depending on genetic predisposition, the length of addiction, the level of tolerance, and environmental and personal stimuli.

Adrenocorticotropic Hormone (ACTH) Theory Yet another theory of dependence suggests that nicotine stimulates the release of the adrenocorticotropic hormone (ACTH) from the "master gland" of the endocrine system (see Chapter 3), causing the release of **beta endorphins** (naturally occurring opiatelike chemicals) that produce mild feelings of **euphoria.** Perhaps this stresslike response mechanism involving ACTH accounts for the increased energy expenditure seen in smokers and thus their tendency to maintain a lower body weight.

Self-Medication Theory Another explanation for the addiction to smoking, called *self-medication,* suggests that nicotine, through the effects of mood-enhancing dopamine, may allow smokers to "treat" feelings of tiredness, lack of motivation, or even depression. In other words, a smoke lifts the spirits, if only briefly. Eventually, however, smokers become dependent on tobacco as a "medication" to make themselves feel better.

Regardless of the mechanism involved, as tolerance to nicotine develops, smoking behavior is adjusted to either maintain arousal or prevent the occurrence of withdrawal symptoms. At some point, however, the desire for constant arousal is probably superseded by the smoker's desire not to experience withdrawal.

Even more impressive (and alarming) than the power of nicotine to cause dependency is the small amount of time needed for it to do so. Instruments designed to assess the time required for the onset of dependence on nicotine—such as Development and Assessment of Nicotine Dependency in Youths (DANDY) and Hooked On Nicotine Checklist (HONC)—have established that beginning smokers (recall that most smokers begin during adolescence) become dependent on cigarettes within three weeks to three months of smoking as few as two cigarettes per day. Males are more likely to be a bit more resistant to dependency, taking a month or two, whereas females can become dependent in just a few days of initial experimentation. Additionally, it is now known that for children who try smoking on a very limited basis (even just one cigarette) and then stop, a "sleeper effect" may be put into place that increases their vulnerability to becoming a smoker within the next three years, in comparison to peers who did not experiment with smoking.[12]

A newly recognized variable in understanding dependence formation in young, light smokers (one to six cigarettes per day) is the rate of nicotine metabolism. Dependence, reflected in withdrawal symptoms, occurs much sooner in individuals whose rate of nicotine breakdown was faster than in those with slower rates.[13]

For the purposes of this discussion on physical dependence, it is important to recognize that, whether through the influence of nicotine on the electrochemical activity of the brain (such as mood-enhancing dopamine), leading to feelings of arousal and euphoria, or to the influence of opiumlike hormones in the central nervous system (CNS) produced under the influence of ACTH, the body initially enjoys these altered-feeling states. But soon the body begins to pay dearly from the manner in which they are introduced. Eventually, the addicted smoker reaches a point where it appears that "you will not live long with cigarettes, but you can't live comfortably without them"—the dilemma of dependence.

 TALKING POINTS A smoker says that she does not consider smoking to be a form of drug use. She becomes angry at the suggestion that cigarettes are part of a drug delivery system. How would you respond to her position?

Nicotine Dependence and Traumatic Head Injury Recent findings related to the consequence of strokes occurring in a very specific area of the brain called the *insula* provide an interesting aside to the discussion of the brain and CNS's role in nicotine dependence. Located in the brain at ear level, the insula is a small area that plays a critical role in the communication of information to the area of the brain where behavioral decisions are formulated. In a smoker whose insula has been damaged by the disruption of blood flow (stroke), nicotine dependence often disappears instantly, and the individual can immediately stop smoking.[14] In other words, damage to this specific area of the brain appears to disrupt the flow of information from other nicotine-sensitive areas of the brain, disrupting the reward system that would otherwise result in the act of smoking. Perhaps in the future there will be a smoking-cessation technology centered on insula function.

Acute Effects of Nicotine on Nervous System Function

In comparison with the more chronic effects of nicotine on the CNS that may eventually result in physical dependence or addiction, nicotine also produces changes of short duration within the brain. Through the use of electroencephalography (EEG) and magnetic resonance imaging (MRI) technology, the location and extent of brain activity can be assessed. This is part of a general arousal pattern signaled by the release of at least four different neurotransmitters. Heavy use of tobacco products, resulting in high levels of nicotine in the bloodstream, eventually produces a blocking effect as more and more receptor sites for these neurotransmitters are filled. The result is a generalized depression of the CNS.

The level of nicotine in the blood associated with normal levels of heavy smoking (one to two packs per day) would not likely produce the depressive effect just described. However, in chain smokers (four to eight packs per day), nicotine levels would be sufficient to have a depressive influence on CNS function. In fact, it has been suggested that chain smoking is driven by the fruitless effort to counter the depressive influence of chronically excessively high levels of nicotine. In contrast to chain smokers, inexperienced smokers, lacking tolerance, can quickly reach a blood level of nicotine sufficient to activate the brain's vomiting centers. This response is a built-in protective mechanism against nicotine poisoning.

The CNS is one of the body's principal control and coordination mechanisms, on which nicotine has both long- and short-term disruptive influences. Therefore, nicotine should be seen for what it is—a powerful psychotropic (mind-altering) drug capable of changing normal brain activity to produce dependence. The delivery system for this drug is the array of tobacco products manufactured and marketed by the tobacco industry.

Non-Nervous-System Acute Effects of Nicotine

Outside the CNS, nicotine affects the transmission of nerve signals at the point where nerves innervate muscle tissue (called the *neuromuscular junction*) by mimicking the action of the neurotransmitter acetylcholine. Nicotine occupies receptor sites at the junction and prevents the transmission of nerve impulses from nerve cell to muscle cell.

Nicotine also causes the release of epinephrine from the adrenal glands (see Chapter 3), which results in an increase in respiration rate, heart rate, blood pressure, and coronary blood flow. These changes are accompanied by the constriction of the blood vessels beneath the skin, a reduction in the motility in the bowel, loss of appetite, and changes in sleep patterns.

Although a lethal dose of nicotine could be obtained through the ingestion of a nicotine-containing insecticide, to "smoke oneself to death" in a single intense period of cigarette use would be highly improbable. In humans, 40–60 mg (0.06–0.09 mg/kg) is a lethal dose. A typical cigarette supplies 0.05–2.5 mg of nicotine, and that nicotine is relatively quickly broken down for removal from the body.

Psychosocial Factors Related to Dependence

Recall that a psychological aspect of dependence (habituation) exists and is important in maintaining the smoker's need for nicotine. Both research and general observation support many of the powerful influences this aspect of dependence possesses, especially for beginning smokers, before the onset of physical addiction. Consequently, in the remainder of this section, we will explore nonphysiological factors that may contribute to the development of this aspect of dependence.

Modeling Behavior Because tobacco use is a learned behavior, it is reasonable to accept that modeling acts as a stimulus to experimental smoking. **Modeling** suggests that susceptible people smoke to emulate, or model their behavior after, smokers whom they admire or with whom they share other social or emotional bonds. Particularly for young adolescents (ages 11–16), smoking behavior correlates with the smoking behavior of slightly older peers and very young adults (ages 18–22), older siblings, and, most important, parents. Negative parental influences on cigarette smoking by their children include their own smoking status and/or their failure to clearly state their disapproval of smoking.[15]

Modeling is particularly evident when smoking is a central factor in peer group formation and peer group association and can lead to a shared behavioral pattern that differentiates the group from others and from adults. Further, when risk-taking behavior and disregard for authority are common to the group, smoking becomes the behavioral pattern that most consistently identifies and bonds the group. Particularly for those young people who lack self-directedness or the ability to resist peer pressure, initial membership in a tobacco-using peer group may become inescapable. The ability to counter peer pressure is a salient component of successful anti-smoking programs for use with older children and younger adolescents.

Key Terms

beta endorphins Mood-enhancing, pain-reducing, opiatelike chemicals produced within the smoker's body in response to the presence of nicotine.

euphoria A complex interplay of physical and emotional states that suggest heightened energy, enhanced mood, and greater resistance to pain and discomfort.

modeling The process of adopting the behavioral patterns of a person one admires or has bonds with.

In addition, when adolescents have lower levels of self-esteem and are searching for an avenue to improve self-image, a role model who smokes is often seen as tough, sociable, and sexually attractive. These three traits have been played up by the tobacco industry in its carefully crafted advertisements.

Manipulation   In addition to modeling as a psychosocial link to tobacco use, cigarette use may meet the beginning smoker's need to manipulate something and at the same time provide the manipulative "tool" necessary to offset boredom, anxiety, or social immaturity. The availability of affordable smoking paraphernalia provides smokers with ways to reward themselves. For others, the ability to take out a cigarette or fill a pipe adds a measure of structure and control to situations in which they might otherwise feel ill at ease. The cigarette becomes a readily available and dependable "friend" to turn to during stressful moments.

Susceptibility to Advertising   The images of the smoker's world portrayed by the media can be particularly attractive. For adolescents, women, minorities, and other carefully targeted groups of adults, the tobacco industry has paired suggestions of a better life with the use of its products. To these users and potential users, the self-reward of power, liberation, affluence, sophistication, or adult status is achieved by using products that they are told are associated with these desired states. Thus, the self-rewarding use of tobacco products becomes a means of hoped-for achievement.

With this multiplicity of forces at work, we can understand why so many who experiment with tobacco use find that they quickly, in combination with genetic predisposition, become emotionally dependent on tobacco. Human needs, both physiological and psychosocial, are many and complex. Tobacco use meets the needs on a short-term basis, whereas dependence, once established, replaces these needs with a different, more immediate set of needs.

For those who question whether tobacco promotion leads to the initiation of smoking in children and young adolescents, a recent reassessment of earlier research indicates that the effect of tobacco promotion is so powerful that, when other environmental factors associated with initiation, such as smoking by parents and peer group and the socioeconomic background of the young persons, are controlled for, exposure to tobacco promotion is the single most powerful environmental factor underlying adolescent smoking. In fact, the association between exposure to tobacco promotion and probability of smoking is so strong that causality is assigned (promotion is said to cause smoking).[16] Once smoking is initiated, dependence in some form is almost a certainty and will prove difficult to overcome.

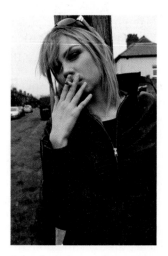

Most smokers pick up the habit as young teens, possibly influenced by older smoking peers and by widespread tobacco advertising and promotions.

Preventing Smoking: Childhood Intervention

Although significant concern centers on the onset of smoking behavior by adolescents in the 11- to 14-year-old age group and later teen years, the decision to smoke (or use other forms of tobacco) may be made at a much earlier age. Accordingly, parents (and other adults) who do not want their children to smoke or use tobacco in other forms should begin educating their children as preschoolers and certainly by school age. The following recommendations, and many additional ones, can be found in *A Parent's Guide to Prevention,* available from the National Clearinghouse for Alcohol and Drug Information.

When dealing with preschool children, it should be remembered that facts are unlikely to be comprehended. Accordingly, the following activities are suggested:

- Set aside regular time when you can give your child your full attention. Playing and reading together builds a strong parent-child bond.

- Point out poisonous and harmful substances that can be found in the home.

- Explain how medicines can be harmful if used incorrectly.

- Provide guidelines that teach the child what kind of behavior is expected.

- Encourage the child to follow instructions.

- Help the child learn decision-making skills; give positive feedback when appropriate decisions have been made.

For children in kindergarten through third grade, new skills and insights need to be developed to deal with drugs, including tobacco products. Adults should attempt to do the following:

- Help the child recognize and understand family rules.
- Discuss how television advertisements try to persuade people to buy their products.
- Practice ways in which the child can say no to other people.
- Develop a "helper" file made up of the names and phone numbers of people the child can turn to when confronted by others who want him or her to try smoking or smokeless tobacco.

As children approach the preteen years, more focused presentations can be made regarding the dangers associated with smoking and the use of other substances. Adults working with children in grades four through six should focus on the following activities:

- Create special times when an adult is available to talk with the child about whatever he or she wants to talk about.
- Encourage participation in a variety of activities that are fun and allow the child to meet new friends.
- Teach the child how drugs, including tobacco products, are promoted and how their messages can be "defused."
- Continue to assist the child in learning how to say no.
- Become acquainted with the parents of the child's friends so that you will be able to work with them in support of a smoke-free community.
- Participate in providing support for supervised activities for children of this age.

Although nothing is certain regarding the decisions that older preadolescents or teens make about beginning to smoke, the activities just listed may be effective in countering the influences of the peer group and the mass media. A recent study provides some insights into the role of parents in helping their young adult children stop smoking. In this study, researchers followed young smokers over time and found that those who managed to stop smoking by their mid-20s were those whose own smoking parents had managed to stop smoking during their children's adolescent years.[17] In a slightly different vein, other studies have suggested that for smoking parents to prevent their children from ever becoming smokers, stopping during their children's childhood years might be more effective.

Perhaps the most innovative attempt to prevent tobacco sales to minors was inherent in a request made by the FDA to allow it to define cigarettes as a drug delivery device (nicotine being the drug). This reclassification was recently approved by Congress. However, at this time, the FDA has utilized its new authority in a very limited manner—approval of new and more graphic health warnings

on cigarette packages, more "honest" manufacturing and accurate labeling of lower-tar and-nicotine cigarettes, and a ban on flavoring cigarettes, including menthol, once used to soften the harsh bite of burning tobacco. If, however, this authority were taken to its fullest extent, the FDA could classify nicotine as a controlled substance and the products containing nicotine for human consumption as "delivery systems," thus relegating cigarettes to a status similar to that of prescription medications.

The FDA's decision to replace current labels with more graphic ones was based in part on similar changes made by Canada and some European countries. These labels were specifically designed to have a positive anti-smoking impact on preadolescents—the age group in which the inclination to smoke is being established.

Tobacco Smoke: The Source of Physiologically Active Compounds

When burned, the tobacco in cigarettes, cigars, and pipe mixtures is the source of an array of physiologically active chemicals, many of which are closely linked to significant changes in normal body structure and function. At the burning tip of the cigarette, the 900°C (1652°F) heat oxidizes tobacco (as well as paper, wrapper, and additives). With each puff of smoke, the body is exposed to approximately 4,700 chemical compounds, hundreds of which are known to be physiologically active, toxic, and carcinogenic. These chemicals have their origins in the tobacco or have been introduced as additives, pesticides, and other agricultural chemicals. An annual 70,000 puffs taken in by the one-pack-a-day cigarette smoker results in an environment that makes the most polluted urban environment seem clean by comparison.

Figure 8-1 shows some of the toxic and carcinogenic compounds in tobacco smoke. In addition to tobacco smoke, these materials, and hundreds of others not shown, are routinely found within many materials used in industrial and residential settings.

Particulate Phase

Cigarette, cigar, and pipe smoke can be described on the basis of two phases: a particulate phase and a gaseous phase. The **particulate phase** includes **nicotine,**

> **Key Terms**
>
> **particulate phase** The portion of the tobacco smoke composed of small suspended particles.
>
> **nicotine** A physiologically active, dependence-producing drug found in tobacco.

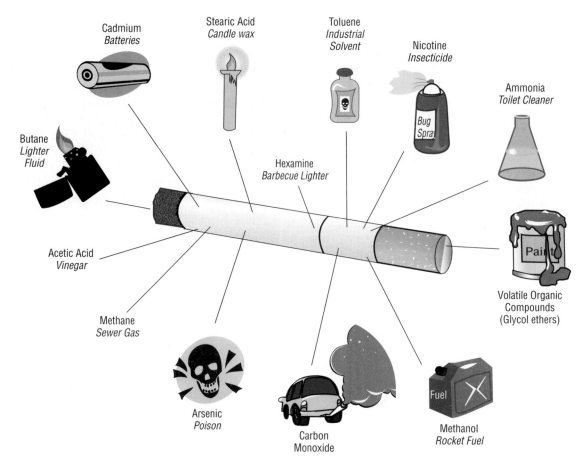

Figure 8-1 Toxic and Carcinogenic Compounds in Tobacco Smoke and Other Sources

water, and a variety of powerful chemicals known collectively as tar. **Tar** includes phenol, cresol, pyrene, DDT, a benzene-ring group of compounds that includes benzo[a]pyrene, and hundreds of additional compounds. A person who smokes one pack of cigarettes per day collects 4 ounces of tar in his or her lungs in a year. Only the gases and the smallest particles reach the small sacs of the lungs, called the *alveoli,* where oxygen exchange occurs. The carcinogen-rich particles from the particulate phase are deposited somewhere along the air passage leading to the lungs.

Gaseous Phase

The **gaseous phase** of tobacco smoke, like the particulate phase, is composed of a variety of physiologically active compounds including carbon monoxide, carbon dioxide, ammonia, hydrogen cyanide, isopyrene, acetaldehyde, and acetone. At least 60 of these compounds in the gaseous phase have been determined to be **carcinogens,** or co-carcinogenic promoters, thus capable of stimulating the development of cancer. Carbon monoxide is, however, the most damaging compound found in this component of tobacco smoke. Its effect is discussed next.

Carbon Monoxide Like any inefficient engine, a cigarette, cigar, or pipe burns (oxidizes) its fuel with less than complete conversion into carbon dioxide, water, and heat. As a result of this incomplete oxidation, burning tobacco forms **carbon monoxide (CO)** gas. Carbon monoxide is one of the most harmful components of tobacco smoke.

Carbon monoxide is a colorless, odorless, tasteless gas that possesses a very strong physiological attraction for hemoglobin, the oxygen-carrying pigment on each red blood cell. When CO is inhaled, it quickly bonds with hemoglobin and forms a new compound, carboxyhemoglobin.[18] In this form, hemoglobin is unable to transport oxygen to the tissues and cells where it is needed.

As mentioned, the presence of excessive levels of carboxyhemoglobin in the blood of smokers leads to shortness of breath and lowered endurance. Because an adequate oxygen supply to all body tissues is critical for normal functioning, any oxygen reduction can have a serious impact on health. Brain function may be eventually reduced, reactions and judgment are dulled, and cardiovascular function is impaired. Fetuses are especially at risk for this oxygen deprivation (hypoxia) because fetal development is so critically dependent on a sufficient oxygen supply from the mother.

Illness, Premature Death, and Tobacco Use

For people who begin tobacco use as adolescents or young adults, smoke heavily, and continue to smoke, premature death is virtually ensured. Two-pack-a-day cigarette smokers can expect to die seven to eight years earlier than their nonsmoking counterparts will. (Only nonsmoking-related deaths that can afflict smokers and nonsmokers alike keep the difference at this level rather than much higher.) Not only will these people die sooner, but they will also probably be plagued with painful, debilitating illnesses for an extended time. Worldwide, it is estimated that smoking is responsible for nearly 5 million premature deaths each year. Figure 8-2 presents an overview of illnesses known to be caused or worsened by tobacco use.

Cardiovascular Disease

Although cancer is now the leading cause of death for Americans under 80 years of age, cardiovascular disease is the leading cause of death among all adults, accounting for 864,500 deaths in the United States in 2007.[18] Tobacco use, and cigarette smoking in particular, is one of the major factors contributing to this cause of death. Although overall progress is being made in reducing the incidence of cardiovascular-related deaths, tobacco use impedes these efforts. So important is tobacco use as a contributing factor in deaths from cardiovascular disease that the cigarette smoker has more than double the risk of experiencing a **myocardial infarction,** the leading cause of death from cardiovascular disease. Smokers also increase their risk of **cardiac arrest** by two to four times. Fully one-third of all cardiovascular disease can be traced to cigarette smoking.

The relationship between tobacco use and cardiovascular disease is centered on two major components of tobacco smoke: nicotine and carbon monoxide.

Nicotine and Cardiovascular Disease The influence of nicotine on the cardiovascular system occurs when it stimulates the nervous system to release norepinephrine. This powerful stimulant increases the heart rate. In turn, an elevated heart rate increases cardiac output, thus increasing blood pressure. The extent to which this is dangerous depends in part on the coronary circulation's ability to supply blood to the rapidly contracting heart muscle. The development of **angina pectoris** and the possibility of sudden heart attack are heightened by this sustained elevation of heart rate, particularly in those individuals with existing coronary artery disease (see Chapter 9).

Nicotine is also a powerful vasoconstrictor of the peripheral blood vessels. As these vessels are constricted by the influence of nicotine, the pressure against their walls increases. Research shows that irreversible atherosclerotic damage to major arteries also occurs with smoking.

For over a decade it has been known that nicotine also increases blood **platelet adhesiveness.**[19] As the platelets become more and more likely to "clump," a person is more likely to develop a blood clot. In people already prone to cardiovascular disease, more rapidly clotting blood is an unwelcome liability. Heart attacks occur when clots form within the coronary arteries or are transported to the heart from other areas of the body.

In addition to other influences on the cardiovascular system, nicotine possesses the ability to decrease the proportion of high-density lipoproteins (HDLs) and to increase the proportion of low-density lipoproteins (LDLs) and very-low-density lipoproteins that constitute the body's serum cholesterol. LDLs appear to support the development of atherosclerosis and are clearly increased in the bloodstreams of smokers. (See Chapter 9 for further information about cholesterol's role in cardiovascular disease.)

Carbon Monoxide and Cardiovascular Disease A second substance contributed by tobacco influences the type and extent of cardiovascular disease found among tobacco users. Carbon monoxide interferes with oxygen transport within the circulatory system.

As described earlier in the chapter, carbon monoxide is a component of the gaseous phase of tobacco smoke and readily joins with the hemoglobin on the red blood cells. Once the hemoglobin on a red cell has accepted

> ### Key Terms
>
> **tar** A chemically rich, syrupy, blackish-brown material obtained from the particulate matter within cigarette smoke when nicotine and water are removed.
>
> **gaseous phase** The portion of the tobacco smoke containing carbon monoxide and many other physiologically active gaseous compounds.
>
> **carcinogens** Environmental agents, including chemical compounds within cigarette smoke, that stimulate the development of cancerous changes within cells.
>
> **carbon monoxide (CO)** A chemical compound that can "inactivate" red blood cells.
>
> **myocardial infarction** Heart attack; the death of heart muscle as a result of a blockage in one of the coronary arteries.
>
> **cardiac arrest** Immediate death resulting from a sudden change in the rhythm of the heart causing loss of heart function.
>
> **angina pectoris** (an **jie** nuh **peck** tor is) Chest pain that results from impaired blood supply to the heart muscle.
>
> **platelet adhesiveness** The tendency of platelets to clump together, thus enhancing the speed at which the blood clots.

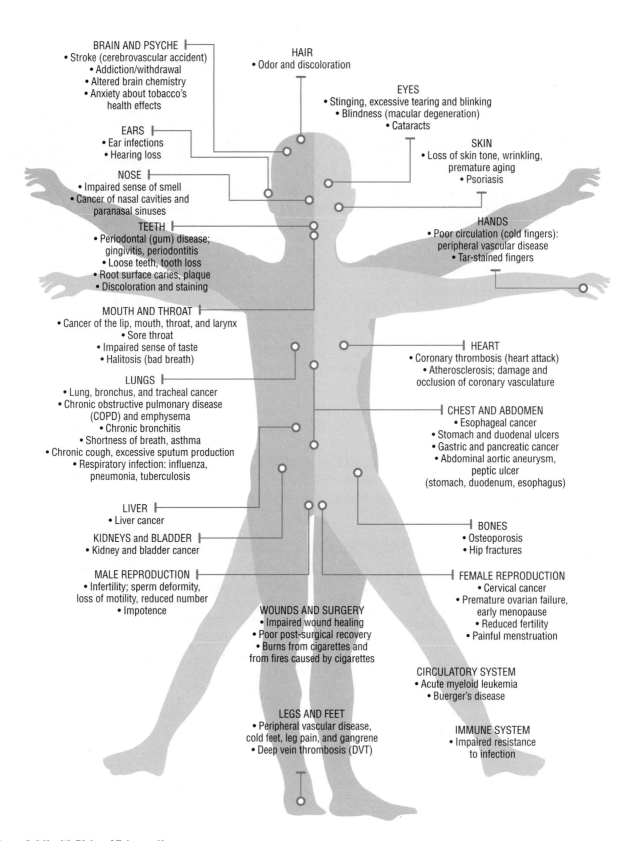

BRAIN AND PSYCHE
• Stroke (cerebrovascular accident)
• Addiction/withdrawal
• Altered brain chemistry
• Anxiety about tobacco's
  health effects

HAIR
• Odor and discoloration

EYES
• Stinging, excessive tearing and blinking
• Blindness (macular degeneration)
• Cataracts

SKIN
• Loss of skin tone, wrinkling,
  premature aging
• Psoriasis

EARS
• Ear infections
• Hearing loss

NOSE
• Impaired sense of smell
• Cancer of nasal cavities and
  paranasal sinuses

HANDS
• Poor circulation (cold fingers):
  peripheral vascular disease
• Tar-stained fingers

TEETH
• Periodontal (gum) disease;
  gingivitis, periodontitis
• Loose teeth, tooth loss
• Root surface caries, plaque
• Discoloration and staining

MOUTH AND THROAT
• Cancer of the lip, mouth, throat, and larynx
• Sore throat
• Impaired sense of taste
• Halitosis (bad breath)

HEART
• Coronary thrombosis (heart attack)
• Atherosclerosis; damage and
  occlusion of coronary vasculature

LUNGS
• Lung, bronchus, and tracheal cancer
• Chronic obstructive pulmonary disease
  (COPD) and emphysema
• Chronic bronchitis
• Shortness of breath, asthma
• Chronic cough, excessive sputum production
• Respiratory infection: influenza,
  pneumonia, tuberculosis

CHEST AND ABDOMEN
• Esophageal cancer
• Stomach and duodenal ulcers
• Gastric and pancreatic cancer
• Abdominal aortic aneurysm,
  peptic ulcer
(stomach, duodenum, esophagus)

LIVER
• Liver cancer

KIDNEYS and BLADDER
• Kidney and bladder cancer

BONES
• Osteoporosis
• Hip fractures

MALE REPRODUCTION
• Infertility; sperm deformity,
loss of motility, reduced number
• Impotence

FEMALE REPRODUCTION
• Cervical cancer
• Premature ovarian failure,
  early menopause
• Reduced fertility
• Painful menstruation

WOUNDS AND SURGERY
• Impaired wound healing
• Poor post-surgical recovery
• Burns from cigarettes and
from fires caused by cigarettes

CIRCULATORY SYSTEM
• Acute myeloid leukemia
• Buerger's disease

LEGS AND FEET
• Peripheral vascular disease,
cold feet, leg pain, and gangrene
• Deep vein thrombosis (DVT)

IMMUNE SYSTEM
• Impaired resistance
to infection

Figure 8-2 Health Risks of Tobacco Use

Source: "How Tobacco Harms You." Reprinted by the permission of the American Cancer Society, Inc. *The Tobacco Atlas, 3rd Edition.* American Cancer Society 2009,
www.cancer.org. All rights reserved.

carbon monoxide molecules, the hemoglobin is transformed into carboxyhemoglobin. So long as smoking continues, these red blood cells remain relatively useless during the remainder of their 120-day lives.

When a person has impaired oxygen-transporting abilities, physical exertion becomes increasingly demanding on both the heart and the lungs. The cardiovascular system will attempt to respond to the body's demand for oxygen, but these responses are themselves impaired as a result of the influence of nicotine on the cardiovascular system. If tobacco does create the good life, as advertisers claim, it also unfortunately lessens the ability to participate actively in that life.

Smoking and Oral Contraceptive Use   Women who smoke and use oral contraceptives, particularly after age 35, are placing themselves at a much greater risk of experiencing a fatal cardiovascular accident (heart attack, stroke, or **embolism**) than are oral contraceptive users who do not smoke. This risk of cardiovascular complications increases further for oral contraceptive users 40 years of age or older. Women who both smoke and use oral contraceptives are four times more likely to die from myocardial infarction (heart attack) than are women who only smoke. Because of this adverse relationship, it is strongly recommended that women who smoke not use oral contraceptives.

Cancer

Over the past 65 years, research from the most reputable institutions in this country and abroad has consistently concluded that tobacco use is a significant factor in the development of virtually all forms of cancer and the most significant factor in cancers involving the respiratory system.

In describing cancer development, the currently used reference is 20 pack-years, or an amount of smoking equal to smoking one pack of cigarettes a day for 20 years. Thus, the two-pack-a-day smoker can anticipate cancer-related tissue changes in as few as 10 years, while the half-pack-a-day smoker may have 40 years to wait. Regardless, the opportunity is there for all smokers to confirm these data by developing cancer as predicted. It is hoped that most people will think twice before disregarding this evidence.

Data supplied by the American Cancer Society (ACS) indicate that during 2010 an estimated 1,529,560 Americans developed cancer.* These cases were nearly equally divided between the sexes and resulted in approximately 569,490 deaths. In the opinion of the ACS, 30 percent of all cancer cases are heavily influenced by tobacco use. Lung cancer alone accounted for about 222,520 of the new cancer cases and 157,300 deaths in

2010. Fully 87 percent of men with lung cancer were cigarette smokers.[20] A genetic link between smoking and lung cancer was established, when mutations to an important tumor suppressor gene, RAD9, came under increased serutiny.[21] If it was necessary to have final "proof" that smoking causes lung cancer, that proof appears to be in hand.

Cancer of the entire respiratory system, including lung cancer and cancers of the mouth and throat, accounted for about 240,610 new cases of cancer and 161,670 deaths.[20] Despite these high figures, not all smokers develop cancer.

Respiratory Tract Cancer   Recall that tobacco smoke produces both a gaseous and a particulate phase. As noted, the particulate phase contains the tar fragment of tobacco smoke. This rich chemical environment contains more than 4,000 known chemical compounds, hundreds of which are known to be carcinogens.

In the normally functioning respiratory system, particulate matter suspended in the inhaled air settles on the tissues lining the airways and is trapped in **mucus** produced by specialized *goblet cells.* This mucus, with its trapped impurities, is continuously swept upward by the beating action of hairlike **cilia** of the ciliated columnar epithelial cells lining the air passages (Figure 8-3). On reaching the throat, this mucus is swallowed and eventually removed through the digestive system.

When tobacco smoke is drawn into the respiratory system, however, its rapidly dropping temperature allows the particulate matter to accumulate. This brown, sticky tar contains compounds known to harm the ciliated cells, goblet cells, and basal cells of the respiratory lining. As the damage from smoking increases, the cilia become less effective in sweeping mucus upward to the throat. When cilia can no longer clean the airway, tar accumulates on the surfaces and brings carcinogenic compounds into direct contact with the tissues of the airway.

At the same time that the sweeping action of the lining cells is being slowed, substances in the tar are stimulating the goblet cells to increase the amount of mucus they normally produce. The "smoker's cough" is the body's attempt to remove this excess mucus.

> ### Key Terms
>
> **embolism** A potentially fatal condition in which a circulating blood clot lodges in a smaller vessel.
>
> **mucus** Clear, sticky material produced by specialized cells within the mucous membranes of the body; mucus traps much of the suspended particulate matter within tobacco smoke.
>
> **cilia (sill** ee uh) Small, hairlike structures that extend from cells that line the air passages.

*Excluding cases of nonmelanoma skin cancer

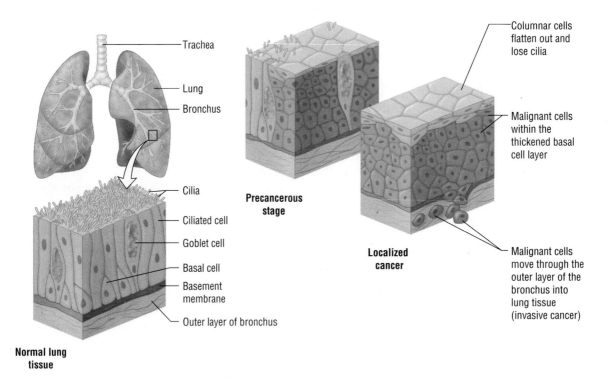

Labels on figure:
Trachea
Lung
Bronchus
Cilia
Ciliated cell
Goblet cell
Basal cell
Basement membrane
Outer layer of bronchus

Normal lung tissue

Precancerous stage

Localized cancer

Columnar cells flatten out and lose cilia

Malignant cells within the thickened basal cell layer

Malignant cells move through the outer layer of the bronchus into lung tissue (invasive cancer)

Figure 8-3 Development of Lung Cancer   Certain tissue changes are associated with lung cancer (bronchogenic carcinoma).

With prolonged exposure to the carcinogenic materials in tar, predictable changes will begin to occur within the respiratory system's basal cell layer (see Figure 8-3). The basal cells begin to display changes characteristic of all cancer cells. In addition, an abnormal accumulation of cells occurs. When a person stops smoking, preinvasive lesions do not repair themselves as quickly as once thought.

By the time lung cancer is usually diagnosed, its development is so advanced that the chance for recovery is very poor. Still, today, only 16 percent of all lung cancer victims survive for five years or more after diagnosis.[20] Most die in a very uncomfortable, painful way.

Cancerous activity in other areas of the respiratory system, including the larynx, and within the oral cavity (mouth) follows a similar course. In the case of oral cavity cancer, carcinogens found within the smoke and within the saliva are involved in the cancerous changes. Tobacco users, such as pipe smokers, cigar smokers, and users of smokeless tobacco, have a higher (4–10 times) rate of cancer of the mouth, tongue, and voice box.

Other Tobacco-Enhanced Cancers   In addition to drawing smoke into the lungs, tobacco users swallow saliva that contains an array of chemical compounds from tobacco. This saliva is retained in the stomach and then passes into the small intestine, where carcinogenic and toxic compounds in the saliva are absorbed into the blood. Contact between this material and the walls of the digestive organs leads to an enhanced risk of cancer in these areas of the gastrointestinal system. Additionally, the breakdown of carcinogens and toxic substances in the liver greatly increases

the development of cancer in this critically important organ. Filtering of the blood by the kidneys eventually concentrates toxic materials in the urinary bladder, leading to increases in kidney and bladder cancer. Smoking may also accelerate the rate of pancreatic cancer development.

As reported earlier in the chapter, documents released in 1997 from within the tobacco industry clearly show that the major tobacco companies were aware of tobacco's role in the development of cancer and had made a concerted effort to deprive the American public access to such knowledge.

Chronic Obstructive Lung Disease

Chronic obstructive lung disease (COLD), also known as chronic obstructive pulmonary disease (COPD), is a disorder in which the amount of air that flows in and out of the lungs becomes progressively more limited. COLD is a disease state that is made up of two separate but related diseases: **chronic bronchitis** and **pulmonary emphysema.**

With chronic bronchitis, excess mucus is produced in response to the effects of smoking on airway tissue, and the walls of the bronchi become inflamed and infected. This produces a characteristic narrowing of the air passages. Breathing becomes difficult, and activity can be severely restricted. With cessation of smoking, chronic bronchitis is reversible.

Emphysema causes irreversible damage to the tiny air sacs of the lungs, the **alveoli.** Chest pressure builds when air becomes trapped by narrowed air passages (chronic bronchitis) and the thin-walled sacs rupture. Emphysema

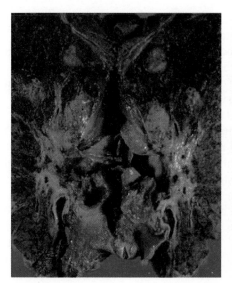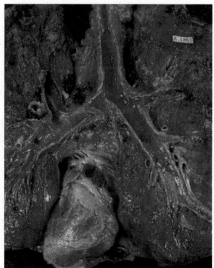

A healthy lung (right) versus the lung of a smoker (left). Smoking causes shortness of breath and "smoker's cough" and can lead to chronic obstructive lung disease.

patients lose the ability to ventilate fully. They feel as though they are suffocating. You may have seen people with this condition in malls and other locations as they walk slowly by, carrying or pulling their portable oxygen tanks.

More than 10 million Americans suffer from COLD. It is responsible for a greater limitation of physical activity than any other disease, including heart disease. COLD patients tend to die a very unpleasant, prolonged death, often from a general collapse of normal cardiorespiratory function that results in congestive heart failure (see Chapter 9). It should be noted that, while cellular changes associated with the formation of lung cancer are generally measured in longer periods of time, depending on the duration and intensity of cigarette use, changes more closely related to COLD require relatively lower levels of smoking before making their first appearance.[22]

Smoking and Body Weight

Although not perceived as a health problem by people who continue smoking to control weight, smoking does appear to minimize weight gain. In studies using identical twins, twins who smoked were 6–8 pounds lighter than their nonsmoking siblings. Current understanding about why smoking results in lower body weight is less than complete. One factor may be an increase in basal metabolic rate (BMR) (see Chapter 6) brought about by the influence of nicotine on nervous system function. However, in spite of the modest level of weight management provided by regular cigarette smoking, the overall increase in morbidity and premature death experienced by smokers is in no way "worth" the benefit of weighing a few pounds less.

Additional Health Concerns

In addition to the serious health problems stemming from tobacco use already described, other health-related changes are routinely seen. These include a generally poor state of nutrition, a decline in insulin sensitivity, a decline in short-term memory, the gradual loss of the sense of smell, and premature wrinkling of the skin. Tobacco users are also more likely to experience strokes (a potentially fatal condition), lose bone mass leading to osteoporosis, experience more back pain and muscle injury, and find that fractures heal more slowly. Further, smokers who have surgery spend more time in the recovery room. Additionally, smokers have a fourfold greater risk of developing serious gum (periodontal) disease, now thought to be a risk factor for cardiovascular disease. Also, smokers may need supplementation for two important water-soluble vitamins: vitamin C and vitamin B.

In a study of the effects of smoking on memory, a 23-year longitudinal study of over 5,000 heavy smokers (two packs per day) identified 100 percent higher rates of Alzheimer's disease and other forms of vascular dementia than were noted in a control group of nonsmokers.[23]

Combining Tobacco and Alcohol Use

Although there are exceptions to every generalization, it is very common to see tobacco and alcohol being used by

---

Key Terms

chronic bronchitis Persistent inflammation and infection of the smaller airways within the lungs.

pulmonary emphysema An irreversible disease process in which the alveoli are destroyed.

alveoli (al **vee** oh lie) Thin, saclike terminal ends of the airways; the sites at which gases are exchanged between the blood and lungs.

the same people, often at the same time. Younger people who use both tobacco and alcohol are also more likely to use additional drugs. Accordingly, both tobacco and alcohol are considered *gateway drugs* because they are often introductory drugs that "open the door" for a more broadly based polydrug use pattern (see Chapter 7).

Beyond the potential for polydrug use initiated by the use of tobacco and alcohol is the simple reality that the use of both tobacco products and alcoholic beverages is associated with a wide array of illnesses and with premature death. As you have seen in this chapter and in Chapter 7 regarding alcohol use, the negative health impact of using both is significant. When use is combined, of course, the risks of living less healthfully and dying prematurely are accentuated.

Risks from Specific Tobacco Products

Most tobacco used today in the United States is in the form of standard machine-produced cigarettes. However, there are other forms of tobacco and variations on the standard cigarette in use by Americans. Products such as bidis, cigars, mentholated cigarettes, and smokeless tobacco have their own special health risks and regulatory challenges.

Before turning to these products, special mention should be made of the unexpectedly high levels of nicotine in the filtered cigarettes that are favored by virtually all smokers of machine-produced cigarettes. New testing technologies have shown that smokers of filtered cigarettes take in almost twice the amount of nicotine as previously believed. Part of the reason for this high level of nicotine intake is that the row of ventilation holes in the filter is obstructed by the lips or fingers of smokers, thus blocking the escape of smoke. Additionally, smokers of filter-tipped

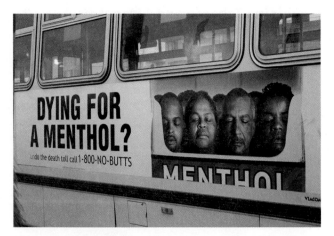

Mentholated cigarettes have been heavily marketed to African American smokers.

low-tar and low-nicotine cigarettes seem strongly inclined to increase their "puff volume" by inhaling more deeply and more often. In combination, these factors help deliver the nicotine loads that keep smokers dependent and the tobacco industry in business.[24]

Nonmanufactured Forms of Cigarettes

Although the vast majority of American cigarette smokers use familiar brand-name manufactured cigarettes produced in this country, small segments of the smoking population use nonmanufactured cigarettes. Nonmanufactured cigarettes (or the supplies for making them) generally are sold in places that might not enforce the legal age restrictions on purchasing manufactured cigarettes. Of course, in terms of dependence and harmfulness, these kinds of cigarettes are no better, if not worse, than manufactured cigarettes. Nonmanufactured cigarettes include bidis and kreteks.

Bidis are small handmade cigarettes, most often imported from the Indian subcontinent, consisting of a small amount of tobacco wrapped in a dried temburni or tendu leaf, and tied with a small length of colorful string. These cigarettes are particularly dangerous to health because the tobacco used is high in tar and nicotine and these cigarettes' inefficient combustion delivers a high level of carbon monoxide.

Kreteks are a popular cigarette from Indonesia. These hand-wrapped cigarettes are made from clove-flavored tobacco or other highly flavored tobacco. A particular health danger of kreteks is that they contain an additive, eugenol, that produces an anesthetic-like numbing in the throat, resulting in a tendency to inhale more deeply, thus delivering more tar and nicotine into the lungs.

Mentholated Cigarettes

Of the 599 additives approved for use in the manufacturing of cigarettes, one of the most familiar, and most popular, was menthol—which imparts a unique taste and "cooling" sensation in the throat. Menthol-flavored cigarettes were on the market for decades and had proven highly attractive to African American male smokers.

Health researchers have speculated that there is a relationship between the long-term smoking of mentholated cigarettes among African American males and the high level of lung cancer in this population. A meta-analysis (a study of other studies) of five large epidemiological studies of African American smokers concluded that the menthol in cigarette tobacco was not a factor in the higher rate of lung cancer in this population.

However, a recent study of cessation among light smokers indicates that it was more difficult to quit smoking mentholated brands than those without menthol.[25] As noted earlier in the chapter, the FDA has banned flavoring in all cigarettes, including mentholated brands.

Water Pipes (Hookahs)

With origins in the Middle East, the hookah consists of a head into which prepackaged shredded tobacco leaves are combined with sweetened flavoring agents (collectively called shisha) and set atop lit charcoal. When one draws a breath through the end of the pipe, the shisha is ignited and smoke travels down a tube-like body of the pipe into a partially filled bowl of water where the smoke is cooled and released into the airspace above the water; it than continues upward through the flexible hose's mouthpiece for movement into the airways. Multiple users may alternately use a single hose/mouthpiece or their own if the water pipe is designed accordingly.

Although the hookah has been in use for centuries, research into its unique potential for serious health-related consequences is a relatively new field of study. One of the many concerns surrounding hookah use is that single periods of use as long as 40–45 minutes can lead to a tobacco smoke exposure period approximating the smoke generated by nearly 100 cigarettes. This hyperextended period of tobacco-based exposure generates nicotine levels 2.5 times higher than those associated with one episode of cigarette use. An analysis of hookah-generated smoke suggests a chemical composition very similar to that of cigarette smoke. When hookah users also smoke cigarettes, the combined use of both sources of tobacco leads to even higher levels of exposure to carcinogenic chemicals, carbon monoxide, and nicotine. The contribution of contaminants from the charcoal

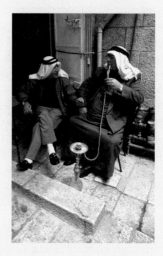

or woodchip-based fuel used to heat the tobacco mixture is unknown. The transmission of infectious agents through shared use of mouthpieces has also been reported.

Although hookah use may be socially integrative, it is far from being safer than cigarettes, and when combined with cigarette use the stage is set for potentially serious negative health consequences.

Source: American Lung Association, Tobacco Policy Trend Alert, 2007. An emerging deadly trend: waterpipe tobacco use. www.lungusa.org.

Pipe and Cigar Smoking

Many people believe that pipe or cigar smoking is a safe alternative to cigarette smoking. Unfortunately, this is not the case. All forms of tobacco present users with a series of health threats (see the box "Water Pipes [Hookahs]").

When compared with cigarette smokers, pipe and cigar smokers have cancer of the mouth, throat, larynx (voice box), and esophagus at the same frequency. Cigarette smokers are more likely than pipe and cigar smokers to have lung cancer, chronic obstructive lung disease (COLD), also called chronic obstructive pulmonary disease (COPD), and heart disease. The cancer risk of death to pipe and cigar smokers is 4 times greater from lung cancer and 10 times greater from laryngeal cancer than it is for nonsmokers.

On the basis of a renewed interest in cigar smoking beginning in the mid-1990s, in addition to clinical evidence appearing in medical journals for decades, the National Cancer Institute commissioned the first extensive study of regular cigar smoking.[24] That report confirmed and expanded on the health risks identified in earlier studies.

In response to the recognition of these risks as reported in journal articles,[25] the FTC required that cigar manufacturers disclose the tobacco content and additives in their products. Most recently, the FTC announced its intention of requiring rotating health warnings to appear on cigars, including two that have been currently agreed on by the FTC and major cigar manufacturers:

Cigars Are Not a Safe Alternative to Cigarettes

Cigar Smoking Can Cause Cancer of the Mouth and Throat, Even If You Don't Inhale

The federal government has also imposed a tax on premium cigars based on price and weight, which can be as high as $0.40.

Smokeless Tobacco Products

As the term implies, *smokeless tobacco,* such as Skoal and Copenhagen, is not burned; rather, it is placed in the mouth. Once in place, the physiologically active nicotine and other soluble compounds are absorbed through the mucous membranes and into the blood. Within a few minutes, chewing tobacco and snuff generate blood levels of nicotine in amounts equivalent to those seen in cigarette smokers.

Chewing tobacco is taken from its foil pouch, formed into a small ball (called a "wad," "chaw," or "chew"), and placed in the mouth. Once in place, the bolus of tobacco is sucked and occasionally chewed, but not swallowed.

Snuff, a more finely shredded smokeless tobacco product, is marketed in small round cans. Snuff is formed into a small mass (or "quid") for dipping or used in pre-packaged pouches. The quid or pouch is placed between the jaw and the cheek; the user sucks the quid or pouch, then spits out the brown liquid.

Although smokeless tobacco would seem to free the tobacco user from many of the risks associated with smoking, chewing and dipping are not without their own substantial risks. The presence of *leukoplakia* (white spots) and *erythroplakia* (red spots) on the tissues of the mouth indicate precancerous changes. In addition, an increase in **periodontal disease** (with the pulling away of the gums from the teeth, resulting in later tooth loss), the abrasive damage to the enamel of the teeth, and the high concentration of sugar in processed tobacco all contribute to dental problems among users of smokeless tobacco. In those who develop oral cancer, the risk is dramatically heightened if the cancer metastasizes from the site of origin in the mouth to the brain.

In the opinion of health experts, the use of smokeless tobacco and its potential for life-threatening disease is very real and should not be disregarded.[26] Consequently, television advertisements have been banned, and the following warnings have been placed in rotation on all smokeless tobacco products:

> WARNING: THIS PRODUCT MAY CAUSE
> MOUTH CANCER
> WARNING: THIS PRODUCT MAY CAUSE GUM
> DISEASE AND TOOTH LOSS
> WARNING: THIS PRODUCT IS NOT A SAFE
> ALTERNATIVE TO CIGARETTE
> SMOKING

Smokeless tobacco is a dangerous product, and little doubt exists that continued use of tobacco in this form is a serious problem to health in all its dimensions. Fortunately, however, the percentage of adults using smokeless tobacco during the previous month is slightly less than reported for cigar use, and this figure too is inversely related to education level. Among high school graduates, 4.4 percent use smokeless tobacco, while only 2.1 percent of college graduates reported use during the previous month.

Whether defined as another form of smokeless tobacco or as a bridge product, the Swedish-developed product *snus* (sounds like *noose*) is being successfully marketed as Camel Snus. The use of snus closely resembles that of other smokeless tobacco products that feature small pouches inserted between the gum and cheek. The attractive features of snus include a flavored taste (available in three flavors), an apparent lack of odor on the breath, and an absence of the need to spit the juicy extract that is common to other forms of smokeless tobacco. The tobacco used in snus is steam-pasteurized, a process that alters the nature of fluid extract in a manner allowing it to be "safely" swallowed. Although legally sold in this country, the European Union banned the sale of snus in 2004 over concerns about its potential for adverse health influences.

Yet to come to the market but reportedly under development are dissolvable nicotine-containing strips (akin to breath-freshening strips), as well as a variety of delivery devices that will, most likely, serve the tobacco industry well as it attempts to tighten its hold on the current nicotine-dependent population and build its base for the future.

E-Cigarettes

E-cigarettes are designed to look like and produce a similar experience to regular cigarettes, yet they contain no tobacco and produce no smoke. An e-cigarette comprises a battery chamber with a glowing indicator light on the end, followed by an atomizer and an inhalation tip that contains a nicotine cartridge. When the user inhales, warmed air passes through the atomizer, where liquid propylene glycol is vaporized into a fine mist that resembles tobacco smoke, then on through the inhalation tip, where synthetic nicotine is released into the "smoke." On exhalation, the purportedly nicotine-free vaporous "smoke" is released into the air. Early testing of e-cigarettes found some familiar carcinogenic agents of regular cigarettes within the vapor, in addition to a nicotine content that is higher than that of traditional tobacco cigarettes. Because these devices can be sold to anyone, including children, the product's appearance and nicotine content suggest a clear gateway device to the future use of real cigarettes, although their price is high at $50–$200 for a starter kit. So far, the FDA has attempted to prevent foreign-manufactured versions of the product from entering the country, but they are still being sold domestically.

Currently, the FDA deems e-cigarettes to be potentially harmful, in a manner akin to cigarettes, to both users and nonusers; and the airline industry has banned their use in plane cabins. Supporting the airlines' prohibition of e-cigarettes in planes was the FDA's 2011 decision to place them in the same category as traditional cigarettes. Thus, the e-cigarette remains a nicotine bridge product, used by smokers to fill the interval during which smoking actual cigarettes is prohibited.

Smoking and Reproduction

In all its dimensions, the reproductive process is impaired by the use of tobacco, particularly cigarette smoke and environmental tobacco smoke in close proximity to pregnant women. Problems can be found in association with infertility, pregnancy, breast-feeding, and the health of the newborn. So broadly based are reproductive problems and smoking that the term *fetal tobacco syndrome* or *fetal smoking syndrome* is regularly used in clinical medicine. Some physicians even define a fetus being carried by a smoker as a "smoker" and, upon birth, as a "former smoker."

Infertility

Recent research indicates that cigarette smoking by both men and women can reduce levels of fertility. Among men, smoking adversely affects blood flow to erectile tissue, reduces sperm motility, and alters sperm shape; it also causes an overall decrease in the number of viable sperm. Among women, the effects of smoking involve abnormal ovum formation, including a lessened ability on the part of the egg to prevent polyspermia, or the fertilization by multiple sperm. Smoking also negatively influences estrogen levels, resulting in underdevelopment of the uterine wall and ineffective implantation of the fertilized ovum. Lower levels of estrogen may influence the rate of transit of the fertilized egg through the fallopian tube, making it arrive in the uterus too early for successful implantation or, in some cases, restricting movement to the point that an ectopic (tubal) pregnancy may develop. Further, the early onset of menopause is associated with smoking.

Problem Pregnancy

The harmful effects of tobacco smoke on the course of pregnancy are principally the result of the carbon monoxide and nicotine to which the mother and her fetus are exposed. Carbon monoxide from the incomplete oxidation of tobacco is carried in the maternal blood to the placenta, where it diffuses across the placental barrier and enters the fetal circulation. Once in the fetal blood, the carbon monoxide bonds with the fetal hemoglobin to form fetal carboxyhemoglobin. As a result of this exposure to carbon monoxide, the fetus is progressively deprived of normal oxygen transport and eventually becomes compromised by chronic hypoxia.

Nicotine also exerts its influence on the developing fetus. Thermographs of the placenta and fetus show signs of marked vasoconstriction within a few seconds after inhalation by the mother. This constriction further reduces the oxygen supply, resulting in hypoxia. In addition, nicotine stimulates the mother's stress response, placing the mother and fetus under the potentially harmful influence of elevated epinephrine and corticoid levels (see Chapter 3). Any fetus exposed to all of these agents is more likely to be miscarried, stillborn, or born prematurely. Even when carried to term, children born to mothers who smoked during pregnancy have lower birth weights and may show other signs of a stressful intrauterine life.

Breast-Feeding

Women who breast-feed their infants and continue to smoke also continue to expose their children to the harmful effects of tobacco smoke. It is well recognized that nicotine appears in breast milk and thus is capable of exerting its vasoconstricting and stress-response influences on nursing infants. Mothers who stop smoking during pregnancy should be encouraged to continue to refrain from smoking while they are breast-feeding.

Neonatal Health Problems

Babies born to women who smoked during pregnancy, on average, are shorter and have a lower birth weight than do children born to nonsmoking mothers. During the earliest months of life, babies born to mothers who smoke experience an elevated rate of death caused by sudden infant death syndrome (SIDS).[27] Statistics also show that infants are more likely to develop chronic respiratory problems, have more frequent colic, be hospitalized, and have poorer overall health during their early years of life. Problems such as those just mentioned may also be seen in children of nonsmoking mothers when they were exposed prenatally to environmental tobacco smoke. In addition, environmental tobacco smoke exposure extending beyond the home and into the workplace may increase the probability of problem pregnancies and neonatal health problems. Recently, the interest in the effects of tobacco smoke on pregnancy has been extended to include behavioral differences in children born to women who smoked during pregnancy.

Parenting, in the sense of assuming responsibility for the well-being of children, begins not at birth, but during the prenatal period. In the case of smoking, this is especially true. Pregnant women who continue smoking are disregarding the well-being of the children they are carrying. Other family members, friends, and coworkers who subject pregnant women to cigarette, pipe, or cigar

> ### Key Terms
>
> **periodontal disease** Destruction of soft tissue and bone that surround the teeth.
>
> **ectopic (tubal) pregnancy** Pregnancy resulting from the implantation of the fertilized ovum within the inner wall of the fallopian tube.
>
> **hypoxia** Oxygenation deprivation at the cellular level.

smoke are, in a sense, exhibiting their own disregard for the health of the next generation.

Involuntary (Passive) Smoking

The smoke generated by the burning of tobacco can be classified as either **mainstream smoke** (the smoke inhaled and then exhaled by the smoker) or **sidestream smoke** (the smoke that comes from the burning end of the cigarette, pipe, or cigar that simply disperses into the air without being inhaled by the smoker). When either form of tobacco smoke is diluted and stays within a common source of air, it can eventually be referred to as **environmental tobacco smoke.** In addition to the definitions just given, the term *environmental tobacco smoke* can also refer to tobacco smoke of any type to which the nonsmoker is exposed. All three forms of tobacco smoke lead to involuntary or passive smoking and can present health problems for both nonsmokers and smokers.

Surprisingly, mainstream smoke accounts for only 15 percent of our exposure to the harmful substances associated with involuntary smoking. Sidestream smoke is responsible for 85 percent of the harmful substances associated with secondhand smoke exposure. Because it is not filtered by the tobacco, the filter, or the smoker's body, sidestream smoke contains more free nicotine and produces higher yields of carbon dioxide and carbon monoxide. Much to the detriment of nonsmokers, sidestream smoke has a much higher quantity of highly carcinogenic compounds, called *N-nitrosamines,* than mainstream smoke has.

Current scientific opinion suggests that smokers and nonsmokers are exposed to very much the same smoke when tobacco is used within a common airspace. The important difference is the quantity of smoke inhaled by smokers and nonsmokers. It is likely that for each pack of cigarettes smoked by a smoker, nonsmokers who must share a common air supply with the smokers involuntarily smoke the equivalent of three to five cigarettes per day. Even today, because of the small size of the particles produced by burning tobacco, environmental tobacco smoke cannot be completely removed from a workplace, restaurant, or shopping mall by the most effective ventilation system.

Health Risks of Passive Smoking

Research indicates that involuntary smoke exposure may have been responsible for 31,000 premature deaths per year from heart disease among nonsmokers in the United States.[28] Other estimates range upward to 53,000 premature deaths when lung cancer and COPD are included. In addition, large numbers of people exposed to involuntary smoke develop eye irritation, nasal symptoms, headaches, and coughs. Furthermore, most nonsmokers dislike the odor of tobacco smoke. Data from

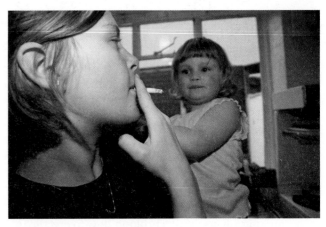

Children exposed to environmental tobacco smoke are at increased risk for wheezing, ear infections, bronchitis, and pneumonia.

1999–2008 indicate that an estimated 88 million persons were exposed to secondhand smoke, although the number is declining annually.[28]

Involuntary smoking poses some threats to nonsmokers within residential settings. Spouses and children of smokers are at greatest risk for involuntary smoking. Scientific studies suggest that nonsmokers married to smokers are more likely to experience heart attacks than nonsmoking spouses of nonsmokers. This said, a recent meta-analysis (reassessment) of earlier studies concluded that an increased risk for CVD exists; however, the risk for nonsmoking spouses is less than once reported.

In spite of what may or may not be the effects of passive smoking on the nonsmoking partners of smokers, the effects of environmental tobacco smoke on the health of children seems well established. The children of parents who smoke are twice as likely as children of nonsmoking parents to experience bronchitis or pneumonia during the first year of life. In addition, throughout childhood, these children will experience more wheezing, coughing, and sputum production than will children whose parents do not smoke. Otitis media (middle ear infection), one of the most frequently seen conditions in pediatric medicine, is also significantly more common in children under age 3 who reside with one or more adults who smoke.

Regarding the relationship between exposure to environmental tobacco smoke and SIDS, a recent comprehensive

---

Key Terms

mainstream smoke Smoke inhaled and then exhaled by a smoker.

sidestream smoke Smoke that comes from the burning end of a cigarette, pipe, or cigar.

environmental tobacco smoke Tobacco smoke, regardless of its source, that stays within a common source of air.

meta-analysis raised important issues about the methodology of nearly 60 earlier studies on smoking and SIDS. Researchers in New Zealand suggest that currently it is difficult to obtain an accurate picture of the relationship. In particular, research needs to better separate the influences of maternal smoking during pregnancy, maternal smoking after pregnancy (in the months immediately following delivery), and other sources of environmental tobacco smoke during the prenatal and postnatal periods.

The Cost of Smoking

The 20.6 percent of the U.S. population that smoke inflict a substantial cost on their nonsmoking neighbors in a multiplicity of ways. In more personal ways, smokers also accrue costs that are less easily documented. They lose some independence (nicotine-based needs will structure many aspects of day-to-day living) and may be socially rejected by the nonsmoking majority, including the significant number of young adults who do not want smokers as their life partners (see the box "The Hidden Cost of Smoking"). Smokers may experience subtle forms of discrimination when they search for employment (smokers miss more days of work, waste an hour per day on smoking breaks, and eventually raise their employer's health insurance expenditures). Smokers often receive lower trade-ins on their vehicles (double detailing is expensive to the dealer) and have a harder time selling their smoke-saturated houses (even freshly baked bread won't hide the odorous evidence that smokers lived in the house).

Smokers' contention that "smoking only hurts smokers" is patently untrue. In fact, the economic costs alone should stimulate those smokers reading this chapter to pay close attention to the discussion of quitting at the end of the chapter.

Stopping What You Started

Experts in health behavior contend that before people will discontinue harmful health behaviors, such as tobacco use, they must appreciate fully what they are expecting of themselves. This understanding grows in relation to the following:

- *Knowledge* of the health risks associated with tobacco use
- *Recognition* that these health risks are applicable to all tobacco users
- *Familiarity* with steps that can be taken to eliminate or reduce these risks
- *Belief* that the benefits to be gained by no longer using tobacco will outweigh the pleasures gained through the use of tobacco
- *Certainty* that one can start and maintain the behaviors required to stop or reduce the use of tobacco

These steps combine both knowledge and desire (or motivation). Being knowledgeable about risks, however, will not always stop behaviors that involve varying degrees of psychological and physical dependence. The 75 percent failure rate thought to be common among tobacco cessation programs suggests that the motivation is not easy to achieve or maintain. In fact, on the basis of information reported by the Hazelden Foundation, for persons who are successful in quitting, approximately 18.6 years elapse between the first attempt to stop and the actual time of quitting. The many health benefits of quitting smoking are shown in Figure 8-4 and Table 8.3.

Smoking Cessation Programs

A variety of smoking cessation programs exist, including those using highly organized formats, with or without the use of prescription or OTC nicotine replacement systems. In past years, most people who managed to quit smoking each year did so by throwing away their cigarettes (going cold turkey) and paying the physical and emotional price while waiting for their bodies to adjust to life without nicotine. Today, however, the use of nicotine replacement products in combination with other smoking cessation approaches, such as the use of prescription medication, is more common. The box "Countdown to

Quit Day" on page 210 highlights strategies to help smokers prepare to quit.

Programs to help people stop their tobacco use are available in a variety of formats, including educational programs, behavior modification, aversive conditioning, hypnosis, acupuncture, and various combinations of these approaches (see the box "Hypnotism" on page 211). Programs are offered in both individual and group settings and are operated by hospitals, universities, health departments, voluntary health agencies, churches, and private practitioners. The better programs will have only limited success rates—20–50 percent as measured over one year (with self-reporting), whereas the remainder will have even poorer results. If results are monitored using the assessment of nicotine breakdown products in the blood, the effectiveness rate of these programs falls even lower, as some "successful" self-reporters are not completely honest in their reporting of cessation. After one year, the success rates of smoking cessation efforts continue to drop, particularly with self-directed efforts (without the involvement

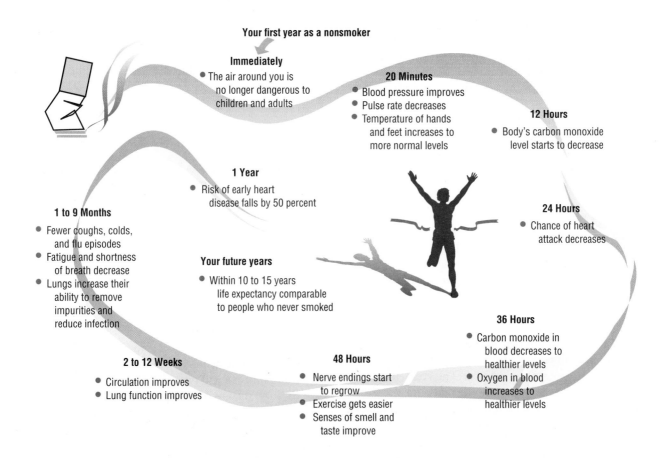

Your first year as a nonsmoker

Immediately
- The air around you is no longer dangerous to children and adults

20 Minutes
- Blood pressure improves
- Pulse rate decreases
- Temperature of hands and feet increases to more normal levels

12 Hours
- Body's carbon monoxide level starts to decrease

1 Year
- Risk of early heart disease falls by 50 percent

24 Hours
- Chance of heart attack decreases

1 to 9 Months
- Fewer coughs, colds, and flu episodes
- Fatigue and shortness of breath decrease
- Lungs increase their ability to remove impurities and reduce infection

Your future years
- Within 10 to 15 years life expectancy comparable to people who never smoked

36 Hours
- Carbon monoxide in blood decreases to healthier levels

2 to 12 Weeks
- Circulation improves
- Lung function improves

48 Hours
- Nerve endings start to regrow
- Exercise gets easier
- Senses of smell and taste improve

- Oxygen in blood increases to healthier levels

Figure 8-4 Benefits of Quitting   The health benefits of quitting smoking begin immediately and become more significant the longer you stay smoke-free.

Sources: Adapted from American Cancer Society, Guide to Quitting Smoking, http://www.cancer.org/Healthy/StayAwayfromTobacco/GuidetoQuittmgSmoking/guide-to, and other sources including the American Lung Association and the Office of the Surgeon General of the United States.

Table 8.3 Ever Wonder What Happens to Your Body the Moment You Stop Smoking?

Within 20 minutes of smoking that last cigarette, the body begins a series of changes that continues for years.

20 Minutes
- Blood pressure drops to normal.
- Pulse rate drops to normal.
- Body temperature of hands and feet increases to normal.

8 Hours
- Carbon monoxide level in blood drops to normal.
- Oxygen level in blood increases to normal.

24 Hours
- Chance of heart attack decreases.

48 Hours
- Nerve endings start regrowing.
- Ability to smell and taste is enhanced.

2 Weeks to 3 Months
- Circulation improves.
- Walking becomes easier.
- Lung function increases up to 30 percent.

1 to 9 Months
- Coughing, sinus congestion, fatigue, and shortness of breath decrease.
- Cilia regrow in lungs, increasing ability to handle mucus, clean the lungs, and reduce infection.
- Body's overall energy increases.

1 Year
- Excess risk of coronary heart disease is half that of a smoker.

5 Years
- Lung cancer death rate for average smoker (one pack a day) decreases by almost half.
- Stroke risk is reduced to that of a nonsmoker 5–15 years after quitting.
- Risk of cancer of the mouth, throat, and esophagus is half that of a smoker's.

10 Years
- Lung cancer death rate similar to that of nonsmokers.
- Precancerous cells are replaced.
- Risk of cancer of the mouth, throat, esophagus, bladder, kidney, and pancreas decreases.

15 Years
- Risk of coronary heart disease is that of a nonsmoker.

Source: From http://my.clevelandclinic.org/tobacco/benefits_of_quitting_tobacco.aspx. Copyright © 2000-2011 Cleveland Clinic. All Rights Reserved. Reprinted with permission.

are increased taxes on cigarettes and the involvement of family, friends, and coworkers. In a study of attrition from ongoing cessation programs, it was noticed that when a spouse (67 percent), friend (36 percent), coworker in a small firm (34 percent), or sibling (25 percent) has quit or will join a program with a smoker, program completion rates increased.[29] Research now indicates that a daily "encouragement" e-mail or tweet from a cessation program leader or supportive friend or family member will have a positive influence on the participant's ability to complete the program and remain smoke-free.

A second effective tool for moving smokers into cessation programs involves taxation. This was clearly effective in New York State when the per-pack state tax on cigarettes was increased from $1.25 to $2.75, raising the price of cigarettes in some areas of the state into the $6.00–$7.00 per pack range and to nearly $10 per pack in New York City. Two states, Rhode Island ($3.46) and Connecticut ($3.00), surpass New York's ($2.75) state excise tax rate, while the lowest rates are found in Missouri ($0.17) and South Carolina ($0.07). The median state excise tax is found in Minnesota ($1.23). Further, during the first month of President Obama's administration, a 62-cent increase in the federal tobacco tax was imposed on each pack of cigarettes. This was done to gain revenue to expand the provision of affordable health care insurance for 11 million children. One hopes that this additional layer of taxation will encourage yet more potential smokers and young smokers to reconsider a trip into dependence.

In a meta-analysis of smoking cessation program success involving African Americans, it was found that there is no statistically significant difference between the success rates of this racial group and others. Of interest, however, was a finding that church-based programs might be more successful in smoking cessation than previously recognized.

Medically Managed Smoking Cessation

Having given a general overview of smoking cessation, your text will give more detailed attention to medically managed cessation programs, such as those conducted by clinics, hospitals, or university student health centers. Because they have a medical affiliation, these programs have access to prescription medication in addition to OTC products, nutritional and exercise expertise, and affiliated behavior therapy. The prescription medications, in particular, are a key component to these programs.

Nonnicotine-based medications are those medications that influence the production, diffusion, or reuptake of neurotransmitters with the CNS that are associated with feelings of hunger, satiety, and the CNS's neurological reward centers. A simple description of synaptic function can be found in Chapter 7. Medication influencing neurotransmitter function includes many of the antidepressants, such as Zyban, Wellbutrin, and Prozac, among others.

of physicians or group-based leadership), often reaching levels as low as 5 percent.

Although not part of most smoking cessation programs, two additional resources found to be effective in aiding smokers to both attempt cessation and succeed

Countdown to Quit Day: A Plan for Smoking Cessation

I started smoking at parties to feel more relaxed. Now I smoke at least a pack a day, and I'm afraid I'm hooked for life. How do I get myself off tobacco?

Make a decision to quit smoking on a particular day during the next week. Then use the following steps to begin preparing yourself for that day.

Five Days Before Quit Day

- Keep a daylong record of each cigarette you smoke. List when you smoked, whom you were with, and why you decided to light up (for example, for stimulation, tension reduction, or social plea-sure, or because you had a craving or wanted something to do with your hands). Once you know why you smoke, you can plan intervention strategies for use during the two-minute periods of craving you will feel during the first weeks of your smoke-free life.
- Contact your physician to help you decide whether to use pre-scription or OTC nicotine replacement therapy. Make sure you understand all directions for its safe and effective use.
- Draw up a contract in which you formally state your intention to quit smoking. Sign and date the contract, and clearly display it in your home or workplace.

Four Days Before Quit Day

- Solicit support from family, friends, and coworkers by shar-ing your intention with them and asking for their help and encouragement.
- Organize your intervention strategies and assemble needed supplies, such as gum, bottled water, diet soda, handwork (for example, needlepoint or wood carving), and walking shoes.

Three Days Before Quit Day

- Review your quitting contract and touch bases with several people in your support group to bolster your resolve.
- Study all nicotine-replacement-therapy product information and any material supplied by your physician.
- Continue preparing your intervention supplies.

- Reschedule your personal calendar and work schedule to minimize situations that could tempt you to smoke during the first several days of your smoke-free life.

Two Days Before Quit Day

- Continue or revisit any earlier tasks that you have not yet finished.
- Practice your intervention strategies as appropriate. For example, map out a safe walking route and practice your deep-breathing exercises.
- Obtain a large glass or other container, such as an empty milk jug, that will serve as a bank into which you will deposit daily the money that you would have otherwise spent on cigarettes.
- If you feel comfortable doing so, construct a yard sign to inform outsiders that your home is a smoke-free environment and to report your daily success toward a smoke-free life.
- Smoke-proof your home and workplace by removing and destroy-ing all materials and supplies associated with tobacco use, saving only enough tobacco products needed for today and tomorrow.

One Day Before Quit Day

- Complete all preparations described, including the almost total removal and destruction of smoking-related materials.
- As the end of the day approaches, review your contract and call a few people in your support network for last-minute words of encouragement.
- Smoke your last cigarette and flush any remaining cigarettes down the toilet.
- Begin your nicotine replacement therapy as directed by your phy-sician or by product insert information.
- Publicly display your yard sign, if you decided to make one.
- Retire for the night and await your rebirth in the morning as a for-mer smoker.

InfoLinks

www.smokefree.gov

A relative newcomer to this group (brand name Chantix) is not a neurotransmitter-influencing medi-cation, like those just described, but rather a drug that blocks the ability of nicotine receptors in various tis-sues of the body to recognize the presence of nicotine, thus depriving it of its dependence-producing potential. Although Chantix is effective in getting users off nico-tine, potentially serious issues related to suicidal thoughts and vivid dreams have resulted in Pfizer, Inc. adding cau-tionary information to the drug's labeling regarding the need to more fully assess its appropriateness for particu-lar individuals.

A second medication is the European drug rimonabant, which was to be marketed in the United States as Acom-plia. This medication was initially approved in Europe for weight loss, but it also showed efficacy in smoking cessa-tion. However, to date, the FDA has denied approval of rimonabant or Acomplia due to concerns over suicidal thoughts in users. The European counterpart to the FDA has removed the medication from the market as well.

Hypnotism: A Solution for Smokers?

In addition to all of the other aids to smoking cessation that are discussed in this chapter, what is the role of hypnosis in helping smokers break away from their dependence on nicotine? Unfortunately, the question is not easily answered because hypnosis is a relatively minor player in smoking cessation, and research to date is relatively limited and often conflicting. Additionally, there is uncertainty and disagreement within the hypnotic community itself, in terms of both technique and the underlying psychophysiological dynamic that occurs, further clouding an understanding of the nature of hypnosis and the hypnotic

state. That said, today, when practiced by medically trained practitioners, such as psychiatrists, hypnosis can be placed among the various other forms of psychotherapy currently practiced. In addition, self-hypnosis techniques using various approaches can move hypnosis out of the clinical realm and into the confines of the self-care movement.

As noted earlier, the efficacy of hypnosis is consistently in question. A host of potential problems exist in designing well-controlled studies, including the tendency to rely on self-reporting of continued cessation of smoking, the limited use of laboratory-based

assessments such as blood serum measurements of carbon monoxide levels or other nicotine substrates, and the unreported uses of other cessation techniques in addition to having been hypnotized. In other studies, however, hypnosis has been shown to be equal to or better than other recognized approaches.

Sources: Ahijevych K, et al., Descriptive outcomes of the American Lung Association of Ohio Hypnotherapy Smoking Cessation Program, *International Journal of Clinical and Experimental Hypnosis*, 48(4), 374–387, October 2000; Elkins G, et al., Intensive hypnotherapy for smoking cessation: a prospective study, *International Journal of Clinical and Experimental Hypnosis*, 54(3), 303–315, July 2006.

Nicotine replacement medications comprise a variety of products, some obtainable only by prescription and others available as OTC products, intended to allow a controlled and less harmful relationship with nicotine than that associated with tobacco products. This form of nicotine replacement therapy (NRT) facilitates a gradual turning down of nicotine dependence, until the individual is virtually free of a tissue-based dependence on tobacco products. A variety of delivery systems are used in NRT, including gum, lozenges, transdermal patches, nasal sprays, and inhalers.

People who are concerned that NRT is simply a trade-off of dependences should remember that while using the therapy the former smoker is no longer being exposed to carbon monoxide and carcinogens, and the step-down feature allows for a gradual return to a totally nicotine-free lifestyle. Therefore, a short period of cross-addiction should be seen as an acceptable cost to recovery.

Prescription Medications Based on Nicotine Receptor Inhibitors

Several newer medications have been recently approved or are still in controlled trials. One such medication, developed in Europe, is marketed in the United States as varenicline (Chantix). Chantix influences nervous system receptors for nicotine to level out the peaks and valleys normally associated with smoking. This leveling-out aids cessation by diminishing the "highly satisfying" character of the first inhalation following a low-nicotine valley and by minimizing the discomfort experienced while in a state of nicotine depletion (a valley). Recall that earlier in the chapter the potential for suicidal thoughts and vivid dreams associated with the use of Chantix led the FDA to require a black box label to be added to the packaging of this smoking cessation drug.

Anti-Smoking Vaccines

The goal of anti-smoking vaccines is to prevent nicotine from reaching nicotine receptors in the brain by conditioning the immune system to attack the nicotine molecules. Research in vaccine development has begun to bear fruit. Clinical trials are currently under way on a vaccine named NicVAX.[30,31] In these trials, subjects will receive four or five immunization shots over a period of many weeks. In response, the immune system should eventually begin producing antibodies (see Chapter 11) against nicotine. The most recent clinical trials of NicVAX report anticipated and necessary antibody formation through week 39, following the five-injection protocol. At least four other vaccines are in earlier stages of development.

Despite the satisfaction of the dependency that continued smoking brings, approximately 80 percent of adult smokers have, on at least one occasion, expressed a desire to quit, and the majority of these have actually attempted to become nonsmokers. Today, with the over-the-counter availability of transdermal nicotine patches, nicotine-containing gum, nicotine inhalers, prescription medications such as antidepressants, and nicotine receptor inhibitors, the number of smokers making concerted and repeated attempts to stop smoking is up considerably. It therefore seems apparent that tobacco use is a source of **dissonance.** This dissonance stems from the need

> ### Key Terms
>
> **dissonance** (**dis** son ince) A feeling of uncertainty that occurs when a person believes two equally attractive but opposite ideas.

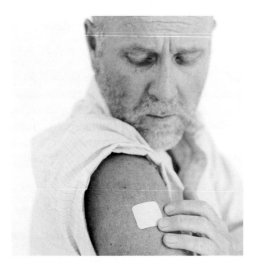

Nicotine patches are one form of nicotine replacement therapy available to help smokers quit.

to deal emotionally with a behavior that is both highly enjoyable and highly dangerous but known to be difficult to stop. The degree to which this dissonance exists probably varies from user to user.

Nicotine Bridge Products

In light of the rapidly expanding restrictions on smoking, how do smokers survive long hours in smoke-free environments? The answer: a nicotine bridge product—a gel, cream, or candylike piece that contains nicotine for absorption through a body surface to maintain an adequate level of titration until cigarettes can be smoked. These OTC products, bearing names such as Ariva and Stonewall, are more convenient, affordable, tasty, and pleasant smelling than the nicotine step-down products used for smoking cessation. Of course, there is concern that these products enable smokers to continue their

nicotine dependence in place of seeking cessation and that they may be nicotine-introductory products if they become too readily available to children.

Tobacco Use: A Question of Rights

For those readers who have found themselves involved (or nearly so) in confrontation situations involving smokers' versus nonsmokers' rights, we hope the following section allows you to see more clearly the positions that you have taken. For those who have somehow remained removed from this discussion, consideration of these issues now may be good preparation for the future. Regardless, consider these two important questions:

1. To what extent should smokers be allowed to pollute the air and endanger the health of nonsmokers?
2. To what extent should nonsmokers be allowed to restrict the personal freedom of smokers, particularly since tobacco products are sold legally?

At this time, answers to these questions are only partially available, but one trend is developing: The tobacco user is being forced to give ground to the nonsmoker. Today, in fact, it is becoming more a matter of where the smoker will be allowed to smoke, rather than a matter of where smoking will be restricted. Smoking is becoming less and less tolerated. The health concerns of the majority are prevailing over the dependence needs of the minority.

 TALKING POINTS You're having a discussion with a friend about life insurance and mention that you get a 10 percent reduction in your annual premium because you're a nonsmoker. Your friend, who is a smoker, becomes annoyed and says that this is just one example of how smokers are penalized. How would you respond?

Taking Charge of Your Health

- Commit yourself to establishing a smoke-free environment in the places where you live, work, study, and recreate.
- Support friends and acquaintances who are trying to become smoke-free.

- Support legislative efforts, at all levels of government, to reduce your exposure to environmental tobacco smoke.
- Be civil toward tobacco users in public spaces, but respond assertively if they infringe on smoke-free spaces.

- Support agencies and organizations committed to reducing tobacco use among young people through education and intervention.

SUMMARY

- The percentage of American adults who smoke has leveled off at approximately one in five (20.6 percent) adults.
- In spite of a reversal on the part of more recent college graduates, cigarette smoking has traditionally been inversely related to the level of formal education.
- A number of demographical variables influence the incidence of tobacco use.
- The tobacco industry continues to aggressively market its products to potential smokers.
- Multiple theories regarding nicotine's role in tobacco dependence have been advanced, including a better understanding of the proportional influences of genetics, environment, and personality.
- Nicotine exerts acute effects both within the central nervous system and on a variety of other tissues and organs.
- Tobacco smoke can be divided into gaseous and particulate phases. Each phase has its unique chemical composition.
- Thousands of chemical components and hundreds of carcinogenic agents are found in tobacco smoke.
- Nicotine and carbon monoxide have predictable effects on the function of the cardiovascular system.

- The development of nearly one-third of all cancers can be attributed to tobacco use, and virtually every form of cancer is found more frequently in smokers than in nonsmokers.
- Chronic obstructive lung disease (COLD), also called chronic obstructive pulmonary disease (COPD), is a likely consequence of long-term cigarette smoking, with early symptoms appearing shortly after beginning regular smoking.
- Smoking alters normal structures and functions of the body, as seen in a wide variety of noncardiovascular and noncancerous conditions, such as infertility, problem pregnancy, and neonatal health concerns. Additional health concerns include the diminished ability to smell, periodontal disease, vitamin inadequacies, and bone loss leading to osteoporosis.
- The use of smokeless tobacco carries its own health risks, including oral cancer.
- The presence of secondhand smoke results in involuntary (or passive) smoking by those who must share a common air source with smokers.
- Stopping smoking can be undertaken in any one of several ways.

REVIEW QUESTIONS

1. What percentage of the American adult population smoke? In what direction has change been occurring?
2. What is the current direction that adolescent smoking is taking?
3. What was the outcome of the class action suit brought by all 50 states, and what was the effect of the Master Tobacco Settlement Agreement (1999) on the ability of the tobacco industry to market its products?
4. What are the two principal dimensions of nicotine dependence? What are specific aspects seen within physical dependence?
5. Identify each of the theories of nicotine dependence discussed in the chapter.
6. How do modeling and manipulation explain the development of emotional dependence on tobacco?
7. In the amount consumed by the typical smoker, what is the effect of nicotine on central nervous system function? How does this differ in chain smokers?
8. What effects does nicotine have on the body outside of the central nervous system? How does the influence of

nicotine resemble that associated with the stress response?
9. What is the principal effect of carbon monoxide on cardiac function?
10. What influences does passive smoking have on nonsmoking adult partners of smokers? On their children?
11. How is the federal government attempting to limit the exposure that children and adolescents currently have to tobacco products and tobacco advertisements?
12. In comparison to cigarettes, what health risks are associated with pipe and cigar smoking?
13. How might concerned parents begin to "tobacco proof" their children to keep them from becoming smokers in the future?
14. What prescription and OTC products are now available to assist smokers in quitting?
15. What percentage of smokers are able to quit, and what is the best way to confirm that quitting has actually occurred?

ANSWERS TO THE "WHAT DO YOU KNOW?" QUIZ

1. False   2. False   3. True   4. False   5. False   6. False   7. True

SOURCE NOTES

1. Centers for Disease Control and Prevention (CDC). Vital signs: current cigarette smoking among adults aged ≥ 18 years—United States, 2009. *Morbidity and Mortality Weekly Report,* 58, 35, September 10, 2010.

2. Centers for Disease Control and Prevention (CDC). State-specific cigarette smoking and smokeless tobacco use among adults—United States, 2009. *Morbidity and Mortality Weekly Report,* 59, 93, November 5, 2010.

3. Tobacco use among adults—United States, 2005. *Morbidity and Mortality Weekly,* 55(42), 1145–48, Table 2, October 27, 2006.

4. Centers for Disease Control and Prevention (CDC). Your risk behavior surveillance—United States, 2007. *Morbidity and Mortality Weekly,* 57(22-4), June 6, 2008.

5. Aldworth J, et al. *Results from the 2005 National Survey on Drug Use and Health: National Findings.* SAMHSA. Department of Health and Human Services (DHHS Publication No. SMA 06-4194), 2006. Centers for Disease Control and Prevention (CDC). Cigarette smoking among adults—United States, 2007. *Morbidity and Mortality Weekly,* 57(45), November 14, 2008.

6. QuickStats: cigarette smoking prevalence among adults aged 18 years who have ever spent 24 hours on the streets, in a shelter, or in a jail or prison, by sex—United States, 2004. *Morbidity and Mortality Weekly,* 55(10), 287, March 17, 2006.

7. Wilson JJ. *Summary of the Attorneys General Master Tobacco Settlement Agreement.* National Conference of State Legislators. March; pages 1–44. www.academic.idayton.edu/health/syllabi/tobacco/summary.htm. 1999.

8. Henriksen L, et al. Industry sponsored anti-smoking ads and adolescent reactance: test of a boomerang effect. *Tobacco Control,* 15(1), 13–18, February 2006.

9. Shiffman S, Paty J. Smoking Patterns and dependence: contrasting chippers and heavy smokers. *Journal of Abnormal Psychology,* 115(3), 509–523, August 2006.

10. Savageau JA, Mowery PD, DiFranza JR. Symptoms of diminished autonomy over cigarettes with non-daily use. *International Journal of Environmental Research and Public Health,* 6(1), 25–35, 2009.

11. Maes HH, et al. Genetic and cultural transmission of smoking initiation: an extended twin kinship model. *Behavior Genetics,* 36(6), 798–808, November 2006.

12. Batra V, et al. The genetic determinants of smoking. *Chest,* 123(5), 1730–39, 2003.

13. Saccone NL, Schwantes-An TH, Wang JC, et al. Multiple cholinergic nicotinic receptor genes affect nicotine dependence risk in African and European Americans. *Genes, Brain, and Behavior,* 105, 9(7), 741–750, 2010.

14. Hefzy H, Silver RW, Silver B. The no-smoking sign insular infarction. *Journal of Neuroimaging,* July 1, 2010 (Epub ahead of print).

15. Gilman SE, et al. Parental smoking and adolescent smoking initiation: an intergenerational perspective on tobacco control. *Pediatrics,* 123(2), e274–e281, February 2009.

16. DiFranza JR, et al. Tobacco Consortium, Center for Child Health Research of the American Academy of Pediatrics. *Pediatrics,* 117(6), 1237–48, June 2006.

17. McGee R, Williams S, Reeder A. Parental tobacco smoking behavior and their children's smoking and cessation in adulthood. *Addiction,* 101(8), 1193–1201, August 2006.

18. Minino AM, Xu J, Kochanek MA, et al. Death in the United States, 2007. *NCHS Data Brief,* 26, December 2009.

19. Padmavathi P, Reddy VD, Maturu P, et al. Smoking-induced alterations in platelet membrane and Na(+)/K(+) – ATPase activity in chronic smokers. *Journal of Atherosclerosis Thrombosis,* 17(6), 619–627, 2010.

20. American Cancer Society. *Cancer Facts and Figures—2010.* Atlanta: American Cancer Society, 2010.

21. Lieberman HB, Bernstock JD, Broustas CG, et al. The role of RAD9 in tumorigenesis. *Journal of Molecular Cell Biology,* 3(1), 39–43, 2011.

22. Strulovivi-Barel Y, Omberg L, O'Mahony M, et al. Threshold of biologic responses of the small airway epithelium to low levels of tobacco smoke. *American Journal of Respiratory Critical Care Medicine,* 182(12), 1524–32, 2010.

23. Rusanen M, Kivipelto M, Quesenberry CP, et al. Heavy smoking in midlife and long-term risk of Alzheimer disease and vascular dementia, *Archives of International Medicine,* October 25, 2010. (Epub ahead of print).

24. *Cigars: Health Effects and Trends.* Cancer Monograph Series (No. 9). National Cancer Institute, 1998.

25. Symm B, et al. Cigar smoking: an ignored public health threat. *Journal of Primary Prevention,* 26(4), 363–375, July 2005.

26. *The Health Consequences of Using Smokeless Tobacco: A Report of the Advisory Committee to the Surgeon General.* U.S. Department of Health and Human Services, Public Health Service. NIH Publication No. 86-2874. 1986.

27. Mitchell EA, Milerad J. Smoking and the sudden infant death syndrome. *Reviews on Environmental Health,* 21(2), 81–103, April–June 2006.

28. Centers for Disease Control and Prevention. Vital signs: nonsmokers' exposure to secondhand smoke—United States, *Morbidity and Mortality Weekly Report,* 59(35), 1–2, 2010.

29. Christakis NA, Fowler JH. The collective dynamics of smoking in a large smoking network. *New England Journal of Medicine,* 358(21), 2249–58, May 22, 2008.

30. Maurer P, Bachmann MF. Vaccination against nicotine: an emerging therapy for tobacco dependence. *Expert Opinion on Investigational Drugs,* 16(11), 1775–83, November 2007.

31. Hatsulami DK, Jorenby DE, Gonzales D, et al. Immunogenicity and smoking-cessation outcomes for a novel nicotine immunotherapeutic. *Clinical Pharmacological Therapy,* 89(3), 392–399, 2011.

Personal Assessment

What Are Your Feelings About Smoking and Relationships?

For several semesters this questionnaire was administered by one of your textbook's authors to students in personal health classes. The instructions are simple: Select the statement that best describes your feelings about smoking as it relates to establishing a meaningful (trusted or true) friendship or life partnership.

1. It would be imperative that the individual be a smoker.
2. It would be desirable but not imperative that the individual be a smoker.
3. It would be a nonissue.
4. It would be desirable but not imperative that the individual be a nonsmoker.
5. It would be imperative that the individual be a nonsmoker.

With your choice in mind, check both the typical pattern of responses and short collection of statements that were appended.

This is a typical pattern of responses from a class of approximately 30 students:

1. 0
2. 1–2
3. 5–7
4. 8–11
5. 18–26

These are comments made by students at each level of selection:

1. "I smoke and probably couldn't stop, so I guess it's best if my best friend is a smoker as well."
2. "I smoke and I want to quit. Having someone who wants to stop smoking will allow us to help each other."
3. "Love and respect are more important than any other aspect of a relationship—more than whether another person smokes."
4. "It's OK, so long as he does not smoke at home, or if he smokes on the patio or in a special room (vented to the outside), and if he tries to quit, and if he does not smoke when with me or our children, or in the car (at any time)."
5. "I can hardly be around anyone who smokes. I sure wouldn't choose a smoker to be my roommate, closest friend, or my wife."

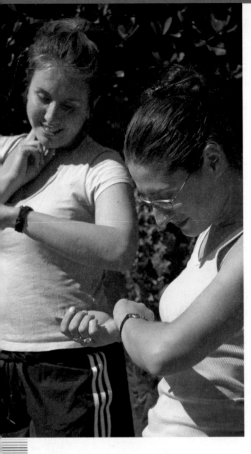

Enhancing Your Cardiovascular Health

What Do You Know About Keeping Your Heart Healthy?

1. About one in every three American adults has some form of cardiovascular disease. True or False?

2. There are more cardiovascular disease risk factors that you can change (such as your cholesterol levels) than ones you cannot change (such as your age). True or False?

3. The risk for a heart attack is the same for a person who smoked a pack a day of cigarettes for 20 years and quit more than a year ago as for the person who has smoked for 20 years and is continuing to smoke a pack a day. True or False?

4. You do not need to have your cholesterol checked until you are 30 years old. True or False?

5. Only health care professionals should use an automated external defibrillator (AED) to assist a person experiencing cardiac arrest. True or False?

6. African Americans have a greater risk of stroke than Caucasians do. True or False?

7. Individuals with diabetes have a greater risk of developing cardiovascular disease than do people of the same age without diabetes. True or False?

Check your answers at the end of the chapter.

If you're a traditional-age college student, you may find it difficult to understand the importance of **cardiovascular** health. Unless you were born with a heart problem, you may think that cardiovascular damage will not occur until you reach your 50s or 60s. During your young adult years, you're much more likely to be concerned about cancer and sexually transmitted diseases.

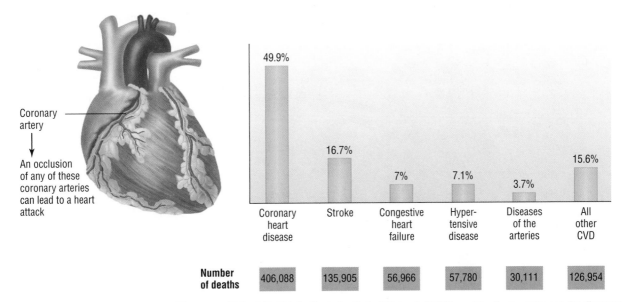

Figure 9-1 Deaths from Cardiovascular Disease Of the 813,804 deaths in the United States in 2007* resulting from cardiovascular diseases, nearly half were attributable to heart disease.

*The most recent year for which statistics are available.

Source: National Center for Health Statistics, reproduced in American Heart Association, Heart disease and stroke statistics–2011 update, *Circulation,* 123, e18–e209, 2011.

Yet autopsy reports on teenagers and young adults who have died in accidents are now showing that relatively high percentages of young people have developed conditions consistent with coronary artery disease; that is, fatty deposits have already formed in their coronary arteries. Since the foundation for future heart problems forms early in life, cardiovascular health is a very important topic for all college students.

Cardiovascular diseases were directly related to 33.6 percent of deaths in the United States in 2005 and contributed to another 21.8 percent.[1] Heart disease, stroke, and related blood vessel disorders combined to kill more than 800,000 Americans in 2007 (see Figure 9-1).[1] This figure represents approximately the same number of deaths that were caused by cancer, accidents, pneumonia, influenza, lung diseases, and diabetes combined. Cardiovascular disease (CVD) causes one out of every three deaths in the United States.[1] Indeed, CVD is our nation's number-one "killer" (see Table 9.1).

There is some good news about CVD. Between 1997 and 2007, the death rates from CVD declined 27.8 percent.[1] The American Heart Association, in its 2011 *Heart and Stroke Statistical Update,* credits this reduction to a combination of changing American lifestyles and medical advances in the diagnosis and treatment of CVD.[1]

This chapter explains how the heart works. It also will help you identify your CVD risk factors and suggest ways you can alter certain lifestyle behaviors to reduce your risk of developing heart disease.

Table 9.1 Estimated Prevalence of Major Cardiovascular Diseases

Hypertension	76,400,000
Coronary heart disease	16,300,000
Stroke	7,000,000
Congestive heart failure	5,700,000
Congenital heart disease*	1,300,000
TOTAL	82,600,000

Note: The sum of the individual estimates exceeds 82,600,000 because many people have more than one cardiovascular disorder. For example, many people with coronary heart disease also have hypertension.

*The prevalence of congenital cardiovascular defects is estimated to range from 650,000 to 1.3 million.

Source: American Heart Association, Heart disease and stroke statistics—2011 update, *Circulation,* 123, e18–e209, 2011.

Normal Cardiovascular Function

The cardiovascular or circulatory system uses a muscular pump to send a complex fluid on a continuous trip through a closed system of tubes. The pump is the heart, the fluid is blood, and the closed system of tubes is the network of blood vessels.

> **Key Terms**
>
> **cardiovascular** Pertaining to the heart *(cardio)* and blood vessels *(vascular).*

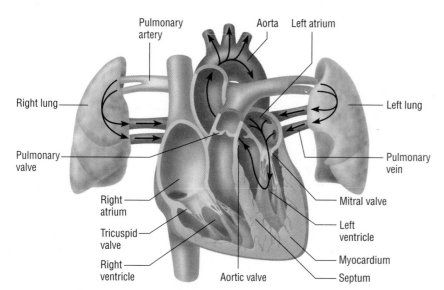

Pulmonary artery
Aorta
Left atrium
Right lung
Left lung
Pulmonary valve
Pulmonary vein
Right atrium
Mitral valve
Tricuspid valve
Left ventricle
Right ventricle
Myocardium
Aortic valve
Septum

Figure 9-2 Circulation Through the Heart
The heart functions like a complex double pump. The right side of the heart pumps deoxygenated blood to the lungs. The left side of the heart pumps oxygenated blood through the aorta to all parts of the body. Note the thickness of the walls of the ventricles. These are the primary pumping chambers.

The Vascular System

The term *vascular system* refers to the body's blood vessels. Although we might be familiar with the arteries (vessels that carry blood away from the heart) and the veins (vessels that carry blood toward the heart), arterioles, capillaries, and venules are also included in the vascular system. Arterioles are the farther, small-diameter extensions of arteries. These arterioles lead eventually to capillaries, the smallest extensions of the vascular system. At the capillary level, exchanges of oxygen, food, and waste occur between cells and the blood.

Once the blood leaves the capillaries and begins its return to the heart, it drains into small veins, or venules. The blood in the venules flows into increasingly larger vessels called *veins.* Blood pressure is highest in arteries and lowest in veins, especially the largest veins, which empty into the right atrium of the heart.

The Heart

The heart is a four-chambered pump designed to create the pressure required to circulate blood throughout the body. About the size of a person's clenched fist, this organ lies slightly tilted between the lungs in the central portion of the **thorax.** The heart does not lie completely in the center of the chest. Approximately two-thirds of the heart is to the left of the body midline, and one-third is to the right.

Two upper chambers, called *atria,* and two lower chambers, called *ventricles,* form the heart.[2] The thin-walled atrial chambers are considered collecting chambers, and the thick-walled muscular ventricles are considered the pumping chambers. The right and left sides of the heart are divided by a partition called the *septum.* Use Figure 9-2 to follow the flow of blood through the heart's four chambers.

For the heart muscle to function well, it must be supplied with adequate amounts of oxygen. The two main

coronary arteries (and their numerous branches) accomplish this. These arteries are located outside the heart (see Figure 9-1). If the coronary arteries are diseased, a heart attack (myocardial infarction) is possible.

The heart contracts and relaxes through the delicate interplay of **cardiac muscle** tissue and cardiac electrical centers called *nodes.* Nodal tissue generates the electrical impulses (i.e. the pacemaker) necessary to contract heart muscle.[3] The heart's electrical activity is measured by an instrument called an *electrocardiograph* (ECG or EKG), which provides a printout called an *electrocardiogram,* which can be evaluated to determine cardiac electrical functioning.

Blood

The average-size man has approximately 5 quarts of blood in his circulatory system. The functions of blood, which are performed continuously, are similar to the overall functions of the circulatory system and include the following:

- Transportation of nutrients, oxygen, wastes, hormones, and enzymes
- Regulation of water content of body cells and fluids
- Buffering to help maintain appropriate pH balance of body fluids

---

Key Terms

thorax The chest; the portion of the torso above the diaphragm and within the rib cage.

coronary arteries Vessels that supply oxygenated blood to heart muscle tissues.

cardiac muscle Specialized muscle tissue that forms the middle (muscular) layer of the heart wall.

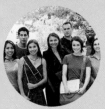

Learning from Our Diversity

Prevention of Heart Disease Begins in Childhood

Youth is one aspect of diversity that is sometimes overlooked. Yet age is important, especially when adults have influence over children's health behavior. Many adults never seriously consider that their health behaviors are imitated by the children around them. When adults care little about their own health, they may also be contributing to serious health issues in young people. Nowhere is this age diversity issue more pronounced than in the area of cardiovascular health.

For many aspects of wellness, preventive behaviors are often best learned in childhood, when they can be repeated and reinforced by family members and caregivers. This is especially true for preventive actions concerning heart disease. Although many problems related to heart disease appear at midlife and later, the roots of heart disease are found early in life.

The most serious childhood health behaviors associated with heart disease are poor dietary practices, lack of physical activity, and cigarette smoking. Unfortunately, America's youth currently shows severe deficiencies in all three areas. Children's diets lack nutrient density and remain far too high in overall fat. Children and teenagers are becoming increasingly overweight and obese. Studies consistently show a decline in the amount of physical activity by today's youth, since television and video games have become the after-school companions for many children. In addition, rates of cigarette smoking continue to rise among school children, especially teenagers. Unfortunately, the problems continue for many young adults when they go to college. The "freshman 15" (gaining 15 pounds or more during the first year of college) has been observed and is attributed to excess food consumption and low levels of physical activity.

These unhealthy behaviors are laying the foundation for coronary artery disease, hypertension, stroke, and other diseases in the future. The focus should be on health measures in childhood that prevent cardiovascular problems rather than treatment of older, already affected people. Parents must make efforts to encourage children to eat more nutritiously and be physically active. Adults should discourage cigarette use by young people. Perhaps the best approach for adults is to set a good example by adopting heart-healthy behaviors themselves. Following MyPlate (see Chapter 5) and exercising regularly are excellent strategies that can be started early in life.

- Regulation of body temperature; the water component in the blood absorbs heat and transfers it

- Prevention of blood loss; by coagulating or clotting, the blood can alter its form to prevent blood loss through injured vessels

- Protection against toxins and microorganisms, accomplished by chemical substances called *antibodies* and specialized cellular elements circulating in the bloodstream

Cardiovascular Disease Risk Factors

As you have just read, the heart and blood vessels are among the most important structures in the human body. By protecting your cardiovascular system, you lay the groundwork for an exciting, productive, and energetic life. The best time to start protecting and improving your cardiovascular system is early in life, when lifestyle patterns are developed and reinforced (see the box "Prevention of Heart Disease Begins in Childhood"). Of course, it's difficult to move backward through time, so the second best time to start protecting your heart is today. Improvements in certain lifestyle activities can pay significant dividends as your life unfolds. (Complete the Personal Assessment at the end of this chapter to determine your risk for heart disease.)

The American Heart Association encourages people to protect and enhance their heart health by examining the 10 cardiovascular risk factors related to various forms of heart disease (see Table 9.2).[3] A *cardiovascular risk factor* is an attribute that a person has or is exposed to that increases the likelihood that he or she will develop some form of heart disease. The first three risk factors are ones you will be unable to change. An additional six risk factors are ones you can change. One final risk factor is thought to contribute to the development of heart disease.

Table 9.2 Risk Factors for Cardiovascular Disease

Factors You Cannot Change
- Increasing age
- Male gender
- Heredity (including race)

Factors You Can Change ("Big Six" Risk Factors)
- Cigarette smoking and secondhand smoke
- Physical inactivity
- Abnormal blood cholesterol levels
- High blood pressure
- Diabetes mellitus
- Abdominal obesity

Contributing Factor
- Individual response to stress

Risk Factors That Cannot Be Changed

The three risk factors that you cannot change are increasing age, male gender, and heredity.[4] However, your knowledge that they might be an influence in your life should encourage you to make a more serious commitment to the risk factors you can change.

Increasing Age Heart diseases tend to develop gradually over the course of one's life. Although we may know of a few people who experienced a heart attack in their 20s or 30s, most of the serious consequences of heart disease are evident in older ages. For example, approximately 81 percent of people who die from heart diseases are age 65 and older.[1]

Male Gender Before age 55, women have lower rates of heart disease than men do. Yet after women move through menopause (typically in their 50s), their rates of heart disease are similar to those of men (see the box "Women and Heart Disease"). It is thought that women are somewhat more protected from heart disease than men because of their natural production of the hormone estrogen during their fertile years.

Heredity Like increasing age and male gender, heredity cannot be changed. By the luck of the draw, some people are born into families in which heart disease has never been a serious problem; others are born into families in which heart disease is quite prevalent. In this latter case, children are said to have a genetic predisposition (tendency) to develop heart disease as they grow and develop throughout their lives. These people have every reason to be highly motivated to reduce the risk factors they can control.

Race is also a consideration related to heart disease. African Americans have moderately high blood pressure at rates twice that of Whites and severe hypertension at rates three times higher than Whites. Hypertension significantly increases the risk of both heart disease and stroke; however, it can be controlled through a variety of methods. It is especially important for African Americans to take advantage of every opportunity to have their blood pressure measured so that preventive actions can be started immediately if necessary.

Risk Factors That Can Be Changed

Six cardiovascular risk factors are influenced largely by our lifestyle choices. These risk factors are cigarette and tobacco smoke, physical inactivity, high blood cholesterol level, high blood pressure, diabetes mellitus, and obesity and overweight.[4] Healthful behavior changes you make for these "big six" risk factors can help you protect and enhance your cardiovascular system.

Getting a Spiritual Lift Through Physical Activity

Pick up almost any book on exercise, and you'll read about the "feel-good" effect. It's what happens when you start doing any type of aerobic activity, such as walking, running, or swimming. First, you'll notice physical changes. You've got more energy. You're sleeping better. Maybe you're even a little less grouchy. In the long term, you will lower your risk for most chronic diseases, including coronary heart disease.

But something else is happening, too. Gradually, your outlook seems more positive. Things you couldn't even think about doing a few weeks ago seem possible. You find yourself thinking about starting to write poetry, figuring out what you want to do with your life, improving your grades, or making new friends. That's the feel-good effect spilling over into all areas of your life.

A few weeks after starting your exercise program, you've dropped a few pounds and your clothes feel more comfortable. But how you think about yourself is changing, too. Maybe you're paying more attention to your appearance. Or you're eating in a healthier way—almost without thinking about it. What's happening is that your self-image is improving. The idea of taking care of yourself is starting to grow, so how you look, what you eat, and how you spend your time are becoming important.

Most health-related organizations (such as the American Heart Association) and government agencies concerned with health (such as the Centers for Disease Control and Prevention) have published recommendations for all individuals to be regularly active.

Joining in physical activities with family or friends offers more than the obvious physical and social benefits. Canoeing, playing volleyball, or backpacking builds connections. You see others in a new way, relate to them differently, gain new insights, and find ways to help others. People and experiences you may have taken for granted take on a new dimension, and you appreciate them more.

Some people get a spiritual lift from the great outdoors. Wilderness hiking, for example, transports you to a different setting. The quietness, beauty, and solitude can be soothing to the soul. You're looking at the sky, trees, and water. You're enjoying a very peaceful time. This feeling may seem to disappear as soon as you get back to your dorm, but it may make the things you need to deal with there a little easier.

To experience this type of spiritual lift, you don't have to become a marathon runner or climb a mountain. Start going for long walks—alone or with a friend. Start a group that plays games, such as basketball, tennis, or volleyball. Try going for an early morning swim. Get into bicycling. The spiritual effects may be hard to measure, but they'll surprise and reward you.

Tobacco Smoke   Smokers have a heart attack risk that is two to four times that of nonsmokers. Smoking cigarettes is the major risk factor associated with sudden cardiac death. In fact, smokers have two to four times the risk of dying from sudden cardiac arrest as nonsmokers do.

Cigarette or tobacco smoke also adversely affects nonsmokers who are exposed to environmental tobacco smoke. Studies suggest that the risk of death caused by heart disease is increased about 30 percent in people exposed to secondhand smoke in the home. Because of the health threat to nonsmokers, restrictions on indoor smoking in public areas and business settings are increasing in every part of the country.

For years, it was believed that if you had smoked for many years, it was pointless to try to quit; the damage to one's health could never be reversed. However, the American Heart Association now indicates that by quitting smoking, regardless of how long or how much you have smoked, your risk of heart disease declines rapidly. For people who have smoked a pack or less of cigarettes per day, within three years after quitting smoking, their heart disease risk is virtually the same as for those who never smoked.

This news is exciting and should encourage people to quit smoking, regardless of how long they have smoked. Of course, if you have started to smoke recently, the healthy approach would be to quit now—before the nicotine controls your life and leads to heart disease, damages your lungs, or causes lung cancer. (For additional information about the health effects of tobacco, see Chapter 8.)

Physical Inactivity   Lack of regular physical activity is a significant risk factor for heart disease. Regular aerobic exercise (discussed in Chapter 4) helps strengthen the heart muscle, maintain healthy blood vessels, and improve the ability of the vascular system to transfer blood and oxygen to all parts of the body. Additionally, physical activity helps increase HDL ("good") cholesterol levels for most people, encourages weight loss and retention of lean muscle mass, and allows people to moderate the stress in their lives.

With all the benefits of physical activity, it amazes health professionals that so many Americans refuse to become regularly active. Some people feel that they don't have enough time or that they must work out strenuously. However, you'll recall from Chapter 4 that only 30 minutes of moderate aerobic activity five times a week can decrease your risk of heart disease. This is not a large price to pay for a lifetime of cardiovascular health. Find a partner and get started! The box "Getting a Spiritual Lift Through Physical Activity" discusses how the benefits of physical activity extend into the spiritual dimension of your life.

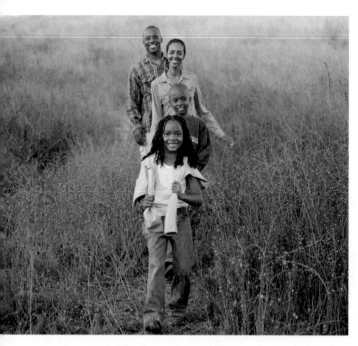

Regular physical activity throughout life helps prevent heart disease and has many other health and functional benefits.

If you are middle-aged or older and have been inactive, it is recommended that you start with light-to-moderate intensity activities, and gradually increase the amounts of activity. However, if you have any known health condition that could be aggravated by physical activity, check with a physician first.

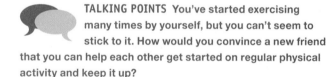

TALKING POINTS You've started exercising many times by yourself, but you can't seem to stick to it. How would you convince a new friend that you can help each other get started on regular physical activity and keep it up?

Abnormal Blood Cholesterol Levels   The third controllable risk factor for heart disease is a high blood cholesterol level. Generally, the higher the blood cholesterol level, the greater the risk for heart disease. When high blood cholesterol levels are combined with other important risk factors, the risks become much greater.

Fortunately, blood cholesterol levels are relatively easy to measure. Many campus health, fitness, and wellness centers provide cholesterol screenings for employees and students. These screenings help identify people whose cholesterol levels (or profiles) may be potentially dangerous. Medical professionals have been able to determine the link between a person's diet and his or her cholesterol levels. People with high blood cholesterol levels are encouraged to consume a heart-healthy diet (see Chapter 5) and to become physically active. In recent years, a variety of cholesterol-lowering drugs have also been developed that are very effective. Cholesterol will be discussed further later in this chapter.

High Blood Pressure   The fourth of the "big six" cardiovascular risk factors is high blood pressure, or *hypertension.* You will soon be reading more about hypertension, but for now, suffice it to say that high blood pressure can seriously damage a person's heart and blood vessels. High blood pressure causes the heart to work much harder, eventually causing it to enlarge and weaken. High blood pressure increases the chances for stroke, heart attack, congestive heart failure, and kidney disease.

When high blood pressure is present along with other risk factors, the risk for stroke or heart attack is increased tremendously. Yet this "silent killer" is easy to monitor and can be effectively controlled using a variety of approaches. This is the positive message about high blood pressure.

Diabetes Mellitus   Diabetes mellitus (discussed in detail in Chapter 10) is a debilitating chronic disease that has a significant effect on the human body. In addition to increasing the risk of developing kidney disease, blindness, and nerve damage, diabetes increases the likelihood of developing heart and blood vessel diseases. At least 65 percent of people with diabetes die of some type of heart or blood vessel disease. The cardiovascular damage is thought to occur because of the abnormal levels of cholesterol and blood fat found in individuals with diabetes. With weight management, exercise, dietary changes, and drug therapy, diabetes can be relatively well controlled in most people. Even with careful management of this disease, diabetic patients are susceptible to eventual heart and blood vessel damage.[5]

Obesity and Overweight   Even if they have no other risk factors, people who are obese are more likely than people who are not obese to develop heart disease and stroke. Obesity, particularly if excess fat is located primarily around the abdomen, places considerable strain on the heart, and it tends to influence both blood pressure and blood cholesterol levels. Also, obesity tends to trigger diabetes in predisposed people. Maintaining body weight within a desirable range minimizes the chance of obesity ever happening. To accomplish this, maintain an active lifestyle and follow the dietary guidelines in Chapter 5.

Metabolic Syndrome   Researchers and clinicians have recently observed that some risk factors seem to group together—most notably, abdominal obesity, abnormal blood lipids, elevated blood pressure, and elevated fasting glucose. This grouping of risk factors has been called *metabolic syndrome.* A person is diagnosed with metabolic syndrome if she or he has three or more of the factors listed in Table 9.3. Individuals with metabolic syndrome (about 34 percent of American adults) are twice as likely to develop coronary heart disease, compared to those without this syndrome.

Table 9.3 Criteria for Metabolic Syndrome

- Enlarged waist circumference
  Men: ≥ 40 inches
  Women: ≥ 35 inches
- Elevated triglycerides
  ≥ 150 mg/dl
- Low HDL cholesterol
  Men: < 40 mg/dl
  Women: < 50 mg/dl
- Elevated blood pressure
  ≥ 130/85 mm Hg
- Elevated fasting glucose (pre-diabetes)
  ≥ 100 mg/dl

Sources: American Heart Association and the National Heart, Lung, and Blood Institute.

Contributing Risk Factors

The American Heart Association identifies other risk factors that may contribute to CVD. These include *individual response to stress, sex hormones, birth control pills,* and *alcohol.* Unresolved stress can encourage negative health dependencies (for example, smoking, poor dietary practices, or underactivity) that lead to changes in blood fat profiles, blood pressure, and heart workload. Female sex hormones tend to protect women from CVD until they reach menopause, but male hormones do the opposite. Birth control pills (see Chapter 13) can increase the risk of blood clots and heart attack, although the risk is small unless the woman also smokes and is over age 35. The consumption of too much alcohol can cause elevated blood pressure and heart failure and lead to stroke, although moderate drinking (no more than one drink per day for women and two drinks per day for men) is associated with lower risk of heart disease.[1]

The news media frequently report on new potential risk factors for heart disease; see the box "Making Sense of Medical Research News" for advice on evaluating medical news reports.

Forms of Cardiovascular Disease

The American Heart Association describes the five major forms of CVD as coronary heart disease, hypertension, stroke, disease of the arteries, and congestive heart failure. A person may have just one of these diseases or a combination of them at the same time. Each form exists in varying degrees of severity. All are capable of causing secondary damage to other body organs and systems.

Coronary Heart Disease

This form of CVD, also known as *coronary artery disease,* involves damage to the vessels that supply blood to the

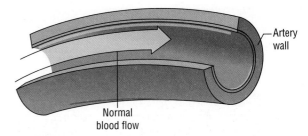

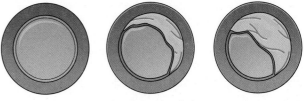

(A) Normal artery

(Artery cross-section)

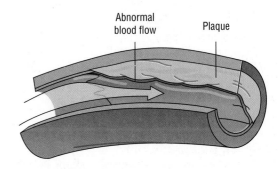

(B) Narrowing of artery due to plaque accumulation

Figure 9-3 Progression of Atherosclerosis This diagram shows how plaque deposits gradually accumulate to narrow the interior space of an artery. Although enlarged here, coronary arteries are only as wide as a pencil lead.

Source: Adapted from National Heart, Lung, and Blood Institute, What causes coronary artery disease? www.nhlbi.nih.gov/health/dci/Diseases/Cad/CAD_Causes.html, May 15, 2007.

heart muscle. The bulk of this blood is supplied by the coronary arteries. Any damage to these important vessels can cause a reduction of blood (and its vital oxygen and nutrients) to specific areas of heart muscle. The ultimate result of inadequate blood supply is a heart attack.

Atherosclerosis The principal cause for the development of coronary heart disease is atherosclerosis (see Figure 9-3). **Atherosclerosis** produces a narrowing of the coronary arteries. This narrowing stems from the long-term buildup of fatty deposits, called *plaque,*

Key Terms

atherosclerosis Buildup of plaque on the inner walls of arteries.

Making Sense of Medical Research News

Have you ever been confused by a medical news report? Does it seem as if the advice from medical research keeps changing? Some of this seeming confusion and conflict stems from the nature of scientific research—the results of many studies done over a long period may be needed to sort out confusing issues of cause and effect. However, some problems in deciphering medical news stem from the way the news is presented by the mass media. News stories may sensationalize research findings by oversimplifying the results, leaving out important caveats, and failing to place the findings in the larger context of other research. To help make more sense out of medical news and determine which study results are most important for you, consider the following types and characteristics of medical research studies:

- *Results published in peer-reviewed scientific journals versus results presented at medical meetings.* Results published in journals have been reviewed by experts who can evaluate the study design and conclusions and help put the findings in context. Leading scientific journals tend to publish the most important studies. Results presented at medical meetings are typically preliminary findings from studies still in progress; they have not yet been reviewed and may never be published due to problems in study design or hypotheses that fail to pan out over the full course of the study.
- *Human studies versus animal or laboratory studies.* Results from animal or laboratory experiments provide important information, but further research is typically needed before the results of such experiments can be applied to humans. See Chapter 10 for more on animal research.
- *Retrospective (backward-looking) studies versus prospective (forward-looking) studies.* Studies that follow subjects going forward in time are generally more accurate and meaningful. Retrospective studies rely on people's memories and past medical records, which may be inaccurate or incomplete.
- *Observational (epidemiological) studies versus interventional studies.* An observational study looks at participants' lifestyle practices and health, comparing people who independently chose a particular health intervention against people who did not. Observational studies are good at showing associations between factors but cannot be used to prove cause-and-effect relationships because other lifestyle factors can influence the results.

An interventional study, also known as a clinical trial, can be used to show causation. The most meaningful type of clinical trial is a *randomized, controlled, double-blind* study. In this type of study, researchers randomly divide participants into a treatment group and a control group for comparison. The treatment group receives an active drug or therapy while the control group receives a placebo, something that seems like the treatment under study. "Double-blind" refers to the fact that neither the participants nor the researchers know who receives the active treatment and who receives the placebo; this study design helps eliminate any possible bias.

- *Size and duration of the research study.* In general, studies that last longer and have more participants are likely to yield more meaningful results. Long study duration is key for research on chronic diseases; for example, a particular dietary change may reduce the risk of heart disease, but this reduction in risk may take 5–10 years to show up.
- *Participant characteristics.* Although this is not always the case, the results of a particular study are more likely to be relevant to you if you share key characteristics with the participants. For example, the results of a study on heart disease prevention in White men over age 65 may have limited relevance for a 25-year-old African American woman.
- *Relative risk versus absolute risk.* News media report on dramatic changes in relative risk—stating, for example, that a particular risk factor doubles your risk for a disease. When evaluating such statements, it is important to also consider your absolute risk of getting the disease. For example, if your absolute risk is only 1 in 100,000, then a doubling of risk would still mean that your overall risk of developing a disease is quite low.

Before you apply the findings from any research study to your own life, it is critical to put the findings into context. Find out what other experts recommend, especially major research associations and federal health agencies. A single study is rarely the final word on a health problem or treatment, and public health recommendations generally take into account all the available research into an issue. Also talk to your health care provider, who can help you make the choices most appropriate for your individual needs and situation.

Sources: Woloshin S, Schwartz LM, Media reporting on research presented at scientific meetings: more caution needed, *Medical Journal of Australia,* 184(11), 576–580, June 5, 2006; Studying research studies: 10 questions you need to ask, *Tufts University Health & Nutrition Letter,* June 2006; Making sense of medical news, *Consumer Reports on Health,* May 2005.

on the inner walls of the arteries. This buildup reduces the blood supply to specific portions of the heart. Some arteries of the heart can become so blocked (occluded) that all blood supply is stopped. Heart muscle tissue begins to die when it is deprived of oxygen and nutrients. This damage is known as **myocardial infarction.** In lay terms, this event is called a *heart attack.*

Cholesterol and Lipoproteins   For many years, scientists have known that atherosclerosis is a complicated disease that has many causes. Some of these causes are not well understood, but others are clearly understood. *Cholesterol,* a soft, fatlike material, is manufactured in the liver and small intestine and is necessary in the formation of sex hormones, cell membranes, bile salts, and nerve fibers. Elevated levels of serum cholesterol (200 mg/dl or more for adults age 20 and older, and 170 mg/dl or more for people below age 20) are associated with an increased risk for developing atherosclerosis.[5]

About 44 percent of American adults age 20 and older exceed the "borderline high" 200 mg/dl cholesterol level. It is estimated that approximately 20 percent of American youth ages 12–19 have "borderline high" cholesterol levels of 170 mg/dl and above; however, the rate is dramatically higher (43 percent) in obese youths. About 16 percent of American adults have a "high" blood cholesterol level, that is, 240 mg/dl or greater.

Initially, most people can help lower their serum cholesterol level by adopting three dietary changes: lowering their intake of saturated fats, lowering their intake of dietary cholesterol, and lowering their caloric intake to a level that does not exceed body requirements. The aim is to reduce excess fat, cholesterol, and calories in the diet while promoting sound nutrition. By carefully following such a diet plan, people with high serum cholesterol levels may be able to reduce their cholesterol levels by 30–55 mg/dl. However, dietary changes do not affect people equally; some will experience greater reductions than others. Some will not respond at all to dietary changes and may need to take cholesterol-lowering medications and increase their physical activity.

Cholesterol is attached to structures called lipoproteins. Lipoproteins are particles that circulate in the blood and transport lipids (including cholesterol).[6] Two major classes of lipoproteins exist: **low-density lipoproteins (LDLs)** and **high-density lipoproteins (HDLs).** A person's total cholesterol level is chiefly determined by the amount of the LDLs and HDLs in a measured sample of blood (see the box "Do You Know Your Cholesterol Levels?"). For example, a person's total cholesterol level of 200 mg/dl could be represented by an LDL level of 130 and an HDL level of 40, or an LDL level of 120 and an HDL level of 60. (Note that other lipoproteins do exist and carry some of the cholesterol in the blood.)

After much scientific study, it has been determined that high levels of LDL are a significant promoter of atherosclerosis. This makes sense because LDLs carry the greatest percentage of cholesterol in the bloodstream. LDLs are more likely to deposit excess cholesterol into the artery walls. This contributes to plaque formation. For this reason, LDLs are often called the "bad cholesterol." High LDL levels are determined partially by inheritance, but they are also clearly associated with smoking, poor dietary habits, obesity, and lack of exercise.

In contrast, high levels of HDLs are related to a decrease in the development of atherosclerosis. HDLs are thought to transport cholesterol out of the bloodstream. Thus, HDLs have been called the "good cholesterol." Certain lifestyle alterations, such as quitting smoking, reducing obesity, increasing physical activity, and

Do You Know Your Cholesterol Levels?

The National Cholesterol Education Program recommends that all Americans age 20 and older have a fasting lipoprotein profile done at least once every five years. Children with a parent who has documented heart disease should be tested before they reach age 20. Most university health and/or wellness centers offer cholesterol screenings throughout the year, often for free for students.

replacing saturated fats with monosaturated fats, help many people increase their level of HDL.

Reducing total serum cholesterol levels is a significant step in reducing the risk of death from coronary heart disease. The National Cholesterol Education Program recommends a therapeutic lifestyle change (TLC) approach to help control LDL cholesterol.[5] The TLCs include specific dietary guidelines, regular physical activity, and weight reduction (if needed). For people with elevated cholesterol levels, a 1 percent reduction in serum cholesterol level yields about a 3 percent reduction in the risk of death from heart disease. Thus, a 10–15 percent cholesterol reduction can reduce risk by 30–45 percent.[4] See Table 9.4 for LDL classifications and current recommended follow-up and Table 9.5 for additional classifications.

Angina Pectoris When coronary arteries become narrowed, chest pain, or *angina pectoris,* is sometimes felt. This pain results from a reduced supply of oxygen to heart muscle tissue. Usually, angina is felt when the coronary artery disease patient becomes stressed or exercises too strenuously. Angina reportedly can range from a feeling of mild indigestion to a severe, viselike pressure in the chest. The pain may extend from the center of the chest to the arms and even up to the jaw. Generally, the more severe the blockage, the more pain is felt.

Key Terms

myocardial infarction Heart attack; the death of part of the heart muscle as a result of a blockage in one of the coronary arteries.

low-density lipoprotein (LDL) The type of lipoprotein that transports the largest amount of cholesterol in the bloodstream; high levels of LDL are related to heart disease.

high-density lipoprotein (HDL) The type of lipoprotein that transports cholesterol from the bloodstream to the liver, where it is eventually removed from the body; high levels of HDL are related to a reduction in heart disease.

Table 9.4 Classification and Recommended Follow-up Based on LDL Cholesterol Level

LDL Cholesterol Level (mg/dl)	Classification	Initiate Therapeutic Lifestyle Changes (TLCs)
< 100	Optimal	—
100–129	Near optimal/ above optimal	If CHD or diabetes is present
130–159	Borderline high	If you have 2 or more risk factors
160–189	High	Yes, and see physician
≥ 190	Very high	Yes, and see physician

Note: The National Cholesterol Education Program (NCEP) recommends that all adults have their LDL cholesterol measured. See http://nhlbi.nih.gov/about/ncep/index.htm.

Source: National Cholesterol Education Program, *The Third Report of the Expert Panel on Detection, Evaluation, and Treatment of High Blood Cholesterol in Adults,* NIH Publication No. 02-5215, 2002.

Table 9.5 Classification of Total Cholesterol, Triglycerides, and HDL Cholesterol

	Normal or Desirable	Borderline-High	High
Total cholesterol	< 200	200–239	≥ 240
Triglycerides	< 150	150–199	≥ 200

	Low	Normal	High (Desirable)
HDL cholesterol	< 40	40–59	≥ 60

Note: All values expressed in mg/dl.

Source: National Cholesterol Education Program, *The Third Report of the Expert Panel on Detection, Evaluation, and Treatment of High Blood Cholesterol In Adults.* NIH Publication No. 02-5215, 2002. (Note: A revised report is scheduled to be released in the spring of 2012.)

However, it is important to note that only 20 percent of heart attacks are preceded by long-standing angina.

Some cardiac patients relieve angina with the drug *nitroglycerin,* a powerful blood vessel dilator. This prescription drug, available in slow-release transdermal (through the skin) patches or small pills that are placed under the patient's tongue, causes a major reduction in the workload of the heart muscle. Other cardiac patients may be prescribed drugs such as **calcium channel blockers** or **beta blockers.**

Arrhythmias Arrhythmias are disorders of the heart's normal sequence of electrical activity that are experienced by more than 2 million Americans. They result in an irregular beating pattern of the heart. Arrhythmias can be so brief that they do not affect the overall heart rate. Some arrhythmias, however, can last for long periods of time and cause the heart to beat either too slowly or too rapidly. A slow beating pattern is called *bradycardia* (fewer than 60 beats per minute), and a fast beating pattern is called *tachycardia* (more than 100 beats per minute).

Hearts that beat too slowly may be unable to pump a sufficient amount for blood throughout the body. The body becomes starved of oxygen, and loss of consciousness and even death can occur. Hearts that beat too rapidly do not allow the ventricles to fill sufficiently. When this happens, the heart cannot pump enough blood throughout the body. The heart becomes, in effect, a very inefficient machine. It beats rapidly but cannot pump much blood from its ventricles. This pattern may lead to ventricular fibrillation, which is the life-threatening, rapid uncoordinated contraction of the heart. Interestingly, whether the heart pumps too slowly or too rapidly, the result is the same: inadequate blood flow throughout the body.

The person most prone to arrhythmia is someone with some form of heart disease, including atherosclerosis, hypertension, or inflammatory or degenerative conditions. The prevalence of arrhythmia tends to increase with age. Certain congenital defects may make a person more likely to have an arrhythmia. Some chemical agents, including high or low levels of minerals (potassium, magnesium, and calcium) in the blood, addictive substances (caffeine, tobacco, other drugs), and various cardiac medications, can all provoke arrhythmias.

Arrhythmias are most frequently diagnosed through an ECG (electrocardiogram), which is a recording of the electrical activity of the heart. After diagnosis, a range of therapeutic approaches can be used, including simple monitoring (if the problem is relatively minor), drug therapy, or use of a pacemaker or implantable defibrillators.

Emergency Response to Heart Crises A *myocardial infarction* (heart attack) need not be fatal. The consequences of any heart attack depend on the location of the damage to the heart, the extent to which heart muscle is damaged, and the speed with which adequate circulation is restored. Injury to the ventricles may well prove fatal unless medical countermeasures are immediately undertaken. The recognition of a heart attack is critical; see the box "Heart Attack Warning Signs."

Cardiopulmonary resuscitation (CPR) is one of the most important immediate countermeasures that trained people can use when confronted with a victim of heart attack. Programs sponsored by the American Red Cross and the American Heart Association teach people how to recognize, evaluate, and manage heart attack emergencies. CPR trainees are taught how to restore breathing and circulation in persons requiring emergency care. Frequently, colleges offer CPR training through courses

I was walking by the track and field and saw a runner in distress. I froze and watched as someone else ran to his aid. How could I tell whether or not this person was having a heart attack? What action should I have taken?

Some heart attacks are sudden and intense—the "movie heart attack," where no one doubts what's happening. But most heart attacks start slowly, with mild pain or discomfort. Often people affected aren't sure what's wrong and wait too long before getting help. Here are signs that can mean a heart attack is happening:

- *Chest discomfort.* Most heart attacks involve discomfort in the center of the chest that lasts more than a few minutes, or that goes away and comes back. It can feel like uncomfortable pressure, squeezing, fullness, or pain.
- *Discomfort in other areas of the upper body.* Symptoms can include pain or discomfort in one or both arms, the back, neck, jaw, or stomach.
- *Shortness of breath* with or without chest discomfort.
- *Other signs* may include breaking out in a cold sweat, nausea, or lightheadedness.

As with men, women's most common heart attack symptom is chest pain or discomfort. But women are somewhat more likely than men to experience some of the other common symptoms, particularly shortness of breath, nausea/vomiting, and back or jaw pain.

Learn the signs, but remember this: Even if you're not sure it's a heart attack, have it checked out. Minutes matter! Fast action can save lives—maybe your own. Don't wait, call 911. Calling 911 is almost always the fastest way to get lifesaving treatment. Emergency medical services staff can begin treatment when they arrive—up to an hour sooner than if someone gets to the hospital by car. The staff is also trained to revive someone whose heart has stopped. Patients with chest pain who arrive by ambulance usually receive faster treatment at the hospital, too.

If you can't access the emergency medical services (EMS), have someone drive you to the hospital right away. If you're the one having symptoms, don't drive yourself, unless you have absolutely no other option.

Cardiac Arrest Strikes Immediately and Without Warning

Here are the signs:

- *Sudden loss of responsiveness* (no response to tapping on shoulders)
- *No normal breathing* (the victim does not take a normal breath when you tilt the head and check for at least five seconds)

If these signs of cardiac arrest are present, tell someone to call 911 and get an automated external defibrillator (AED) if one is available and *begin CPR immediately.*

If you are alone with an adult who has these signs of cardiac arrest, call 911 and get an AED (if one is available) before you begin CPR. Use an AED as soon as it arrives.

Source: American Heart Association. 2010. *Heart Attack, Stroke, and Cardiac Arrest Warning Signs.* Reprinted with permission. www.americanheart.org. Copyright © 2010 American Heart Association.

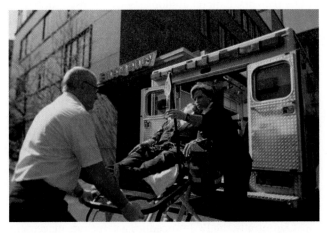

Emergency response teams help keep cardiac patients alive during transit to a medical facility.

in various departments. We encourage students to take a course and become certified. Additionally, members of the public are encouraged to obtain training in the use of automated external defibrillators (AEDs). These devices are now found in most public buildings and can markedly improve the chances of resuscitating a victim.

Diagnosis and Coronary Repair   Once a person's vital signs have stabilized, further diagnostic examinations can reveal the type and extent of damage to heart muscle. Initially, an ECG might be taken, which may be able to identify areas of ischemia (insufficient blood flow) or damage to the heart muscle. Another test that may be used is an echocardiography. This procedure can also

---

Key Terms

calcium channel blockers Drugs that prevent arterial spasms; used in the control of blood pressure and the long-term management of angina pectoris.

beta blockers Drugs that reduce the workload of the heart, which decreases occurrence of angina pectoris and helps control blood pressure.

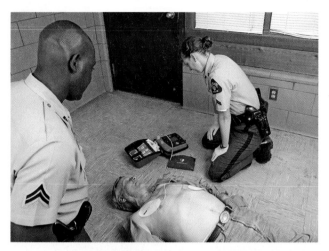

Automated external defibrillators (AEDs) are becoming more common in many places. With only a few hours of training, individuals can learn how to use an AED and become the first responders to an emergency situation. This action can be lifesaving for individuals experiencing a heart attack.

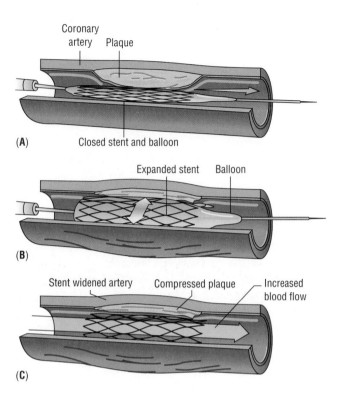

Figure 9-4 Percutaneous Coronary Intervention (A) A "balloon" is surgically inserted into the narrowed coronary artery. (B) The balloon is inflated, compressing plaque and fatty deposits against the artery walls. (C) A stent is left in place to prevent the artery from narrowing again at this site.

Source: Adapted from National Heart, Lung, and Blood Institute, What is coronary angioplasty? www.nhlbi.nih.gov/health/dci/Diseases/Angioplasty/Angioplasty_WhatIs.html, May 15, 2007.

detect ischemia. The diagnostic ability of both of these tests is improved if used in conjunction with exercise (that is, stress ECG or stress echocardiography). This test analyzes the electrical activity of the heart. *Heart catheterization,* also called *coronary arteriography,* is a minor surgical procedure that starts with placement of a thin plastic tube into an arm or leg artery. This tube, called a *catheter,* is guided through the artery until it reaches the coronary circulation, where a *radiopaque dye* is then released. X-ray films called *angiograms* record the progress of the dye through the coronary arteries so that areas of blockage can be easily identified.

Bypass Surgery Once the extent of damage is identified, a physician or team of physicians can decide on a medical course of action. Currently popular is an extensive form of surgery called **coronary artery bypass surgery.** An estimated 232,000 patients had bypass surgeries in 2007.[1] The purpose of such surgery is to detour (bypass) areas of coronary artery obstruction, usually by using a section of an artery from the patient's chest (the internal mammary artery) and grafting it from the aorta to a location just beyond the area of obstruction. Multiple areas of obstruction result in double, triple, or quadruple bypasses.

Percutaneous Coronary Intervention (PCI) An alternative to bypass surgery, **percutaneous coronary intervention (PCI)** involves the surgical insertion of a doughnut-shaped "balloon" directly into the narrowed coronary artery (see Figure 9-4). When the balloon is inflated, plaque and fatty deposits are compressed against the artery walls, widening the space through which blood flows. The balloon usually remains in the artery for less than one minute.

Renarrowing of the artery will occur in about one-quarter of PCI patients. Balloon angioplasty can be used for blockages in the heart, kidneys, arms, and legs. The decision whether to have PCI or bypass surgery can be a difficult one to make. Approximately 622,000 PCI procedures were performed in 2007.[1]

The FDA approved a device for clearing heart and leg arteries called a *motorized scraper.* Inserted through a leg artery and held in place by a tiny inflated balloon, this motor-driven cutter shaves off plaque deposits from inside the artery. A nose cone in the scraper unit stores the plaque until the device is removed.

The use of laser beams to dissolve plaque that blocks arteries has been slowly evolving. The FDA has approved three laser devices for use in clogged leg arteries.

Commonly, the PCI procedure will include placement of a **stent** (a small mesh device) to keep the artery open.

Heart Transplants and Artificial Hearts For almost 40 years, surgeons have been able to surgically replace a person's damaged heart with that of another human being. Although very risky, these transplant operations have added years to the lives of a number of patients who otherwise would have lived only a short time. In 2009, 2,211 heart transplants were performed in the United States.[1]

Artificial hearts have also been developed and implanted in humans. These hearts have extended the lives of many patients, but they have kept them unpleasantly tethered with tubes and wires to large power source machines. However, a major medical breakthrough took place in July 2001, when the world's first self-contained artificial heart was successfully implanted into a 59-year-old patient.

Aspirin Studies released a decade ago highlighted the role of aspirin in reducing the risk of heart attack in men with no history of previous attacks. Specifically, the studies concluded that for men with hypertension, elevated cholesterol levels, or both, taking one aspirin per day was a significant factor in reducing their risk of heart attack. Aspirin works by making the blood less able to clot. This reduces the likelihood of blood vessel blockages. Presently, opinions differ regarding the age at which this preventive action should begin. The safest advice is to check with your physician before starting aspirin therapy. Recent research now indicates that aspirin therapy is also beneficial for women.[7]

Alcohol For years, scientists have been uncertain about the extent to which alcohol consumption is related to a reduced risk for heart disease. The current thinking is that moderate drinking (defined as no more than two drinks per day for men and one drink per day for women) is related to a lower heart disease risk. However, the benefit is much smaller than proven risk reduction behaviors such as stopping smoking, reducing cholesterol level, lowering blood pressure, and increasing physical activity. Experts caution that heavy drinking increases cardiovascular risks and that nondrinkers should not start to drink just to reduce heart disease risk.

Hypertension

Just as your car's water pump recirculates water and maintains water pressure, your heart recirculates blood and maintains blood pressure. When the heart contracts, blood is forced through your arteries and veins. Your blood pressure is a measure of the force that your circulating blood exerts against the interior walls of your arteries and veins.

Measuring and Evaluating Blood Pressure Blood pressure is measured with a *sphygmomanometer*. This instrument is attached to an arm-cuff device that can be inflated to stop the flow of blood temporarily in the brachial artery. This artery is a major supplier of blood to the lower arm. It is located on the inside of the upper arm, between the biceps and triceps muscles.

A health professional using a stethoscope will listen for blood flow while the pressure in the cuff is released. Two pressure measurements will be recorded: The **systolic pressure** is the highest blood pressure against the vessel walls during the heart contraction, and the **diastolic pressure** is the lowest blood pressure against the vessel walls when the heart relaxes (between heartbeats). Expressed in units of millimeters of mercury displaced on the sphygmomanometer, blood pressure is recorded as the systolic pressure over the diastolic pressure—for example, 116/82.

Although a blood pressure of less than 120/80 is considered "normal" for an adult, lower values do not necessarily indicate a medical problem. In fact, many young college women of average weight will indicate blood pressures that seem to be relatively low (100/60, for example), yet these lowered blood pressures are quite "normal" for them.

What Is Hypertension? Hypertension refers to a consistently elevated blood pressure. Generally, treatment for high blood pressure begins when a person has a systolic reading of 140 or above or a diastolic reading of 90 or above (see Table 9.6). People with prehypertension are advised to adopt lifestyle measures to prevent any further elevation in their blood pressure. Approximately 76 million American adults and children have hypertension. The American Heart Association reports that African Americans, Hispanic Americans, and American Indians have higher rates of high blood pressure than White Americans.[1] In contrast, Asian/Pacific Islanders have significantly lower rates of hypertension.[1]

Causes and Effects of Hypertension Although the causes of 90–95 percent of the cases of hypertension

---

Key Terms

coronary artery bypass surgery Surgical procedure designed to improve blood flow to the heart by providing new routes for blood to take around points of blockage.

percutaneous coronary intervention (PCI) Any of a group of procedures used to treat patients suffering from an obstruction in an artery; typically involves inserting a slender, balloon-tipped tube into an artery of the heart.

stent A device inserted inside a coronary artery during a percutaneous coronary intervention (PCI) to prevent the artery from narrowing at that site.

systolic pressure Blood pressure against blood vessel walls when the heart contracts.

diastolic pressure Blood pressure against blood vessel walls when the heart relaxes.

Table 9.6 Blood Pressure Classification

Blood Pressure (mm Hg)	Normal	Prehypertension	Hypertension
Systolic (top number)	Less than 120	120–139	140 or higher
Diastolic (bottom number)	Less than 80	80–89	90 or higher

Note: High blood pressure, or hypertension, is defined in an adult as a systolic pressure of 140 mm Hg or higher and/or a diastolic pressure of 90 mm Hg or higher. Blood pressure is measured in millimeters of mercury (mm Hg).

Source: National Heart, Lung, and Blood Institute, *The Seventh Report of the Joint National Committee on Prevention, Detection, Evaluation, and Treatment of High Blood Pressure.* NIH Publication No. 03-5233, December 2003. (Note: A revised report is scheduled to be released in the spring of 2012.)

are not known, the health risks produced by uncontrolled hypertension are clearly understood. Throughout the body, long-term hypertension makes arteries and arterioles become less elastic and thus incapable of dilating under a heavy workload. Brittle, calcified blood vessels can burst unexpectedly and produce serious strokes (brain accidents), kidney failure (renal accidents), or eye damage **(retinal hemorrhage).** Furthermore, it appears that blood clots are more easily formed and dislodged in a vascular system affected by hypertension. Thus, hypertension can be a cause of heart attacks. Hypertension is a potential killer.

Ironically, despite its deadly nature, hypertension is referred to as "the silent killer" because people with hypertension often are not aware that they have the condition. They cannot feel the sensation of high blood pressure. The condition does not produce dizziness, headaches, or memory loss unless one is experiencing a medical crisis. It is estimated that approximately 20 percent of the people who have hypertension do not realize they have it.[8] Many who are aware of their hypertension do little to control it. Less than half of people who have hypertension control it adequately, generally through dietary control, regular exercise, relaxation training, and drug therapy.

Prevention and Treatment   Hypertension is not thought of as a curable disease; rather, it is a controllable disease. Once therapy is stopped, the condition returns. As a responsible adult, use every opportunity you can to measure your blood pressure on a regular basis.

Weight reduction, physical activity, moderation in alcohol use, and sodium restriction are often used to reduce hypertension. For overweight or obese people, a reduction in body weight may produce a significant drop in blood pressure. Physical activity helps lower blood pressure by expending calories (which may lead to weight loss in those who are overweight or obese) and through other physiological changes that affect the circulation. Moderation

in alcohol consumption (no more than one to two drinks daily) helps reduce blood pressure in some people.

The restriction of sodium (salt) in the diet also helps some people reduce hypertension. Interestingly, this strategy is effective only for those who are **salt sensitive** — estimated to be about 25 percent of the population. Reducing salt intake would have little effect on the blood pressure of the rest of the population. Nevertheless, since our daily intake of salt vastly exceeds our need for salt, the general recommendation to curb salt intake still makes good sense. Indeed, the 2020 Dietary Guidelines for Americans now recommend a sodium intake of at most 1,500 mg per day for people over age 50, African Americans, and anyone with hypertension, diabetes, or chronic kidney disease.

Many of the stress reduction activities discussed in Chapter 3 are receiving increased attention in the struggle to reduce hypertension. In recent years, behavioral scientists have reported the success of meditation, biofeedback, controlled breathing, and muscle relaxation exercises in reducing hypertension. Look for further research findings in these areas in the years to come.

There are literally dozens of drugs available for use by people with hypertension. Unfortunately, many patients refuse to take their medication on a consistent basis, probably because of the mistaken notion that "you must feel sick to be sick." Nutritional supplements, such as calcium, magnesium, potassium, and fish oil, have not been proven to be effective in lowering blood pressure.

 TALKING POINTS   You're having a regular physical examination, and your doctor remarks that your blood pressure puts you in the category of "prehypertension." What questions would you ask about managing this condition?

Stroke

Stroke is a general term for a wide variety of crises (sometimes called *cerebrovascular accidents* [*CVAs*] or brain attacks) that result from blood vessel damage in the brain. African Americans have a much greater risk of stroke than White Americans do, probably because African Americans have a greater likelihood of having hypertension than do White Americans. Data for 2007 indicate that 135,952 deaths and 610,000 new cases of stroke occurred.[1] Just as the heart muscle needs an adequate blood supply, so does the brain. Any disturbance in the proper supply of oxygen and nutrients to the brain can pose a threat.

Perhaps the most common form of stroke results from the blockage of a cerebral (brain) artery. Similar to coronary occlusions, **cerebrovascular occlusions** can be started by a clot that forms within an artery, called a *thrombus,* or by a clot that travels from another part of the body to the brain, called an *embolus* (see Figure 9-5 A and B).

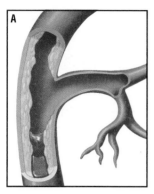

Thrombus
A clot that forms within a narrowed section of a blood vessel and remains at its place of origin.

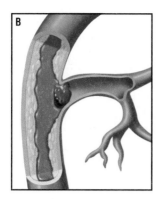

Embolus
A clot that moves through the circulatory system and becomes lodged at a narrowed point within a vessel.

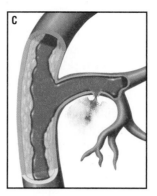

Hemorrhage
The sudden bursting of a blood vessel.

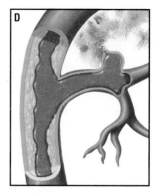

Aneurysm
A sac formed when a section of a blood vessel thins and balloons; the weakened wall of the sac can burst, or rupture, as shown here.

Figure 9-5 Causes of Stroke

Table 9.7 Recognizing Warning Signs of Stroke

The American Heart Association says these are the warning signs of stroke:

- Sudden numbness or weakness of the face, arm, or leg, especially on one side of the body
- Sudden confusion, trouble speaking or understanding
- Sudden trouble seeing in one or both eyes
- Sudden trouble walking, dizziness, loss of balance or coordination
- Sudden, severe headache with no known cause
- Individual response to stress

If you or someone with you has one or more of these signs, don't delay! Immediately call 911 so an ambulance (ideally with advanced life support) can be sent for you. Also, check the time so you'll know when the first symptoms appeared. It's very important to take immediate action. If given within three hours of the start of symptoms, a clot-busting drug can reduce long-term disability for the most common type of stroke.

Source: American Heart Association. 2010. *Heart Attack, Stroke, and Cardiac Arrest Warning Signs.* Reprinted with permission. www.americanheart.org. Copyright © 2010 American Heart Association.

---

understood, although there seems to be a relationship between aneurysms and hypertension. It is quite possible that many aneurysms are congenital defects. In any case, when a cerebral aneurysm bursts, a stroke results.

A person who reports any warning signs of stroke (see Table 9.7) or any ministroke, called a **transient ischemic attack (TIA),** will undergo a battery of diagnostic tests, which could include a physical examination, a search for possible brain tumors, tests to identify areas of the brain affected, use of the electroencephalogram, cerebral arteriography, and use of the **computed axial tomography (CT) scan** or **magnetic resonance imaging (MRI) scan.** Many additional tests are also available.

Key Terms

retinal hemorrhage Uncontrolled bleeding from arteries within the eye's retina.

salt sensitive Term used to describe people whose bodies overreact to the presence of sodium by retaining fluid and thus experience an increase in blood pressure.

cerebrovascular occlusions Blockages to arteries supplying blood to the cerebral cortex of the brain; strokes.

transient ischemic attack (TIA) Strokelike symptoms caused by temporary spasm of cerebral blood vessels.

computed axial tomography (CT) scan An x-ray procedure designed to illustrate structures within the body that would not normally be seen through conventional x-ray procedures.

magnetic resonance imaging (MRI) scan An imaging procedure that uses a powerful magnet to generate images of body tissues.

The resultant accidents (cerebral thrombosis or cerebral embolism) cause more than 87 percent of all strokes. The portion of the brain deprived of oxygen and nutrients can literally die.

A second type of stroke can result from an artery that bursts to produce a crisis called *cerebral hemorrhage* (see Figure 9-5 C). Damaged, brittle arteries can be especially susceptible to bursting when a person has hypertension.

A third form of stroke is a *cerebral aneurysm.* An aneurysm is a ballooning or outpouching on a weakened area of an artery (Figure 9-5 D). Aneurysms may occur in various locations of the body and are not always life-threatening. The development of aneurysms is not fully

Treatment of stroke patients depends on the nature and extent of the damage. Some patients require surgery (to repair vessels and relieve pressure) and acute care in the hospital. Others undergo drug treatment, especially the use of anticoagulant drugs, including aspirin and tissue plasminogen activators (TPA, the "clot buster" drug).

The advancements made in the rehabilitation of stroke patients are amazing. Although some severely affected patients have little hope of improvement, our increasing advancements in the application of computer technology to such disciplines as speech and physical therapy offer encouraging signs for stroke patients and their families.

Other Cardiovascular Diseases

A number of less common conditions can affect the functioning of the cardiovascular system. These include congenital heart disease, rheumatic heart disease, congestive heart failure, and peripheral artery disease.

Congenital Heart Disease A congenital defect is one that is present at birth. The American Heart Association estimates that each year about 36,000 babies are born with a congenital heart defect. In 2007, 3,547 children (mostly infants) died of congenital heart disease.[1]

A variety of abnormalities may be produced by congenital heart disease, including valve damage, holes in the walls of the septum, blood vessel transposition, and underdevelopment of the left side of the heart. All of these problems ultimately prevent a newborn from adequately oxygenating tissues throughout the body. A bluish skin color (cyanosis) is seen in some infants with such congenital heart defects. These infants are sometimes referred to as *blue babies*.

The cause of congenital heart defects is not clearly understood, although one cause, *rubella*, has been identified. The fetuses of mothers who contract the rubella virus during the first three months of pregnancy are at great risk of developing *congenital rubella syndrome (CRS)*, a catch-all term for a wide variety of congenital defects, including heart defects, deafness, cataracts, and mental retardation. Other hypotheses about the development of congenital heart disease implicate environmental pollutants; maternal use of drugs, including alcohol, during pregnancy; and unknown genetic factors.

Treatment of congenital defects usually requires surgery, although some conditions may respond well to drug therapy. Defective blood vessels and certain malformations of the heart can be surgically repaired. This surgery is so successful that many children respond quite quickly to the increased circulation and oxygenation. Many are able to lead normal, active lives.

Rheumatic Heart Disease **Rheumatic heart disease** is the final stage in a series of complications started by a streptococcal infection of the throat (strep throat) that is not effectively treated. The symptoms of strep throat include these:

- Sudden onset of sore throat, particularly with pain when swallowing
- Fever
- Swollen, tender glands under the angle of the jaw
- Headache
- Nausea and vomiting
- Tonsils covered with a yellow or white pus or discharge

This bacterial infection, if untreated, can result in an inflammatory disease called *rheumatic fever* (and a related condition, *scarlet fever*). Rheumatic fever is a whole-body (systemic) reaction that can produce fever, joint pain, skin rashes, and possible brain and heart damage. A person who has had rheumatic fever is more susceptible to subsequent attacks. Rheumatic fever tends to run in families. Some 3,201 Americans died from rheumatic fever and rheumatic heart disease in 2007.[1]

Damage from rheumatic fever centers on the heart's valves. For some reason, the bacteria tend to proliferate in the heart valves. Defective heart valves may fail either to open fully (*stenosis*) or to close fully (*insufficiency*). Diagnosis of valve damage might initially come when a physician hears a backwashing or backflow of blood (a **murmur**). Further tests—including chest x-rays, cardiac catheterization, and echocardiography—can reveal the extent of valve damage. Once identified, a faulty valve can be replaced surgically with a metal or plastic artificial valve or a valve taken from an animal's heart.

Congestive Heart Failure **Congestive heart failure** is a condition in which the heart lacks the strength to continue to circulate blood normally throughout the body.

Key Terms

rheumatic heart disease Chronic damage to the heart (especially heart valves) resulting from a streptococcal infection within the heart; a complication associated with rheumatic fever.

murmur Atypical heart sound that suggests a backwashing of blood into a chamber of the heart from which it has just left.

congestive heart failure Inability of the heart to pump out all the blood that returns to it; can lead to dangerous fluid accumulations in veins, lungs, and kidneys.

peripheral artery disease (PAD) Atherosclerotic blockages that occur in arteries that supply blood to the legs and arms.

Table 9.8 Definitions of Poor, Intermediate, and Ideal Cardiovascular Health for Each Metric in the AHA 2020 Goals

	Level of Cardiovascular Health for Each Metric		
	Poor	**Intermediate**	**Ideal**
• Current smoking			
Adults aged > 20 y	Yes	Former ≤ 12 mo	Never or quit > 12 mo
Children aged 12–19 y	Tried prior 30 d	. . .	Never tried; never smoked whole cigarette
• BMI			
Adults aged > 20 y	≥ 30 kg/m²	25–29.9 kg/m²	< 25 kg/m²
Children aged 2–19 y	> 95th percentile	85th–95th percentile	< 85th percentile
• Physical activity			
Adults aged > 20 y	None	1–149 min/wk moderate or 1–74 min/wk vigorous or 1–149 min/wk moderate + vigorous	150+ min/wk moderate or 75+ min/wk vigorous or 150+ min/wk moderate + vigorous
Children aged 12–19 y	None	> 0 and < 60 min of moderate or vigorous every day	60+ min of moderate or vigorous every day
• Healthy diet score			
Adults aged > 20 y	0–1 components	2–3 components	4–5 components
Children aged 5–19 y	0–1 components	2–3 components	4–5 components
• Total cholesterol			
Adults aged > 20 y	≥ 240 mg/dl	200–239 mg/dl or treated to goal	< 200 mg/dl
Children aged 6–19 y	≥ 200 mg/dl	170–199 mg/dl	< 170 mg/dl
• Blood pressure			
Adults aged > 20 y	SBP ≥ 140 or DBP ≥ 90 mm Hg	SBP 120–139 or DBP 80–89 mm Hg or treated to goal	< 120/< 80 mm Hg
Children aged 8–19 y	> 95th percentile	90th–95th percentile or SBP ≥ 120 or DBP ≥ 80 mm Hg	< 90th percentile
• Fasting plasma glucose			
Adults aged > 20 y	≥ 126 mg/dl	100–125 mg/dl or treated to goal	< 100 mg/dl
Children aged 12–19 y	≥ 126 mg/dl	100–125 mg/dl	< 100 mg/dl

Note: . . . Indicates no definition for this stratum; AHA, American Heart Association; BMI, body mass index; SBP, systolic blood pressure; DBP, diastolic blood pressure.

Source: Lloyd-Jones DM, et al., Defining and setting national goals for cardiovascular health promotion and disease reduction: the American Heart Association's strategic impact goal through 2020 and beyond, *Circulation,* 121, 586–613, 2010.

In 2007, 56,966 people died from congestive heart failure.[1] During congestive heart failure, the heart continues to work, but it cannot function well enough to maintain appropriate circulation. Venous blood flow starts to "back up." Swelling occurs, especially in the legs and ankles. Fluid can collect in the lungs and cause breathing difficulties and shortness of breath, and kidney function may be damaged.

Congestive heart failure can result from heart damage caused by congenital heart defects, lung disease, rheumatic fever, heart attack, atherosclerosis, or high blood pressure. Generally, congestive heart failure is treatable through a combined program of rest, proper diet, modified daily activities, and the use of appropriate drugs. Without medical care, congestive heart failure can be fatal.

Diseases of the Arteries **Peripheral artery disease (PAD),** also called *peripheral vascular disease (PVD),* is a blood vessel disease characterized by pathological changes to the arteries and arterioles in the extremities (primarily the legs and feet but sometimes the hands). PAD affects approximately 8 million Americans. These changes result from years of damage to the peripheral blood vessels. Important causes of PAD are cigarette smoking, a high-fat diet, obesity, and sedentary occupations. In some cases, PAD is aggravated by blood vessel changes resulting from diabetes.

PAD severely restricts blood flow to the extremities. The reduction in blood flow is responsible for leg pain or cramping during exercise, numbness, tingling, coldness, and loss of hair in the affected limb. The most serious consequence of PAD is the increased likelihood of developing ulcerations and tissue death. These conditions can lead to gangrene and may eventually necessitate amputation.

The treatment of PAD consists of multiple approaches and may include efforts to improve blood lipid levels (through diet, exercise, or drug therapy), reduce hypertension, reduce body weight, and eliminate smoking. Blood vessel surgery is also a possible treatment approach.

Additional Conditions   Besides the cardiovascular diseases already discussed, the heart and blood vessels are also subject to other pathological conditions. Tumors of the heart, although rare, occur. Infectious conditions involving the pericardial sac that surrounds the heart (*pericarditis*) and the innermost layer of the heart (*endocarditis*) are more commonly seen. In addition, inflammation of the veins (*phlebitis*) is troublesome to some people. Some young people have hypertrophic cardiomyopathy, an enlarged heart usually caused by genetic factors. This condition results in obstructed blood flow to the heart muscle and can lead to sudden death.

Cardiovascular Health Goals

The American Heart Association recently issued the following revised 10-year goal: "*By 2020, to improve the cardiovascular health of all Americans by 20%, while reducing deaths from cardiovascular disease and stroke by 20%.*"[1] In conjunction with this report, the American Heart Association is launching a major initiative for prevention of cardiovascular disease by establishing seven key health behaviors and factors to promote achievement of the 2020 goals. Its definition of "ideal cardiovascular health" is the absence of cardiovascular disease and the simultaneous presence of optimal levels of all seven health behaviors (lean body mass, avoidance of smoking, participation in physical activity, and healthy dietary intake) and health factors (total cholesterol, blood pressure, and fasting blood glucose). To help guide people toward ideal cardiovascular health, the American Heart Association developed a method to evaluate the level (poor, intermediate, ideal) of each of these health behaviors and factors (see Table 9.8).

Taking Charge of Your Health

- Complete the Personal Assessment to determine your risk for heart attack and stroke.

- Review MyPlate in Chapter 5, and make changes to your diet so that it is more "heart healthy."

- Follow the surgeon general's recommendations and engage in a moderate amount of physical activity daily or begin an aerobic exercise program that is appropriate for your current fitness level.

- If you are a smoker, resolve to quit smoking. Visit your physician to talk about safe and effective approaches. Begin putting your plan into action.

- Develop a plan to lower your dietary intake of saturated fat to keep your blood cholesterol level low.

- Have your blood pressure checked, and review your weight, physical activity, alcohol intake, and salt intake to determine whether you can make changes in any of these areas.

- If you are overweight or obese, develop a plan to combine dietary changes and increased physical activity to lose weight gradually but steadily.

SUMMARY

- Cardiovascular disorders are responsible for more disabilities and deaths than any other disease.
- The cardiovascular system consists of the heart, blood, and blood vessels. This system performs many functions.
- Our overall health depends on the health of the cardiovascular system.
- A cardiovascular risk factor is an attribute that a person has or is exposed to that increases the likelihood of heart disease.
- The "big six" risk factors are tobacco smoke, physical inactivity, high blood cholesterol level, high blood pressure, diabetes mellitus, and abdominal obesity. These are controllable risk factors.
- Increasing age, male gender, and heredity are risk factors that cannot be controlled.

- Four contributing risk factors to heart disease are individual response to stress, sex hormones, birth control pills, and alcohol overconsumption.
- The major forms of cardiovascular disease include coronary artery disease, hypertension, stroke, diseases of the arteries, and congestive heart failure. Each disease develops in a specific way and may require a highly specialized form of treatment.
- Atherosclerosis is the pathophysiological process that results in the narrowing of coronary arteries.
- It is important to recognize the warning signs of both heart attacks and strokes.

REVIEW QUESTIONS

1. Identify the principal components of the cardiovascular system. Trace the path of blood through the heart and cardiovascular system.
2. What are some of the important functions of blood?
3. Define cardiovascular risk factor. What relationship do risk factors have to cardiovascular disease?
4. Identify those risk factors for cardiovascular disease that cannot be changed. Identify those risk factors that can be changed. Identify the risk factors that can be contributing factors.

5. What are the five major forms of cardiovascular disease? For each of these diseases, describe what the disease is, its cause (if known), and its treatment.
6. Describe how high-density lipoproteins differ from low-density lipoproteins.
7. What problems does atherosclerosis produce?
8. Why is hypertension referred to as "the silent killer"?
9. What are the warning signals of stroke?
10. What is peripheral artery disease?

ANSWERS TO THE "WHAT DO YOU KNOW?" QUIZ

1. True   2. True   3. False   4. False   5. False   6. True   7. True

Visit the Online Learning Center (**www.mhhe.com/hahn11e**), where you will find tools to help you improve your grade including practice quizzes, key terms flashcards, audio chapter summaries for your MP3 player, and many other study aids.

SOURCE NOTES

1. American Heart Association. Heart disease and stroke statistics—2011 update, *Circulation*, 123, e18–e209, 2011.
2. Thibodeau GA, Patton KT. *Structure and Function of the Human Body* (11th ed.). St. Louis, MO: Mosby-Year Book, 2000.
3. Brubaker PH, Kaminsky LA, Whaley MH. *Coronary Artery Disease.* Champaign, IL: Human Kinetics, 2002.
4. American Heart Association. Risk factors and coronary heart disease. www.heart.org/HEARTORG/Conditions/ HeartAttack/Understand-Your-Risk-of-Heart-Attack_ UCM_002040_Article.jsp.

5. American Diabetes Association. Standards of medical care in diabetes. *Diabetes Care,* 33, S11–S61, 2010.
6. National Cholesterol Education Program. *The Third Report of the Expert Panel on Detection, Education, and Treatment of High Blood Cholesterol in Adults.* NIH Publication No. 02-5215, 2002.
7. U.S. Preventative Services Task Force. Aspirin for the primary prevention of cardiovascular events. *Annals of Internal Medicine,* 150, 405–410, 2009.
8. National Heart, Lung, and Blood Institute. www.nhlbi.nih.gov/ guidelines/hypertension/index.htm. July 21, 2003.

Personal Assessment

What Is Your Risk for Heart Disease?

Coronary Disease Risk Prediction Score Sheet for Men Based on Total Cholesterol Level

For steps 1–6, determine the points for your characteristics and record these in the summary box (step 7). Using your point total, determine your risk score in step 8. Step 9 allows you to compare your risk level with that of the average person of your age. (*If you are younger than 30 years old, use the 30–34 age group.*) Ideally, you want your value to be at or below the "low risk" score.

Step 1

Age	
Years	Points
30–34	−1
35–39	0
40–44	1
45–49	2
50–54	3
55–59	4
60–64	5
65–69	6
70–74	7

Step 2

Total Cholesterol		
(mg/dl)	(mmol/L)	Points
<160	≤4.14	−3
160–199	4.15–5.17	0
200–239	5.18–6.21	1
240–279	6.22–7.24	2
≥280	≥7.25	3

Key	
Color	Risk
green	Very low
white	Low
yellow	Moderate
orange	High
red	Very high

Step 3

HDL Cholesterol		
(mg/dl)	(mmol/L)	Points
<35	≤0.90	2
35–44	0.91–1.16	1
45–49	1.17–1.29	0
50–59	1.30–1.55	0
≥60	≥1.56	−2

Step 4

Blood Pressure					
Systolic (mm Hg)	Diastolic (mm Hg)				
	<80	80–84	85–89	90–99	≥100
<120	0				
120–129		0 pts			
130–139			1 pt		
140–159				2 pts	
≥160					3 pts

Note: When systolic and diastolic pressures provide different estimates for point scores, use the higher number.

Step 5

Diabetes	
	Points
No	0
Yes	2

Step 6

Smoker	
	Points
No	0
Yes	2

Risk estimates were derived from the experience of the NHLBI's Framingham Heart Study, a predominantly Caucasian population in Massachusetts, USA.

Step 7 (sum from steps 1–6)

Adding Up the Points	
Age	———
Total Cholesterol	———
HDL Cholesterol	———
Blood Pressure	———
Diabetes	———
Smoker	———
Point Total	———

Step 8 (determine CHD risk from point total)

CHD Risk	
Point Total	10 Yr CHD Risk
≤−1	2%
0	3%
1	3%
2	4%
3	5%
4	7%
5	8%
6	10%
7	13%
8	16%
9	20%
10	25%
11	31%
12	37%
13	45%
≥14	≥53%

Step 9 (compare to men of the same age)

Comparative Risk		
Age (years)	Average 10 Yr CHD Risk	Low* 10 Yr CHD Risk
30–34	3%	2%
35–39	5%	3%
40–44	7%	4%
45–49	11%	4%
50–54	14%	6%
55–59	16%	7%
60–64	21%	9%
65–69	25%	11%
70–74	30%	14%

* Low risk was calculated for a man the same age, normal blood pressure, total cholesterol 160–199 mg/dl, HDL cholesterol 45 mg/dl, nonsmoker, no diabetes.

Source: www.nhlbi.nih.gov/about/framingham/risktmen.pdf.

Coronary Disease Risk Prediction Score Sheet for Women Based on Total Cholesterol Level

For steps 1–6, determine the points for your characteristics and record these in the summary box (step 7). Using your point total, determine your risk score in step 8. Step 9 allows you to compare your risk level to that of the average person of your age. (*If you are younger than 30 years old, use the 30–34 age group.*) Ideally, you want your value to be at or below the "low risk" score.

Step 1

Age	
Years	Points
30–34	−9
35–39	−4
40–44	0
45–49	3
50–54	6
55–59	7
60–64	8
65–69	8
70–74	8

Step 2

Total Cholesterol		
(mg/dl)	(mmol/L)	Points
<160	≤4.14	−2
160–199	4.15–5.17	0
200–239	5.18–6.21	1
240–279	6.22–7.24	1
≥280	≥7.25	3

Key	
Color	Risk
green	Very low
white	Low
yellow	Moderate
orange	High
red	Very high

Step 3

HDL Cholesterol		
(mg/dl)	(mmol/L)	Points
<35	≤0.90	5
35–44	0.91–1.16	2
45–49	1.17–1.29	1
50–59	1.30–1.55	0
≥60	≥1.56	−3

Step 4

Blood Pressure					
Systolic	Diastolic (mm Hg)				
(mm Hg)	<80	80–84	85–89	90–99	≥100
<120	−3 pts				
120–129		0 pts			
130–139			0 pts		
140–159				2 pts	
≥160					3 pts

Note: When systolic and diastolic pressures provide different estimates for point scores, use the higher number.

Step 5

Diabetes	
	Points
No	0
Yes	4

Step 6

Smoker	
	Points
No	0
Yes	2

Risk estimates were derived from the experience of the NHLBI's Framingham Heart Study, a predominantly Caucasian population in Massachusetts, USA.

Step 7 (sum from steps 1–6)

Adding Up the Points	
Age	_____
Total Cholesterol	_____
HDL Cholesterol	_____
Blood Pressure	_____
Diabetes	_____
Smoker	_____
Point Total	_____

Step 8 (determine CHD risk from point total)

CHD Risk	
Point Total	10 Yr CHD Risk
≤−2	1%
−1	2%
0	2%
1	2%
2	3%
3	3%
4	4%
5	4%
6	5%
7	6%
8	7%
9	8%
10	10%
11	11%
12	13%
13	15%
14	18%
15	20%
16	24%
≥17	≥27%

Step 9 (compare to women of the same age)

Comparative Risk		
Age (years)	Average 10 Yr CHD Risk	Low* 10 Yr CHD Risk
30–34	<1%	<1%
35–39	1%	<1%
40–44	2%	2%
45–49	5%	3%
50–54	8%	5%
55–59	12%	7%
60–64	12%	8%
65–69	13%	8%
70–74	14%	8%

*Low risk was calculated for a woman the same age, normal blood pressure, total cholesterol 160–199 mg/dl, HDL cholesterol 55 mg/dl, nonsmoker, no diabetes.

Source: www.nhlbi.nih.gov/about/framingham/risktwomen.pdf.

TO CARRY THIS FURTHER . . .

Were you surprised with your score on this assessment? What were the factors that gave you the most points? See how changing those factors will lower your risk of heart disease.

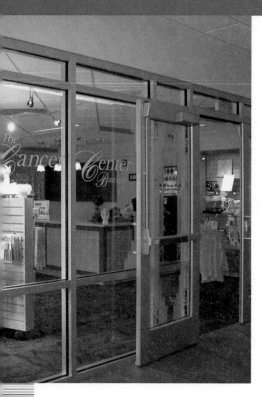

Living with Cancer and Other Chronic Conditions

What Do You Know About Cancer and Other Chronic Conditions?

1. The incidence of cancer is highest during childhood but declines with age. True or False?

2. Lung cancer is the leading cause of cancer deaths in both adult males and adult females. True or False?

3. Clear strategies, based on lifestyle changes, now exist to prevent nearly all cancers. True or False?

4. Type 1 diabetes mellitus and type 2 diabetes mellitus are exactly the same condition, except that one form requires the use of insulin (from outside the body) and the other does not. True or False?

5. Irritable bowel syndrome becomes defined as irritable bowel disease if more than one year of treatment does not result in significant improvement. True or False?

6. Multiple sclerosis (MS) is a chronic condition of the nervous system, although its cause lies in the abnormal functioning of the immune system. True or False?

7. Alzheimer's disease is a condition reflecting changes to the brain's ability to use neurotransmitters in the normal manner. True or False?

Check your answers at the end of the chapter.

Most people can attest to the disruptive influence an illness can have on their ability to participate in day-to-day activities. When we are ill, school, employment, and leisure activities are replaced by periods of lessened activity and even periods of bed rest or hospitalization. When an illness is chronic, the effect of being ill may extend over long periods, perhaps even an entire lifetime. People with chronic illness must eventually find a balance between day-to-day function and the continuous presence of their condition. Cancer is usually a chronic illness.

In spite of our understanding of its relationship to human health and our ceaseless attempts to prevent and cure it, progress in the "war on cancer" has been relatively limited. In this regard, cancer is an "expensive" condition, in terms of both its human consequences and its monetary costs. However, concurrent with these costs are clear declines in the rate at which both breast and lung cancer are being diagnosed in the United States, and the survival rate for some types of cancer has significantly improved over the past several decades. Conversely, on the world stage, the picture is increasingly darker; in 2010, cancer became the leading cause of death, and cancer-related mortality is expected to double to 15 million by 2020.[1] In this country, it is estimated that 4,529,560 people developed cancer in 2010.* Once diagnosed, approximately 68 percent (adjusted for other causes of death) of this group will be alive 5 years later.[2] This 5-year period, called *relative survivability,* includes "persons who are living 5 years after diagnosis, whether disease free, in remission, or under treatment with evidence of another cancer."[2] Understandably, the term *cured* is used guardedly since an initially diagnosed case of cancer can affect survivability beyond the end of the 5-year time period. Regardless of survivability, for those who develop cancer, the physical, emotional, and social costs will be substantial.

No single explanation can be given for why progress in eliminating cancer has been so limited. It is a combination of factors, including the aging of the population, continued use of tobacco, the high-fat American diet, the continuing urbanization and pollution of our environment, the lack of health insurance for an estimated 46 million Americans to pay for early diagnosis and proper treatment,[3] or simply our delayed recognition of cancer's true role in deaths once ascribed to other causes. Regardless, we continue to be challenged to control this array of abnormal conditions that we collectively call cancer. There is, however, increasing optimism that with a greater understanding of cancer genetics, new pharmacological agents, and the development of vaccines to prevent and treat cancers, real progress will finally be made.

That said, however, perhaps the final answer to reality of cancer is most succinctly stated in Siddhartha Mukherjee's *The Emperor of All Maladies: A Biography of Cancer.*[4]

 TALKING POINTS A close friend justifies her high-cancer-risk lifestyle by saying that "everyone will die of something." How would you counter this point?

*This figure does not include the majority of noninvasive cancers (carcinoma *in situ*), nor the million or more squamous cell and basal cell skin cancers.

Cancer: A Problem of Cell Regulation

Just as a corporation depends on individuals to staff its various departments, the body depends on its basic units of function, the cells. Cells band together as tissues, such as muscle tissue, to perform a prescribed function. Tissues in turn join to form organs, such as the heart, and organs are assembled into the body's several organ systems, such as the cardiovascular system. Such is the "corporate structure" of the body.

If individuals and cells are the basic units of function for their respective organizations, the failure of either to perform in a prescribed, dependable manner can erode the overall organization to the extent that it might not be able to continue. Cancer, the leading cause of death among adults under 80 years of age,[5] is a condition reflecting cell dysfunction in its most extreme form. In cancer, the normal behavior of cells ceases.

Cell Regulation

Most of the body's tissues lose cells over time. This continual loss requires that replacement cells come from areas of young and less specialized cells. The process of specialization required to turn the less specialized cells into mature cells is controlled by genes within the cells. On becoming specialized, these newest cells copy, or replicate, themselves. These two processes are carefully monitored by the cells' **regulatory genes.** Failure to regulate specialization and replication results in abnormal, or potentially cancerous, cells.

In addition to genes that regulate specialization and replication, cells also have genes designed to repair mistakes in the copying of genetic material (the basis of replication) and genes to suppress the growth of abnormal cells should it occur. Thus, repair genes and tumor suppressor genes (now separated into one of two subgroups of suppressor genes—caretaker genes [CTs] and gatekeeper genes [GKs]—that control cell death[6]), such as the *p53* gene (altered or missing in half of all cancers), can also be considered regulatory genes in place to prevent the development of abnormal cells. Should these genes fail to function properly, resulting in the development of malignant (cancerous) cells, the immune system (see Chapter 11) will ideally recognize their presence and remove them before a clinical (diagnosable) case of cancer can develop.

Because, when they are not working properly, replication, specialization, repair, and suppressor genes can

> **Key Terms**
>
> **regulatory genes** Genes that control cell specialization, replication, DNA repair, and tumor suppression.

become cancer-causing genes, or **oncogenes,** these four types of genes can also be referred to as **proto-oncogenes,** or potential oncogenes.[7] Beyond the involvement of the regulatory genes just discussed, nonregulatory genes too may hold oncogenic potential, resulting in an even wider array of cancer stimulators. Today over 200 different oncogenes have been identified, and significantly more may be discovered in the near future. Further, multiple oncogenes may be involved in the development of a particular form of cancer, and variations within an oncogene can be identified within a particular malignant tumor.

How normal genes become oncogenes is a question that cannot be completely answered at this time. Regardless, abnormal cells produce abnormal proteins, and the absence of normal proteins alters the body's ability to function appropriately, from the molecular to the organ system level.

Oncogene Formation

All cells have proto-oncogenes, so what events alter otherwise normal genes, including critically important regulatory genes, causing them to become cancer-causing genes? Three mechanisms—genetic mutations, viral infections, and carcinogens—have received much attention.

Genetic mutations develop when dividing cells miscopy genetic information. If the gene that is miscopied is a gene that controls specialization, replication, repair, or tumor suppression (a proto-oncogene), the oncogene that results will allow the formation of cancerous cells. A variety of factors, including aging, free radical formation, and radiation, are associated with the miscopying of the complex genetic information that constitutes the genes found within the cell, including those intended to prevent cancer.

Radiation from technological sources plays an increasingly greater role in the development of cancer, particularly as medical imaging technology and radioactive isotopes play an inordinately important role in the diagnosis and treatment of illnesses. Of particular concern are the high levels of the radiation generated by computer-aided tomography (CAT) scans.[8] Table 10.1 compares the amount of exposure generated by diagnostic imaging to that received on a daily basis from ambient or background radiation.

In both animals and humans, cancer-producing infectious agents, such as the feline leukemia virus in cats and the human immunodeficiency virus (HIV) and multiple forms of the human papillomavirus (HPV) in humans (see Chapter 11), have been identified. These viruses seek out cells of a particular type, such as cells of the immune system, or the lining of the cervix, and substitute some of their genetic material for some of the cells', thus converting them into virus-producing cells. In so doing, they convert proto-oncogenes into oncogenes.

Table 10.1 Average Radiation Dose to Entire Body (millisieverts)

Natural background (U.S.) per year	3.1
Airport scanner (backscatter method)	0.0001
Natural gas cooking per year	0.0004
Arm x-ray	0.001
Bone density x-ray	0.001
Highway travel per year	0.004
Dental x-ray	0.005
Domestic airline flight (five hours)	0.017
Smoking one pack of cigarettes per day for a year	0.36
Mammogram	0.4
Fukushima emergency workers per *hour*	1.0
Brain CT scan	2.0
Thyroid scan (nuclear medicine)	4.8
Brain scan (nuclear medicine)	6.9
Pelvis CT scan	10
Coronary CT angiography	16
Astronaut on space station for one year	72

Source: National Council on Radiation Protection and Measurements, RadiologyInfo.org.

Once converted into oncogenes, the altered genes are passed on through cell division.

A third possible explanation for the development of proto-oncogenes into oncogenes involves the presence of environmental agents known as *carcinogens.* Over an extended period, carcinogens, such as chemicals found in tobacco smoke, polluted air and water, toxic wastes, and even high-fat foods, may convert proto-oncogenes into oncogenes. These carcinogens may work alone or in combination with co-carcinogenic promoters (see Figure 8-1) to alter the genetic material, including regulatory genes, within cells. Thus, people might develop lung cancer only if they are exposed to the right combination of carcinogens over an extended period.

You may already see that some of the specific risk factors in each area—such as radiation in the development of mutations, sexually transmitted viruses in cancers of the reproductive tract, and smoking-introduced carcinogens in the development of lung cancer—can be moderated by adopting health-promoting behaviors.

In light of the complexity of cancer, some people in the scientific community believe that cancer can never be truly prevented. Rather, they feel that the ability to stop and then reverse cancerous changes at an early stage of development is more likely than is the prevention of this complex disease process. However, this text addresses the concepts of prevention in the belief that prevention-based practices reflect our personal contribution to the war on cancer.

The Cancerous Cell

Compared with noncancerous cells, cancer cells function in similar and dissimilar ways. It is the dissimilar aspects that often make them unpredictable and difficult to manage.

Perhaps the most unusual aspect of cancerous cells is their infinite life expectancy. Specifically, it appears that cancerous cells can produce an enzyme, *telomerase,* that blocks the cellular biological clock that informs normal cells that it is time to die.[9] In spite of this ability to live forever, cancer cells do not necessarily divide more quickly than normal cells do. In fact, they can divide at the same rate or even on occasion at a slower rate.

In addition, cancerous cells do not possess the *contact inhibition*[9] (a mechanism that influences the number of cells that can occupy a particular space at a particular time) of normal cells. In the absence of this property, cancer cells accumulate, altering the functional capacity of the tissue or organ they occupy. Further, the absence of *cellular cohesiveness*[9] (a property seen in normal cells that "keeps them at home") allows cancer cells to spread through the circulatory or lymphatic system to distant points via **metastasis** (see Figure 10-1). Interestingly, once migrating cancer cells arrive at a new area of the body, they "rediscover" their cellular cohesive capabilities. Adding to an understanding of cancer's spreading ability is a newly recognized role of pre-invasive lesions, or disruptions in the basal layer of cells at the site of tumor formation, which allow for early outward migration of malignant cells. A final unique characteristic of cancerous cells is their ability to command the circulatory system to send them additional blood supply to meet their metabolic needs and to provide additional routes for metastasis. This *angiogenesis*[9] capability of cancer cells makes them extremely hardy compared with noncancerous cells.

Cancers can be "staged" into four general categories in terms of their extent and severity:[2]

- *In situ* cancers are early cancers present only in cells in the layer of tissue of the cancer's origin.

- Localized cancers are limited to the organ in which the cancer began.

- Regional cancers have spread beyond the original site (the primary tumor) to nearby lymph nodes, organs, and/or tissues.

- Distant cancers have spread from the primary site to distant organs or lymph nodes.

The stage of a cancer strongly influences survivability; in general, *in situ* and localized cancers have higher survival rates than regional and distant cancers. Staging also affects treatment decisions. For example, *in situ* cancer of the colon is typically treated with surgery to remove a small section of colon tissue,

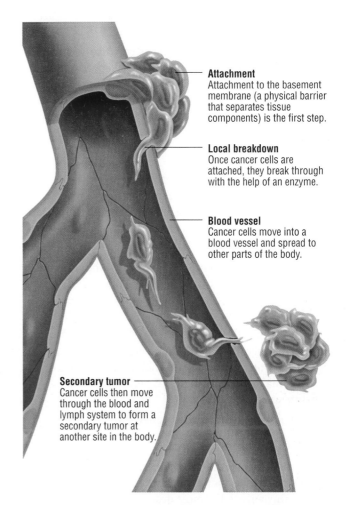

Attachment
Attachment to the basement membrane (a physical barrier that separates tissue components) is the first step.

Local breakdown
Once cancer cells are attached, they break through with the help of an enzyme.

Blood vessel
Cancer cells move into a blood vessel and spread to other parts of the body.

Secondary tumor
Cancer cells then move through the blood and lymph system to form a secondary tumor at another site in the body.

Figure 10-1 How Cancer Spreads   Locomotion (movement) is essential to the process of metastasis (spread of cancer). Scientists have identified a protein that causes cancer cells to grow arms, or pseudopodia, enabling them to move to other parts of the body.

Source: National Cancer Institute, *Horizons of Cancer Research,* NIH Pub. No. 89–3011 © 1989.

while more advanced cases of colon cancer that have spread to distant sites are treated with more extensive surgery—removal of an entire section of the colon as well as tumors in other parts of the body—along with chemotherapy and/or radiation.

> ### Key Terms
>
> **oncogenes** Faulty regulatory genes that are believed to activate the development of cancer.
>
> **proto-oncogenes** (pro toe **on** co genes) Normal regulatory genes that may become oncogenes.
>
> **metastasis** (muh **tas** ta sis) The spread of cancerous cells from their site of origin to other areas of the body.

Benign Tumors

Noncancerous, or **benign,** tumors can also form in the body. These **tumors** are usually enclosed by a membrane and do not spread from their point of origin. Benign tumors can be dangerous when they crowd out normal tissue within a confined space.

Types of Cancer

Cancers are named according to the types of cells or tissues from which they originate. Although physicians routinely use these labels, another set, to be described later, is more familiar to laypersons:

- *Carcinoma.* Found most frequently in the skin, nose, mouth, throat, stomach, intestinal tract, glands, nerves, breasts, urinary and genital structures, lungs, kidneys, and liver; approximately 85 percent of all malignant tumors are classified as carcinomas

- *Sarcoma.* Formed in the connective tissues of the body; bone, cartilage, and tendons are the sites of sarcoma development; only 2 percent of all malignancies are of this type

- *Melanoma.* Arises from the melanin-containing cells of skin; found most often in people who have had extensive sun exposure, particularly a deep, penetrating sunburn; although once rare, the incidence of this cancer has increased markedly in recent years; remains among the most deadly forms of cancer

- *Neuroblastoma.* Originates in the immature cells found within the central nervous system; neuroblastomas are rare; usually found in children

- *Adenocarcinoma.* Derived from cells of the endocrine glands

- *Hepatoma.* Originates in cells of the liver; although not thought to be directly caused by alcohol use, seen more frequently in people who have experienced **sclerotic changes** in the liver

- *Leukemia.* Found in cells of the blood and blood-forming tissues; characterized by abnormal, immature white blood cell formation; several forms are found in children and adults

- *Lymphoma.* Arises in cells of the lymphatic tissues or other immune system tissues; includes lymphosarcomas and Hodgkin's disease; characterized by abnormal white cell production and decreased resistance

Figure 10-2 presents information about the estimated new cases of cancer and deaths from cancer at various sites in both men and women.[2] Table 10.2 on page 244 shows that cancer incidence and mortality rates vary among different racial and ethnic groups.[2]

Cancer at Selected Sites in the Body

A second and more familiar way to describe cancer is on the basis of the organ site at which it occurs. The following discussion relates to some of these more familiar sites. A lack of space, in combination with the wide array of human cancers, limits the number of specific malignancies that can be described. Remember, also, that regular screening procedures can lead to early identification of cancer at these sites.

Skin Cancer

In the footnote in Figure 10-2, you will see that the American Cancer Society (ACS) excludes two of the three forms of skin cancer and reports statistics only for melanoma, the least common form of skin cancer but the most serious of the three forms. However, when all three forms (melanoma, basal cell, and squamous cell) are taken into account, skin cancer is the most common kind of cancer, with an estimated number of more than 1 million new cases in 2010.[2] When combined with recurrent cases, nearly 2 million Americans were treated for these two forms of skin cancer in 2010. On the basis of this prevalence, this textbook covers skin cancer first.

Thanks largely to our desire for a fashionable tan, many teens and adults have spent more time in the sun (and in tanning booths) than their skin can tolerate. As a result, skin cancer, once common only among people who had to work in the sun, is occurring with alarming frequency. In 2010, more than 1 million Americans developed basal or squamous cell skin cancer and 68,130 cases of highly dangerous malignant melanoma were diagnosed.[2]

Deaths from skin cancer do occur, with 11,790 estimated in 2010. About 75 percent of these deaths were the result of malignant melanoma.

Risk Factors Severe sunburning during childhood and chronic sun exposure during adolescence and younger adulthood are largely responsible for the "epidemic" of skin cancer being reported. The current emphasis on screening for skin cancer may also be increasing the

Key Terms

benign Noncancerous; localized nonmalignant tumors contained within a fibrous membrane.

tumor Mass of cells; may be cancerous (malignant) or noncancerous (benign).

sclerotic changes (skluh **rot** ick) Thickening or hardening of tissues.

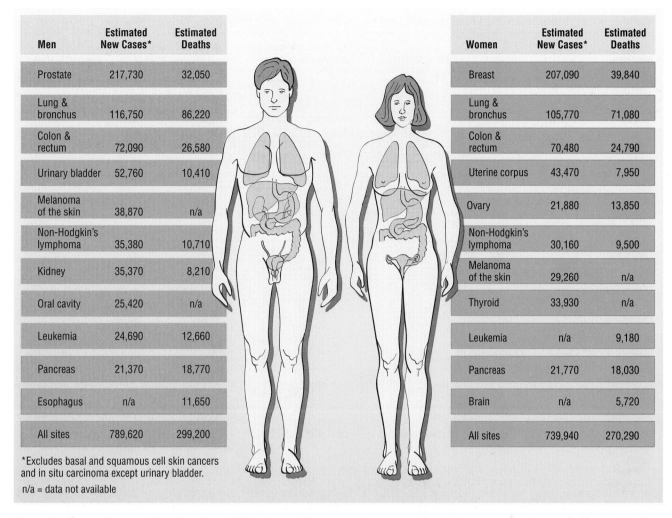

Men	Estimated New Cases*	Estimated Deaths
Prostate	217,730	32,050
Lung & bronchus	116,750	86,220
Colon & rectum	72,090	26,580
Urinary bladder	52,760	10,410
Melanoma of the skin	38,870	n/a
Non-Hodgkin's lymphoma	35,380	10,710
Kidney	35,370	8,210
Oral cavity	25,420	n/a
Leukemia	24,690	12,660
Pancreas	21,370	18,770
Esophagus	n/a	11,650
All sites	789,620	299,200

*Excludes basal and squamous cell skin cancers and in situ carcinoma except urinary bladder.

n/a = data not available

Women	Estimated New Cases*	Estimated Deaths
Breast	207,090	39,840
Lung & bronchus	105,770	71,080
Colon & rectum	70,480	24,790
Uterine corpus	43,470	7,950
Ovary	21,880	13,850
Non-Hodgkin's lymphoma	30,160	9,500
Melanoma of the skin	29,260	n/a
Thyroid	33,930	n/a
Leukemia	n/a	9,180
Pancreas	21,770	18,030
Brain	n/a	5,720
All sites	739,940	270,290

Figure 10-2 Cancer Cases and Deaths These 2010 estimates of new cases of cancer and deaths from cancer reveal some significant similarities between men and women. Note that lung cancer is the leading cause of cancer deaths for both sexes.

Source: American Cancer Society, *Cancer Facts and Figures 2010.* Atlanta: American Cancer Society, Inc.

incidence of early-stage cancer being reported. Occupational exposure to some hydrocarbon compounds can also cause skin cancer.

In spite of the progress reported by the American Academy of Dermatology, Americans continue to seek natural sources of sun or tanning salons for cosmetically related tanning, or they find that their exposure cannot be avoided owing to the nature of their jobs. In regard to "purposeful tanning" either outdoors or indoors, recent research has given some credibility to the contention that tanning is emotionally "addictive."[10] In fact, people (most frequently younger women) who are so compulsive about tanning that they do so multiple times per week are now being described as "tanorexics." During 2011, legislative bodies in several states discussed laws that would restrict adolescents from visiting tanning salons. Researchers are now beginning to see this factor as a detrimental player in ongoing efforts to persuade the public to increase their avoidance of ultraviolet radiation exposure.

Prevention Prevention of skin cancer should be a high priority for people who enjoy the sun or must work outdoors. The use of sunscreen with a sun protection factor (SPF) of 15 or greater is very important. In addition, parents can help their children prevent skin cancer later in life by restricting their outdoor play from 11 a.m. to 2 p.m. Further, it should be noted that in response to concerns over tanning and sunburns during childhood, products intended to protect children from the sun, such as high-quality sunglasses, ultraviolet (UV) blocking summer clothing and swim wear, stroller covers, and spray-on sunscreen with an SPF of 70 or higher, are now appearing in stores.

Note that controversy abounds within the scientific community as to both the effectiveness of sunscreens and the form of sunscreen used (organic versus inorganic). New technologies are under development and the current controversy may eventually be resolved, but in the meantime practicing dermatologists continue to recommend their use. However, users are reminded that the level of

Table 10.2 Incidence and Mortality Rates* by Site, Race, and Ethnicity, United States, 2002–2006

Incidence	White	African American	Asian American and Pacific Islander	American Indian and Alaska Native[†]	Hispanic/Latino[‡]
All sites					
Males	550.1	626.0	334.5	318.4	430.3
Females	420.0	389.5	276.3	265.1	326.8
Breast (female)	123.5	113.0	81.6	67.2	90.2
Colon & rectum					
Males	58.2	68.4	44.1	38.1	50.0
Females	42.6	51.7	33.1	30.7	35.1
Kidney & renal pelvis					
Males	19.7	20.6	9.0	16.6	18.2
Females	10.3	10.6	4.5	10.6	10.3
Liver & bile duct					
Males	8.0	12.5	21.4	8.9	15.9
Females	2.8	3.8	8.1	4.6	6.2
Lung & bronchus					
Males	85.9	104.8	50.6	57.9	49.2
Females	57.1	50.7	27.6	41.3	26.5
Prostate	146.3	231.9	82.3	82.7	131.1
Stomach					
Males	8.9	16.7	17.5	9.4	14.3
Females	4.2	8.5	9.8	4.7	8.6
Uterine cervix	7.9	11.1	7.6	6.6	12.7

Mortality	White	African American	Asian American and Pacific Islander	American Indian and Alaska Native[†]	Hispanic/Latino[‡]
All sites					
Males	226.7	304.2	135.4	183.3	154.8
Females	157.3	183.7	95.1	140.1	103.9
Breast (female)	23.9	33.0	12.5	17.6	15.5
Colon & rectum					
Males	21.4	31.4	13.8	20.0	16.1
Females	14.9	21.6	10.0	13.7	10.7
Kidney & renal pelvis					
Males	6.1	6.0	2.4	9.0	5.2
Female	2.8	2.7	1.2	4.2	2.4
Liver & bile duct					
Males	6.8	10.8	15.0	10.3	11.3
Females	2.9	3.9	6.10	6.5	5.1
Lung & bronchus					
Males	69.9	90.1	36.9	48.0	33.9
Females	41.9	40.0	18.2	33.5	14.4
Prostate	23.6	56.3	10.6	20.0	19.6
Stomach					
Males	4.8	11.0	9.6	9.8	8.3
Females	2.4	5.3	5.8	4.6	4.8
Uterine cervix	2.2	4.6	2.2	3.4	3.1

*Per 100,000, age adjusted to the 2000 US standard population.

[†]Data based on Contract Health Service Delivery Areas, comprising about 55 percent of the U.S. American Indian/Alaska Native population; for more information, please see: Espey DK, Wu XC, Swan J, et al., Annual report to the nation on the status of cancer, 1975–2004, featuring cancer in American Indians and Alaska Natives.

[‡]Persons of Hispanic/Latino origin may be of any race.

Source: Edwards BK, Ward E, Kohler BA, et al., Annual report to the nation on the status of cancer, 1975–2006, *Cancer*, 16, 544–573, 2010.

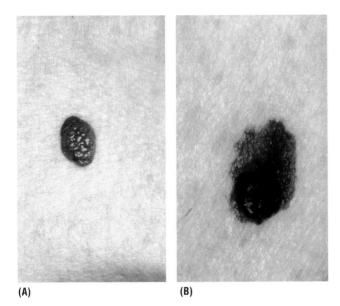

(A)   **(B)**

Figure 10-3 Normal Mole Versus Malignant Melanoma   A: Normal mole. This type of lesion is often seen in large numbers on the skin of young adults and can affect any body site. Note its symmetrical shape, regular borders, uniform color, and relatively small size (actual size is about 6 millimeters). **B:** Malignant melanoma. Note its asymmetrical shape, irregular borders, uneven color, and relatively large size (actual size is about 2 centimeters).

protection provided is not doubled by simply doubling the SPF—for example, a sunscreen carrying an SPF of 30 does not provide twice the protection provided by a product with an SPF of 15. Today it is believed that an SPF above 50 is unnecessary, and the FDA has altered the labeling standard for sunscreens, making 50+ the highest SPF that can be used on a product's label.

Early Detection   Although many doctors do not emphasize this point enough, the key to the successful treatment of skin cancer is early detection. For basal cell or squamous cell cancer, a pale, waxlike, pearly nodule or red, scaly patch may be the first symptom. Other types of skin cancer may be indicated by a gradual change in the appearance of an existing mole. A physician should be consulted if such a change is noted. Melanoma usually begins as a small, molelike growth that increases progressively in size, changes color, ulcerates, and bleeds easily. To help detect melanoma, the American Cancer Society recommends using the following guidelines:[2] **A** for asymmetry, **B** for border irregularity, **C** for color (change), and **D** for a diameter greater than 6 mm.

Figure 10-3 shows a mole that would be considered harmless and one that clearly demonstrates the ABCD characteristics just described. The box "Self-Examination for Melanoma" shows how to make a regular inspection of the skin.

Table 10.3 lists cancer's seven warning signs.

Table 10.3   Cancer's Seven Warning Signs

Listed below are the seven warning signs of cancer, which the acronym CAUTION will help you remember.

1. **C**hange in bowel or bladder habits
2. **A** sore that does not heal
3. **U**nusual bleeding or discharge
4. **T**hickening or lump in the breast or elsewhere
5. **I**ndigestion or difficulty in swallowing
6. **O**bvious change in a wart or mole
7. **N**agging cough or hoarseness

If you have a warning sign for more than five days, see your doctor!

Treatment   When nonmelanoma skin cancer is found, an almost 100 percent cure rate can be expected. Treatment of these skin cancers can involve surgical removal by traditional excising or laser vaporization, destruction by burning or freezing, or destruction using x-ray therapy. When the more serious melanomas are found at an early stage, a high cure rate (99 percent) is accomplished using the same techniques. However, when malignant melanomas are more advanced, extensive surgery and chemotherapy are necessary. The five-year survival rate for regionalized forms of the disease drops to 63 percent, and, unfortunately, long-term disease recovery is uncommon (15 percent).[2]

In addition to "regular" skin cancer and malignant melanoma, a second form of highly lethal skin cancer, *Merkel cell carcinoma,* is beginning to receive much needed attention.[11] This infrequently seen form of cancer first appears as a painless bump that can be mistaken for a cyst. If not excised at an early point, a biopsy performed, and then treated aggressively with radiation, this malignancy has a very high mortality rate.

Lung Cancer

Lung cancer is one of the most lethal and frequently diagnosed forms of cancer. Primarily because of the advanced stage of the disease at the time symptoms first appear, only 16 percent of all people with lung cancer (all stages) survive 5 years beyond diagnosis.[2] By the time a person is sufficiently concerned about having a persistent cough, blood-streaked sputum, and chest pain, it is often too late for treatment to be effective. This failure to be able to diagnose lung cancer in its earlier stages could, however, begin to change. Currently, the National Cancer Institute is studying the efficacy of *spiral CT scans* in detecting lung tumors earlier than can be done by conventional chest X-rays. Although this technology has resulted in earlier recognition of masses, there at first appeared to be little improvement in survivability that could be directly attributed to this spiral CT technology. A longitudinal study, the National Lung Screening Trial, that was completed in 2010 did, however, show a modest reduction in deaths among those who had received CT scans versus

Self-Examination for Melanoma

Through a routine physical exam, my brother found out he has melanoma. How should I check myself for this condition?

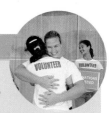

How to look for melanoma

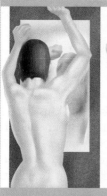 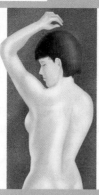 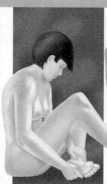 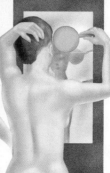 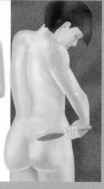

1. Examine your body front and back in the mirror, then right and left sides with arms raised.

2. Bend your elbows and carefully look at your palms, forearms, and under your upper arms.

3. Look at the backs of your legs and feet, the spaces between your toes, and the soles of your feet.

4. Examine the back of your neck and scalp with a hand mirror. Part your hair for a closer look.

5. Finally, check your back and buttocks with a mirror.

What to look for
Potential signs of malignancy in moles or pigmented spots:

Asymmetry

One half unlike the other half

Irregularity Border

Border irregular or poorly defined

Color

Color varies from one area to another; shades of tan, brown, or black

Diameter

Diameter larger than 6 mm, as a rule (diameter of a pencil eraser)

Source: Based on information from the American Academy of Dermatology.

---

conventional chest x-rays.[12] Currently, little third-party (insurance and Medicare) coverage exists for this form of lung cancer screening.

Risk Factors Today it is known that genetic predisposition is important in the development of lung cancer. Perhaps, in fact, the majority of people who develop this form of cancer have an inherited "head start." When people who are genetically at risk also smoke, their level of risk for developing lung cancer is significantly greater than it is for nonsmokers. Of particular interest at this time are multiple genes on chromosome 3. Damage to three tumor suppressors on this chromosome is found in virtually every case of small-cell lung cancer and 90 percent of cases of nonsmall-cell lung cancer. Most of the remaining lung cancer cases appear in people who smoke but are not genetically predisposed.

Cigarette smoking is unquestionably the single most important behavioral factor in the development of lung cancer. For men who smoke, the rate of lung cancer is 23 times higher than it is for men who do not smoke. For women who smoke, the rate is 13 times higher than for women who do not smoke. Smokers account for 87 percent of all reported cases of lung cancer, and lung cancer itself accounts for at least 28 percent of all cancer-caused deaths.[2]

Since 1987, lung cancer has exceeded breast cancer as the leading cause of cancer death in women, although more new cases of breast cancer than lung cancer are diagnosed each year. The incidence of lung cancer in men has shown a gradual decline over the last several years that parallels their declining use of tobacco products. In contrast to men, in women the rate of lung cancer development has remained relatively constant over the last several years. Women tend to develop a different form of lung

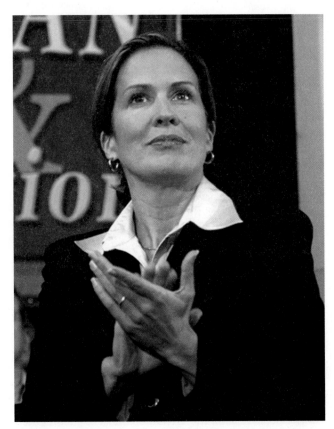

In August 2005, shortly after the death of her husband (actor Christopher Reeve) following a tragic equestrian accident, Dana Reeve shocked the nation by announcing that she had contracted a highly lethal form of lung cancer. Neither Mrs. Reeve nor her husband had been smokers. She died of the disease in March 2006.

cancer than men, suggesting that they might absorb toxins more completely than men do. Also, among nonsmokers, women are more likely to develop lung cancer, although recent studies have challenged this conclusion. The tumor type found in women may also be estrogen-sensitive, as is true for forms of breast cancer, in comparison to the primary type developed by men.[13] On a cautious note, in March 2011, it was reported that during the period 2003–2007, deaths from lung cancer in women dropped by 1.6 percent—a small but positive reduction following a plateau in the years prior to the period of study.

Environmental agents, such as radon, asbestos, beryllium, uranium, and air pollutants, make a smaller contribution to the development of lung cancer. Radon alone may be the principal causative agent in most lung cancer found in nonsmokers.

Prevention The preceding information clearly suggests that not smoking or quitting smoking and avoiding secondhand tobacco smoke (see Chapter 8) are the most important factors in the prevention of lung cancer. In addition, place of residence, particularly as it relates to air pollution, is a long-suspected risk factor for lung cancer. Nonsmokers who are considering living with a smoker or working in a confined area where secondhand tobacco smoke is prevalent should carefully consider the risk of developing lung cancer. A recent study does, however, lessen concern over moderate alcohol use and the risk of developing lung cancer.

Treatment The prognosis for surviving lung cancer remains extremely guarded. Depending on the type of lung cancer, its extent, and factors related to the patient's overall health, various combinations of surgery, radiation, and chemotherapy remain the physicians' primary approach to treatment. Today, for persons with early-stage lung cancer, chemotherapy, following surgery, has increased survivability slightly. Additionally, new medications that primarily shrink tumors are available. Experimental vaccines (LBLP25, TGF_beta2 antisense gene vaccine, GVAX) now in the early stages of testing have shown encouraging results in patients with nonsmall-cell lung cancer, the most common form of the disease.

In addition to progress being made in vaccine development, new medications are in various stages of clinical trials, including crizotinib, for use in cases of advanced lung cancer. Tumor shrinkage was evident in over 60 percent of the patients taking the drug; whether this reduction in tumor size equates with life extension has not yet been determined.[14]

In spite of the new vaccines and medications mentioned, in combination with older approaches to treating lung cancer, such as surgery, radiation, and chemotherapies, the level of improvement in survivability from lung cancer is nearly static (with some regional variability). In the opinion of experts, significant improvement cannot occur in the absence of even more aggressive reductions in smoking, particularly among women.[15]

Colorectal Cancer

Colorectal cancer—cancer of the colon (large intestine) and the rectum (terminal portion of the large intestine)—is the third most common kind of new cancer (excluding skin cancers) in both males and females; the second leading cause of cancer deaths in males (behind lung cancer); and the third leading cause of cancer deaths in females (behind lung and breast cancers; see Figure 10-2). Fortunately, when diagnosed in a localized state, colorectal cancer has a relatively high survival rate (91 percent when localized and 70 percent for all stages).[2]

Risk Factors Underlying the development of colorectal cancer are at least two potentially important areas of risk: genetic susceptibility and dietary patterns. Genes have recently been discovered that lead to familial colon cancer and familial polyposis (abnormal tissue growth that occurs before the formation of cancer) and are believed to be responsible for the tendency of colorectal cancer to run in families. Dietary risk factors include diets that are high in saturated fat from red meat and possibly too low in fruits and vegetables, which contain antioxidant vitamins and fiber. In regard to fiber's ability to prevent colorectal cancer, however, the ability of dietary fiber, when taken in supplement form, is in question. In addition to familial and dietary links to an increased risk of colorectal cancer, alcohol use and smoking (alone or in combination) also appear related, particularly in terms of age of onset. In persons who regularly drink and/or smoke, colorectal cancer may appear years earlier than in people who do not. This pattern was particularly noted in males.[16]

Prevention   Small outpouchings in the lower intestinal tract wall, called *polyps,* are frequently important in the eventual development of colorectal cancer. Prompt removal of polyps has been shown to lower the risk of colorectal cancer. Further, some evidence indicates that the development of colorectal cancer may be prevented or slowed through regular exercise, an increase in dietary calcium intake, and long-term folic acid supplementation. Additionally, oral contraceptive use may be protective for women.

Recently, the belief that the consistent use of a low-dose (81-mg) aspirin could reduce polyp formation was strongly disputed and is no longer recommended by the American Cancer Association for this purpose (although low-dose aspirin therapy is recommended in conjunction with cardiovascular disease prevention). Having said this about aspirin's relationship to colorectal cancer, it should be noted that a 2010 meta-analysis of five European studies, over a 20-year period and involving 14,000 persons, demonstrated a strong preventive effect from the use of low-dose (81-mg) aspirin over a period of 6 years.[17]

Again, routine screening for colorectal cancer should be considered a form of prevention, much as PSA testing is for prostate cancer and mammography is for breast cancer.

Early Detection   Symptoms of colorectal cancer include bleeding from the rectum, blood in the stool, and a change in bowel habits. In addition, a family history of inflammatory bowel disease, polyp formation, or colorectal cancer should make one more alert to symptoms.[2] In people over age 50, any sudden change in bowel habits that lasts 10 days or longer should be evaluated by a physician. The American

Cancer Society's recommendations for colorectal cancer screening, beginning at age 50—including fecal occult blood tests, flexible **sigmoidoscopy** examinations, double-contrast barium enema examinations, and **colonoscopy** examinations—are detailed in Table 10.4. However, on the basis of information gleaned from recent studies, smokers and regular users of alcohol could expect recommendations for earlier screening, beginning at age 45.

In 2008, additional colorectal cancer screen recommendations introduced by other medical organizations broadened the basic guidelines issued by the American Cancer Society (see page 249). Principal among these were recommendations by the U.S. Preventive Services Task Force regarding (1) discontinuation of *routine* colorectal screen for adults ages 76–85 (although remaining responsive, via examination, to episodic signs of disease) and (2) discontinuation of all screening for persons over 85.[18]

A second alternative viewing technique of the colon and rectum is the use of computerized axial tomography (CT) scanning of the lower intestinal tract. Although adequately effective, this procedure also requires the preparation whose fear causes so many people to disregard the need for any colorectal screening. Additionally, some important limitations are recognized, as well as the risk of radiation exposure produced by the procedure. On the positive side, the virtual colonoscopy (computed tomography colonography, or CTC) is capable of identifying extracolonic (outside the colon) abnormalities, including solid masses.[19]

It should also be noted that the digital stool-sample test, used as the only stool-sample test by many doctors and taken during physical examinations, as well as the newer test to find traces of cancer cell DNA in the stool, have both been found to be less effective than previously believed.

Treatment   When one or more of these screening procedures suggests the possibility of disease within the lower intestinal tract, a careful visual evaluation of the entire length of the colon will be undertaken. During colonoscopy, areas of concern can be biopsied and the presence of a malignancy confirmed. Upon diagnosis, a localized and noninvasive malignancy will be removed surgically. When an invasive tumor is identified, supportive treatment with radiation or chemotherapy is necessary. Metastatic cancer requires chemotherapy.

Breast Cancer

Surpassed only by lung cancer, breast cancer is the second leading cause of death from cancer in women. It is the third leading cause of cancer deaths overall. Nearly one in eight women will develop breast cancer in her lifetime, resulting in an estimated 207,090 new invasive cases and 39,840 deaths in 2010. In men, an estimated 1,970 new cases and 390 deaths occurred in 2010 (see the box "Breast Cancer: A Rare Diagnosis in Men" on

---

Key Terms

sigmoidoscopy Examination of the sigmoid colon (lowest section of the large intestine), using a short, flexible fiber-optic scope.

colonoscopy (co lun **os** ko py) Examination of the entire length of the colon, using a flexible fiber-optic scope to inspect the structure's inner lining.

Table 10.4 Screening Guidelines for the Early Detection of Cancer

Cancer Site	Population	Test or Procedures	Frequency
Breast	Women, age 20+	Breast self-examination	Beginning in their early 20s, women should be told about benefits/limitations of breast self-examination. Women should know how their breasts normally feel and report any breast change promptly to their health care provider.
		Clinical breast examination	Clinical breast exams should be part of a periodic health exam every three years for women in their 20s and 30s, and every year for women 40+.
		Mammography	Yearly mammograms are recommended starting at age 40.
Colon and rectum	Men and women, age 50+	Flexible sigmoidoscopy or	Every five years, starting at age 50.
		Colonoscopy or	Every 10 years, starting at age 50.
		Double-contrast barium enema (DCBE) or	Every five years, starting at age 50.
		CT colonography (virtual colonoscopy)	Every five years, starting at age 50.
		Fecal occult blood test or	Yearly starting at age 50.
		Stool DNA test (sDNA)	Starting at age 50. Discuss interval with health care provider.
Prostate	Men, age 50+	Prostate-specific antigen test (PSA) with or without digital rectal exam (DRE)	Men without symptoms and with at least a 10-year life expectancy should make an informed decision with their health care provider regarding prostate cancer screening beginning at age 50. Men at a higher risk should make an informed decision at age 40.
Cervix	Women, age 18+	Pap test	Cervical cancer screening should begin yearly approximately three years after a woman begins having vaginal intercourse, but no later than 21 years of age.
Endometrial	Women, at menopause	At the time of menopause, women of average risk should be informed about risks and symptoms of endometrial cancer and strongly encouraged to report any unexpected bleeding or spotting to their health care provider.	
Cancer-related checkup	Men and women, age 20+	A cancer-related checkup should be performed during periodic health examinations to check for cancers of the thyroid, testicles, ovaries, lymph nodes, oral cavity, and skin, as well as health counseling about tobacco use, sun exposure, diet and nutrition, risk factors, sexual practices, and environmental and occupational exposure.	

Source: Based on information in *American Cancer Society, Cancer Facts and Figures 2010*. Atlanta: American Cancer Society.

page 250).[2] As women age, their risk of developing breast cancer increases. Early detection is the key to complete recovery. Today, 98 percent of women whose breast cancer is localized (confined to the breast) survive more than five years.

Most recently, it has been reported that the actual rate of new cases of breast cancer has declined. According to data from 2006 (the last year for which actual versus estimated numbers of new cases of various forms of cancer are known), an annual decline of 2 percent in new breast cancer cases was reported. Initial interpretation of this dramatic finding relates to a sharp decline in the use of hormone replacement therapy (HRT) and a disturbing decline in the use of mammograms.[2]

Risk Factors   Although all women and men are at some risk of developing breast cancer, the following groups of women have a higher risk:

- Women whose menstrual periods began at an early age, or whose menopause occurred late (although the former may be more important than the latter is)

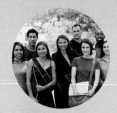

Learning from Our Diversity

Breast Cancer: A Rare Diagnosis in Men

With all the attention given to breast cancer in women—in the news, by physicians, and by research foundations—you may be surprised to learn that men are also diagnosed with this condition. For every 100 women who develop breast cancer, however, only one case is reported among men. Estimates for the year 2010 suggest that no more than 1,970 American men will develop breast cancer. When compared to the 207,090 cases anticipated in women during the same year, the rarity of breast cancer in men becomes apparent.[2]

The typical male breast cancer victim is usually older than 60 and often has a family history of the disease. The *BRCA2* tumor suppressor gene mutation is also found within the victim's genetic lineage. In some cases, the male breast cancer victim has the inherited condition of Klinefelter's syndrome, in which a second X (or female) sex chromosome is present. The extra sex chromosome produces enhanced estrogen within the male body, resulting in adolescent development of prominent breasts and a higher risk of breast cancer later in life.

Other conditions, such as various forms of liver disease, also result in higher levels of estrogen and, eventually, a greater risk of male breast cancer.

In most ways, male breast cancer is very similar in type to that seen in women. Infiltrating ductal cancer, ductal carcinoma *in situ,* and a form of cancer arising from the ducts immediately beneath the nipple (Paget's disease) have been reported. Because of this close similarity to female breast cancer, medical management of male breast cancer closely parallels that seen in women. Surgery (a modified radical mastectomy), chemotherapy, external radiation, and hormonal therapy are used alone or in combination. The latter therapy may include not only drugs to block the influence of estrogen on estrogen-sensitive cancer cells but removal of testicles as well. As with virtually all forms of cancer, early diagnosis and treatment are of critical importance.

Source: American Cancer Society & *Cancer Facts & Figures—2010.*

- Women who had no children, had their first child later in life, or did not breast-feed
- Women who have used hormone replacement therapy (HRT), particularly combined estrogen and progestin or combined estrogen and testosterone
- Women who have a high degree of breast density (high level of glandular tissues relative to fat) or biopsy-established hyperplasia
- Women whose diets are high in saturated fats, who are sedentary, or who are obese after menopause (particularly central body cavity obesity; see Chapter 6)
- Women who carry the *BRCA1* and/or *BRCA2* mutated tumor suppressor genes, or women with a strong family history of breast cancer

As mentioned, significant concern exists regarding the long-term use of hormone replacement therapy and the development of breast cancer in postmenopausal women. Many physicians are now advising that HRT be used only on a very short-term basis to relieve the symptoms of menopause, rather than the much longer period of time previously deemed appropriate.

While initial concerns about the risk of breast cancer in postmenopausal women were centered on the use of HRT medication combining estrogen and progesterone, recent attention is being directed to those using HRTs that combine estrogen and testosterone. These medications, often compounded (formulated) by pharmacists on the directions of a physician, may increase the risk of more invasive breast cancer.

The effects of environmental pollutants and regional influences have also been investigated as causative factors in the development of breast cancer. Environmental pollutants vary from region to region and are influenced by a number of factors, including the type of industrial and agricultural activity in a particular area. A wide array of regional factors may be involved, including the genetic background of people in a given area and lifestyle differences involving diet, alcohol consumption, and exercise patterns.

The role of genetic predisposition in the development of breast cancer has also received considerable attention. For example, a small percentage (perhaps 5 percent) of women with breast cancer have inherited or developed mutations in one or both of two tumor suppressor genes (proto-oncogenes), *BRCA1* and *BRCA2*. Discovered in 1994 and 1995, respectively, and currently the focus of extensive research, more than 200 mutations in these genes have been identified. In a study involving 5,000 Ashkenazi Jews (Jews of Central and Eastern European descent) living in the Washington, DC, area, mutation in the *BRCA1* gene resulted in a 56 percent greater chance of developing breast cancer by age 70 (versus a 13 percent greater risk for people without a mutated version of the gene).[20] In the years since these genes' identification, studies have been ongoing in an attempt to more accurately define the level of risk for developing breast cancer among women who carry one or both *BRCA1* or *BRCA2* mutations, regardless of race or other aspects of ethnicity.[21] Both of these genes are also associated with increased risk of developing ovarian cancer (see page 257) and, perhaps, prostate cancer in men.

Other genetic links to breast cancer have been identified. For example, one involves an increased risk for breast cancer development in Black women. The gene

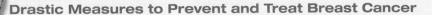

Drastic Measures to Prevent and Treat Breast Cancer

When a combination of risk factors for breast cancer exists, including having a mother or sister who has developed breast cancer, having a high prevalence of breast cancer in family members over time, being a carrier of a breast cancer–related mutated gene, or having already had breast cancer, an increasing number of young women are electing to undergo prophylactic mastectomy. This decision was made in 2008 by actress Christina Applegate.

In Ms. Applegate's case, a number of risk factors coalesced by an early age, including having a mother who had breast cancer, the identification of herself as a *BRCA1* carrier, an early-stage malignancy in one breast, and suspicious masses removed from the other breast. Driven by these realities, she made the decision to have removed not only the breast in which cancer had already been diagnosed, but the other breast as well.

As mentioned in the textbook, the *BRCA1/2* genes also bear a heightened relationship to ovarian cancer and to prostate cancer in males. Perhaps after some time and based upon careful monitoring, including MRIs, women who have had a preventive mastectomy, such as Ms. Applegate, might also consider bilateral removal of the ovaries.

---

in question is *BPI*, a gene that, if shut off, allows cancer cells to establish cellular immortality. Two additional gene mutations play important roles in the development of breast cancer and provide direction in the treatment of this cancer. These are the *p53* tumor suppressor gene and the *HER-2* gene. Other mutated genes also play cancer-promoting roles, including one that influences the synthesis of estrogen, a hormone that stimulates the development of some forms of breast cancer.

Prevention   As already discussed, a variety of risk factors are thought to be important in the development of most cases of breast cancer. Accordingly, some degree of prevention is possible when factors such as diet; alcohol use; physical activity level; decisions about contraception, pregnancy, and breast-feeding; occupational exposure to toxins; and even place of residence are considered.

For women who have a primary family history of breast cancer (sisters, mother, or grandmothers with the disease) and who have been found to carry one or both of the *BRCA* genes discussed, an extreme form of prevention is also possible— **prophylactic mastectomy.** In this surgical procedure, both noncancerous breasts are removed, in an attempt to eliminate the possibility of future cancer development (see the box "Drastic Measures to Prevent and Treat Breast Cancer").

At the present time, pharmacological prevention represents the newest approach to reducing the incidence of breast cancer. Intended for women with a high risk for the development of breast cancer (**Gail Score** higher than 1.66), two estrogen-related approaches are presently available.[22] The first involves the use of one of two medications (estrogen receptor modulators) that block the ability of estrogen to bind with potentially malignant breast cells whose future progression toward malignancy would be "fueled" by access to estrogen. The first of the two drugs is tamoxifen (Nolvadex) and the second is raloxifene (Evista). Both medications have relatively similar side effects, and both carry some risks for potentially serious conditions, such as blood clots, endometrial (uterine wall) cancer, cataracts, and strokes. A woman

considering chemoprevention will be carefully screened in terms of selecting the specific medication most compatible with her biomedical profile.

The third class of medications used in breast cancer chemoprevention are collectively known as aromatase inhibitors and function by decreasing the amount of estrogen produced in the body, rather than by blocking its availability to breast cells. Although not approved for use by premenopausal women, in postmenopausal women the aromatase inhibitors have been used in both treatment and chemoprevention of breast cancer. The principal risks in using this class of medication relate to fractures and the development of osteoporosis.

Early Detection: Breast Self-Examination   For several decades, a fundamental component of early detection of breast cancer has been breast self-examination (BSE). Generally recommended for women 20 years of age and older, the procedure was to be performed during the menstrual period or on the day immediately following the end of the menstrual period, when estrogen levels are at their lowest and cystic activity in breast tissue is minimal (or on the same day of each month by postmenopausal women). The proper technique is illustrated in the box "Breast Self-Examination." Although BSE is an easily learned technique, today its role as the primary method of detecting breast cancer in its earliest stage has been usurped by clinical breast examination (CBE)

Key Terms

prophylactic mastectomy   Surgical removal of the breasts to prevent breast cancer in women who are at high risk of developing the disease.

Gail Score   A numerical expression of the risk of developing invasive breast cancer, based on several variables, such as age at first menstrual period, age at first live birth, results of previous biopsies, and a family history of breast cancer. A score of 1.66 percent reflects a high level of risk.

Breast Self-Examination

I've never felt confident about doing a breast self-exam. What is the proper technique?

- Lie down and place your right arm behind your head. The exam is done while lying down, not standing up. This is because when you are lying down, your breast tissue spreads evenly over your chest wall and is as thin as possible, making it much easier to feel all the breast tissue.

- Use the finger pads of the three middle fingers on your left hand to feel for lumps in the right breast. Use overlapping, dime-size circular motions of the finger pads to feel the breast tissue.

- Use three different levels of pressure to feel all the breast tissue. Light pressure is needed to feel the tissue closest to the skin, medium pressure to feel a little deeper, and firm pressure to feel the tissue closest to the chest and ribs. A firm ridge in the lower curve of each breast is normal. If you're not sure how hard to press, talk with your doctor or nurse. Use each pressure level to feel the breast tissue before moving on to the next spot.

- Move around the breast in an up-and-down pattern starting at an imaginary line drawn straight down your side from the underarm and moving across the breast to the middle of the chest bone (sternum or breastbone). Be sure to check the entire breast area, moving downward until you feel only ribs and up to the neck or collarbone (clavicle). There is some evidence that the up-and-down pattern (sometimes called the vertical pattern) is the most effective pattern for covering the entire breast without missing any breast tissue.

- Repeat the exam on your left breast, using the finger pads of your right hand.

- While standing in front of a mirror with your hands pressing firmly down on your hips, look at your breasts for any changes of size, shape, contour, dimpling, pulling, or redness or scaliness of the nipple or breast skin. (Pressing your hands down on your hips contracts the chest wall muscles and enhances any breast changes.) Continue to look for changes with your arms down at your sides, and then with your arms raised up over your head with your palms pressed together.

- Examine each underarm while sitting up or standing and with your arm only slightly raised so you can easily feel in this area. Raising your arm straight up tightens the tissue in this area and makes it difficult to examine it.

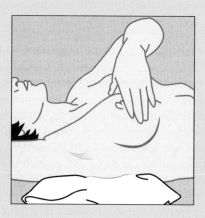
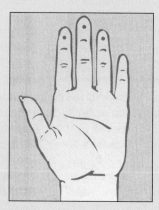
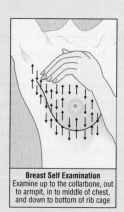

Breast Self Examination
Examine up to the collarbone, out to armpit, in to middle of chest, and down to bottom of rib cage

performed by a physician during scheduled checkups and by mammography and other imaging technologies. However, CBE also has been a source of some concern because of the inconsistencies among clinicians in performing the procedure. Steps have now been taken to correct this, and the American Cancer Society continues to strongly endorse its role in early breast cancer detection. Additionally, during physician visits in which CBE has been done, the ACS recommends that women review, with their clinicians, their own BSE techniques.

In any case, monthly BSE can be viewed as an adjunct to regularly scheduled breast examinations conducted by a physician (CBE) and to the routine use of mammography.

Early Detection: Mammography Although researchers once disagreed about the age at which women should begin routine mammography and the extent to which mammography is effective in finding masses in dense breast tissue, today mammograms are physicians' best tool for the early detection of breast cancer. Accordingly, the ACS recommends that mammography begin at age 40.

Whether women begin routine mammography at 40, as advised by the ACS, or earlier, particularly for women with previous symptoms or a family history of breast disease, women should continue these examinations on an annual basis. Recommendations regarding mammography for older women (age 65 and older) are, however, a bit more individually determined and should be discussed annually with physicians. For older women, overall health status and expectations for reaching a normal life expectancy are weighed relative to the lessening cost-effectiveness of mammography.

Because of the important role routine mammography plays in the early identification of breast lesions, the Mammography Quality Standards Act (MQSA) is a valuable step toward ensuring that mammography is performed by experienced technicians, using correctly calibrated equipment, and interpreted by skilled radiologists. Every woman should be certain that her mammography is being performed in an MQSA-certified facility. Table 10.4 on page 249 provides screening guidelines for breast and other cancers.

In February 2011, the FDA announced the approval of three-dimensional (3-D) mammography (aka digital breast tomosynthesis). Early studies indicate a modest (7 percent) improvement in identifying cancerous breast tumors over two-dimensional digital mammography.[23]

Treatment The modern treatment of breast cancer involves a compliant interplay of the patient (and her family) with a variety of medical care professionals to deliver the most effective treatment available for the type and stage of the disease. Central to the team are, among others, the radiologist, general surgeon, pathologist, plastic-reconstructive surgeon, radiation oncologist, chemotherapy oncologists, a large array of technical support staff, and those providing continuous patient care. Not every position named will be involved with every breast cancer patient, but all constitute the clinical resources available in a major cancer center.

If it can be assumed there is a "typical" case of breast cancer, it will most often involve a combination of major treatment modalities, including surgery, radiation therapy, chemotherapy, reconstructive surgery (if elected), and a period of rehabilitation, often using physical therapy or a tailored exercise program to maintain strength and flexibility in the shoulder girdle. In some cases, maintenance chemotherapy may continue well beyond the more familiar treatment period.

In the interest of brevity, only selected aspects of the postsurgical treatment protocol will be briefly described.[24]

Chemotherapy involves the use of drugs delivered intravenously or in pill form for the purpose of killing (in one or more manners) portions of a tumor that were incapable of being adequately addressed by surgery or cells that may have migrated to a location beyond the primary tumor site.

Radiation therapy, in a wide array of forms including brachytherapy, gamma knife therapy, and stereotactic radiosurgery, is intended to kill malignant cells during specific stages of cell division in which their genetic material is particularly vulnerable to the effects of radiation. The rapid replication rate of cancer cells makes radiation more effective in killing cancer cells than neighboring exposed cells above, below, and near the treatment field, such as those of skin, glandular tissue, vascular tissue, nervous tissue, and underlying musculature. Radiation physicists are routinely engaged in the planning of the type and extent of radiation to use.

Hormone therapy, similar in some ways to chemotherapy, is, as the name implies, directed at reducing the presence of a hormone, such as estrogen or, less commonly, progesterone, needed by the cancer cells, or by altering the ability of receptors on the surface of the cancer cells to interface with needed hormones despite their normal level within the body.

Targeted therapy involves the formulation of drugs tailored to the uniqueness of the proteins manufactured by breast cancer patients' own cancer cells. The drugs Herceptin, Gleevec, and Avastin represented the current frontier of cancer therapy until January 2011, when the FDA withdrew Avastin's approval (used in combination with Taxol), when its manufacturer could not demonstrate sufficient prolongation of life, to justify the several adverse cardiovascular conditions traced to its use. These included heart attack, stroke, severe hypertension, and other noncardiovascular side effects.

Prostate Cancer

Unlike their female counterparts, males do not have anatomically separate urinary and reproductive systems, as both utilize the urethra as a passageway out of the body—urine and the ejaculate, respectively. From a structural perspective, the prostate, an accessory gland of the reproductive system, encompasses an important segment of the urethra, the *prostatic portion*. From a functional perspective, the prostate supplies approximately 30 percent of the ejaculate's makeup, in the form of a milky-white fluid that is rich in important excretions needed for sperm survivability.[7]

Clearly, the prostate is not lacking in value to the normal functioning of both body systems. That said, the majority of recognition that the prostate receives in the eyes of both the public and the medical community is in relation to prostate cancer—the most prevalent form of cancer in males, and the second leading cause of cancer deaths. Today, considerable uncertainty exists regarding prevention, identification, and treatment, as well as minimizing side effects stemming from treatment-related decisions. Accordingly, your authors have decided to refer you to a comprehensive exploration of these issues as they are discussed in "Special Section: Prostate Cancer," found in *Cancer Facts & Figures—2010*. This information can be accessed through your textbook's Online Learning Center (OLC) or at the American Cancer Society's website at www.cancer.org.

Having assigned the American Cancer Society's comprehensive "Special Section: Prostate Cancer," readers

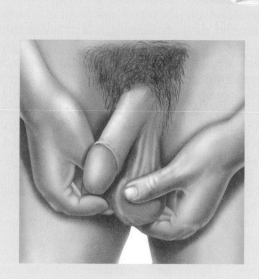

should be aware that two important studies relating, in part, to prostate screening were released in scientific journals and reported to the general public via many media. The European Randomized Study of Screening for Prostate Cancer (ERSPC) and the Prostate, Lung, Colorectal, Ovarian Cancer (PLCO) studies reached conflicting conclusions regarding the use of the **prostate-specific antigen (PSA) test** in screening for prostate cancer. Interestingly, how and what the media reported very likely did little to aid in clarifying the role of screening for this prevalent form of cancer.[25]

Testicular Cancer

Cancer of the testicle is among the least common forms of cancer; however, it is the most common solid tumor in men ages 15–34. Awareness of this type of cancer was raised in 1996 and 1997, when seven-time winner of the tour de France Lance Armstrong was diagnosed with testicular cancer. For Armstrong, chronic fatigue and abdominal discomfort were the first symptoms of the disease. The American Cancer Society estimates that in 2010 testicular cancer was diagnosed in 8,040 men and caused the deaths of 310.

Risk Factors   Risk factors for testicular cancer are variable, ranging from family history to environmental factors. The disease is more frequently seen in White Americans and in men whose testicles were undescended during childhood. Additional risk factors, such as difficulty during the mother's pregnancy, elevated temperature in the groin, and mumps during childhood, have been reported. The incidence of this cancer has been increasing in recent decades, while a corresponding drop in sperm levels has also been observed. Although no single explanation can be given for these changes, environmental factors such as agricultural pesticide toxicity may be involved. Once pesticides are concentrated in the tissues of the human body, during pregnancy they mimic estrogen. This, in turn, may lead to testicular dysgenesis syndrome, or the failure of the testicles to develop normally. The suspicion that testicular cancer is linked to vasectomies appears to be unfounded.

Prevention   Because risk factors for testicular cancer are so variable, prevention is limited to regular self-examination of the testicles. Symptoms such as fatigue, abdominal discomfort, and enlargement of the testicle should be reported to a physician, since these can be associated with other disease processes. A male infant with one or both testicles in the undescended position (resulting in an empty scrotum) should be seen promptly by a physician so that corrective procedures can be undertaken.

Early Detection   In addition to the fatigue and abdominal distress reported by Armstrong, symptoms of testicular cancer include a small, painless lump on the side or near the front of the testicle; a swollen or enlarged testicle; and a heaviness or dragging sensation in the groin or scrotum. The importance of testicular self-examination, as well as early diagnosis and prompt treatment, cannot be overemphasized for men in the at-risk age group of 15 to 34 years; see the box "Testicular Self-Examination" for a description of the proper technique.

Treatment Depending on the type, stage, and degree of localization of the tumor, surgical intervention generally includes removal of the testicle, spermatic cord, and regional lymph nodes. Chemotherapy and radiation might also be used. The highly publicized recovery of Lance Armstrong (and his subsequent accomplishments in professional biking) made the "Einhorn Regimen" (a combination of three chemotherapy agents) one of the chemotherapy protocols most widely recognized by the general public. Today, treatment is very effective, with 95 percent of all testicular cancer patients surviving five years and 99 percent surviving five years when the cancer was localized at the time of diagnosis.[26] It should be noted, however, that concern exists regarding the development of other forms of cancer, such as leukemia, later in life.

Cervical Cancer

In 2010 an estimated 12,300 new cases of cancer of the cervix (the anatomical neck of the uterus) occurred in the United States.[2] Fortunately, the death rate from cervical cancer has dropped greatly since 1950, largely because of the **Pap test.** This test screens for precancerous cellular changes (called *cervical intraepithelial neoplasia,* or *CIN*) and malignant cells. If malignant cells are found, it is hoped that they represent only cancer *in situ* (at the site of origin), rather than a more advanced invasive stage of the disease. Unfortunately, this simple and relatively inexpensive screening test is still underused, particularly in women over age 60, the group in which cervical cancer is most frequently found.

Today, refinements in laboratory techniques and the incorporation of computerization have enhanced the diagnostic precision of the Pap test. ThinPrep represents the former, while PAPNET and FocalPoint have enhanced the technologist's ability to identify abnormal cells.

Risk Factors Because of the clear association between sexually transmitted infections and cervical cancer, risk factors for this form of cancer include early age of first intercourse, large number of sex partners, history of infertility (which may indicate chronic pelvic inflammatory disease), and clinical evidence of *human papillomavirus* infections (see Chapter 11). For patients with previous HPV infections or whose sexual history suggests a higher risk for HPV, a Pap-plus (a combination of the liquid Pap and the HPV test) test has been shown to be effective in detecting the DNA from four HPVs that are known to be cancer causing, while being as easy to use as the traditional Pap test. Today the test is approved only for identifying HPV infection, but it is also capable of detecting both chlamydia and gonorrhea. The first effective vaccine against the HPV variants associated with cervical cancer became available in 2006. This vaccine (Gardasil) and the forms of HPV against which it protects are described in greater detail in Chapter 11. In 2008 the FDA extended the approved use of the Gardasil vaccine to include prevention against cancer of the vagina and the vulva (the external area adjacent to the vaginal opening).[27] In 2009, a second vaccine, Cervarix, also designed to prevent infection from HPVs associated with cervical cancer, was approved by the FDA for use in females ages 10–25.[2]

In addition to sexual history, cigarette smoking and socioeconomic factors are risk factors for cervical cancer. The latter most likely relates to less frequent medical assessment, including infrequent Pap tests.

Prevention Sexual abstinence is the most effective way of reducing the risk of developing cervical cancer (for example, Catholic nuns have extremely low rates of cervical cancer). However, abstinence is unlikely to be the choice for most women; other alternatives include fewer sexual partners, more careful selection of partners to minimize contact with those at high risk, the use of condoms, and the use of spermicides. In addition, regular medical assessment, including annual Pap tests (and the Pap-plus test), represents prevention through early detection. The HPV vaccines will further increase prevention.

Early Detection At this time, the importance of women having Pap tests for cervical cancer performed on a regular basis cannot be overemphasized. However, the specific scheduling of cervical screening is undergoing adjustment. For young, sexually active women, initial screening using the Pap test (preferably in combination with the Pap-plus) should be undertaken within three years of first exposure. For young women not sexually at risk, or for women who have had a hysterectomy, the initial screening with the Pap test can be determined in consultation with health care providers. Once initiated,

---

Key Terms

prostate-specific antigen (PSA) test A blood test used to identify prostate-specific antigen, an early indicator that the immune system has recognized and mounted a defense against prostate cancer.

Pap test A cancer screening procedure in which cells are removed from the cervix and examined for precancerous changes.

---

however, following three consecutive annual negative tests, the interval between tests may be increased upon discussion with health care providers.

In addition to the tests just recommended, studies reported in *The Lancet Oncology* suggest that in comparison to cytology-based Pap tests that look for evidence of precancerous changes in cervical cells, testing for DNA from the HPVs associated with the development of cervical cancer may provide even earlier evidence of cervical cancer susceptibility.[28]

The Pap tests are not perfect, however. About 7 percent will be false negatives, resulting in a 93 percent accuracy rate.

For many women with an abnormal Pap test, visual assessment (colposcopy) of the cervix will be performed. Traditional colposcopy technology generates some false negatives. A newer technology, the Luma Cervical Imaging System, has enhanced the ability of clinicians to visually identify signs of tissue change.

In addition to changes discovered by a Pap test, symptoms that suggest potential cervical cancer include abnormal vaginal bleeding between periods and frequent spotting.

Treatment   Should precancerous cellular changes (CIN) be identified, treatment can include one of several alternatives. Physicians can destroy areas of abnormal cellular change using cryotherapy (freezing), electrocoagulation, laser destruction, or surgical removal of abnormal tissue. More advanced (invasive) cancer of the cervix can be treated with a hysterectomy combined with other established cancer therapies. A combination of radiation and chemotherapy is the most effective treatment for cervical cancer.

Uterine (Endometrial) Cancer

The American Cancer Society estimates that in 2010, 43,470 cases of uterine cancer (cancer within the inner wall of the body of the uterus, rather than within the cervix or neck of the uterus) were diagnosed in American women. In addition, 7,950 women died of the disease.[2] Although African Americans have a lower incidence of uterine cancer than White women do, their death rate is nearly twice as high.

Risk Factors   Unlike cervical cancer, in which a strong viral link has been identified, the principal risk factor related to the development of endometrial cancer is a high estrogen level. Accordingly, the following factors are related to higher levels of estrogen and, thus, to the development of endometrial cancer:

- Early menarche (early onset of menstruation)
- Late menopause (prolonged exposure to estrogen)
- Lack of ovulation (infertility)

- Never having given birth
- Estrogen replacement therapy (ERT not moderated with progesterone)
- Obesity
- Use of tamoxifen (a drug used in breast cancer therapy)
- History of polycystic ovary syndrome
- Hereditary nonpolyposis colon cancer

To some degree, endometrial cancer is seen more frequently in people who are diabetic or hypertensive, or who have gallbladder disease.

Prevention   The risk factors associated with high levels of estrogen are areas in which prevention might be targeted. In addition, regular gynecological care that includes pelvic examination is a principal factor in minimizing the risk of uterine cancer. Pregnancy and the use of oral contraceptives both provide some protection from endometrial cancer.[2]

In recent years, there has been growing interest in using foods high in phytoestrogens, such as soy, coffee, and orange juice, to protect against uterine cancer by moderating estrogen levels. Most recently, however, an assessment of circulating enterolactone, the main form of dietary phytoestrogens in Western diets, failed to show a protective role against uterine cancer in ranges associated with normal dietary intake.[29]

Early Detection   Compared with cervical cancer, which is routinely identified through Pap tests, endometrial cancer is much more likely to be suspected on the basis of symptoms (irregular or postmenopausal bleeding) and confirmed by biopsy. Although more invasive, biopsy is a more effective method than ultrasound to diagnose uterine cancer. However, when a saline infusion is coupled with sonography, visual inspection of the inner wall of the uterus is improved to the extent that diagnosis accuracy surpasses that of random punch biopsy.[30]

Treatment   The treatment for early or localized endometrial cancer is generally surgical removal of the uterus (hysterectomy). Other therapies, such as radiation, chemotherapy, and hormonal therapy, may then be added to the treatment regimen. However, in terms of hormone replacement therapy (HRT), in which estrogen is combined with a synthetic progesterone, the FDA, the National Institute on Aging, and various medical associations now advise that no woman 65 or older with an intact uterus use HRT owing to several concerns, including an increased risk for endometrial cancer. For women who are undergoing menopause and experiencing troublesome symptoms such as night sweats and hot flashes, HRT should be used in the smallest doses that provide relief and for the shortest duration of time possible.

Ovarian Cancer

Since the death in 1989 of actress Gilda Radner, a star in the early years of *Saturday Night Live,* public awareness of ovarian cancer has increased in the United States. The American Cancer Society estimates that in 2010 there were 21,880 new cases diagnosed, and 13,850 women died of the disease.[2] Most cases develop in women over age 40 who have not had children or began menstruation at an early age. The highest rate is in women over age 60. Today ovarian cancer causes more deaths than does any other form of female reproductive system cancer.

For a relatively small percentage of all women (10 percent), the inheritance of either the *BRCA1* or *BRCA2* suppressor gene mutation (see page 250) significantly increases the risk of developing both breast and ovarian cancer. Today it is estimated that about 20 percent of all cases of ovarian cancer stem from these genetic mutations.

Beyond the 20 percent of cases attributed to genetic mutations, what might account for the majority of ovarian cancers? A number of studies, with varying degrees of assurance, suggest that decades of HRT used to counter symptoms of menopause, maintain bone mass, and provide hormonal protection from heart disease could be responsible for the majority of ovarian cancer. As mentioned in conjunction with endometrial cancer, today HRT is used, and then for only the briefest period of time.

Prevention   Methods of preventing or lowering the risk of developing ovarian cancer are very similar to those recommended for breast cancer. These include using oral contraceptives, giving birth and breast-feeding (for at least three months), reducing dietary fat intake, abstaining from alcohol use, and performing regular physical activity.

For the small group of women with a strong family history of ovarian cancer, a **prophylactic oophorectomy** should be seriously considered. In this surgical procedure, both ovaries are removed. Carefully monitored HRT is then used to provide the protective advantages of estrogen in maintaining cardiovascular health and bone density.

Early Detection   Because of its vague symptoms, ovarian cancer has been referred to as a *silent cancer.* Women in whom ovarian cancer has been diagnosed often report that the only symptoms of their cancer's presence were digestive disturbances, gas, urinary incontinence, stomach distention, and a crampy abdominal pain over a few short weeks. The latter should be medically evaluated immediately.

Three ovarian cancer tests are now available for use in early detection and progress monitoring of ovarian therapy. OvaSure is a new screening test that the developer believes can identify a developing tumor in the ovary months or even a few years before it would have become invasive. Although approved by the FDA, OvaSure is undergoing evaluation based on the level of its ability to function as intended.

The two remaining tests, CA125 and HE4, are now used to monitor the progress and effectiveness of therapies by determining the levels of antibodies against the ovarian cancer cells at various points in the treatment protocol and during follow-up, although they were used as screening tests as well.

For women with a strong family history of ovarian cancer (four primary family members who have had breast or ovarian cancer, with two or more cases occurring before age 50) or women of Ashkenazi Jewish descent (see page 250), genetic screening and transvaginal ultrasound screening are likely to be recommended. These women may also be referred for participation in one of several prevention trials now under way.

Treatment   At this time, treatment of ovarian cancer requires surgical removal of the ovary, fallopian tubes, and uterus, followed by aggressive use of chemotherapy. Use of the chemotherapeutic drug Taxol results in a 50 percent survival rate 19 months after the completion of therapy. Most recently, use of an experimental three-drug combination and a two-drug therapy, delivered directly into the abdominal cavity, has extended survival rates beyond those capable of being achieved only a decade ago. Today, the American Cancer Society reports survival rates at five years following diagnosis at 57 percent for younger women and 30 percent for those over age 65. With the addition of young women to the data, the overall one-year survival rate is 75 percent, with the five-year rate at 46 percent. If ovarian cancer is diagnosed in the very earliest stage of development, the five-year survival rate is 94 percent.

Pancreatic Cancer

Pancreatic cancer is one of the most lethal forms of cancer, with a survival rate of only 6 percent five years after diagnosis.[2] Because of this gland's important functions in both digestion and metabolic processes related to glucose utilization (see the discussion of diabetes mellitus on page 263), its destruction by a malignancy leaves the body in a state incompatible with living.

In 2010 an estimated 43,140 new cases of pancreatic cancer were diagnosed and 36,800 deaths occurred.[2]

Key Terms

prophylactic oophorectomy   Surgical removal of the ovaries to prevent ovarian cancer in women at high risk of developing the disease.

Chapter Ten   Living with Cancer and Other Chronic Conditions

Risk Factors Pancreatic cancer is more common in men than women, occurs more frequently with age, and develops most often in African American men. Smoking is clearly a risk factor for this form of cancer, with smokers more than twice as likely to develop the disease. Other risk factors have been tentatively suggested, such as chronic inflammation of the pancreas (pancreatitis), diabetes mellitus, alcohol-induced liver deterioration (cirrhosis), obesity, and high-fat diets. A meta-analysis (a restudy of earlier studies) assessed whether the long-term use of nonsteroidal anti-inflammatory drugs is a risk factor for the development of pancreatic cancer. No clear link was found between the use of these medications, including aspirin, and an enhanced risk of pancreatic cancer.[31]

Prevention Not smoking or using smokeless tobacco and abstaining from alcohol use are the most effective steps toward preventing this form of cancer. Further, reducing the risk of type 2 diabetes mellitus, through weight loss and exercise, would also make an important contribution to prevention. Annual medical examinations are, of course, associated with overall cancer prevention.

The role of dietary and supplemental vitamin D use is currently being assessed. Preliminary findings from a group of studies that included nearly 120,000 men and women suggest a positive role for vitamin D in the prevention of pancreatic cancer.[32] A second study examined the relationship between ultraviolet B radiation and several cancers and found an inverse relationship between the levels of solar radiation received and the incidence of several cancers, including pancreatic cancer.[33] UV radiation is a facilitator of the production of vitamin D_3, so a speculative inference can be drawn regarding a protective role for this vitamin in minimizing the development of this form of cancer. A more recent study based on serum vitamin D levels found a small inverse relationship between those levels and the incidence of pancreatic cancer.[34] At this time, however, there are no recommendations to increase vitamin D intake as a preventive measure for pancreatic cancer.

Early Detection Early detection of this cancer is difficult because of the absence of symptoms until late in its course. Perhaps for people with a history of chronic pancreatitis, physicians might consider routine ultrasound assessment or computerized axial tomography scans (CT scans). Once symptoms appear, a biopsy is performed.

Treatment At this time there is no effective treatment for pancreatic cancer. Surgical removal of malignant sites within the gland, in addition to radiation and chemotherapy, is usually tried. Certainly, if a particular patient with pancreatic cancer qualifies, enrollment in a clinical trial would be worth consideration.

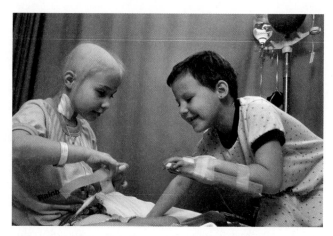

Chemotherapy involves the use of chemical agents given by mouth or injection to treat or control cancer. Chemotherapy typically affects rapidly dividing cells, which include cancer cells but also healthy cells in the blood, hair, and lining of the gastrointestinal tract. If healthy cells are damaged, side effects such as nausea and hair loss can occur.

Lymphatic Cancer

An estimated 74,030 new cases of lymphoma (8,490 cases of Hodgkin's disease and 65,540 cases of non-Hodgkin's lymphoma) were diagnosed in 2010. The number of deaths from both forms of lymphoma was near 21,530. The incidence of Hodgkin's disease has declined over the last 40 years, while the incidence of non-Hodgkin's disease has nearly doubled, but is now holding steady.[2]

Risk Factors Risk factors for lymphoma are difficult to determine. Some possible factors are a general reduction in immune protection, exposure to toxic environmental chemicals such as pesticides and herbicides, the use of some biologics in the treatment of autoimmune conditions (see Chapter 11), and viral infections.[2] As you will learn in Chapter 11, the virus that causes AIDS (HIV) is a leukemia/lymphoma virus that was initially called HTLV-III (human T-cell leukemia/lymphoma virus-type III). A related leukemia/lymphoma virus, HTLV-I, is also suspected in the development of lymphatic cancer. The Epstein-Barr virus (EBV) may also play a role in lymphatic cancer development, as well as the hepatitis C virus.

Prevention Beyond limiting exposure to toxic chemicals and sexually transmitted viruses, few recommendations can be made about prevention. Again, early detection and diagnosis can serve as a form of prevention, since early-stage cancer is more survivable than advanced disease.

Early Detection Unlike other cancers, the early symptoms of lymphoma are diverse and similar to symptoms of other illnesses, most of which are not serious. These symptoms include enlarged lymph nodes (frequently a sign of any infection that the immune system is fighting), fever, itching, weight loss, and anemia.

Treatment   Although surgery (beyond a biopsy) is usually not associated with the treatment of lymphoma, a variety of other therapies are employed. Depending on the stage and type of lymphoma, therapy may involve only radiation treatment of localized lymph nodes, as is seen in non-Hodgkin's lymphoma. Radiation combined with chemotherapy is generally used in the treatment of late-stage non-Hodgkin's lymphoma. More recently, other therapies, including more aggressive chemotherapy, monoclonal antibody therapy, and bone marrow and stem cell transplantation, in combination with either high-dose or low-dose radiation, have been employed with non-Hodgkin's lymphoma.

After completion of therapy, one-year survival rates for Hodgkin's disease are near 92 percent and near 80 percent for non-Hodgkin's lymphoma. By the end of five years, these rates have dropped to 81 percent and 56 percent, respectively.[2] Lower rates of survival are seen at 10 years and beyond.

Status of the "War on Cancer"

Along with the issues of unhealthy lifestyle choices and the absence of a comprehensive national medical care system to provide wide-ranging services in an affordable manner, also negatively influencing our efforts to win the war on cancer are factors such as the ongoing financial recession (that technically ended in 2010), the near-static military conflicts that cost annually hundreds of millions of dollars to sustain, and the near record unemployment that reduces tax revenues at all levels of government. It is, therefore, unlikely that adequate funds will be available to sustain (let alone expand) the research and development required to win the war on cancer.

Prevention Through Risk Reduction

Because cancer will probably continue to be the leading cause of death among adults under the age of 80, you should explore ways to reduce your risk of developing cancer. The following factors, which could make you vulnerable to cancer, can be controlled or at least recognized:

- *Know your family history.* You are the recipient of the genetic strengths and weaknesses of your biological parents and your more distant relatives. If you are able to determine that cancer is prevalent in your family medical history, you cannot afford to disregard this fact. It may be appropriate for you to be screened for certain types of cancer more often or at a younger

age. The importance of family history was clearly seen in our discussion of the *BRCA1/BRCA2* inheritance pattern and related decisions about prophylactic mastectomy and prophylactic oophorectomy.

- *Select and monitor your occupation carefully.* Because of recently discovered relationships between cancer and occupations that bring employees into contact with carcinogenic agents, you must be aware of the risks posed by certain job selections and assignments. Worksites where you will come into frequent contact with pesticides, strong solvents, volatile hydrocarbons, and airborne fibers could pay well but also shorten your life. The importance of this point is evident in reviewing the current list of environmental carcinogens studies funded by the National Cancer Institute. Included are studies that focus on indoor air pollution (tobacco smoke, cooking oils), dust (cotton, grain, plastic, wood), organic solvents (benzene, carbon tetrachloride, toluene, xylene, chlordane), organophosphates (diazinon, dichlorvos, malathion, triazines, cyaniazine), polybrominated biphenyls, polychlorinated biphenyls, fumigants (ethylene), water pollutants (chloride, phosphene, fluoride), petroleum products (diesel fuel, gasoline, jet fuel), radiation (radon, neutron therapy, and reactor accidents), biological agents (chlamydia, HIV/HPV, helicobacter, hepatitis B and C), and radioisotopes (iodine and radium).

- *Do not use tobacco products.* You may want to review Chapter 8 on the overwhelming evidence linking all forms of tobacco use (including smokeless tobacco) to the development of cancer. Smoking is so detrimental to health that it is considered the number-one preventable cause of death along with obesity.

- *Monitor environmental exposure to carcinogens.* When one considers carcinogenic concerns related to types of employment, residential radon levels, ozone depletion leading to increased exposure to solar radiation, and environmental tobacco smoke, one realizes that the environment holds great potential as a source of carcinogenic exposure. To the extent to which it is possible to select the environment in which you will reside, work, and recreate, you should add selecting a low-risk environment to your list of cancer-prevention activities.

- *Follow a sound diet.* As mentioned in conjunction with folic acid and colorectal cancer, and high-fat diets and prostate cancer, dietary patterns are known to play both a causative and a preventive role in cancer. Review Chapter 5 for information about dietary practices and the incidence of various diseases, including cancer. In that chapter, emphasis was placed on the role of fruits and vegetables as excellent sources of nutrients, as well as important cancer-protective compounds known as phytochemicals.

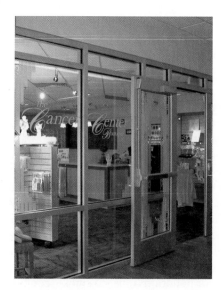

Today the care of cancer patients extends beyond the diagnosis and treatment of the disease to include services designed to improve the emotional well-being of patients and enhance the role of their support groups. The Cancer Center Boutique, a part of Ball Memorial Hospital's Cancer Center, plays an important role in this process.

Consider these simple modifications to familiar food items that can be made in support of overall health:

- For breakfast: Toast whole-grain bread and top with reduced-fat peanut butter and a sliced banana.
- For lunch: Order salads, vegetable soups, or stir-fried vegetables when eating out.
- For dinner: Add broccoli, green beans, corn, or peas to a casserole.
- As a snack: Store cleaned, cut-up vegetables in the fridge at eye level and keep a low-fat or fat-free dip on hand.

Should research demonstrate an even clearer role for nutrients, **chemoprevention** may become an even more widely practiced component of cancer prevention. Chemoprevention is not limited to food items and dietary supplements but can also involve pharmaceutical agents, such as aspirin, estrogen replacement therapy, and hormone replacement therapy.

- *Control your body weight.* For women, obesity is related to a higher incidence of cancer of the uterus, ovary, and breast because obesity correlates with

high estrogen levels. Maintaining a desirable body weight could improve overall health and lead to more successful management of cancer should it develop. For example, obesity makes biopsies and surgeries more difficult to perform, prolongs recovery time, and may diminish the desired effects of some chemotherapy agents.

- *Exercise regularly.* Chapter 4 discusses in detail the importance of regular moderate exercise to all aspects of health, including reducing the risk of chronic illnesses. Moderate exercise increases the body's ability to deliver oxygen to its tissues and thus to reduce the formation of cancer-enhancing free radicals during incomplete oxidation of nutrients. Moderate exercise also stimulates the production of enzymes that remove free radicals.
- *Limit your exposure to the sun.* It is important to heed this message even if you enjoy many outdoor activities. Particularly for people with light complexions, the radiation received through chronic exposure to the sun may foster the development of skin cancer. Of course, the same advice is given in light of the substantial concern that exists regarding tanning bed use and the development of skin cancers, including melanoma.
- *Consume alcohol in moderation if at all.* People who consume a lot of alcohol have an increased prevalence of several types of cancer, including cancer of the oral cavity, larynx, and esophagus. Whether this results directly from the presence of carcinogens in alcohol or is more closely related to the alcohol user's tendency to smoke has not yet been established.

Chronic Health Conditions

In addition to the two most widely recognized chronic health problems of adulthood—cardiovascular disease and cancer—adults can experience an array of other chronic health conditions. What all these chronic conditions have in common is the ability to cause significant change in the lives of people—on the part of both the affected person and his or her family members and friends (see the box "Chronic Illness—The End or a Turning Point?").

Some of these conditions are seen in early adulthood, such as lupus and Crohn's disease. Others, such as type 2 diabetes, generally do not appear until nearer middle age, although today it is appearing at much younger ages. However, some chronic diseases seen during adulthood have their origins in childhood, such as type 1 diabetes.

Systemic Lupus Erythematosus

Systemic lupus erythematosus (SLE), or simply *lupus,* is perhaps the most familiar of a class of chronic conditions known as **autoimmune** disorders, or connective tissue

Most people diagnosed with a chronic illness go through a period of serious adjustment. For college students, the necessary adaptations feel particularly burdensome because so few of their peers are faced with equal demands. Not only must self-care routines be changed, but the help of others may be necessary to carry out that care. The limitations imposed by a chronic illness restrict the activities and behavior of the affected individual and his or her family and friends. Financial matters (including the ability to afford medications), the need to see physicians frequently, and insurance issues add to the person's stress. When their lives change so profoundly, young people can feel isolated and singled out in a negative way.

People respond to the diagnosis of a chronic illness in various ways. Frequently, their first reaction is denial. When this occurs, care may be delayed. At the same time, school and work performance and relationships begin to suffer from the internalized stress. Eventually, though, denial gives way to anger, which is often directed at others. Common targets of this anger are people close to the ill person, such as family and friends. Then the anger broadens to include the world or a God (for "letting these things happen"). Eventually, the demands

of the illness, combined with a sense of futility, give way to acceptance. At this stage, the individual's resourcefulness surfaces as he or she looks within for untapped sources of strength. Gradually, the person becomes open to the assistance offered by others, begins to discover new interests and abilities, and realizes that life is not over—just different.

The decision to accept the chronic condition often brings a sense of inner peace and allows for a new approach to living. People who believe that they will not be given a burden too great for them to bear may rise to the challenge and find a level of strength that they—and others—didn't know they had. With acceptance comes new learning experiences. The person begins to understand the limitations of the body, to appreciate what true friendships are, and to recognize the importance of emotional resources once taken for granted. Even more significant is the realization that the spiritual dimension of health is bountiful. As the daily challenges of the illness continue, the person realizes that his or her personal beliefs and values have not only survived but are even stronger.

---

diseases. Collectively, these conditions reflect a concentrated and inappropriate attack by the body's immune system on its own tissues, which then serve as *self-antigens* (see Chapter 11 for a discussion of the immune response).

The name *systemic lupus erythematosus* reflects the widespread (systemic, or systemwide) destruction of fibrous connective tissue and other tissues and the appearance in some patients of a reddish rash (erythematosus) that imparts a characteristic "mask" to the face. Lupus is most often seen in women who developed the condition during young adulthood, although it is now known that autoantibodies may first appear in the blood as much as a decade before the first observable symptoms of SLE appear.[35] The course of the condition is gradual, with intermittent periods of inflammation, stiffness, fatigue, pleurisy (chest pain), and discomfort over wide areas of the body, including muscles, joints, and skin. Similar changes may also occur with tissue of the nervous system, kidneys, and heart.[35] Additionally, decreased bone mineral density, leading to osteopaenia and osteoporosis, can become evident even in children with lupus.[36] Diagnosis is made on the basis of symptoms and several laboratory tests.

Why the immune system turns on the body in such an aggressive manner is not fully understood. It is likely, however, that a combination of genetic predisposition and an earlier viral infection or environmental exposure may be involved. Episodes (called *flares*) of lupus often follow exposure to the sun, periods of fatigue, or an infectious disease; all these should be avoided to the fullest extent possible. Management of the condition generally may involve long-term (and low-dose) use of prednisone

(a corticosteroid) or newer medications, such as hydroxychloroquine and azathioprine, may be employed.

Irritable Bowel Syndrome (IBS) and Inflammatory Bowel Disease (IBD)

Although these conditions have strikingly similar labels, they are different in several important ways. IBS is a *syndrome*—the presence of an array of symptoms in the absence of a single definable disease. IBD involves more definitive pathological processes that give rise to more discernible conditions. IBS and IBD are both significantly more common in females than in males, and both can coexist in the same person.

IBS is characterized by highly uncomfortable episodes of spasticity-based pain, diarrhea, or constipation that are localized to the colon, or large intestine. *Spastic colon* is an older term used frequently by the general public to describe this condition. Fortunately for many diagnosed with IBS, the drug Zelnorm has proven effective in reducing the frequency and duration of symptoms by helping to coordinate the nerve and muscle activity of the colon, although currently the safety of this drug is in question. As distressing as this condition can be, it is important to remember that IBS is nonprogressive, is localized to the colon, causes no damage to the colon, can be controlled with noninvasive measures, and is never fatal. Diet, stress management, and medication can help control the alienating and embarrassing issues associated with IBS.

In comparison to IBS, IBD is a more highly defined pathological progress that involves invasive, inflammatory changes to the gastrointestinal tract. Two recognizable diseases that fall under the label *IBD* are ulcerative colitis (UC) and Crohn's disease (CD).

Treatments for ulcerative colitis depend on the severity and duration of symptoms, but they focus on promptness of diagnosis and initiation of treatment, minimization of complications (such as anemia and malabsorption of nutrients), maintenance of normal growth (when dealing with young children), and establishment of remission, in which symptoms and disease progression are significantly minimized. Treatment options include dietary changes, enteral (tube) feeding, "gut rest," antidiarrheal medications, and the use of corticosteroids when symptoms have been present for a longer duration. Inflammation is identified through abnormal bloodwork results or visual changes seen through a colonoscopy. Removal of the colon, known as a colectomy, may be the only "cure" for this condition. Patients with ulcerative colitis have a significantly elevated risk of developing colon cancer.

Unlike ulcerative colitis, Crohn's disease can occur anywhere along the course of the gastrointestinal tract ("from tip to tail"), from the mouth and lips to the anus. This condition involves clear pathological changes within the gastrointestinal tract and, unlike ulcerative colitis, is the only form of IBD that can penetrate the wall of the gastrointestinal tract. At times, persons with Crohn's disease can develop **fistulas**, open pathways between the gastrointestinal wall and neighboring structures, such as the vagina and urinary bladder.

Crohn's disease is increasingly treated with immunosuppressive drugs. These drugs produce antibodies, aimed principally against tumor necrosis factor (TNF), and are intended to counter the immune system's inappropriate destruction of elements within the intestinal wall (see Chapter 11 for additional information on immune system function). Because they suppress the immune system, these powerful drugs must be monitored carefully and patients should take extra caution to avoid exposure to colds, flu, and other opportunistic infections. Also of considerable concern is the possibility that persons taking TNF drugs will develop fungal infections, including histoplasmosis, which could be fatal if not treated.[37] Surgery is often needed to remove the colon and parts of the small intestine when inflammation does not respond to treatment with diet and drugs.

Along with the inflammatory changes that happen to the GI tract in persons with IBD, there are "extraintestinal manifestations" involving the eyes, skin, and joints. There might also be side effects related to the medications.

Although the etiology of IBD is not completely known, there are strong indications that genetic mutations underlie its development, leading to the establishment of an autoimmune reaction to proteins within the gastrointestinal wall. It has also been found that there are family patterns of IBS and IBD, further suggesting that genetically based etiologies are in play.

Though there are no known cures for IBS or IBD, neither condition is generally considered to be fatal.

 TALKING POINTS You learn that two young women who are your coworkers have recently been diagnosed with lupus and Crohn's disease, respectively. How can you be supportive of them? What should you say to them about their conditions, particularly on days when it is obvious that they are not feeling well?

Multiple Sclerosis

For proper nerve conduction to occur in the brain and the spinal cord, an insulating sheath of myelin must surround the neurons. In the progressive disease multiple sclerosis (MS), the cells that produce myelin are destroyed and myelin production ceases. Eventually, the vital functions of the body can no longer be carried out. The cause of MS is not fully understood. Research continues to focus on virus-induced autoimmune mechanisms in which T cells attack viral-infected, myelin-producing cells. At this time a large number of viruses have been discovered in the cerebrospinal fluid (CSF) of persons with MS and other neurological disorders, and these viruses generally have not been found in persons without these conditions. Among the most actively accessed viruses are herpes simplex virus 1 (HSV-1), herpes simplex virus 2 (HSV-2), Epstein-Barr virus (EBV), varicella zoster virus (VZV), human cytomegalovirus (HCMV), human herpes virus 6 (HHV-6), and the JC virus (JCV). The number of viruses found in the patient depends on the patient's form of MS. However, the virus most commonly found in the spinal fluid of persons with progressive MS (regardless of type) and others with neurological disorders is the varicella zoster virus (VZV), making it a suspect in the etiology of multiple sclerosis.[38] Some immune system evidence of this virus can be found in about 90 percent of all Americans, but not at the levels associated with MS.

Usually, MS first appears during the young adult years. It may take one of four forms, depending on the interplay of periods of stabilization (remitting), renewed deterioration (relapsing), continuous deterioration (progressive), or combinations of all of these. The initial symptoms are often visual impairment, prickling and burning in the extremities, or an altered **gait.** Deterioration of nervous system function occurs in various forms during the course of MS. In the most advanced stages of MS, movement is greatly impaired, and mental deterioration

Key Terms
fistula An open pathway between the gastrointestinal wall and other internal organs; often caused by Crohn's disease.
gait Pattern of walking.

Support groups are composed of people who come together to help one another through the demands of a chronic health condition. These groups have traditionally been organized by institutions in the local health care community, such as hospitals; by the local affiliates of national organizations, such as the American Cancer Society; or by citizens who have the same chronic condition. Today, however, more and more support group members are connected not by physical proximity but by the Internet.

Health self-help groups on the Internet develop in one of two ways. The first occurs when a brick-and-mortar organization, such as a national agency or health care institution, develops a support group for its homepage. The second way is for a person with the condition (or a family member of that person) to organize an online group, utilizing various social networking sites, such as Facebook, BlackPlanet, DailyStrength, and Disaboom. Today the Internet, Wi-Fi, smart phones, and notebook/netbook computers have added a new dimension to the enhanced well-being of persons with chronic conditions.

You can find a health support group simply by surfing the Net. Or you can be referred to a site by a health care professional, friend, family member, colleague, or someone with a similar condition. You can also go to the homepage of a medical institution or a national agency to find out if it provides a support group link.

For someone with a newly diagnosed chronic condition, the initial contact with a support group may be made to get information about the condition and its treatment. For others, it is a way of connecting with other people who have the condition. Web support groups provide windows to the outside world, particularly for those whose conditions limit their mobility and social contacts. The Internet support group transcends the restrictions of various diseases to make new connections possible.

Note that online support groups' members are rarely physicians or other highly trained health professionals, so you shouldn't rely on this source for specific technical information. Instead, your main sources of information about medical management of a chronic condition should be your health care providers.

---

may be present. It should be noted, however, that MS may be a "silent epidemic" among children, including those younger than 10 years of age. To facilitate a more timely diagnosis of MS, children showing mild tremors or reporting intermittent dimming of vision should be seen by a pediatric neurologist. It is currently estimated that over 20,000 American children may have early-onset MS.

Treatment of MS involves reducing the severity of the symptoms and extending the periods of remission. Today a variety of therapies are used, including immune-targeted biologics, steroid drugs, drugs that relieve muscle spasms, injection of nerve blockers, and physical and occupational therapy.

At the heart of modern treatment of MS are several biologics, all of which were developed since 1993, some as recently as 2006. Among these are four *immunomodulating biologics:* Avonex, Betaseron, Extaria, and Rebif (all of which are versions of interferon alpha and beta and taken by injection); Copaxon and Tysabri (which use different avenues to modify the activity of the immune system, and are taken by injection and infusion, respectively); and an *immunosuppressant biologic,* Novantrone (initially developed for the treatment of cancer, taken four times per year, by infusion). Gilenya, the first oral medication approved for the treatment of MS, has also joined the growing list of therapeutics. The goals of these therapies are to reduce the frequency of attacks, reduce the accumulation of lesions in the brain and spinal cord, and slow the accumulation of disabilities. Encouraging news was reported by researchers at Northwestern University who were able to reverse some MS deterioration by implanting bone marrow stem cells that were taken from patients before the chemotherapy-based suppression of their immune systems.[39] For more information on stem cells and the controversy surrounding stem cell research, visit the book's Online Learning Center at www.mhhe.com/hahn11e.

Additional medications are available to address complications of MS, such as spasticity. Deterioration of motor control, particularly as it relates to gait (walking and balance) control, is a serious problem for many persons with MS. A recently approved medication, Ampyra, is now available to treat this symptom.[40] An extended-release version is nearing the end of clinical trials.

In addition to drug therapy, psychotherapy is an important adjunct to the treatment of MS. Profound periods of depression often accompany the initial diagnosis of this condition. Emotional support is helpful in dealing with the progressive impairments associated with most forms of the condition (see the box "Support Is Just a Click Away").

Diabetes Mellitus

Currently, headlines carry the news that American youths are rapidly developing a high risk for type 2 diabetes mellitus and its associated heart disease and other health problems. In response, the CDC launched SEARCH for Diabetes in Youth, a campaign intended to find children and adolescents with a set of prediabetes markers, referred to as *metabolic syndrome.* For most individuals with metabolic syndrome, contributing factors have been a childhood marked by faulty dietary practices and gross inactivity, in combination with a genetic predisposition for diabetes (see Chapter 9 for more information on metabolic syndrome). Additionally, the American Diabetes Association issued new guidelines to hone diagnostic criteria and the pharmacological treatment of children, adolescents, and young adults with type 2 diabetes mellitus.[41]

Type 2 Diabetes In people who do not have diabetes mellitus, the body's need for energy is met through the "burning" of glucose (blood sugar) within the cells. Glucose is absorbed from the digestive tract and carried to the cells by the blood system.[7] Passage of glucose into the cell is achieved through a transport system that moves the glucose molecule across the cell's membrane. Activation of this glucose transport mechanism requires the presence of the hormone insulin. Specific receptor sites for **insulin** can be found on the cell membrane. In addition to its role in the transport of glucose into sensitive cells, insulin is required for the conversion of glucose into glycogen in the liver and the formation of fatty acids in adipose cells. Insulin is produced in the cells of the islets of Langerhans in the pancreas. The release of insulin from the pancreas corresponds to the changing levels of glucose within the blood.[7]

In adults, and tragically in a rapidly increasing percentage of children and adolescents, with a **genetic predisposition** for developing type 2 diabetes, a trigger mechanism (most likely obesity) begins a process through which the body cells become increasingly less sensitive to the presence of insulin, although a normal (or slightly greater than normal) amount of insulin is produced by the pancreas. The growing ineffectiveness of insulin in getting glucose into cells results in the buildup of glucose in the blood. Elevated levels of glucose in the blood lead to *hyperglycemia*, a hallmark symptom of type 2 diabetes.

In response to this buildup, the kidneys begin the process of filtering glucose from the blood. Excess glucose then spills over into the urine. This removal of glucose in the urine results in frequent urination, a second important symptom of type 2 diabetes. Increased thirst, a third symptom of developing diabetes, results in response to the movement of fluid from extracellular spaces into the circulatory system to maintain homeostasis.[5]

For many adults with diabetes or with a prediabetic status often referred to as having "glucose intolerance" or "insulin resistance," dietary modification (with an emphasis on monitoring total carbohydrate intake, not just sugar), weight loss, and regular exercise is the only treatment

required to maintain an acceptable glucose level. Weight loss will improve the condition by "releasing" more insulin receptors, and exercise increases the actual number of receptor sites. With better insulin recognition, the affected person can better maintain glucose levels.

For people whose condition is more advanced, dietary modification, increased activity, and weight loss are not sufficient, and a hypoglycemia agent must be used. Increasingly, very aggressive management, including hypoglycemic agents and insulin, successfully reduces risks associated with the disease. Until 2010, the use of oral medications was common, with nearly 80 percent of patients taking them, and less than 25 percent using insulin. However, with FDA-advised restrictions on the use of Avandia (and related medications), use of insulin may return to pre-2007 levels.

In addition to genetic predisposition and obesity, unresolved stress appears to be involved in the development of hyperglycemic states. Although stress alone probably cannot produce a diabetic condition, it is likely that stress can create a series of endocrine changes that can lead to a state of hyperglycemia.

Diabetes in both of its principal forms can cause serious damage to virtually all of the body's organ systems, but particularly the cardiovascular, nervous, and renal systems. For the 23.6 million Americans with diagnosed diabetes, the estimated 5.7 million not yet diagnosed, as well as the 57 million who have various components of metabolic syndrome,[42] future levels of health will be determined by prompt diagnosis and treatment, subsequent daily monitoring, and compliance with suggested lifestyle adjustments. Perhaps no single group of Americans is more susceptible to the development of type 2 diabetes mellitus than Hispanic Americans of Mexican descent.

As mentioned previously, self-monitoring of glucose levels is a critical component of diabetes management. To this end, the American Diabetes Association has fine-tuned its recommendations regarding self-monitoring. When using plasma glucose (glucometer) monitoring, the following glucose levels are applicable for the general adult population:

- 90–130 mg/dl before meals and 110–150 mg/dl at bedtime
- Less than 180 mg/dl one to two hours after meals

Modified values are assigned by the ADA for use in monitoring plasma glucose levels in children and in pregnant women. Modified glucose levels for children reflect needs for blood glucose related to development of the nervous system. For pregnant women, adjusted levels relate to the development of a transitory form of diabetes known as gestational diabetes, although this latter form of diabetes does not bode well for the later development of type 2 diabetes.

Key Terms

insulin A pancreatic hormone required by the body for the effective metabolism of glucose (blood sugar).

genetic predisposition An inherited tendency to develop a disease process if necessary environmental factors exist.

Common Complications of Diabetes

- Cataract formation
- Glaucoma
- Blindness
- Dental caries
- Stillbirths/miscarriages
- Neonatal deaths
- Congenital defects
- Cardiovascular disease
- Kidney disease
- Gangrene
- Impotence
- Cognitive decline (before age 65)

A second set of indices for monitoring diabetes involves the amount of glycated (think "sugar-coated") hemoglobin (A1C or HbA1C) in the blood (hemoglobin is the oxygen-carrying pigment on the surface of red blood cells). Once taken, the results give a picture of the average glucose in the blood over a two- to three-month period. The American Association of Clinical Endocrinologists considers 6.5 mg/dl or less as the upper limit of normal, while the American Diabetes Association considers the upper limit as 7 mg/dl or less. A reading above 7 mg/dl is reflective of glucose intolerance or insulin insensitivity.

Perhaps the most distressing aspect of this situation is the increasing number of young children, most often overweight or obese, accompanied by an equally overweight parent, presenting in pediatric offices across the country. Many of these children already have two or three of the five "metabolic syndrome" risk factors. As these children with "diabesity" progress into adulthood, the number of persons with type 2 diabetes mellitus could increase to 50 million by mid-century.

Type 1 Diabetes A second type of diabetes mellitus is insulin-dependent diabetes mellitus, or type 1 diabetes. The onset of this condition generally occurs before age 35, most often during childhood. In contrast to type 2 diabetes, in which insulin is produced but is ineffective because of insensitivity, in type 1 diabetes, the body does not produce insulin at all. Destruction of the insulin-producing cells of the pancreas by the person's immune system (possibly in combination with a genetic predisposition) accounts for this sudden and irreversible loss of insulin production.

In most ways, the two forms of diabetes are similar, with the important exception being that type 1 diabetes mellitus requires the use of insulin from an outside source, whereas some persons with type 2 diabetes mellitus may require supplemental insulin in order to adequately overcome the insulin insensitivity that is the hallmark of type 2 diabetes. Today insulin is taken by injection (one to four times per day), through the use of an insulin pump that provides a constant supply of insulin to the body, by a transdermal patch, or through nasal inhalation. An insulin pill, now under development, will hopefully be available within the next few years. The use of a glucometer, a highly accurate device for measuring the amount of glucose in the blood, allows for sound management of this condition and a life expectancy that is essentially normal. With both forms of diabetes mellitus, sound dietary practice, weight management, planned activity, and control of stress are important for keeping blood glucose levels within normal ranges. Without good management of diabetes mellitus, several serious problems can result, including blindness, gangrene, kidney disease, and heart attack; see the box "Common Complications of Diabetes." It has also been recently found that people with diabetes have an increased risk for the development of cognitive decline, including Alzheimer's disease, before the age of 65, adding yet another significant health concern for the rapidly expanding diabetic population.[43] People who cannot establish good control are likely to live a shorter life than those who can.

Double Diabetes, or Type 3 Diabetes Most recently, a "third" form of diabetes has appeared in the medical literature. This form is seen in children with type 1 diabetes mellitus, who usually have normal insulin receptors but must take exogenous insulin. In these children, most likely because of their metabolic syndrome, the body loses its ability to recognize the exogenous insulin, leading to the development of type 2 diabetes mellitus. When both forms of diabetes mellitus coexist, the child has *double diabetes,* or *type 3 diabetes mellitus.*

Sickle-Cell Trait and Sickle-Cell Disease

Among the hundreds of human diseases, few are found almost exclusively in a particular racial or ethnic group. Such is the case, however, for the inherited condition *sickle-cell trait/sickle-cell disease.* In the United States, sickle-cell abnormalities are virtually unique to African Americans.

Of all the chemical compounds found in the body, few occur in as many forms as hemoglobin, which helps bind oxygen to red blood cells. Two forms of hemoglobin are associated with sickle-cell trait and sickle-cell disease. African Americans can be the recipients of either form of this abnormal hemoglobin. Those who inherit the trait form do not develop the disease but can transmit the gene for abnormal hemoglobin to their children. In the past, those who inherited the disease form faced a shortened life characterized by periods of pain and impairment. Today, however, with effective screening and new therapeutic approaches to treatment, life expectancy is being extended. Central to this progress has been the implantation of stem cells into young sickle-cell victims that have been taken from the bone marrow of compatible donors, particularly siblings. In the future, technological advances will likely allow the use of embryonic stem cells, although probably not in the United States, and cells taken from unrelated donors.

About 8 percent of all African Americans have the gene for sickle-cell trait; they experience little impairment, but they can transmit the abnormal gene to their children. For about 1.5 percent of African Americans, sickle-cell disease is a painful, incapacitating, and life-shortening disease.

In the fully expressed disease form, red blood cells are elongated, crescent-shaped (sickled), and unable to pass through the body's minute capillaries. The body responds to the presence of these abnormal red blood cells by removing them very quickly. This sets the stage for anemia. Thus, the condition is often called *sickle-cell anemia*. In addition to anemia, the disease form of the condition can cause many serious medical problems, including impaired lung function (including pulmonary hypertension), congestive heart failure, gallbladder infections, bone changes, and abnormalities of the eye and skin.

If a key exists for preventing sickle-cell trait and disease, it lies in genetic counseling and testing in preparation for reproduction or in the use of **in vitro** fertilization followed by genetic testing of the embryo before implantation. At present, both of these preventive approaches are very expensive and limited in availability. However, further research and testing could make these methods more affordable and increase their availability to people who are at high risk.

Alzheimer's Disease

Although it affects slightly less than 2 percent of the elderly, **Alzheimer's disease (AD)** is an incapacitating, emotionally painful, and costly affliction. It is the best known of the dementia disorders, affecting an estimated 5 million adults. Today, more than ever before, it is *the* disease associated with aging. Recently, the concept of

"predementia" changes was introduced, although only initial research has been completed. A very tentative estimate of 1 million newly afflicted middle-aged people per year has been suggested.

The first signs of Alzheimer's disease are often subtle and may be confused with mild depression. Initially, the person might have difficulty answering questions such as "What is today's date?" Over the next several months, greater memory loss, evident deterioration of driving skills, confusion, and *dementia* (or loss of normal thought processes) occur. In the advanced stages, people with Alzheimer's disease become incontinent, show infantile behavior, and finally become incapacitated as brain tissue is destroyed. With advanced Alzheimer's disease, institutionalization becomes necessary.

In the current classification system for AD, two principal categories are used, *early-onset AD* (before age 65) and *late-onset AD* (after age 65). Early-onset AD, encompassing types 1, 3, and 4, accounts for approximately 25 percent of all AD patients and is an inherited form of the disease. Chromosomes 1, 14, and 21 have been identified as factors in this form of the disease. Late-onset AD, designated as type 2, the most prevalent form of the disease, is less clearly understood from a genetic point of view, although chromosome 19 is believed to be involved. Chromosomes 9, 10, and 12 are also drawing attention. Perhaps as many as 20 specific genes, found on these and other chromosomes, have recently been hypothesized to be involved in the development of AD.

Alzheimer's disease is difficult to diagnose because its symptoms are similar to those of other types of dementia. It is only after the person's death, if an autopsy is performed, that the characteristic changes in the brain can be used to make a definitive diagnosis. As a practical matter, a probable diagnosis of Alzheimer's disease is made by the process of elimination. Newer medical imaging technologies, such as MRI, have become so refined that it is now *almost* possible to confirm the diagnosis of Alzheimer's disease before death. An example of this is the recent development of a new double-contrast medium, Amyvid (florbetapir), that, upon injection, produces PET scan images of amyloid plaque with extremely high definition. This technology not only makes a definitive diagnosis possible before death but also allows the progression of the disease to be more accurately seen.[44]

Medications to cure Alzheimer's disease do not exist at this time. However, three drugs (Razadyne [galantamine], Exelon [rivastigmine], and Aricept [donepezil]) provide temporary improvement in intellectual function during the early stages of the disease by inhibiting the breakdown of acetylcholine, whose diminished availability is the basis of the disease. A newer medication, memantine, used in treating moderate-to-severe AD, functions by blocking glutamate, a substance capable of damaging neurons. Of all AD drugs, donepezil is most widely used, while galantamine influences receptors for

---

> **Key Terms**
>
> **in vitro** Outside the living body, in an artificial environment.
>
> **Alzheimer's disease (AD)** Gradual development of memory loss, confusion, and loss of reasoning; eventually leads to total intellectual incapacitation, brain degeneration, and death.

three other neurotransmitters, as well as nicotine receptors, all of which play roles in the disease.

At this time, a wide array of studies attempting to link behavioral patterns to the prevention of cognitive decline with aging and the development of AD are under way. Among these are studies assessing the role of fatty acids (particularly n-3 omega fatty acid) in preventing cognitive decline, the role of exercise (particularly walking) in improving cognitive capabilities in aging adults, and the contributions of regular light alcohol consumption in protecting against Alzheimer's-like conditions. Additional studies in the same vein include those related to the effectiveness of nonsteroidal anti-inflammatory drugs (NSAIDs) in preventing cognitive decline, the ability of antioxidant vitamins (carotenes, vitamin C, and vitamin E) to prevent dementia, and the role of the Mediterranean diet (see Chapter 5), as well as reductions in dietary fats, and steps needed to reduce the growing incidence of metabolic syndrome (prediabetes) that is developing at alarming rates in this country and around the world.

Chronic Conditions and a Sense of Well-Being

Now that we have given ample consideration to several types of cancer and selected chronic conditions, return to Chapter 1 to review Figures 1-1, 1-2, and 1-3. In doing so, you can more fully appreciate the potentially negative impact that a chronic, demanding, and potentially life-shortening condition like cancer (or any of the other chronic conditions discussed in the chapter) can have on a person's quest for a sense of well-being. Recall that resources from all dimensions of health are needed to engage in the activities required to fulfill role responsibilities. Chronic conditions diminish the quantity and quality of these resources, requiring that, in some cases, roles be relinquished. For example, the CEO of a company may be forced to take a reduced leadership role to deal with the effects and treatment of her condition, or a father may similarly be unable to meet all the demands placed on him by his children.

As a person with cancer or another chronic condition becomes less capable of meeting role fulfillment, over time the growing inability to meet role expectations can minimize progress in fulfilling the even larger developmental expectation of his or her life-cycle stage. As this occurs, the chronically ill victim's sense of well-being, normally fueled by the knowledge that progress can be sustained, is lessened. Further, because of the reciprocity that exists between all of the elements depicted in Figures 1-1, 1-2, and 1-3, resource deterioration continues, often at an accelerated pace, and a sense of life satisfaction declines further. For cancer victims or others whose prognosis is poor, a sense of despair can develop to the extent that both death and dying may become the central focus of their remaining time.

Taking Charge of Your Health

- Monitor your work, home, and recreational environments to determine whether they are placing you at risk for cancer.
- Perform regular self-examinations for forms of cancer that can be detected through this technique.

- Undergo the recommended cancer screening procedures for your age and sex.
- Stay attuned to media reports about chronic conditions so that you can make informed choices.

- Support agencies devoted to the prevention of chronic health conditions.
- If you have a chronic condition, participate actively in your own treatment.

SUMMARY

- Cancer is a condition in which the body is unable to control the specialization, replication, and repair of cells or the suppression of abnormal cell formation.
- A variety of agents, including genetic mutations, viruses, and carcinogens, stimulate the conversion of regulatory genes (proto-oncogenes) into oncogenes.
- Cigarette smoking is a principal player in the development of nearly 30 percent of all forms of cancer.
- Early detection based on self-examination and screening is the basis for the early identification of several cancers.

- Systemic lupus erythematosus (SLE) is an autoimmune condition in which the immune system fails to recognize the body's own connective tissues and instead interprets them as being foreign.
- Irritable bowel syndrome and inflammatory bowel disease reflect differing levels of hypersensitivity on the part of the immune system to tissues of the gastrointestinal tract.
- Multiple sclerosis (MS) results from a continuing attack by the immune system on cells within the nervous system

that produce myelin, the insulating material critical in the functioning of the brain and spinal cord.
- Types 1 and 2 diabetes mellitus are metabolic disorders involving difficulties in the production or recognition of insulin, thus depriving the body of its normal ability to manage blood glucose utilization. Type 3 diabetes is the combination of types 1 and 2 in the same individual.
- Sickle-cell disease is an inherited abnormality involving the presence of two recessive genes that result in the production of abnormal hemoglobin, thus reducing oxygen-carrying capacity. Sickle-cell trait involves the presence of a single recessive gene for the disease condition, resulting in the person's being a carrier of the condition.
- Alzheimer's is a disease that results, over time, in a profound state of dementia in which the brain is unable to continue producing a neurotransmitter critical to cognitive functioning.

REVIEW QUESTIONS

1. What is the relationship between regulatory genes, including tumor suppressor genes, in the development of cancer? Why are regulatory genes called both proto-oncogenes and oncogenes?
2. What properties do cancer cells possess that are lacking in normal cells?
3. What are the principal factors that contribute to the development of lung cancer? Of breast cancer? When should regular use of mammography begin, and which women should begin using it earliest?
4. What are the steps for effective self-examination of the breasts and testicles? What is the new status of breast self-examination?
5. What signs indicate the possibility that a skin lesion has become cancerous?
6. What are the problems that arise with SLE, and how is this autoimmune condition managed?
7. What critically important material within the nervous system is eroded by the immune system in conjunction with multiple sclerosis? What are the consequences of losing the ability to continue production of this material?
8. How are type 1 and type 2 diabetes similar, and how are they clearly different conditions? What is "metabolic syndrome," and how does it relate to type 2 diabetes mellitus?
9. What racial group is most susceptible to sickle-cell trait/ disease? What is sickle-cell trait/disease? How could genetic counseling be used in the prevention of this condition?
10. In terms of Alzheimer's disease, what is the cause of its victims' cognitive decline? How effective are current medications used in the treatment of AD?

ANSWERS TO THE "WHAT DO YOU KNOW?" QUIZ

1. False   2. True   3. False   4. False   5. False   6. True   7. True

Visit the Online Learning Center (www.mhhe.com/hahn11e), where you will find tools to help you improve your grade including practice quizzes, key terms flashcards, audio chapter summaries for your MP3 player, and many other study aids.

SOURCE NOTES

1. World Health Organization. Boyle P, Levin B. *World Cancer Report—2008*, February 2009.
2. American Cancer Society. *Cancer Facts & Figures—2010.*
3. DeNavas-Walt C, Proctor B, Smith J. *Income, Poverty, and Health Insurance Coverage in the United States: 2007.* U.S. Census Bureau, August 2008.
4. Mukherjee S. *The Emperor of All Maladies: A Biography of Cancer.* New York: Scribner, 2010.
5. Jemal A, et al. Trends in the Leading Causes of Death in the United States, 1997–2002. *Journal of the American Medical Association,* 294(10), 1255–59, September 14, 2008.
6. Zhao Y, Epstein RJ. Unexpected functional similarities between gatekeeper tumour suppressor genes and proto-oncogenes revealed by systems biology. *Journal of Human Genetics,* March 3, 2011 (Epub ahead of print).
7. Buonaguro FM, Lewis GK, Pelicci P. Introducing infectious agents and cancer. *Infectious Agents and Cancer,* 1, 1, September 14, 2006.
8. Neumann R, Bluemke D. Tracking radiation exposure from diagnostic devices at the NIH. *Journal of the American College of Radiology,* 7(2), 87–89, 2010.
9. Schwad M (ed.). *Encyclopedia of Cancer* (Vols. 1–4, 2nd ed.). New York: Springer, 2008.
10. Harrington CR, Beswick C, Leitenberger J, et al. Addictive-like behaviors to ultraviolet light among frequent indoor tanners. *Clinical and Experimental Dermatology,* 36(l), 33–38, 2011.
11. Louafi A, et al. Merkel Cell Carcinoma: study of 24 cases and review of the literature. *Annales de chirurgie plastique et esthétique,* February 2009 (Epub ahead of print).
12. Berle DR, Berg CD, Bloack WC, et al. The National Lung Screening Trial: overview and study design. *Radiology,* 258(l), 243–253, 2011.
13. Henschke CI, et al. Survival of patients with stage 1 lung cancer detected on CT screening. *New England Journal of Medicine,* 355(17), 1763–71, October 26, 2006.
14. Ou SH, Bazhenova L, Camidge DR, et al. Rapid and dramatic radiographic and clinical response to an ALK inhibitor (crizotinib, PF02341066) in an ALK translocation-positve patients with non-small cell lung cancer. *Journal of Thoracic Oncology,* 5(12), 2044–46, 2010.
15. Jemal A, et al. Annual report to the nation of the status of cancer, 1975–2005, featuring trends in lung cancer, tobacco use, and tobacco control. *Journal of the National Cancer Institute,* 100(23), 1672–98, December 3, 2008.
16. Acott AA, et al. Association of tobacco and alcohol use with earlier development of colorectal cancer: Should we modify screening guidelines? *American Journal of Surgery,* 196(6), 915–919, December 2008.

17. Rothwell PM, Wilson M, Elwin CE, et al. Long-term effect of aspirin on colorectal cancer incidence and mortality: 20-year follow-up of five randomized trials. *Lancet,* 376(9754), 1741–50, 2010.

18. Whitlock EP, et al. Screening for colorectal cancer: a targeted, updated systematic review for the U.S. preventive services task force. *Annals of Internal Medicine,* 149(9), 638–656, November 4, 2008.

19. Veerappan GR, Ally MR, Choi JH, et al. Extracolonic findings on CT colonography increases yield of colorectal cancer screening. *American Journal of Roentgenology,* 195(3), 677–686, 2010.

20. Krainer M, et al. Differential contributions of BRCA1 and BRCA2 to early-onset breast cancer. *New England Journal of Medicine,* 336(20), 1416–21, 1997.

21. Hansen TO, Jonson L, Albrechtsen A, et al. Large BRCA1 and BRCA2 genomic rearrangement in Danish high risk breast-ovarian cancer families. *Breast Cancer Research and Treatment,* 115, 315–323, 2009.

22. *Breast Cancer Chemoprevention: Medicines That Reduce Breast Cancer Risk.* Updated January 2009. Mayo Foundation. www.mayoclinic.com/health/breast-cancer/WO00092.

23. D'Orsi CJ, Newell MS. On the frontline of screening for breast cancer. *Seminars in Oncology,* 38(1), 119–127, 2011.

24. *Breast Cancer Treatment.* Updated January 2011. Mayo Foundation. www.mayoclinic.org/breast-cancer/treatment.html.

25. Lawrentschuk N, Daljeet N, Trottier G. An analysis of world media reporting of two recent large randomized prospective trials investigating screening for prostate cancer. March 29, 2011 (Epub ahead of print).

26. American Cancer Society. Survival rates for testicular cancer. *British Journal of Urology,* 2011. www.cancer.org/cancer/testicularcancer/overviewguide/testicular-cancer-overview.

27. U.S. Food and Drug Administration. FDA News. FDA approves expanded use of Gardasil to include preventing certain vulvar and vaginal cancers. September 12, 2008. www.fda.gov/bbs/topics/NEWS/2008/NEW01885.html.

28. Giorgi Rossi P, Ronco G. HPV types in early-onset cervical cancer. *Lancet Oncology,* 12(2), 1048–56, 2010.

29. Zeleniuch-Jacquotte A, et al. Circulating enterolactone and risk of endometrial cancer. *International Journal of Cancer,* 119(10), 2376–81, November 15, 2006.

30. Moschos E, Ashfaq R, McIntire D, et al. Saline-infusion sonography endometrial sampling compared with endometrial biopsy in diagnosing endometrial pathology. *Obstetrics and Gynecology,* 113(4), 881–887, 2009.

31. Larsson SC, et al. Aspirin and nonsteroidal anti-inflammatory drug use and risk of pancreatic cancer: a meta-analysis. *Cancer Epidemiology Biomarkers Prevention,* 15 (12), 2561–64, 2006.

32. Skinner HG, et al. Vitamin D intake and the risk of pancreatic cancer in two cohort studies. *Epidemiology, Biomarkers and Prevention,* 15(9), 1688–95, September 2006.

33. Boscoe FP, Schymura MJ. Solar Ultraviolet-B exposure and cancer incidence and mortality in the United States, 1993–2002. *BMC Cancer,* 6, 264, November 10, 2006.

34. Bulathsinghala P, Syrigos KN, Saif MW. Role of vitamin D in the prevention of pancreatic cancer. *Journal of Nutrition and Metabolism.* Epub January 9, 2011.

35. Kasper, et al. *Harrison's Principles of Internal Medicine* (17th ed.). New York: McGraw-Hill, 2008.

36. Compeyrot-Lacassagne S, et al. Prevalence and etiology of low bone mineral density in juvenile systemic lupus erythematosus. *Arthritis and Rheumatism,* 56(6), 1966–73, June 2007.

37. Information for Healthcare Professionals. Cimzia (Certolizumab Pegol), Embrel (Etanercept), Humira (Adalimumab), and Remicade (Infliximab). U.S. Food and Drug Administration. Center for Drug Evaluation and Research, September 4, 2008. www.fda.gov/CDER/drug/InfoSheets/HCP/TNF_blockersHCP.htm.

38. Ordonez G, Martinez-Palomo A, Corona T. Varicella zoster virus in progressive forms of multiple sclerosis. *Clinical Neurology and Neurosurgery,* 112(8), 653–657, 2010.

39. Burk RK, et al. Autologous non-myeloablative haemopoietic stem cell transplantation in relapsing-remitting multiple sclerosis: a phase I/II study. *Lancet Neurology,* 8(3), 244–253, March 2009. Epub January 29, 2009.

40. Goodman AD, Brown TR, Edwards KR. A phase 3 trial of extended release dalfampridine in multiple sclerosis. *Annals of Neurology,* 68(4), 494–502, 2010.

41. Clinical Practice Recommendations 2010. Standards of Medical Care in Diabetes 2010. American Diabetes Association. *Diabetes Care,* 33, Supp. 1, 2010.

42. Libman IM, Becker JD. Coexistence of type 1 and type 2 diabetes mellitus: "double" diabetes? *Pediatric Diabetes,* 4(2), 110–113, June 2006.

43. Xu W, et al. Mid- and late-life diabetes in relation to the risk of dementia: a population-based twin study. *Diabetes,* 58(1), 71–77, January 2009. Epub October 2008.

44. Clark CM, Schneider JA, Bedell BJ, et al. Use of florbetapir-PET for imaging beta-amyloid pathology. *Journal of the American Medical Association,* 305(3), 275–283, 2011.

Personal Assessment

Thinking About Chronic Illness

Not all personal assessment needs to focus on some behavior and then generate a score that indicates your level of compliance. Rather, a personal assessment can be helpful by simply asking you to think about how you feel about a particular trait, situation, or characteristic, such as those related to being chronically ill. Consider the following scenarios:

1. You have recently been diagnosed with a chronic illness that, though treatable, is not curable and is progressive in nature. As you leave the physician's office and the reality sets in, what thoughts are in your mind?

2. Many illnesses and injuries cause significant changes in appearance. A student in your health/wellness class looks noticeably different than he or she did earlier in the semester. You overhear some of your classmates making insensitive comments. How might you respond?

3. You have recently been diagnosed with a condition that, due to a weakened immune system, has forced you to drop out of school, leave your job, and go on disability. Now homebound, how do you keep up with your responsibilities as a partner and parent, your activities and hobbies, and even your own sense of self?

4. Your condition of multiple sclerosis has progressed to the point where you cannot walk safely—the frequency of falls has prompted your neurologist to insist that you use a walker. Now, a formerly "silent condition" is visible to everyone. To what extent will you comply with your physician's advice?

5. You have a condition that has affected your optic nerve and impaired your vision to the point that you can no longer drive. You live in a somewhat isolated area, and your friends seem to have forgotten you. How will

you fill your time? To what extent will social networking sites, text messaging, and e-mails help you to feel connected?

6. Along with the diagnosis of your chronic illness comes the news that you will never be able to have your own biological children. You have always dreamt of being a parent. Will you look into alternative forms of parenting, such as adoption, surrogacy, or foster parenting? Even though this may not be a biological child, to what extent will you still feel fulfilled as a parent?

7. You have had Crohn's disease for years, and the disease's progression has caused malabsorption, anemia, and diarrhea accompanied by many "accidents." Going into surgery, you expect a resection of the colon; however, waking up in recovery, you discover that you have an ileostomy. Your surgeon explains that the colon was too diseased to salvage and as a consequence, the end of the small intestine has been brought through the abdominal wall to form a stoma (or opening). This opening will be "bagged" to collect your bodily waste. You'll have to develop a new way of going to the bathroom, learn how to change your ostomy bag, and modify your wardrobe to accommodate your appliance. How will you adjust to an ileostomy?

8. Your life used to be so different. You took part in every activity. You ran half-marathons. Now, due to your chronic illness, all of those things you enjoyed you can no longer do. Your vision, dexterity, motor skills, and ability to eat, drink, excrete waste, talk, write, and type are all compromised. So many changes have happened to your body, yet the length of your life will not be significantly shortened. At what point would you consider ending your life?

11

Preventing Infectious Diseases

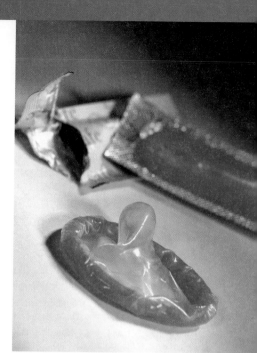

What Do You Know About Infectious Diseases?

1. Infectious diseases follow a predictable pathway as they move from an infected person to a soon-to-be infected person. *True or False?*

2. The immune system can be "armed" to fight infectious disease by only one process—contracting the particular disease and then recovering from it. *True or False?*

3. Nosocomial infections are most often contracted in large public gatherings, such as an indoor sports arena. *True or False?*

4. On the college campus, the student group most susceptible to contracting bacterial meningitis is graduate students. *True or False?*

5. Because of concerns over tampon misuse, health officials are strongly encouraging women to discontinue the use of internal sanitary protection products (tampons). *True or False?*

6. Today the American public seems less interested in the HIV/AIDS pandemic than it was in the past. *True or False?*

7. The most effective way to avoid contracting STDs is through abstaining from sexual activity. *True or False?*

Check your answers at the end of the chapter.

In the nineteenth century, infectious diseases were the leading cause of death. These deaths came after exposure to the organisms that produced such diseases as smallpox, tuberculosis (TB), influenza, whooping cough (pertussis), typhoid, diphtheria, and tetanus. However, since the early 1900s, improvements in public sanitation, the widespread use of antibiotic drugs, and vaccinations have considerably reduced the number of people who die from infectious diseases. People now die more often from chronic disease processes.

Today, however, we have a new respect for infectious diseases. By the end of 2009, an estimated 33.3 million people worldwide were living with HIV/AIDS,[1] with long-range projections pointing to 70 million in the absence of effective prevention programs. We are witnessing a resurgence of TB. We recognize the role of pelvic infections in infertility. We also know that failure to fully immunize children has laid the

Table 11.1 Pathogens and Common Infectious Diseases

Pathogen	Description	Representative Disease Processes
Viruses	Smallest common pathogens; nonliving particles of genetic material (DNA) surrounded by a protein coat; requires host cells for growth and replication	Rubeola, mumps, chicken pox, rubella, influenza, warts, colds, oral and genital herpes, shingles, AIDS, genital warts
Prion	Potentially self-replicating protein, lacking both DNA and RNA, virus-like in size	Creutzfeldt-Jakob disease, Gerstmann-Straussler-Scheinker syndrome, "mad cow" disease (bovine spongiform encephalopathy)
Bacteria	One-celled microorganisms with sturdy, well-defined cell walls; three distinctive forms: spherical, rod shaped, and spiral shaped	Tetanus, strep throat, scarlet fever, gonorrhea, syphilis, chlamydia, toxic shock syndrome, Legionnaires' disease, bacterial pneumonia, meningitis, diphtheria, Lyme disease
Fungi	Plantlike microorganisms; molds and yeasts	Athlete's foot, ringworm, histoplasmosis, San Joaquin Valley fever, candidiasis
Protozoa	Single-cell, nucleated, primitive, parasitic animal-like organisms, capable of mobility	Malaria, amebic dysentery, trichomoniasis, vaginitis
Rickettsia	A type of bacteria, with many virus-like characteristics, that requires host cells for growth and replication	Typhus, Rocky Mountain spotted fever, rickettsialpox
Parasitic worms	Many-celled relatively simple animals; represented by tapeworms, leeches, and roundworms	Dirofilariasis (dog heartworm), elephantiasis, onchocerciasis

Source: From Barbara Hamann, *Disease: Identification, Prevention and Control*, 3/e, © 2007 The McGraw-Hill Companies, Inc. Used with permission.

groundwork for a return of whooping cough, measles, polio, and other serious childhood diseases. In fact, some experts suggest that because of HIV/AIDS and the emergence and reemergence of infectious diseases, today's young adults may have a lower life expectancy than did the generation immediately ahead of them.

Several new types of infectious disease have appeared such as the NDM-1 bacterium (first identified in New Delhi) and the KPC bacterium (which produces an enzyme that now inactivates multiple antibiotics that once were effective).[2]

Infectious Disease Transmission

Infectious diseases can generally be transmitted from person to person, although the transfer is not always direct. Infectious diseases can be especially dangerous because they can spread to large numbers of people, producing **epidemics** or **pandemics.** The following sections explain the process of disease transmission and the stages of infection.

Pathogens

For a disease to be transferred, a person must come into contact with the disease-producing agent, or **pathogen,** such as a virus, bacterium, or fungus. When pathogens enter our bodies, the pathogens can sometimes resist body defense systems, flourish, and produce an illness. We commonly call this an *infection.* Because of their small size, pathogens are sometimes called *microorganisms* or *microbes.*[3] Table 11.1 describes infectious disease agents and some of the illnesses they produce.

Chain of Infection

The movement of a pathogenic agent through the various links in the chain of infection (see Figure 11-1) explains how diseases spread. Not every pathogenic agent moves all the way through the chain of infection, because various links in the chain can be broken. Therefore, the presence of a pathogen creates only the potential for causing disease.

Agent The first link in the chain of infection is the disease-causing **agent.** Whereas some agents are highly **virulent** and lead to serious infectious illnesses such as HIV, which causes AIDS, others produce far less serious infections, such as the common cold. Through mutation, some pathogenic agents, particularly viruses, can become more virulent.

Key Terms

epidemic A highly significant increase in the number of cases of an infectious illness existing within the same time period in a given geographical area.

pandemic An epidemic that has crossed national boundaries, thus achieving regional or international status (HIV/AIDS is a pandemic).

pathogen A disease-causing agent.

agent The causal pathogen of a particular disease.

virulent (**veer** yuh lent) Capable of causing disease.

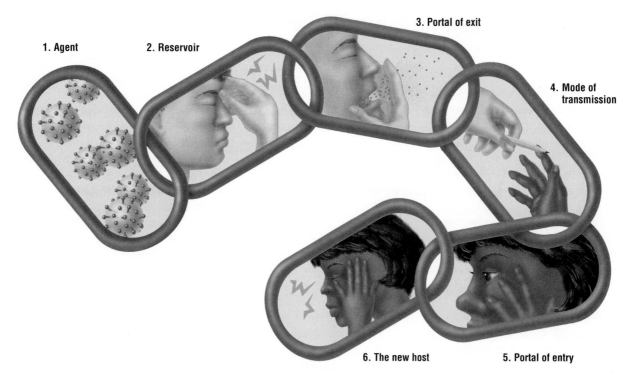

1. Agent **2. Reservoir** **3. Portal of exit** **4. Mode of transmission** **6. The new host** **5. Portal of entry**

Figure 11-1 The Chain of Infection   The example above shows a rhinovirus, which causes the common cold, being passed from one person to another. (1) The *agent* (pathogen) is a rhinovirus; (2) the *reservoir* is the infected person; (3) the *portal of exit* is the respiratory system (coughing); (4) the *mode of transmission* is the indirect hand contact; (5) the *portal of entry* is the mucous membranes of the uninfected person's eye; (6) the virus now has a *new host*.

Reservoir   Infectious agents require the support and protection of a favorable environment to survive. This environment forms the second link in the chain of infection and is called the *reservoir.* For many of the most common infectious diseases, the reservoirs are the bodies of people who are already infected. Here the agents thrive before being spread to others. These infected people are, accordingly, the hosts for particular disease agents. In some infectious illnesses, a person's reservoir status may be restored after treatment and apparent recovery from the original infection. This is because some pathogens, particularly viruses, can remain sequestered (hidden), emerging later to give rise to another infection. The herpes viruses are often sequestered.

For other infectious diseases, however, the reservoirs are the bodies of animals. Avian (bird) flu is a much discussed animal-reservoir disease. The infected animals are not always sick and do not always show symptoms similar to those seen in infected people.

The third type of reservoir in which disease-causing agents can live is a nonliving environment, such as the soil. The spores of the tetanus bacterium, for example, can survive in soil for up to 50 years, entering the human body in a puncture wound.

Portal of Exit   For pathogenic agents to cause diseases and illnesses in others, they must leave their reservoirs.

Thus, the third link in the chain of infection is the *portal of exit,* or the point at which agents leave their reservoirs.

The principal portals of exit are familiar—the digestive, urinary, respiratory, and reproductive systems, and the blood, especially with infectious diseases that infect humans.

Mode of Transmission   The fourth link in the chain of infection is the *mode of transmission,* or the way in which pathogens move from reservoirs to susceptible hosts. Two principal methods are direct transmission and indirect transmission.

We see three types of direct, human-to-human transmission. These include contact between body surfaces (such as kissing, touching, and sexual intercourse), droplet spread (inhalation of contaminated air droplets), and fecal-oral spread (feces on the host's hands are brought into contact with the new host's mouth), as could occur when changing the diaper of an infected infant.

Indirect transmission between infected and uninfected people occurs when infectious agents travel by means of nonhuman materials. Vehicles of transmission include inanimate objects (known as *fomites*), such as water, food, soil, towels, clothing, and eating utensils.

Infectious agents can also be indirectly transmitted through vectors. *Vectors* are living things, such as insects, birds, and other animals, that carry diseases from human to human. An example of a vector is the deer tick, which transmits Lyme disease.

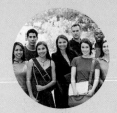

Learning from Our Diversity

Infectious Disease: A Challenge for Older Adults

It's not always easy for young adults in excellent health to recover quickly and completely from some infectious diseases. Later in life, the recovery often becomes much more difficult and in some cases impossible. For a variety of reasons, older adults do not recover from infectious conditions with the same resiliency as they once did.

Central to this issue is the gradual degradation of the immune system over time. For reasons not fully understood, the immune system loses both its ability to recognize the presence of pathogens that have entered the body and its ability to mount an effective response against them. Whether this reduced level of immune protection is a "programmed" aspect of aging (all human life does end at some point in time) or whether it reflects a process that is preventable (perhaps through lifestyle modifications) remains hotly debated. Perhaps no group of older adults is at greater risk because of a compromised immune system than are those with AIDS.

In addition to the normal aging of their immune systems, older adults are generally afflicted with a variety of chronic conditions. The presence of multiple chronic illnesses (known as *comorbidity*) places the body under great stress, which also undermines the immune system. The combined effects of these conditions result in damage to different organ systems of the body—most importantly, the cardiovascular system, the respiratory system, and the renal system. Any time these systems are compromised by the effects of illness, either chronic or acute, the body becomes particularly vulnerable to infectious agents that routinely exist in our environment.

Compounding this situation is the inability of many older adults to understand the potential seriousness of infections at this stage of their lives. In addition, a lack of social support, isolation from health care facilities, and the inability to afford expensive prescription medication together make important medical care less available at a time when it could be effective.

When these factors are combined, as they are for many older adults, serious and even fatal infectious conditions become a reality. Therefore, anyone who is responsible for the health and well-being of older persons needs to understand their susceptibility to infectious conditions and recognize the fact that timely and competent care is of critical importance.

Airborne indirect transmission includes the inhalation of infected particles that have been suspended in an air source for an extended time. Unlike droplet transmission, in which both infected and uninfected people must be in close physical proximity, noninfected people can become infected through airborne transmission by sharing air with infected people who were in the same room hours earlier. Viral infections such as German measles can be spread this way.

Portal of Entry   The fifth link in the chain of infection is the *portal of entry*. As with the portals of exit, portals of entry have three primary methods that allow pathogenic agents to enter the bodies of uninfected people. These are through the digestive, respiratory, and reproductive systems. In addition, a break in the skin provides another portal of entry. In most infectious conditions, the portals of entry are the same systems that served as the portals of exit from the infected people. In HIV, however, we see cross-system transmission. Oral and anal sex allow infectious agents to pass between the warm, moist tissues of the reproductive and digestive systems.

The New Host   All people are, in theory, at risk for contracting infectious diseases and thus could be called susceptible hosts. In practice, however, factors such as overall health, acquired immunity, health care services, and health-related behavior can affect susceptibility to infectious diseases (see the box "Infectious Disease: A Challenge for Older Adults").

Stages of Infection

When a pathogenic agent assaults a new host, a reasonably predictable sequence of events begins. That is, the disease moves through five distinctive stages.[3] You may be able to recognize these stages of infection each time you catch a cold.

1. *The incubation stage.* This stage lasts from the time a pathogen enters the body until it multiplies enough to produce signs and symptoms of the disease. The duration of this stage can vary from a few hours to many months, depending on the virulence of the organisms, the concentration of organisms, the host's level of immune responsiveness, and other health problems. This stage has been called a *silent stage.* The pathogen can be transmitted to a new host during this stage, but this is not likely. A host may be infected during this stage but not be infectious. HIV infection is an exception to this rule.

2. *The prodromal stage.* After the incubation stage, the host may experience a variety of general signs and symptoms, including watery eyes, runny nose, slight fever, and overall tiredness for a brief time. These symptoms are nonspecific and may not be severe enough to force the host to rest. During this stage, the pathogenic agent continues to multiply. Now the host is capable of transferring pathogens to a new host, but this is not yet the most infectious stage of an infectious disease. One should practice

self-imposed isolation during this stage to protect others. Again, HIV infection is different in this stage.

3. *The clinical stage.* This stage, also called the *acme* or *acute stage,* is often the most unpleasant stage for the host. At this time, the disease reaches its highest point of development. Laboratory tests can identify or analyze all of the clinical (observable) signs and symptoms of the particular disease. The likelihood of transmitting the disease to others is highest during this peak stage; all of our available defense mechanisms are in the process of resisting further damage from the pathogen.

4. *The decline stage.* The first signs of recovery appear during this stage. The infection is ending or, in some cases, falling to a subclinical level. People may suffer a relapse if they overextend themselves.

5. *The recovery stage.* Also called the *convalescence stage,* this stage is characterized by apparent recovery from the invading agent. The disease can be transmitted during this stage, but this is not probable. Until the host's overall health has been strengthened, he or she may be especially susceptible to another (perhaps different) disease pathogen. Fortunately, after the recovery stage, further susceptibility to the pathogenic agent is typically lower because the body has built up immunity. This buildup of immunity is not always permanent; for example, many sexually transmitted diseases can be contracted repeatedly.

We will discuss HIV/AIDS later in the chapter; for now, however, we need to note that this critically important pandemic infectious disease does not easily fit into the five-stage model of infectious diseases just presented. In individuals infected with HIV, there is an initial asymptomatic *incubation stage,* followed by a *prodromal stage* characterized by generalized signs of immune system inadequacy. However, once the level of specific protective cells of the immune system declines to the point that the body cannot be protected from opportunistic diseases, and the label AIDS is assigned, the five-stage model becomes less easily applied.

Body Defenses: Mechanical and Cellular-Chemical Immune Systems

Much as a series of defensive alignments protect a military installation, so too is the body protected by sets of defenses. These defenses can be classified as either mechanical or cellular-chemical. Mechanical defenses are first-line defenses, because they physically separate the internal body from the external environment. Examples include the skin, the mucous membranes that line the respiratory

Are Americans Too Clean?

Infectious disease specialists are increasingly concerned about the widespread popularity and availability of antimicrobial cleaning products and the contribution they may be making to the development of antibiotic-resistant "super bugs." In fact, it is estimated that approximately 75 percent of all liquid hand soaps and nearly 30 percent of all bar soaps contain either triclocarban or triclosan, antibacterial chemicals to which pathogenic agents are already showing resistance.

As concern about our increasing reliance on antimicrobial products grows, we are reminded of the first personal hygiene rule that most Americans were taught as children at home and in school: Wash your hands thoroughly with soap and *hot water!* Even today, microbiologists remind us that nothing is more effective in cleaning our bodies, our homes, and our workplaces than "old-fashioned" soap and hot water.

and gastrointestinal tracts, earwax, the tiny hairs and cilia that filter incoming air, and even tears. These defenses serve primarily as a shield against foreign materials that may contain pathogenic agents. These defenses can, however, be disarmed, such as when tobacco smoke kills the cilia that protect the airways, resulting in chronic bronchitis, or when contact lenses reduce tearing, leading to irritation and eye infection (see the box "Are Americans Too Clean?").

The second component of the body's protective defenses is the cellular-chemical system or, more commonly, the **immune system.** The immune system is far more specific than the mechanical defenses. Its primary mission is to eliminate microorganisms, foreign protein, and abnormal cells from the body. A wellness-oriented lifestyle, including sound nutrition, effective stress management, and regular exercise, supports this important division of the immune system. The microorganisms, foreign protein, or abnormal cells that activate this cellular component are collectively called *antigens.*[4]

Divisions of the Immune System

Closer examination of the immune system, or cellular-chemical defenses, reveals two separate but highly cooperative groups of cells. One group of cells originates in the

> **Key Terms**
>
> **immune system** The system of cellular and chemical elements that protects the body from invading pathogens, foreign protein, and abnormal cells.

fetal thymus gland and has become known as *T cell–mediated immunity,* or simply **cell-mediated immunity.** The second group of cells that makes up cellular immunity are the B cells (bursa of Fabricius), which are the working units of **humoral immunity.** [5] Cellular elements of both cell-mediated and humoral immunity can be found within the bloodstream, the lymphatic tissues of the body (including those within the gastrointestinal system), and the fluid that surrounds body cells. In addition to the two major divisions of the immune system, a variety of antibodies, phagocytes (large white cells) such as natural killer (NK) cells, monocytes and macrophages, granulocytes (including neutrophils, eosinophils, and basophiles), and important large protein complexes called *complement* function in ways both independent of cell-mediated immunity and humoral immunity and in cooperation with these two major divisions of the immune system. When viewed collectively, these components directly eat antigens (phagocytosis), release caustic chemicals that degrade antigens, and send out chemical messengers that support cellular and humoral responses.

Although we are born with the structural elements of both cell-mediated and humoral immunity, developing an immune response requires that components of these cellular systems encounter and successfully defend against specific antigens. When the immune system has done this once, it is, in most cases, primed to respond quickly and effectively if the same antigens appear again. This initial confrontation produces a state of **acquired immunity (AI).** [4] Acquired immunity develops in different ways.

- **Naturally acquired immunity (NAI)** develops when the body is exposed to infectious agents. Thus, when we catch an infectious disease, we fight the infection and in the process become immune (protected) from developing that illness if we encounter these agents again. For example, when a child catches chicken pox and then recovers, it is unlikely that the child will develop a subsequent case of chicken pox. Before the advent of immunizations, this was the only way of developing immunity.

- **Artificially acquired immunity (AAI)** occurs when the body is exposed to weakened or killed infectious agents introduced through vaccination or immunization. As in NAI, the body fights the infectious agents and records the method of fighting the agents. Young children, older adults, and adults in high-risk occupations should consult their physicians about immunizations.

- **Passively acquired immunity (PAI),** a third form of immunity, results when extrinsic antibodies are introduced into the body. These antibodies are for a variety of specific infections, and they are produced outside the body (either in animals or by the genetic manipulation of microorganisms). When introduced into the human body, they provide immediate protection until the body can develop a more natural form of immunity. This form of short-term but immediate protection is provided when the emergency room staff administers a tetanus-toxoid "booster." Note that in PAI no actual pathogenic agents are introduced into the body—only the antibodies against various forms of disease-causing agents.

Regardless of how infectious agents are acquired, either through NAI or through AAI, the result is an "arming" of the body's own immune system. This process is frequently labeled as *active immunity.* This contrasts to PAI, in which the body "borrows" another's immune elements, without actual involvement of the body's own immune system. This latter case is called *passive immunity.*[6]

In addition to the forms of immunity just described, unborn infants are also provided with a period of short-term immunity via the biological mother's immune system elements crossing the placental barrier (see Chapter 13), and then following birth via breast milk. This *maternal immunity,* however, gradually deteriorates but is concurrently being replaced by the child's own increasingly functional immune system.

Collectively, these forms of immunity can provide important protection against infectious disease.

> **Key Terms**
>
> **cell-mediated immunity** Immunity provided principally by the immune system's T cells, both working alone and in combination with highly specialized B cells; also called *T cell–mediated immunity.*
>
> **humoral immunity** Immunity responsible for the production of critically important immune system elements known as *antibodies;* also called *B cell–mediated immunity.*
>
> **acquired immunity (AI)** A form of immunity resulting from exposure to foreign protein (most often wild, weakened, or killed pathogenic organisms).
>
> **naturally acquired immunity (NAI)** A type of acquired immunity resulting from the body's response to naturally occurring pathogens.
>
> **artificially acquired immunity (AAI)** A type of acquired immunity resulting from the body's response to pathogens introduced into the body through immunizations.
>
> **passively acquired immunity (PAI)** A temporary immunity achieved by providing antibodies to a person exposed to a particular pathogen.
>
> **antibodies** Chemical compounds produced by the body's immune system to destroy antigens and their toxins.

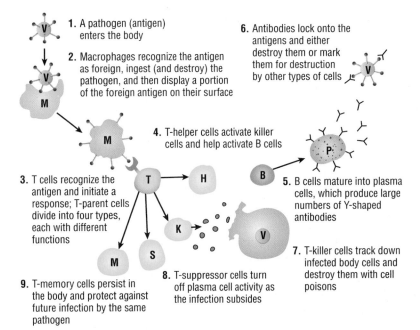

Figure 11-2 The Immune Response Cellular and chemical elements act together to destroy pathogens and guard against repeat infections such as the viral (V) infected cell shown.

1. A pathogen (antigen) enters the body

2. Macrophages recognize the antigen as foreign, ingest (and destroy) the pathogen, and then display a portion of the foreign antigen on their surface

3. T cells recognize the antigen and initiate a response; T-parent cells divide into four types, each with different functions

4. T-helper cells activate killer cells and help activate B cells

5. B cells mature into plasma cells, which produce large numbers of Y-shaped antibodies

6. Antibodies lock onto the antigens and either destroy them or mark them for destruction by other types of cells

7. T-killer cells track down infected body cells and destroy them with cell poisons

8. T-suppressor cells turn off plasma cell activity as the infection subsides

9. T-memory cells persist in the body and protect against future infection by the same pathogen

The Immune Response

Fully understanding the function of the immune system requires a substantial understanding of human biology and is beyond the scope of this text. Figure 11-2 presents a simplified view of the immune response.

When antigens (whether microorganisms, foreign proteins, or abnormal cells) are discovered within the body, various types of white blood cells confront and destroy some of these antigens. Principal among these blood cells are the *macrophages* (very large white blood cells) that begin ingesting antigens as they are encountered. In conjunction with this "eating" of antigens, macrophages display segments of the antigen's unique protein coat on their outer surface. Now in the form of macrophage/antigen complexes, macrophages transport their captured antigen identifiers to awaiting T cells, whose recognition of the antigen will initiate the full cell-mediated immune response. This involves the specialization of "basic" T cells into four forms: T-helper cells, T-killer cells, T-suppressor cells, and T-memory cells.

Once T-helper cells have been derived from the "parent" T cells by the presence of the macrophage/antigen complex, they notify a second component of cellular immunity, the T-killer cells. T-killer cells produce powerful chemical messengers that activate specific white blood cells that destroy antigens through the production of caustic chemicals called *cytotoxins,* or "cell poisons." In addition to the T-helper cells' activation of T-killer cells, T-helper cells play a critical role in the activation of B cells, principal players in the expression of humoral immunity.

Activation of the humoral immunity component of the overall immune response involves the T-helper cells' ability to construct a working relationship among themselves, the macrophage/antigen complexes (mentioned earlier), and the small B cells. Once these three elements have been constituted into working units, the B cells are transformed into *plasma cells.* Plasma cells then utilize the information about the antigen's identity to produce massive numbers of **antibodies.** On release from the plasma cells, these antibodies then circulate throughout the body and capture free antigens in the form of *antigen/antibody complexes.*[6] The "captured" antigens are now highly susceptible to a variety of white blood cells that ingest or chemically destroy these infectious agents.

To ensure that the response to the presence of the antigen can be appropriately controlled, a third group of T cells, the T-suppressor cells, have been formed by the activation of T-parent cells. These T-suppressor cells monitor the outcome of the humoral response (antibody formation) and, when comfortable with the number of antibodies produced, turn off further plasma cell activity. The fourth group of specialized T cells, the T-memory cells, record this game plan for fighting the antigen invasion so that any subsequent similar invasion will be quickly fought.

An additional group of cells that operate independently from the T cell/B cell interplay just described are the *natural killer* (NK) cells. These immune cells continuously patrol the blood and intracellular fluids looking for abnormal cells, including cancer cells and viral-infected cells. When these are found, the NK cells attack them with destructive cytotoxins in a process called *lysing.*[6] (Can you think of a popular household sanitizing product that uses a version of *lysing* in its brand name?)

Without a normal immune system employing both cellular and humoral elements, we would quickly fall victim to serious and life-shortening infections and malignancies. As you will see later, this is exactly what occurs in many people infected with HIV.

Emerging medical technology holds promise for repairing damaged immune systems. Perhaps in the not too distant future, *adult stem cells* can be harvested from other areas of the body of a person whose immune system has been compromised, or from the body of a carefully matched donor, and used to return a damaged immune system to a normal level of functioning. A second form of immune system repair involves harvesting *cord blood (stem) cells* taken from the umbilical cord blood collected and "banked" at birth.[7] After careful matching, these cells can be transplanted into a recipient in anticipation that they will specialize into the cell type needed by the damaged or diseased immune system. It is important to note that considerable controversy now surrounds the use of stem cells obtained from embryonic or fetal tissue sources, and the use of federal funds to create new stem cell lines was prohibited during the eight years of George W. Bush's presidency. However, very shortly after the inauguration of President Barack Obama in 2009, the restriction on the use of federal funds was lifted. In spite of the lifting of restrictions on embryonic stem cell research imposed by the Dickey-Wicker Amendment (DWA) (1966), legal challenges remain at various levels of the court system, both federal and state. Additionally, an interesting component of the DWA relates to the use of parthenotes (ova stimulated to begin cellular development without having been fertilized) as a source of stem cells. Since parthenotes contain only 23 chromosomes (22X), they cannot be defined as human. Thus, stem cell researchers question their inclusion in the original DWA restrictions.[8]

Immunizations

Although the incidence of several childhood communicable diseases is at or near the lowest level ever, we are risking a resurgence of diseases such as measles, polio, diphtheria, and rubella. The possible increase in childhood infectious illnesses is based on the disturbing finding that by mid-decade only 81 percent of American preschoolers were adequately immunized, which was principally due to the failure of many parents to complete their children's immunization programs. Based on 2009 data that were reported by the National Immunization Survey (NIS), approximately 90 percent of children between 19 and 35 months of age had received their scheduled immunizations, while 99 percent had received at least one round of the scheduled immunizations.

Vaccinations against several potentially serious infectious conditions are available and should be given. These include the following:

- *Diphtheria.* A potentially fatal illness that leads to inflammation of the membranes that line the throat, to swollen lymph nodes, and to heart and kidney failure
- *Whooping cough.* A bacterial infection of the airways and lungs that results in deep, noisy breathing and coughing

- *Hepatitis B.* A viral infection that can be transmitted sexually or through the exchange of blood or bodily fluids; seriously damages the liver
- *Hepatitis A.* A viral infection contracted by consuming contaminated food or water, or from fecal contaminated hands
- *Haemophilus influenzae type B.* A bacterial infection that can damage the heart and brain, resulting in meningitis, and can produce profound hearing loss
- *Tetanus.* A fatal infection that damages the central nervous system; caused by bacteria found in the soil
- *Rubella (German measles).* A viral infection of the upper respiratory tract that can cause damage to a developing fetus when the mother contracts the infection during the first trimester of pregnancy
- *Measles (red measles).* A highly contagious viral infection leading to a rash, high fever, and upper-respiratory-tract symptoms
- *Polio.* A viral infection capable of causing paralysis of the large muscles of the extremities
- *Mumps.* A viral infection of the salivary glands
- *Chicken pox.* A varicella zoster virus spread by airborne droplets, leading to a sore throat, rash, and fluid-filled blisters
- *Meningococcal infection.* A bacterial infection of the membranes covering the brain; begins with flulike symptoms
- *Pneumococcal infection.* A bacterium capable of causing infections, including pneumonia, and heart, kidney, and middle-ear infections
- *Childhood diarrhea.* Caused by a rotavirus, this form of diarrhea is responsible for 55,000–70,000 hospitalizations, and 20–60 deaths, annually of infants and young children.

Parents of newborns should take their infants to their family care physicians, pediatricians, or well-baby clinics operated by county health departments to begin the immunization schedule. The immunization schedules for children 0–6 years of age and for persons ages 7–18 years of age posted on the Online Learning Center (www.mhhe.com/hahn11e) are recommended by the American Academy of Pediatrics, the American Academy of Family Physicians, and the Centers for Disease Control and Prevention. As children quickly discover, and parents already know, most of today's immunizations are administered by injection. To improve compliance with the immunization schedule (some parents have a fear of "shots" resulting from early childhood experiences and thus avoid completing the schedule), researchers are attempting to develop a single immunization that would combine many individual vaccines. In addition, research is being conducted on new delivery systems, including a skin patch, nasal spray, and vaccine-enriched foods, such as potatoes.

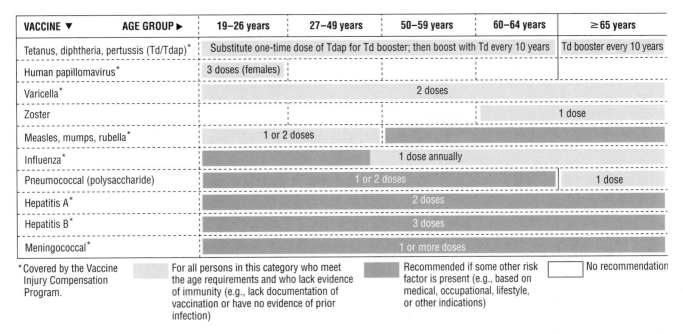

VACCINE ▼　AGE GROUP ▶	19–26 years	27–49 years	50–59 years	60–64 years	≥65 years
Tetanus, diphtheria, pertussis (Td/Tdap)*	Substitute one-time dose of Tdap for Td booster; then boost with Td every 10 years				Td booster every 10 years
Human papillomavirus*	3 doses (females)				
Varicella*	2 doses				
Zoster				1 dose	
Measles, mumps, rubella*	1 or 2 doses		1 dose		
Influenza*		1 dose annually			
Pneumococcal (polysaccharide)	1 or 2 doses				1 dose
Hepatitis A*	2 doses				
Hepatitis B*	3 doses				
Meningococcal*	1 or more doses				

*Covered by the Vaccine Injury Compensation Program.

[light gray] For all persons in this category who meet the age requirements and who lack evidence of immunity (e.g., lack documentation of vaccination or have no evidence of prior infection)

[dark gray] Recommended if some other risk factor is present (e.g., based on medical, occupational, lifestyle, or other indications)

[white] No recommendation

Figure 11-3 Immunizations Recommended for Adults For additional information, visit www.cdc.gov/nip.

Source: Centers for Disease Control and Prevention, Recommended Adult Immunization Schedule—United States, January 2010: MMWR Quick Guide.

In recent years, concern has arisen regarding the role of childhood immunizations in the development of other serious childhood physical and emotional health problems, such as type 1 diabetes mellitus, asthma, autism, and sudden infant death syndrome (SIDS). At this time, studies investigating the possible relationship between recommended immunizations and the conditions mentioned previously have found no demonstrable cause-and-effect relationships. For persons interested in more in-depth information regarding adverse affects and contraindications associated with immunizations, see the Vaccine Adverse Events Reporting System (VAERS), administered by the Food and Drug Administration (FDA) and the CDC. It is in the public domain. Like other reporting systems, the VAERS has limitations; however, information from a wide array of research studies can be readily obtained through the system.[9]

Although immunization is universally viewed as important for infants and children, adults have immunization needs that can be unmet. Accordingly, the CDC's National Immunization Program now provides an immunization schedule for adults. It recommends immunizations that should be updated or initially received by adults (see Figure 11-3) (see the Online Learning Center for more information on the Adult Immunization Schedule). Adults are particularly underprotected in regard to diphtheria and tetanus.

On a final note, as mentioned above, some persons were, or still are, concerned that a causative relationship exists between the MMR childhood immunization and the development of autism. Regardless of the sincerity of this concern, over a decade of research has consistently found no evidence of a causative relationship between the childhood immunization protocol, particularly as it relates to the MMRP (now MMR) vaccine, and the development of autism. To this end, in 2009 the U.S. Court of Claims found against parents who sought compensation from the government's Vaccine Injury Compensation Program, and in February 2011, the U.S. Supreme Court ruled against the parents of a child with autism in their attempt to obtain compensation from vaccine manufacturers. Both rulings were based on the absence of supporting evidence showing causation.

Causes and Management of Selected Infectious Diseases

This section focuses on some of the common infectious diseases and some diseases that are less common but serious. You can use this information as a basis for judging your own disease susceptibility.

Nosocomial Infections

Although the classroom, residence hall, home, worksite, and virtually any place where people gather in large numbers and in close proximity would seem "ideal" places to contract an infectious disease, a better place might come as a surprise—any place where nosocomial infectious agents call "home." Nosocomial infections are infections spread in conjunction with the delivery of health care services—most often from providers to patients or from patients to other patients. Persons who are hospitalized are particularly vulnerable to the development of a potentially fatal nosocomial infection. Recent examples of these infectious agents include *Clostridium difficile (C-diff)*, most often contracted by hospitalized persons who are on antibiotics; methicillin-resistant *Staphylococcus aureus* (MRSA), the so-called flesh eating bacterium; and a collection of infectious agents (HIV, hepatitis C, and syphilis) transplanted in conjunction with the use of untested "stolen" human tissue supplied to hospitals by unethical tissue banks. Returning briefly to MRSA, it should be noted that the rate of hospital-acquired infections has gradually declined since 2007, but the rate of community-acquired MRSA infections is increasing annually. This is most often seen among athletes who participate in contact sports, which suggests that the locker room/practice field provides a favorable environment for this bacterium.[10]

Each year approximately 2.2 million persons develop an infection directly linked to the health care system, including 780,000 in association with operations. Contact with infectious agents occurs in a variety of ways, including the failure of personnel to wash or glove their hands properly prior to conducting examinations, the use of contaminated medical equipment such as endoscopes and catheters, failure to maintain sterile operating areas during surgery, the widespread use of central-lines (catheters implanted directly into a large vein near the collarbone), the use of intravenous medications contaminated during their manufacture, and even the clothing of physicians and other staff members. To counter the risk of nosocomial infections, hospitals increasingly are utilizing monitors (aka germ cops) to shadow the clinical staff to make certain that subtle miscues in treatment procedures do not "open doors" for infectious agents to become established.

Two factors make today's nosocomial infections particularly serious. The first, of course, is that these infections strike people who by virtue of being institutionalized are less than healthy. Second is the fact that the organisms most frequently associated with these infections are among the most pathogenic with which we have contact.

Because of the potential seriousness of nosocomial infections, persons entering the health care arena should discuss infection control with their physician.

The Common Cold

The common cold, an acute upper-respiratory-tract infection, must reign as humankind's supreme infectious disease. Also known as **acute rhinitis,** this highly contagious viral infection can be caused by an array of viruses, including rhinoviruses (the most common cause of colds), respiratory synctial viruses, para-influenza viruses, human metapneumoviruses, and adenoviruses. Colds are particularly common when people spend time in crowded indoor environments, such as classrooms. So common is the cold that over 1 billion cases occur each year in this country. The average American adult has 2–4 colds per year, while children have 6–10.

The signs and symptoms of a cold are fairly predictable. Runny nose, watery eyes, general aches and pains, a listless feeling, and a slight fever all may accompany a cold in its early stages. Eventually, the nasal passages swell, and the inflammation may spread to the throat. Stuffy nose, sore throat, and coughing may follow (see Table 11.2). The senses of taste and smell are blocked, and appetite declines.

When you notice the onset of symptoms, you should begin managing the cold promptly. After a few days, most of the cold's symptoms subside. In the meantime, you should isolate yourself from others, drink plenty of fluids, eat moderately, and rest.

At this time there is no effective way to prevent colds. Some of the many OTC cold remedies can help you manage a cold. These remedies will not cure your cold but may lessen the discomfort associated with it. Nasal decongestants, expectorants, cough syrups, and aspirin or acetaminophen can give some temporary relief. In light of the information regarding the treatment of colds given in Table 11.2 and discussed earlier, it is critically important to know that the FDA has determined that the use of OTC cold medications is inappropriate (and potentially fatal) for children under 2 years of age.[11] Recommendations for older children are currently under review. Particularly when using cold medication, you should follow these important points[11]:

- Check the "active ingredients" section of the DRUG FACTS label.
- Be very careful if you are giving more than one OTC cough and cold medication to a child.
- Carefully follow the directions in the DRUG FACTS part of the label.
- Only use the measuring spoons or cups that come with the medicine or those made for measuring drugs.
- Choose childproof safety caps and store medications out of the reach of children.
- Never use a cough or cold medication to sedate a child or make him or her sleepy.

Giving young children fluids, the passage of time, and TLC is a safer alternative, and will reduce the likelihood of a visit to a hospital's emergency room.

If a cold persists, as evidenced by prolonged chills, fever above 103°F, chest heaviness or aches, shortness of breath, coughing up of rust-colored mucus, or persistent

Table 11.2 Is It a Cold or the Flu?

Symptoms	Cold	Flu
Fever	Rare	Usual; high (100°F–102°F); occasionally higher, especially in young children); lasts 3–4 days
Headache	Rare	Common
General aches, pains	Slight	Usual; often severe
Fatigue, weakness	Sometimes	Usual; can last up to 2–3 weeks
Extreme exhaustion	Never	Usual; at the beginning of the illness
Stuffy nose	Common	Sometimes
Sneezing	Usual	Sometimes
Sore throat	Common	Sometimes
Chest discomfort, cough	Mild to moderate; hacking cough	Common; can become severe
Complications	Sinus congestion, middle-ear infection, asthma	Pneumonia, bronchitis; can be life threatening
Prevention	Wash your hands often; avoid close contact with anyone with a cold	Annual vaccination; antiviral drugs—see your physician
Treatment	Antihistamines, decongestants, nonsteroidal anti-inflammatory medicines	Antiviral medications—see your physician

Note: The need to consult a physician as the result of complications that might arise during the course of a cold or flu is not unknown. During the course of a cold, any of the following should be called to the attention of a physician: (1) when a cold fails to resolve within 5 to 7 days, (2) when an elevated temperature develops (above 103°F), or (3) when a "deep chest" cough develops that produces either a brownish-tinged sputum or does not respond to OTC cough medication. Similar complications can occur in conjunction with the flu and require consultation with a physician. In addition, prolonged vomiting and diarrhea also should be called to the attention of a physician. Upon contracting the flu, children, older adults, pregnant women, and all persons with chronic conditions such as diabetes mellitus, cardiovascular diseases, and malignancies should be carefully monitored and complications should be promptly reported to a physician.
Source: National Institute of Allergy and Infectious Diseases, Is it a cold or the flu? 2008.

sore throat or hoarseness, you should contact a physician. Because we now consider colds to be transmitted most readily by hand contact, you should wash your hands frequently.

Seasonal Influenza

Influenza is also an acute contagious disease caused by viruses. Some influenza outbreaks have killed thousands and even millions of people, such as the influenza pandemics of 1889–1890, 1918–1919, 1957, and 2003–2004. The viral strains that produce this infectious disease have the potential for more severe complications than the viral strains that produce the common cold. The viral strain for a particular form of influenza enters the body through the respiratory tract. After brief incubation and prodromal stages, the host develops signs and symptoms not just in the upper respiratory tract but throughout the entire body. These symptoms include fever, chills, cough, sore throat, headache, gastrointestinal disturbances, and muscular pain (see Table 11.2).

Antibiotics are generally not prescribed for people with influenza, except when the patient has a possible secondary bacterial infection. Physicians may recommend only aspirin, fluids, and rest. Parents are reminded not to give aspirin to children because of the danger of Reye's syndrome. Reye's syndrome is an aspirin-enhanced complication of influenza in which central nervous system changes can occur, including brain swelling.

For a person hoping to avoid the debilitating symptoms of flu, four antiviral vaccines are currently approved by the FDA: Tamiflu, Relenza, Symmetrel, and Flumadine. Unfortunately, the 2008–2009 flu season, although mild by past standards, revealed that the A-H1N1 virus was rapidly becoming resistant to Tamiflu. Relenza (available only for nasal inhalation) was an effective substitute for Tamiflu, except for persons unable to use an inhalant because of respiratory problems and asthma. For these persons, use of the two remaining medications was their only option. On an encouraging note, new antiviral medications are in clinical trials. The influenza vaccine is formulated one year in advance of the flu season in which it will be used, so its composition is based on the types of flu viruses seen in Asia during the prior year.

Most young adults can cope with the milder strains of seasonal influenza that appear each winter or spring. However, pregnant women and older people—especially older people with additional health complications, such as heart disease, kidney disease, emphysema, and chronic bronchitis—are not as capable of handling this viral attack. People who regularly come into contact with the general public, such as teachers, should also consider annual flu shots.

Today the pool of eligible recipients of seasonal influenza vaccine has become almost inclusive. Revised recommended guidelines issued in 2006 and revised in 2010 now approve the influenza vaccine for people 6 months of age and older. Receipt of the vaccine is deemed

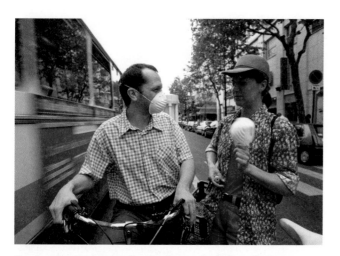

During the 2009 swine flu pandemic, the value of wearing masks as a means of minimizing disease transmission was debated. The couple shown above reflect the uncertainty of the extent to which masks are effective in preventing the spread of the flu virus.

particularly important for people at risk of complications should they experience an episode of the flu and for a variety of persons who "simply can't afford to have the flu." This latter and sizable group once included persons with specific chronic conditions, as well as teachers, people in the public service sector, health care providers, and military personnel. Today, with the exception of infants under 6 months of age, every person is strongly advised to receive the vaccine formulated for each year. However, based on data from the beginning of the 2009–2010 flu season, approximately 33 percent had received the vaccine, 15 percent fully intended to get the vaccine but had yet to do so, and 25 percent said they probably would. Thus, over a quarter of the eligible population most likely did not receive the flu vaccine, leaving a sizable number in the "at risk" pool.

Data for the 2011–2012 flu season have yet to be analyzed. The vaccine that was used was a trivalent vaccine comprised of two A viral strains (California and Perth) and one B strain (Brisbane). A high level of compliance could result in 160 million Americans protected from this virulent infectious viral disease.

In June 2003, the FDA approved the sale of Flumist, a nasal spray inhalation delivery system for influenza vaccine. Its use is approved for people ages 2–49. Its use is not, at this time, recommended for persons most in need of the highest level of protection. Yet another delivery system for immunizations (including flu) is under development. The microneedle system employs a Band-Aid-like skin patch in which are embedded hundreds of tiny needles, each capable of releasing a small amount of vaccine under the outermost layer of skin. Needles dissolve once their vaccine has been released.

Avian (Bird) Influenza and Novel-H1N1 (Swine) Influenza

In 2003, the World Health Organization (WHO) became aware of the presence of a virus that was not among the predictable viral strains that make up the seasonal human flu viruses. An apparently modified version of a virus that was formerly limited to avian species (principally in Near Eastern countries) was now beginning to spread to humans via contact with the excrement of chickens and ducks. In an attempt to stem transmission of the A-H5N1 virus, millions of chickens and ducks were destroyed, principally in China, Korea, Japan, Vietnam, and Indonesia.

As the avian flu virus began migrating into other areas of the world, reports surfaced of cases in the Near East, Middle East, Asia, Europe, Africa, and, to a very limited extent, North America. By August 2009, 438 cases had been reported and 262 deaths had occurred. Although some isolated cases of A-H5N1 influenza in humans suggest that the virus has developed some potential for human-to-human transmission, that capability seems limited.

Today, however, the concern regarding an avian flu pandemic has been significantly replaced with the existence of a Stage 6 pandemic of novel-H1N1 (swine) influenza that began in Mexico in March 2009. Although the H1N1 virus is routinely found in pigs in North America, this virus is distinctly different, having incorporated genetic material from other viruses, including a swine virus common to European and Asian swine, the avian virus (H5N1), and one or more human flu viruses, and is thus known as novel H1N1.

The novel-H1N1 virus is easily spread from an infected person to other people (new hosts) via respiratory inhalation (coughing and sneezing) or by handling a contaminated object such as a towel and then touching the nose or mouth. The novel-H1N1 infection presents with a variety of symptoms, including cough, fever, sore throat, runny nose, chills, body aches, and lethargy. Symptoms range from minimal to severe. Fortunately, it appears that the majority of infected persons recover, although as with seasonal flu, deaths have occurred. Current antiviral medications shorten the duration of symptoms and reduce their discomfort, but will not prevent infection.

Given the virulence of the novel-H1N1 virus, and the rapidity with which it spread within North America and throughout the world, the world health community began immediate formulation and production of preventive vaccines, guidelines for immunizing various segments of the population (for which school facilities were pressed into use), and periods of home isolation for those infected. By August 2009, more than 180,000 cases of swine flu had been reported and 1,799 deaths had occurred, although the WHO acknowledges that these numbers are likely understated because of its backlog of information.

Two influenza pandemics in a decade! The avian (bird) flu in 2003 and novel-H1N1 (swine) flu in 2009 remind us of both the virility that viruses are capable of as they mutate in order to better sustain their reservoirs and the extent to which large segments of the world's population are connected in ways both beneficial and detrimental. Today neither pandemic receives coverage in the media. That said, we are reminded that complacency can be a major mistake when it comes to virally induced illness. On the other hand, labeling outbreaks too quickly as pandemics also carries the potential for provoking overreaction both in the general public and within the scientific community.

Tuberculosis

Experts considered *tuberculosis (TB)*, a bacterial infection of the lungs resulting in chronic coughing, weight loss, and sometimes death, to be under control in the United States until the mid-1980s. The number of cases surged then, however, with a peak of 26,283 cases in 1992. The number has declined since then, with 12,898 cases reported in 2008, a 49 percent decline from 1992.[12] In 2009, 11,540 cases were reported, with 60 percent of these found in newly arrived immigrants,[13] most often from Mexico, India, Vietnam, and the Philippines. In response, in 2009, federal agencies initiated the development of a comprehensive plan to better monitor and manage TB within the United States.[14]

Today, three forms of drug-resistant TB have emerged, including monodrug-resistant TB; multiple-drug-resistant (MDR) TB, from which only 50 percent recover; and most recently, extensively drug-resistant (XDR) TB. Mortality from XDR TB is virtually 100 percent. In a recent assessment of reports from various parts of the world, the CDC reported that in the industrialized nations, 6–7 percent of the MDR TB cases are of the XDR TB form. The rate of XDR TB infection remains relatively low in the United States. However, there could be nearly 180,000 total cases in Africa, the former Soviet Union, and parts of Asia. Globally, tuberculosis, in all of its forms, is estimated to number 9 million cases, claiming 2 million lives annually.

Tuberculosis thrives in crowded places where infected people are in constant contact with others, because TB is spread by coughing. This includes prisons, hospitals, public housing units, and even college residence halls. In such settings, a single infected person can spread the TB agents to many others.

When healthy people are exposed to TB agents, their immune systems can usually suppress the bacteria well enough to prevent symptoms from developing and to reduce the likelihood of infecting others. When the immune system is damaged, however, such as in some older adults, malnourished people, and those who are infected with HIV, the disease can become established and eventually be transmitted to other people at risk.

Also helpful in curbing TB's role in international mortality would be a prompter, more sensitive diagnostic test. In this regard, progress is being made. The CDC has recommended adopting the QuantiFERON-TB Gold test (QFT Gold). Although this test is more expensive than the traditional tuberculin-based skin test for detecting active TB in persons once vaccinated with BCG,[15] it requires only a single blood draw and no return trip to a clinic for assessment, and it yields more accurate results (fewer false positives).

Pneumonia

Pneumonia is a general term that describes a variety of infectious respiratory conditions. There are bacterial, viral, fungal, rickettsial, mycoplasmal, and parasitic forms of pneumonia. However, bacterial pneumonia is the most common form and is often seen with other illnesses that weaken the body's immune system. In 2009 in the United States, there were an estimated 43,500 cases and 5,000 deaths.[16]

In children under the age of 5 years, pneumococcal disease, in addition to pneumonia, is annually responsible for an array of other infectious conditions, including 4.9 million cases of otitis media (middle-ear infection), 700 cases of meningitis, 17,000 cases of bacterial blood infections, and 200 deaths.[17]

In spite of the prevalence and potential severity of pneumococcal disease in young children, the incidence of this infectious condition is beginning to recede as a larger percentage of children gain the protection provided by the polyvalent immunization (PCV-7), introduced into the childhood immunization schedule in 2000, and more recently with the PCV-13 vaccine. Although other factors are certainly involved, such as less exposure of children to parental smoking and more children being breast-fed, the immunization of children for bacterial pneumonia is an important factor in the nearly 30 percent drop in childhood middle-ear infections,[18] resulting in fewer emergency room visits.

Older adults with a history of chronic obstructive lung disease, cardiovascular disease, diabetes, or alcoholism often encounter a potentially serious midwinter form of pneumonia known as *acute (severe) community-acquired pneumonia*. Characteristics of this condition are the sudden onset of chills, chest pain, and a cough producing sputum.

As the number of older Americans grows, recommendations regarding immunization against pneumococcal pneumonia have been established and vaccination programs undertaken. Today, the recommendation for an adult initial pneumonia vaccination is age 65, with starting ages as early as 19 years for people with specific health conditions or those who work in high-risk settings. The cost-effectiveness of pneumonia immunizations for older adults, and particularly for minority older adults, is well established.

The first known drug-resistant strains of pneumonia have been identified in this country. As a result, some experts are calling for an even more comprehensive vaccination plan for older adults.

Mononucleosis

College students who contract **mononucleosis ("mono")** can be forced into a long period of bed rest during a semester when they can least afford it. Other common diseases can be managed with minimal disruption, but given the overall weakness and fatigue seen in many people with mono, they sometimes require a month or two of rest and recuperation.

Mono is a viral infection in which the body produces an excess of mononuclear leukocytes (a type of white blood cell). After uncertain, perhaps long, incubation and prodromal stages, the acute symptoms of mono can appear, including weakness, headache, low-grade fever, swollen lymph glands (especially in the neck), and sore throat. Mental fatigue and depression are sometimes reported as side effects of mononucleosis. After the acute symptoms disappear, the weakness and fatigue usually persist—perhaps for a few months.

Mono is diagnosed by its characteristic symptoms. The Monospot blood smear can also be used to identify the prevalence of abnormal white blood cells. In addition, an antibody test can detect activity of the immune system that is characteristic of the illness.

This disease is most often caused by an Epstein-Barr virus (EBV), so antibiotic therapy is not recommended. Treatment usually includes bed rest and the use of OTC remedies for fever (aspirin or acetaminophen) and for sore throat (lozenges). Corticosteroid drugs can be used in extreme cases. Rupture of the spleen is an occasional, but serious, consequence of the condition, particularly in persons who are too physically active during their recovery. Adequate fluid intake and a well-balanced diet are also important in the recovery stages of mono. Fortunately, the body tends to develop NAI to the mono virus, so repeat infections of mono are unusual. However, persons on immunosuppressant drugs are more likely to experience a recurrence of mononucleosis or other EBV-related infections.

The best preventive measures are the steps that you can take to increase your resistance to most infectious diseases: (1) eat a well-balanced diet, (2) exercise regularly, (3) sleep sufficiently, (4) use health care services appropriately, (5) live in a reasonably healthful environment, and (6) avoid direct contact with infected people.

Chronic Fatigue Syndrome

Chronic fatigue syndrome (CFS) may be the most perplexing "infectious" condition physicians see. First identified in 1985, this mononucleosis-like condition is most often seen in women in their 40s and 50s. Examinations of the first people with CFS revealed antibodies to the Epstein-Barr virus. Thus, observers assumed CFS to be an infectious viral disease (and initially called it *chronic Epstein-Barr syndrome*).

Since its first appearance, the condition has received a great deal of attention regarding its exact nature. Today, opinions vary widely as to whether CFS is a specific viral infection, a condition involving both viral infections and nonviral components, or some other disorder. Perhaps the most creditable explanation involves a more complex causation for CFS. This model suggests involvement of emotional, environmental, and infectious factors, all influencing the stress response (see Chapter 3), in association with a possible genetic predisposition.

Regardless of its cause or causes, CFS is extremely unpleasant for its victims. Because there is no definitive diagnosis (or treatment) for CFS, a probable diagnosis will be based on a medical history featuring exercise-induced malaise, nonrefreshing sleep, impairment of memory, muscle pain, multiple joint pain, unusual headaches, sore throat, and tenderness in the neck or swollen lymph nodes in the armpits. In combination, these characteristic markers of CFS will be chronic in nature and clearly disabling (see the box "Living with a Chronic Infectious Disease—Life Is Not Over, Just Different").

Most recently, attention has shifted to the role of XMRV (xenotropic murine leukemia virus) in the etiology of CFS and prostate cancer.[19] Some studies have consistently found evidence of the virus in the spinal fluid of persons with CFS, raising the question of whether it is the cause of CFS or an after-effect. Conversely, other studies have failed to find XMRV, in persons with either CFS or prostate cancer.

In recent years, it has been noted that another chronic condition, *fibromyalgia,* appears in a manner similar to CFS. As in CFS, the person with fibromyalgia demonstrates fatigue, inefficient sleep patterns, localized areas of tenderness and pain, morning stiffness, and headaches. The onset of this condition, like that of CFS, can follow periods of stress, infectious disease, physical trauma such as falls, or thyroid dysfunction, or in conjunction with a connective tissue disorder.

Bacterial Meningitis

Since approximately 1995, a formerly infrequently seen but potentially fatal infectious disease, *meningococcal meningitis,* has appeared on college campuses, suggesting that college students are currently at greater risk of contracting the disease than are their noncollege peers. Particularly interesting is the fact that among college students, the risk of contracting this infection on campus is highest for those students living in residence halls, suggesting that close living quarters and contact with students from other parts of the world favor transmission of the bacteria. Since many colleges and universities require that first-year students reside in residence halls, it is in this group that the incidence of meningococcal meningitis is highest. Additionally, this group of students is most likely to be in large-section lecture classes and take meals in large dining facilities. Annually, about 150 cases of meningococcal meningitis occur on American college campuses, resulting in 15 deaths per year. Understandably, more and more colleges and universities are requiring, as a condition of admission, documentation of immunization against bacterial meningitis. Some people, however, have questioned the cost-effectiveness of immunizing all entering students. Skepticism about cost-effectiveness aside, now the NIH advises an initial single immunization at 14 or 15 years of age, with a second booster immunization at 16, to better ensure a full 10 years of maximum protection during the critical years of risk. Having near 90 percent coverage in this age group ensures that the "herding effect" should protect the small minority that remain unimmunized. In April 2011, the FDA approved a revised bacterial meningitis vaccine schedule that will more broadly protect the youth population.[20] According to the adjusted schedule, the first application should take place at ages 9–23 months.

Meningococcal meningitis is a bacterial infection of the thin membranous coverings of the brain. In its earliest stages, this disease can easily be confused with the flu. Symptoms usually include a high fever, severe headache, stiff neck, nausea with vomiting, extreme tiredness, and the formation of a progressive rash. For about 10 percent of people who develop this condition, the infection is fatal, often within 24 hours. Therefore, the mere presence of the symptoms just described signals the need for immediate medical evaluation. If done promptly, treatment is highly effective.

Lyme Disease

Lyme disease is an infectious disease that has become a significant health problem in eastern, southeastern, upper midwestern, and West Coast states, with 27,444 cases in 2007. In 2009, Lyme disease was reported in two diagnostic categories, *probable* and *confirmed,* to

---

Key Terms

mononucleosis ("mono") A viral infection characterized by weakness, fatigue, swollen glands, sore throat, and low-grade fever.

chronic fatigue syndrome (CFS) An illness that causes severe exhaustion, fatigue, aches, and depression; mostly affects women in their 40s and 50s.

Lyme disease A bacterial infection transmitted by deer ticks.

better detail the disease's prevalence and spread. That year 29,959 confirmed cases and 8,509 probable cases were reported to the CDC.[21] The increase most likely reflects widening geographical distribution of the disease, a greater awareness of its symptoms by the general public, and more consistent reporting by physicians. Ten states, eight of which are in the Northeast, are routinely assessed during the tick season, as the vast majority of cases continue to come from this region.[22] This bacterial disease results when infected black-legged ticks (also called deer ticks), usually in the nymph (immature) stage, attach to the skin and inject the infectious agent as they feed on a host's blood. The deer ticks become infected by feeding, as larvae, on infected white-footed mice.

The symptoms of Lyme disease vary but typically appear within 30 days as small red bumps surrounded by a circular red rash at the site of bites. The red rash has been described as being like a "bull's-eye" in appearance—a pale center surrounded by a reddish margin. However, in some persons, this characteristic rash does not appear; thus, other symptoms must be recognized so that diagnosis is not delayed. Flulike symptoms, including chills, headaches, muscle and joint aches, and low-grade fever, may accompany this acute phase. A chronic phase develops in about 20 percent of untreated infected persons. This phase may produce disorders of the nervous system, heart, or joints. Fortunately, Lyme disease can be treated with antibiotics. Unfortunately, however, no immunity develops, so infection can recur.

Some people who were treated for Lyme disease, but who continue to report a variety of symptoms or simply lethargy, have chronic Lyme disease. They are placed on prophylactic antibiotic therapy, often without an explanation of the negative consequences of doing so.

In contrast to that approach, other physicians will first order blood tests to determine the presence and level of antibodies for the causative agent (*B. burgdorferi*) in the blood before beginning any prophylactic antibiotic treatment. If the antibody titers are very low or nonexistent, treatment will be restricted to symptomatic protocols, with reassurance that patients no longer have Lyme disease. For both acute and chronic Lyme disease, the ideal is never to have become the new host for an infected deer tick. Lyme disease prevention is thus described.

People who live in tick-prone areas, including near small urban/suburban wood lots, and participate in outdoor activities can encounter the nearly invisible tick nymphs. These people should check themselves frequently to be sure that they are tick-free. They should tuck shirts into pants, tuck pants into socks, and wear gloves and hat when possible. They should shower after coming inside from outdoors and check clothing for evidence of ticks. Pets, particularly dogs who enjoy outdoor play and then return indoors, can carry infected ticks into the house.

If you find ticks, carefully remove them from the skin with tweezers and wash the affected area. Prevention is very important. Repellants containing DEET or permethrin are effective in repelling ticks; they should be used according to directions on the label. A vaccine for Lyme disease was withdrawn from the market in 2002.

Hantavirus Pulmonary Syndrome

Since 1993, a small but rapidly growing number of people have been dying of extreme pulmonary distress caused by the leakage of plasma into the lungs. In the initial cases, the people lived in the Southwest, had been well until they began developing flulike symptoms over one or two days, then quickly experienced difficulty breathing, and died only hours later. Epidemiologists quickly suspected a viral agent such as the *hantavirus,* known to exist in Asia and, to a lesser degree, in Europe, where the infection leads to death by hemorrhage.[23] Exhaustive laboratory work led to the culturing of the virus and confirmed that all of these patients had been infected with an American version of the hantavirus.

Today hantavirus pulmonary syndrome has been reported in areas beyond the Southwest, including most of the western states and some of the eastern states. The common denominator in all these areas is the presence of deer mice. It is now known that this common rodent serves as the reservoir for the virus. In fact, so common is the mouse that in 2000 the National Park Service began warning hikers, campers, and off-road bikers that hantavirus probably existed in every national park and that caution should be taken to avoid high-risk sites. During the period 2001–2008, 16 cases of hantavirus were reported in California; of those cases, 4 died due to the extremely rapid accumulation of fluid in the lungs (pulmonary congestion).[24]

The virus moves from deer mice to humans when people inhale dust contaminated with dried, virus-rich rodent urine or saliva-contaminated materials, such as nests. If you must remove rodent nests from a house, barn, or shed, wear rubber gloves, pour disinfectant or bleach on the nests and soak them thoroughly, and finally, pick up the nests with a shovel and burn them or bury them in holes that are several feet deep. This said, prevention is a better alternative to removing nests and can be accomplished by sealing up holes in structures, trapping and disposing of deer mice in an effective manner, and cleaning up sources of food that would otherwise attract mice.

Because there is no vaccine for hantavirus pulmonary syndrome, people who likely have been exposed to the infected excrement of deer mice should seek early evaluation of flulike symptoms.

West Nile Virus

First detected in New York City in 1999, the *West Nile virus* was, by the summer of 2000, identified in six eastern states. In 2007, the CDC reported a total of 3,630 cases of West Nile virus (WNV), of which 1,227 involved neurological involvement (WNND) and 2,350 reported principally fever (WNF) as their primary symptom. There were 117 deaths from West Nile virus infections, principally in older adults and the chronically ill, and in all cases from the WNND form of the disease. In 2008, 1,370 cases were initially reported, a substantial drop from the 2007 total. A number of variables were determined to have caused this decline, including drier weather conditions, better screening of homes, improved mosquito control, and more consistent use of mosquito repellents by the general public. Unfortunately, it was learned in early 2009 that the 2008 figures were underreported because of defects in widely used testing kits. By 2010, the number of new cases had dropped to 981 (601 WNND and 380 WNF), with 45 deaths reported.[25]

This vector-borne infectious virus is transmitted from a reservoir, most often birds, by mosquitoes that in turn infect humans. Human-to-human transmission (via mosquitoes) apparently does not occur, although the CDC has reported a very small number of cases of virus transmission in conjunction with infected transplanted tissue. West Nile virus infection involves flulike symptoms, including fever, headache, muscle ache, fatigue, and joint pain. In young children, persons with immune systems weakened by HIV, and older adults, West Nile virus infection may involve encephalitis (WNND), a potentially fatal inflammation of the brain. Physicians recommend that any unusual neurological symptoms be considered as a possible West Nile infection.

Additional aspects of the disease were reported to the CDC, including the presence of the virus in blood transfusions. (Today, clinically recovered patients cannot give blood for 60 days following dismissal.) The West Nile virus has also been isolated from breast milk, and cases of prenatal transmission have been confirmed. There is currently no human vaccine approved for use, although development is ongoing.

Tampon-Related Toxic Shock Syndrome

Toxic shock syndrome (TSS) made front-page headlines in 1980, when the CDC reported a connection between TSS and the presence of a specific bacterial agent (*Staphylococcus aureus*) in the vagina associated with the use of tampons. Today, TSS is more clearly differentiated into two categories, toxic shock-like syndrome (TSLS) and staphylococcal toxic shock syndrome

---

Key Terms

toxic shock syndrome (TSS) A potentially fatal condition caused by the proliferation of certain bacteria in the vagina that enter the general blood circulation.

(STSS), the form of TSS associated with tampon use. The former (TSLS) is caused by other infectious agents that are contracted through surgery, burns, influenza, insect bites, and other forms of wounds.

Superabsorbent tampons can irritate the vaginal lining three times more quickly than regular tampons do. This vaginal irritation is aggravated when the tampon remains in the vagina for a long time (more than five hours). When this irritation begins, the staphylococcal bacteria (which are usually present in the vagina) have relatively easy access to the bloodstream. When these bacteria proliferate in the circulatory system, their resultant toxins produce toxic shock syndrome, leading to symptoms including fever (102°F or above), headache, nausea, sore throat, muscle aches, a sunburn-like rash, bloodshot eyes, reduced urination, and peeling of the skin on the hands and soles of the feet. A woman with STSS can die, usually as a result of cardiovascular failure, if left untreated. Fortunately, less than 10 percent of women diagnosed as having STSS associated with tampon use will die.

To minimize the risk of STSS, all premenopausal women, particularly those new to the use of tampons, should consider these recommendations for safe tampon use: (1) tampons should not be the sole form of sanitary protection used, and (2) tampons should not remain in place for too long. Women should change tampons every few hours and intermittently use sanitary napkins. Tampons should not be used during sleep. Some physicians recommend that tampons not be used at all if a woman wants to be extraordinarily safe from STSS.

Hepatitis

Hepatitis is an inflammatory process in the liver that can be caused by several viruses. Types A, B, C (once called non-A and non-B), D, and E have been recognized. Hepatitis can also be caused indirectly from abuse of alcohol and other drugs. General symptoms of hepatitis include fever, nausea, loss of appetite, abdominal pain, fatigue, and jaundice (yellowing of the skin and eyes).

Type A hepatitis is often associated with consumption of fecal-contaminated food, such as raw shellfish raised in fecal-contaminated water, raw vegetables field-washed in contaminated water, or contaminated drinking water. Poor sanitation, particularly in the handling of food and diaper-changing activities, has produced outbreaks in child care centers. Experts once estimated that up to 200,000 people per year contracted this viral infection. However, this figure has been declining significantly since childhood immunizations were introduced in 2005, and the asymptomatic childhood reservoir is disappearing. Given that 20,000 new cases are reported annually, it must be assumed that the infected pool is still sizable and will remain so until the vaccinated population has grown considerably larger. Until then, unvaccinated children, once infected, will remain asymptomatic until they are older than 6 years of age.[26] In 2005 it was recommended that all children between 1 and 2 years of age be immunized against hepatitis A. Today that recommendation is in place, with the first immunization given at 12 months and the second by 18 months of age. Persons who contract hepatitis A generally develop acquired immunity, thus preventing a recurrence.

Type B hepatitis (HBV) is spread in various ways, including sexual contact, intravenous drug use, tattooing, body piercing, and even sharing electric razors. On the basis of these modes of transmission, college students should be aware of the potential risk that they too carry for HBV infection. Beyond the risk factors just identified, medical and dental procedures are also a potential means of transmitting the virus, including patient-to-practitioner and practitioner-to-patient transmission. Chronic HBV infection has been associated with liver cirrhosis and is the principal cause of liver cancer. An effective immunization for hepatitis B is now available; thus, the incidence of HBV in children and adolescents has dropped by one-fifth since 1999. However, an increase has been noted in people over 19 years of age. Although it is given during childhood, it should be seriously considered for older unvaccinated people and college students. In 2002 the American Academy of Pediatrics recommended that all newborns be immunized before leaving the hospital. Adults too should seriously consider being immunized against hepatitis B, particularly if they are likely to have multiple sex partners, have sex partners from high-risk groups, or are caregivers to an infected person. For those who suspect that they might be infected, a diagnostic test and treatment protocols are available for both acute (up to six months following infection) and chronic forms of HBV. Untreated chronic hepatitis results in approximately 3,000 deaths annually from liver diseases including liver cancer.

Hepatitis C is contracted in ways similar to hepatitis B (sexual contact, tainted blood, in association with tattooing and piercing, and shared needles). In the absence of immunization, the pool of infected people is in excess of 4.1 million, and the death rate is expected to climb. In recent years, a dual-drug therapy for HCV involving multiple forms of interferon in combination with the drug ribavirin was the preferred treatment. However, In April 2011, within a two-day period, the FDA approved two new drugs, boceprevir and telaprevir, each of which will be combined with one or two older medications to form two updated treatment protocols designed to alter the mechanisms through which HCV damages hepatic (liver) cells.[27] In the absence of screening, and thus treatment, many infected persons can remain asymptomatic for decades, but by this time liver failure or liver cancer may be too established for treatment options to be successful. In June 2010, the FDA approved a rapid diagnostic test for HCV to be used with persons who show early signs of being infected; the test is not, however, approved for mass screenings.

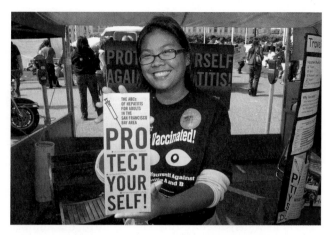

Effective vaccines are available for both hepatitis A and hepatitis B.

The newly identified type D (delta) hepatitis is very difficult to treat and is found almost exclusively in people already suffering from type B hepatitis, since the hepatitis D virus requires the presence of the hepatitis B virus in order to gain full pathogenicity. This virus, like type B hepatitis and HIV, makes unprotected sexual contact, including anal and oral sex, very risky. Hepatitis E, associated with water contamination, is rarely seen in this country other than in people returning from hepatitis E virus–endemic areas of the world.

Often overlooked is the fact that, when combined, the number of persons in this country with undiagnosed hepatitis B and C infections would surpass the number infected with HIV by a factor of five.[28]

AIDS

Acquired immunodeficiency syndrome (AIDS) has become the most devastating infectious disease in recent history, and it is virtually certain to be among the most devastating diseases in history unless a cure is forthcoming. Setting aside for the present the international scope of the HIV/AIDS epidemic, statistics for the United States alone paint a distressing picture. For the period 2006–2009 (using the 40 states with confidential name-based reporting processes), 42,011 people were newly diagnosed as HIV-positive, 878,366 transitioned from being HIV-positive to having AIDS since its initial recognition in the early 1980s, and 594,496 succumbed to HIV/AIDS.[29] See the Online Learning Center (www.mhhe.com/hahn11e) for a table of the estimated number of persons living with HIV/AIDS by race/ethnicity, sex, and transmission category in 34 states with confidential name-based reporting.

Cause of AIDS AIDS is the disease caused by HIV, a virus that attacks the T-helper cells of the immune system (see pages 277–278). When HIV attacks T-helper cells, people lose the ability to fight off a variety of infections that would normally be easily controlled. Because these infections develop while people are vulnerable, they are collectively called *opportunistic infections.* HIV-infected (HIV-positive) patients become increasingly vulnerable to infection by bacteria, protozoa, fungi, and several viruses. A variety of malignancies also develop during this period of immune system vulnerability.

Today, experts tend to assign the label of HIV positive with AIDS to HIV-infected people when their level of CD4 T-helper cells drops below 200 cells per μL (microliter) of blood, regardless of whether specific conditions are present. (CD4 cells are the type of cells most often infected and destroyed by HIV.) That said, in terms of treatment trials reported in 2010, CD4 cell categories ranging from as low as 50 per μL to as high as 350–500 per μL, and 500–799 per μL were employed; this indicates that newer treatment protocols are not bound by traditional clinical standards.[30]

Spread of HIV   HIV cannot be contracted easily. The chances of contracting HIV through casual contact with HIV-infected people at work, school, or home are extremely low or nonexistent. HIV is known to be spread only by direct sexual contact involving the exchange of bodily fluids (including blood, semen, and vaginal secretions), the sharing of hypodermic needles, transfusion of infected blood or blood products, and perinatal transmission (from an infected mother to a fetus or newborn baby). For HIV to be transmitted, it must enter the bloodstream of the noninfected person, such as through needles or tears in body tissues lining the rectum, mouth, or reproductive system. Current research also indicates that HIV is not transmitted by sweat, saliva, tears, or urine, although the virus may be found in very low concentrations in these fluids. The virus cannot enter the body through the gastrointestinal system because digestive enzymes destroy it. However, transmission can occur in conjunction with breast-feeding infants. A second exception involves the transmission of HIV between infected persons and their uninfected sex partners during episodes of unprotected oral sex when the uninfected persons have evident gingivitis and bleeding gums. In 2010 a patient contracted HIV in conjunction with an infected transplanted kidney.

Women are at much greater risk than men of contracting HIV through heterosexual activity because of the higher concentration of lymphocytes in semen (±10 million lymphocytes/tsp) than in vaginal secretions (±1,200 thousand lymphocytes/tsp). This susceptibility is evidenced in part by the increasing percentage of women with AIDS who were infected through heterosexual contact—from 8 percent in 1981, to 19 percent in 1993, and 72 percent in 2007. Women under age 25 contract the virus principally through heterosexual contact.

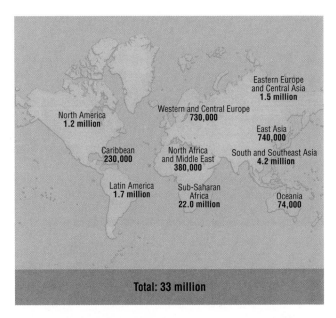

Figure 11-4 HIV/AIDS Worldwide Statistics: Adults and Children Estimated to Be Living with HIV/AIDS at the End of 2007   For every person counted in these statistics, there is a face and a story. What are you doing to protect yourself from HIV/AIDS?

Source: Joint United Nations Programme on HIV/AIDS (UNAIDS) and World Health Organization (WHO), *2008 Report on the Global AIDS Epidemic.* Geneva: UNAIDS, www.unaids.org.

HIV/AIDS on the World Stage   In comparison to one and a half decades of media attention directed primarily to HIV/AIDS in the United States, since the late 1990s, attention has been increasingly drawn toward the "AIDS crisis" that is occurring in other regions of the world. Principal among these are Africa, the Indian subcontinent, and areas of Asia and Latin America. Figure 11-4 depicts the strikingly disproportionate number of cases in sub-Saharan Africa in comparison to other regions of the world. This helps explain the urgency being expressed on the part of the international community, including the industrialized nations, world relief agencies, and the pharmaceutical industry, as well as philanthropic foundations and celebrities.

The extent to which the international scope of the HIV/AIDS crisis can be ameliorated seems highly uncertain, at best. In the absence of a vaccine to immunize against HIV, the limited availability of effective prevention programs, and the prohibitive cost of the antiretroviral medication required to manage declining health, time may be running out for those now infected and those likely to soon join them.

On AIDS Day 2008, a small debate took place, challenging two aspects of the global AIDS epidemic. The first challenge was directed toward concerns that data supporting the extent of the global scope of the epidemic have been overstated in recent years, given treatment and prevention efforts. The second concern

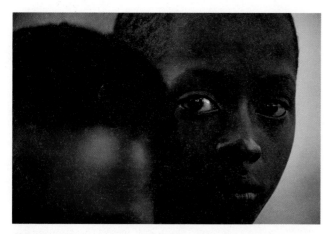

These children are among the thousands of orphaned children in Africa fending for themselves following the death of their parents from AIDS.

expressed was related to the $200 million spent annually by UNAIDS (the umbrella WHO organization) being misdirected by disregarding the treatment and prevention of pneumonia, a condition that kills more children annually than AIDS, measles, and malaria combined. Further evidence of this redirection of funds, from both governmental and private sources, was seen in 2010 and 2011 when public attention was directed toward the eradication of malaria and polio. The latter has been absent from the United States and other developed countries since the end of the 1950s, when effective vaccines became available.

Diagnosis of HIV Infection   HIV infection is diagnosed through a clinical examination, laboratory tests for accompanying infections, and an initial screening test. Should the initial screening test produce a negative result, persons at risk for infection should be rescreened in three to six months. For persons reluctant to present themselves for screening in a clinical setting, home screening tests are also available. Regardless, once initial screening has been undertaken, to eliminate the small chance of a false positive having occurred, more sensitive tests can be administered, including the enzyme-linked immunosorbent assay (ELISA) and Western blot test. Although expensive and not completely reliable, even more recently developed tests are now available. One of these tests identifies the existence of viral mutations known to be drug resistant, while another helps determine whether a particular drug will function in suppressing the contracted viral strain. This information helps physicians structure treatment protocols.

The Course of HIV Infection   Some newly infected people experience flulike symptoms within a month or two after exposure to HIV. The symptoms usually disappear within a few weeks and are typically mistaken for another

illness. During this period, people carry high levels of HIV in their blood and genital fluids and are very infectious. The immune system fights back, which reduces the HIV level in the body; this immune response also produces the antibodies that can be detected through testing. Unlike most infections, however, the immune system is unable to clear HIV from the body despite a strong immune response.

The next stage of HIV infection—an asymptomatic stage—may last from a few months to more than 12 years. In Western countries, the average time between infection and the appearance of symptoms is about 10–12 years in untreated individuals. The length of the asymptomatic stage may be influenced by such factors as age, gender, overall health status, access to health care, and the particular strain of HIV causing the infection. During this period, the virus is actively multiplying and killing cells of the immune system, and the HIV-positive individual can transmit the infection. This long incubation period is one of the key reasons why widespread testing is recommended; if people know they are infected, they can take steps to avoid transmitting HIV to others. To counter the reality of such a lengthy incubation period, the American College of Physicians now strongly encourages that all patients 13 years of age and older be screened for HIV, with rescreening being determined on a case-by-case basis.

As the status of the immune system worsens, symptoms begin to appear, including enlarged lymph nodes, loss of energy, frequent fevers and sweats, and persistent infections. As described earlier, a diagnosis of AIDS is made when a person develops one of the AIDS-defining conditions or the level of CD4 T-helper cells drops below 200 per μL of blood (healthy adults typically have CD4 counts over 1,000). People with AIDS are vulnerable to many opportunistic infections and may become very ill.

Treatment of HIV Infection   Although no treatment currently exists to cure HIV infection, drugs are available to help reduce the level of HIV in the body, prevent opportunistic infections, and improve chances for survival. Decisions about treatment are usually made on the basis of blood tests and symptoms. CDC guidelines recommend treatment when a person has an AIDS-defining condition or when CD4 cell counts are low and viral counts are high. Currently, there is considerable discussion regarding initial antiviral medications when the CD4 T-helper cell count reaches a level of 350 μL, or even at 800 μL; earlier recommendations delayed initiation of treatment at levels as low as 250 μL and even 200 μL. Today initial or modified antiviral treatments can be altered relative to CD4 T-helper cell counts depending on the viral load and its relative rate of increase.

Currently, different classes of drugs are used to treat HIV-infected persons. One major class prevents the virus from duplicating itself inside infected CD4 T-helper cells.

A second major class blocks HIV entry into the cells. Combinations of drugs are taken, a treatment approach referred to as highly active antiretroviral therapy, or HAART. Since the introduction of HAART, death rates from AIDS have declined for patients who can stick to treatment regimens and tolerate the side effects of the drugs (see the box "From Fear to Hope, and Now Benign Neglect—AIDS in the News").

Drug Resistance in HIV Infection Consistent with other pathogenic agents, both bacterial and viral, the HIV virus has the ability to develop drug resistance during the course of HIV/AIDS treatment and might already be drug resistant at the time of transmission.

In comparison to these apparently "wild" drug-resistant viruses, it is now recognized that in 10–20 percent of the persons under treatment a resistant-related mutation will develop within a portion of the virus pool infecting their body. These drug-resistant viruses diminish the antiretroviral therapy's ability to sustain manageable levels of CD4 cells and to keep the viral load at the lowest levels possible. Unfortunately, the percentage of people who will develop an antiretroviral-resistant status is rising.

Today, trials are under way, using newly developed technology, to develop a test that would be much faster than previous tests in detecting the mutated viruses. Additionally, a newly approved test that measures the levels of antiviral drugs in hair can be used to accurately predict the long-term success of the antiviral treatment being used.

Prevention of HIV Infection Can HIV infection be prevented? The answer is a definite yes. HIV infection rates on college campuses are considered low (approximately 0.2 percent), but students can be at risk. Every person can take several steps to reduce the risk of contracting and transmitting HIV. All these steps require understanding one's behavior and the methods by which HIV can be transmitted. Some appropriate steps for college-aged people are abstinence, safe sex, sobriety, and communication with potential sex partners. To ensure the greatest protection from HIV, one should abstain from sexual activity. Other than this, the box "Reducing Your Risk of Contracting HIV" lists recommendations for safe sex, sobriety, and the exchange of honest, accurate information about sexual histories.

TALKING POINTS In a job interview with a representative from a large pharmaceutical company, you are asked about your feelings regarding the affordability of HIV/AIDS medications in third world countries. What would your response be?

Sexually Transmitted Diseases

Sexually transmitted diseases (STDs) were once called venereal diseases (for Venus, the Roman goddess of love). Today the term *venereal disease* has been superseded by the broader terms *sexually transmitted disease* or *sexually transmitted infection*. Despite the preference some instructors might have for the new term (STI), your text will retain the older designation (STD), as it is the term used by the CDC (the terms are interchangeable). Experts currently emphasize the successful prevention and treatment of STDs rather than the ethics of sexuality. Thus, one should consider the following points: (1) By age 25 years, approximately one-third of all adults will have contracted a sexually transmitted disease—most often chlamydia, herpes simplex, or human papillomavirus infection; (2) a person can have more than one STD at a time; (3) the symptoms of STDs can vary over time and from person to person; (4) the body develops little immunity for STDs; and (5) STDs can predispose people to additional health problems, including infertility, birth defects in their children, cancer, and long-term disability. In addition, the risk of HIV infection is higher when sex partners are also infected with STDs.

Most STDs are treated with an array of antibacterial, antiviral, and antifungal prescription medication; for more information on specific treatments, visit the Online Learning Center. The latest treatment guidelines,[31] published by the CDC in 2010, serve as the basis of this online information.

This section focuses on the STDs most frequently diagnosed among college students: chlamydia, gonorrhea, human papillomavirus infection, herpes simplex, syphilis, and pubic lice. Complete the Personal Assessment at the end of this chapter to determine your risk of contracting an STD.

Chlamydia (Nonspecific Urethritis)

Chlamydia is thought to be the most prevalent STD in the United States today. Chlamydia infections occur an estimated 3 times more frequently than does gonorrhea and up to 10 times more frequently than syphilis. In 2009, 1,224,160 cases were reported by the CDC. Because of its high prevalence in sexually active adolescents (782,013 cases in 2007), they should be screened for chlamydia twice a year, even in the absence of symptoms. Because chlamydia frequently accompanies gonorrheal infections, a dual therapy is often appropriate when gonorrhea is found. Sexually active people in the 15- to 24-year age range should also be considered for routine screening, particularly if they have a history of multiple sex partners and have not practiced a form of barrier contraception (see Figure 11-5).

Chlamydia trachomatis is the bacterial agent that causes the chlamydia infection. Chlamydia is the most common cause of nonspecific urethritis (NSU). NSU describes infections of the **urethra** and surrounding tissues that are not caused by the bacterium responsible for gonorrhea. About 80 percent of men with chlamydia display gonorrhea-like signs and symptoms, including painful urination and a whitish pus discharge from the penis. As in gonorrheal infections and many other STDs, most women report no overt signs or symptoms. A few women might exhibit a mild urethral discharge, painful urination, and swelling of vulval tissues. The recommended treatment for chlamydia is antibiotics; visit

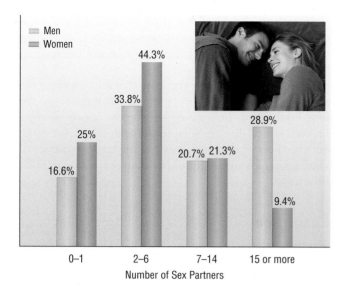

Figure 11-5 Number of Lifetime Sex Partners Among Adults Ages 20–59 Years The fewer the number of partners you've had, the lower your risk of contracting HIV or an STD. How many partners have you had, and how accurate is your count? People may be less than truthful when answering sensitive questions. In addition, researchers have found that the methods used by men and women to calculate or estimate their number of sex partners tend to lead to underestimation by women and overestimation by men.

Source: National Center for Health Statistics. Drug use and sexual behaviors reported by adults: United States, 1999–2002. *Advance Data from Vital and Health Statistics*, 384, 2007; Lovers and liars: How many sex partners have you really had? University of Michigan News Service, February 13, 2006. www.umich.edu/news/index.html?Releases/2006/Feb06/r021306d.

the Online Learning Center for more information. The infected person should carefully comply with instructions to abstain from sexual intercourse.

Both sex partners should receive treatment to avoid the ping-pong effect—the back-and-forth reinfection that occurs among couples when only one partner receives treatment. Furthermore, as with other STDs, having chlamydia once does not effectively confer immunity.

Unresolved chlamydia can lead to the same negative health consequences that result from untreated gonorrheal infections. In men the pathogens can invade and damage the deeper reproductive structures (the prostate gland, seminal vesicles, and Cowper's glands). Sterility can result. The pathogens can spread further and produce joint problems (arthritis) and heart complications (damaged heart valves, blood vessels, and heart muscle tissue).

In women the pathogens enter the body through the urethra or the cervical area. If the invasion is not properly treated, it can reach the deeper pelvic structures, producing a syndrome called **pelvic inflammatory disease (PID).** The infection may attack the inner uterine wall (endometrium), the fallopian tubes, and any surrounding structures to produce this painful syndrome. A variety of further

complications can result, including sterility, ectopic (tubal) pregnancies, and **peritonitis.** Infected women can transmit a chlamydia infection to the eyes and lungs of newborns during a vaginal birth. Detecting chlamydia and other NSUs early is of paramount concern for both men and women.

Human Papillomavirus

The appearance of another STD, **human papillomavirus (HPV),** is unwanted news. Because HPV infections are generally asymptomatic, the exact extent of the disease is unknown. A recent study of women across a wide age range found that among those 20–24 years of age, nearly 45 percent had been infected with HPV; and among women across the study's entire age range (14–59 years of age), 27 percent were infected with one or more forms of HPV. HPV-related changes to the cells of the cervix are found in nearly 5 percent of the Pap tests taken from women under age 30. Researchers currently believe that risk factors for HPV infection in women include (1) sexual activity before age 20, (2) intercourse with three or more partners before age 35, and (3) intercourse with a partner who has had three or more partners. The extent of HPV infection in men is even less clearly known, but it is probably widespread. It has even been suggested that virtually all sexually active persons will have acquired some form of HPV during their lifetime.

HPV infection is alarming because some of the nearly 100 strains of the virus are strongly associated with precancerous changes to cells lining the cervix, illustrating the importance of the new viral Pap-plus test (see Chapter 10). Additionally, visible genital warts (cauliflower-like,

---

Key Terms

sexually transmitted diseases (STDs) Infectious diseases that are spread primarily through intimate sexual contact.

chlamydia The most prevalent sexually transmitted disease; caused by a nongonococcal bacterium.

urethra (yoo **ree** thra) The passageway through which urine leaves the urinary bladder.

pelvic inflammatory disease (PID) An acute or chronic infection of the peritoneum or lining of the abdominopelvic cavity and fallopian tubes; associated with a variety of symptoms or none at all, and a potential cause of sterility.

peritonitis (pare it ton **eye** tis) Inflammation of the peritoneum, or lining of the abdominopelvic cavity.

human papillomavirus (HPV) Sexually transmitted viruses, some of which are capable of causing precancerous changes in the cervix; causative agent for genital warts.

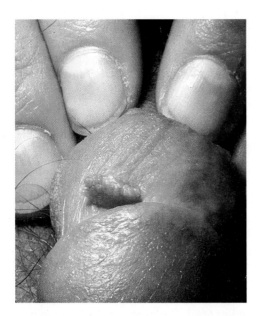

Figure 11-6 Human Papillomavirus Infection (Genital Warts)

raised, pinkish-white lesions) are associated with viral forms 6 and 11, while viral forms 16, 18, 31, 33, and 35 foster changes in other areas (see Figure 11-6). Found most commonly on the penis, scrotum, labia, and cervix, and around the anus, these lesions represent the most common symptomatic viral STD in this country. Although most genital wart colonies are small, they may become very large and block the anus or birth canal during pregnancy.

Treatment for HPV, including genital warts, may involve patient-applied gels or creams or physician-administered cryotherapy, topical medication, or surgery. Regardless of treatment, however, the viral colonies will probably return. One should use condoms to attempt to prevent transmission of HPV.

As noted in Chapter 10, in conjunction with cervical cancer, Gardasil and Cervarix, vaccines effective for HPV 6 and 11 (genital warts) and 16 and 18 (cervical cancer), have been approved for use by the FDA. The current recommendation calling for the inoculation of young women between the ages of 9 and 26, and older if just beginning sexual activity, is being strongly encouraged by the health care community. The CDC recommends that the preferred (or most reasonable) age for receiving the initial vaccination is between ages 11 and 12. In states that are considering mandatory inoculation as a part of required school-based immunizations, controversy abounds. With approximately 7 percent of children sexually active by age 13, and nearly 25 percent by age 15, when is young too young? Some experts suggest that when girls clearly display signs of sexual maturation, including the onset of menstruation, then the inoculation is appropriate. The need for an eventual booster has not yet been determined, but current recommendations suggest a booster might be needed in about 10 years following initial vaccination

to sustain an effective level of protection. By mid-2009, about 30 percent of young women ages 13–17 years had received a vaccine (3 million out of 10 million girls in that age range).

Additional vaccines are under development, some intended for use in newly infected patients, some for long-established infections but before clear changes in the cervical-lining cells occur, and others for more advanced cervical cancer. Most of the last two classes of vaccines are for treatment rather than prevention of HPV infections.

Gonorrhea

Another extremely common (301,174 cases reported in 2009) STD, *gonorrhea* is caused by a bacterium (*N. gonorrhoeae*). The incidence of gonorrhea rose 18 percent between 1997 and 2001, perhaps, in part, because of decreasing fear of HIV/AIDS brought about by the effectiveness of the protease inhibitors being widely reported at that time. However, since 2001 the reported cases of gonorrhea have declined; but in 2005 a marked upturn was reported over the 2004 level, and by 2007 the level had increased by 4.9 percent over the 2005 level. But a decline was noted between 2007 and 2009.

In men this bacterial agent can produce a milky-white discharge from the penis, accompanied by painful urination. About 80 percent of men who contract gonorrhea report varying degrees of these symptoms. This figure is approximately reversed for women: only about 20 percent of women are symptomatic and thus report varying degrees of frequent, painful urination, with a slimy yellow-green discharge from the vagina or urethra. Oral sex with an infected partner can produce a gonorrheal infection of the throat (pharyngeal gonorrhea). Gonorrhea can also be transmitted to the rectal areas of both men and women.

An interesting finding relative to gonorrhea in adolescents suggests that the incidence of gonorrhea within the adolescent population correlates closely with the consumption of beer, suggesting that alcohol consumption fosters a higher level of high-risk sexual behavior, including earlier onset of sexual activity, an increased number of partners, and less selectivity in choosing those partners. With heavy consumption of beer on many college campuses, this finding does not bode well for the highly asymptomatic female population.

Although prevalent in other areas of the world, drug-resistant strains of gonorrhea are not extensive in the United States. However, a clear increase in drug-resistant strains has been reported along the West Coast; in various Pacific areas, such as Hawaii and other Pacific islands; and in Asia. Infected persons who might have contracted the disease while in these areas should report this information to their physicians. An alternative treatment plan for persons with drug-resistant strains of gonorrhea appears in the Online Learning Center.

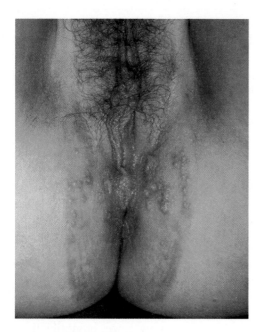

Figure 11-7 Severe Herpes Infection

Testing for gonorrhea is included as a part of prenatal care so that infections in mothers can be treated before they give birth. If the birth canal is infected, newborns can easily contract the infection in the mucous membranes of the eye.

Herpes Simplex

Public health officials think that the sexually transmitted genital herpes virus infection rivals chlamydia as the most prevalent STD. To date, about 45 million Americans have been diagnosed, although the asymptomatic (thus undiagnosed) population could increase this figure substantially. *Herpes* is really a family of more than 50 viruses, some of which produce recognized diseases in humans (chicken pox, **shingles,** mononucleosis, and others). One subgroup, called herpes simplex 1 virus (HSV-1), produces an infection called *labial herpes* (oral or lip herpes). Labial herpes produces common fever blisters or cold sores around the lips and oral cavity. Herpes simplex 2 virus (HSV-2) is a different strain that produces similar clumps of blisterlike lesions in the genital region (see Figure 11-7). Laypeople call this second type of herpes the STD type, but both types produce identical clinical pictures. About 5–30 percent of cases are caused by HSV-1. Oral-genital sexual practices most likely account for this crossover infection.

Herpes appears as a single sore or as a small cluster of blisterlike sores. These sores burn, itch, and (for some) become very painful. The infected person might also report swollen lymph glands, muscular aches and pains, and fever. Some patients feel weak and sleepy when they have blisters. The lesions may last from a few days to a few weeks. Viral shedding lasts a week on average; then the blisters begin scabbing, and new skin is formed. Even when the patient has become asymptomatic, viral transmission is still possible.

Herpes is an interesting virus for several reasons. It can lie dormant for long periods. For reasons not well understood but perhaps related to stress, diet, or overall health, the viral particles can be stimulated to travel along the nerve pathways to the skin and then create an active infection. Thus, herpes can be considered a recurrent infection. Fortunately for most people, recurrent infections are less severe than the initial episode and do not last as long. Treatment options with antiviral drugs for HSV-1 and HSV-2 can be found at the Online Learning Center. Because herpes may occur at intervals following initial treatment, two equally effective treatment choices exist. One is to treat each recurrence as it arises (episodic recurrent treatment), and the second is to attempt to suppress recurrence through continuous use of medication (daily suppressive therapy). Additionally, physicians may recommend other medications for relief of various symptoms. Genital herpes is almost always diagnosed through a clinical examination.

Currently, the best method of preventing herpes infection is to avoid all direct contact with a person who has an active infection. Do not kiss someone with a fever blister—or let them kiss you (or your children) if they have an active lesion. Do not share drinking glasses or eating utensils. Check your partner's genitals. Do not have intimate sexual contact with someone who displays the blisterlike clusters or rash. (Condoms are only marginally helpful and cannot protect against lesions on the female vulva or the lower abdominal area of men.) Be careful not to infect yourself by touching a blister and then touching any other part of your body.

Although there is currently no cure for genital herpes, antiviral medication can be effectively employed. Intended as prophylactic medications (to be taken daily), these antiviral medications do reduce the number and duration of viral shedding episodes. Certainly, the sex partners of persons infected with HSV-2 need to be fully aware of and involved in the management of this sexually transmitted infection. Infected persons can best accomplish this communication by becoming educated about their condition, determining the appropriate point in the relationship to introduce this important information, answering in an honest manner questions asked by the new partner, and,

> **Key Terms**
>
> **shingles** Painful fluid-filled skin eruptions along underlying sensory nerve pathways—due to reactivation of once-sequestered herpes zoster (chicken pox) viruses.

finally, developing a mutually agreed-upon plan regarding all aspects of sexual intimacy during periods of potential disease transmission.

Syphilis

Like gonorrhea, *syphilis* is caused by a bacterium (*Treponema pallidum*) and is transmitted almost exclusively by sexual intercourse. The chance of contracting syphilis during a single sexual encounter with an infected partner is about 30 percent. Syphilis takes a well-established course after it is contracted. Moist, warm tissue, such as that lining the reproductive, urinary, and digestive tracts, offers an ideal environment for the agent.

If contracted during an episode of unprotected coitus, syphilis incubates without symptoms for 10–90 days, followed by the characteristic primary stage of the disease, which lasts 1–5 weeks. A small, raised, painless sore called a chancre forms. This highly infectious lesion is not easily identified in 90 percent of women and 50 percent of men; thus, these people generally do not seek treatment. The chancre heals in 4–8 weeks.

The extremely contagious secondary stage of the disease occurs 6–12 weeks after initial infection. The infectious agents are now systemic, so symptoms may include a generalized body rash, a sore throat, or a patchy loss of hair. A blood test (VDRL) will be positive, and treatment can be effectively administered. If untreated, the second stage subsides within 2–6 weeks. A pregnant woman can easily transmit syphilis to her fetus during this stage. Congenital syphilis often results in stillbirth or an infant born with a variety of life-threatening complications. Early treatment of infected pregnant women can prevent congenital syphilis.

After the secondary stage subsides, an extended period of noninfectiousness occurs. The infectious agents remain dormant within the body cells, and the infected person displays few clinical signs during this stage. This latent stage of 15–30 years was, in the past, often unrecognized, thus masking the relationship between contraction of the disease and the earlier clinical stage, and the latter terminal manifestation of the untreated disease difficult to connect. During late-stage syphilis, tissue damage is profound and irreversible. The person suffers damage to the cardiovascular system, central nervous system, eyes, and skin, and death from the effects of the disease is likely.

The incidence of syphilis, a CDC-reportable disease, is far lower than that of gonorrhea. In 1950 a record 217,558 cases of syphilis were reported in this country. The number of cases then fell steadily to fewer than 80,000 cases in 1980. From 1980 through 1990, the incidence climbed, reaching nearly 140,000 cases in 1990. Another decline then began, and in 1993 the number of cases dropped to 101,259. In 2000 the CDC reported that syphilis had fallen to the lowest level (5,972) in 42 years. By 2005, however,

reported cases of primary syphilis had risen to 8,724. In 2009 the CDC reported 13,997 new cases of syphilis. It should be noted that it was recently concluded that about 20 percent of the persons tested for syphilis received false-positive reports due to oversensitivity or improper assessment of test results.[32] This suggests that the size of the increases recently reported should be smaller.

Whether the upward trend in the number of reported cases of primary syphilis continues remains to be seen. As has been true for most of the last few decades, a high percentage of cases have been associated with HIV infections, largely among gay men in several larger cities. Observers have noted an alarming increase in infant syphilis in children born to mothers who use drugs and support their habit through sexual activity.

For specific information on the antibiotics used in the treatment of syphilis, see the Online Learning Center's section on the treatment of STDs. It is important to note that the medications listed could become less efficacious with the increasing prevalence of antibiotic-resistant syphilis in some areas of the country since the late 1990s.

Pubic Lice

Three types of lice infect humans: the head louse, the body louse, and the pubic louse, all of which feed on the blood of the host. Except for the relatively uncommon body louse, these tiny insects do not carry diseases. They are, however, very annoying.

Pubic lice, also called *crabs,* attach themselves to the base of the pubic hairs, where they live and lay their eggs (nits). These eggs move into a larval stage after one week; after two more weeks, they develop into mature adult crab lice.

People usually notice they have a pubic lice infestation when they suffer intense itching in the genital region. Prescription and OTC creams, lotions, and shampoos are usually effective in killing both the lice and their eggs, although some reports suggest that lice are becoming resistant to OTC treatments.

The following are specific steps to be taken in the eradication of pubic lice:[33]

- Wash the infested area; towel dry.
- Follow label directions in using lice medications. Dry with a clean towel.
- Following application of lice medications, remove nits from hair shafts with your fingernails.
- Put on clean underwear and clothing after treatment.
- Machine wash all clothing and bedding used by the infected person during the two to three days before treatment (use hot wash cycle for at least 20 minutes).
- Dry-clean clothing that is not washable and store in plastic bags for two weeks.

- Inform sex partners that they are at risk of infestation and that they should be examined and treated.
- Do not have sex until treatment is completed.
- Repeat treatment in 7–10 days if lice are still found.

Bed Bugs

Very likely your parents, as young children, before being put to bed, heard the "Good night; don't let the bed bugs bite," warning even though bed bugs were nonentities during their childhood. They are, however, a part of today's reality.

Similar in appearance and biologically related to pubic lice, bed bugs are back with a vengeance since the EPA removed propoxur from the list of approved inside pesticides due to its carcinogenic potential. Now hotels, motels, movie theaters, campgrounds, airlines, railroads, taxi services, and university residences struggle to keep you and the bed bugs from finding each other. Their hiding places are in the folds of bedding, under the edges of carpets, on draperies, in coat closets, in the seams of your clothing. They will hitch rides in your luggage, backpack, or purse, and the fabric of car seats. Class distinction is not a factor, as bed bugs want only the availability of a human skin surface through which they can obtain a life-sustaining blood meal.

Since bed bugs are not vectors for any infectious conditions, their bites do not transmit pathogenic organisms. That said, the red, slightly inflamed area surrounding bite marks will likely itch, and by scratching these areas, you could infect yourself with a pathogenic organism. Should that happen, keep your hands clean and away from these areas, seek medical care for any clear evidence of infection, and report your exposure to a person affiliated with the location you suspect of harboring the bugs. Professional exterminators will, hopefully, soon have an effective and approved pesticide, but be prepared to spend a sizable amount of time and money ridding your living space and personal items of these new roomies.

Vaginal Infections

Three common pathogens produce uncomfortable *vaginal infections*. The first is the yeast or fungus pathogen *Candida (Monilia) albicans,* which produces the yeast infection often called *thrush.* These organisms, commonly found in the vagina, seem to multiply rapidly when some unusual stressor (pregnancy, use of birth control pills or antibiotics, diabetes) affects a woman's body. This infection, now called *vulvovaginal candidiasis (VVC),* is signaled by a white- or cream-colored vaginal discharge that resembles cottage cheese. Vaginal itching and vulvar swelling are also commonly reported. Current treatment is based on the use of one of several prescription and OTC azole drugs. For women who have

recurrent VVC, some degree of prophylactic suppression of candidiasis seems possible. As has been recommended for all STDs discussed here, the Online Learning Center provides an extensive listing of recommended and alternative prescription-based medications now used in the treatment of STDs. When OTC medications exist for use in treating sexually transmitted infections, such as those used with vaginal infections, they too will be listed.

One should first consult with a physician before using these new products for the first time. Men rarely report this monilial infection, although some may report mildly painful urination or a barely noticeable discharge at the urethral opening or beneath the foreskin of the penis.

A second type of sexually transmitted vaginal infection is somewhat less easily described in terms of a clearly defined pathogenic agent. Rather, bacterial vaginosis (BV) reflects an imbalance in the normal relationship between all vaginal flora, leading to some bacterial forms gaining a level of pathogenicity sufficient to allow the formation of abnormal symptoms. Included among these signs of microbial imbalance are abnormal vaginal discharge, a strong fishlike odor (most often following intercourse), burning during urination, and clinical indicators that can be ascertained by visual inspection by a physician and laboratory test results.[34]

BV is considered an STD because it is rarely seen in women who are celibate or who have had a very limited number of sex partners. Increased risk is associated with having a new sex partner, having had multiple sex partners, having used an intrauterine device (IUD), and frequent douching. Directly or indirectly, having BV seems to increase the risk of contracting HIV, contracting other STDs, and developing pelvic inflammatory disease (PID). Bacterial vaginosis is usually treated with antibiotics (see the Online Learning Center). In some cases, the condition resolves itself with changes in sexual practices.

The protozoan *Trichomonas vaginalis,* a third STD-related pathogenic agent, also produces a vaginal infection. This parasite can be transmitted through sexual intercourse or by contact with contaminated (often damp) objects, such as towels, clothing, or toilet seats, that may contain some vaginal discharge. In women, this infection, called *trichomoniasis,* or "trich," produces a foamy, yellow-green, foul-smelling discharge that may be accompanied by itching, swelling, and painful urination. Although topically applied treatments for trichomoniasis are available, they have limited effectiveness. Only one highly effective oral medication is currently on the market. Men infrequently contract trichomoniasis but may harbor the organisms without realizing it. They also should be treated to minimize reinfection of partners.

The vagina is warm, dark, and moist, an ideal breeding environment for a variety of organisms. Unfortunately, some highly promoted commercial products seem to increase the incidence of vaginal infections. Among these are tight panty hose (without cotton panels), which tend to increase the vaginal temperature, and commercial vaginal douches, which can alter the acidic level of the vagina. Both of these products might promote infections. Avoiding public bathrooms when possible is also a good practice. Of course, if you notice any unusual discharge from the vagina, you should report this to your physician.

Cystitis and Urethritis

Cystitis, an infection of the urinary bladder, and *urethritis,* an infection of the urethra, occasionally can be caused by a sexually transmitted organism. Such infections can also be caused by the organisms that cause vaginitis and organisms found in the intestinal tract. A culture is required to identify the specific pathogen associated with a particular case of cystitis or urethritis. The symptoms are pain when urinating, the need to urinate frequently, a dull ache above the pubic bone, and the passing of blood-streaked urine.

Physicians can easily treat cystitis and urethritis with antibiotics when the specific organism has been identified. The drug Monurol, which requires only a single dose, has proved effective. Few complications result from infections that are treated promptly. If cystitis or urethritis is left untreated, the infectious agent could move upward in the urinary system and infect the ureters and kidneys. These upper-urinary-tract infections are more serious and require more extensive evaluation and aggressive treatment. Therefore, one should obtain medical care immediately upon noticing symptoms.

Urinary tract infections in men not related to the gonorrhea bacterium are extremely common. These cases of nongonococcal urethritis (NGU) are sexually transmitted in predictable ways, with a discharge from the penis and pain on urination being the symptoms that bring men into treatment. Recently, it has been established that NGU is also transmitted in conjunction with oral sex, when the recipient's penis is exposed to infectious agents from the mouth of his partner.

Preventing cystitis and urethritis depends to some degree on the source of the infectious agent. One can generally reduce the incidence of infection by urinating completely (to fully empty the urinary bladder) and by drinking ample fluids to flush the urinary tract. Drinking cranberry juice has been found to reduce urinary tract infections. Prevention of urinary tract infections cannot be disregarded, from both medical and cost perspectives. As noted, untreated cystitis and urethritis can be the basis of serious damage to the kidneys. These two infections combined are the second greatest cause of antibiotic use—which is both costly and increasingly losing effectiveness.

 TALKING POINTS Honesty regarding past sexual experiences is a critical issue in the decision to introduce sexual intimacy into a relationship. What questions would you feel comfortable being asked by another person, and what questions would you be prepared to ask that person?

Sexually Transmitted Diseases, Health, Role Fulfillment, and a Sense of Well-Being

In recalling Figures 1-1, 1-2, and 1-3, in which a more broadly based perception of health was depicted, it should be easy to understand that a sexually transmitted disease (both acute and chronic) can interfere with the competent fulfillment of role expectations. Particularly for those who "push the sexual envelope" in terms of the number and types of partners, various types and degrees of impairment may become hindrances to undertaking the daily tasks that are demanded by various roles and may eventually compromise the degree to which self-identity, emotional independence, social interconnectivity, and the assumption of responsibility for the well-being of self and others can be accomplished. If health is, as your text contends, a reflection of your resourcefulness for living life well, then STDs contribute nothing that is positive to that list.

Taking Charge of Your Health

- Because microorganisms develop resistance to antibiotics, continue taking all such medications until gone, even when the symptoms of the infection have subsided.

- Check your current immunization status to make sure you are protected against preventable infectious diseases.

- If you are a parent, take your children to receive their recommended immunizations as necessary.

- Because of the possibility of contracting HIV/AIDS and sexually transmitted diseases, incorporate disease prevention into all of your sexual activities.

- Use the Personal Assessment at the end of this chapter to determine your risk of contracting a sexually transmitted disease.

- If you have ever engaged in high-risk sexual behavior, get tested for HIV.

SUMMARY

- A variety of pathogenic agents are responsible for infectious conditions.
- A chain of infection with six potential links characterizes every infectious condition.
- One can acquire immunity for some diseases through both natural and artificial means. Children and adults should be immunized according to a schedule.
- The common cold and influenza produce many similar symptoms but differ in their infectious agents, incubation period, prevention, and treatment.
- Tuberculosis and pneumonia are potentially fatal infections of the respiratory system.
- Bacterial meningitis, a potentially fatal infection of the linings that cover the brain, is of increasing concern on college campuses.

- Hantavirus pulmonary syndrome is caused by a virus carried by deer mice; human-to-human transmission has also been reported.
- Hepatitis B (serum hepatitis) is a viral infectious condition that produces serious liver damage. Other varieties are hepatitis A, C, D, and E.
- HIV/AIDS is a widespread, incurable viral disease transmitted through sexual activity, through intravenous drug use, in infected blood products, or across the placenta during pregnancy.
- There are a variety of sexually transmitted diseases, many of which do not produce symptoms in most infected women and many infected men.

REVIEW QUESTIONS

1. Describe the six links in the chain of infection.
2. What are the two principal chemical-cellular components of the immune system, and how do they cooperate to protect the body from infectious agents, foreign protein, and abnormal cells?
3. What are nosocomial infections, and in what settings are these infections most likely to develop?
4. How are the common cold and influenza similar? How do they differ in their causative agents, incubation period, prevention, and treatment?
5. Why is bacterial meningitis of greater concern on the college campus than elsewhere?
6. Why is outdoor activity a risk factor for contracting Lyme disease?

7. What role do birds play in the transmission of the West Nile virus? What insect is the vector?
8. How is hepatitis B transmitted, and which occupational group is at greatest risk of contracting this infection? How do forms A, C, D, and E compare with hepatitis B?
9. How is HIV transmitted? How are HIV/AIDS currently treated, and how effective is the treatment? In what areas of the world does the HIV/AIDS epidemic seem virtually unchecked? In terms of STD prevention, how can sexual practices be made safer?
10. Why are women more often asymptomatic for STDs than men?

ANSWERS TO THE "WHAT DO YOU KNOW?" QUIZ

1. True   2. False   3. False   4. False   5. False   6. True   7. True

Visit the Online Learning Center (**www.mhhe.com/hahn11e**), where you will find tools to help you improve your grade including practice quizzes, key terms flashcards, audio chapter summaries for your MP3 player, and many other study aids.

SOURCE NOTES

1. Worldwide HIV and AIDS Statistics. *UNAIDS: Report on the Global AIDS Epidemic. 2010.* (Overview brochure on 2011 high-level meeting on AIDS). www.unaids.org/en/aboutunaids/unitednationsdeclarationsandgoals/2011highlevelmeetingonaids/.
2. Walsh TR, Weeks J, Livermore DM, et al. Dissemination of NDM-1 positive bacteria in the New Delhi environment and its implications for human health: an environmental point prevalence study. *Lancet Journal of Infectious Disease,* April 6 (Epub ahead of print).
3. Hamann B. *Disease Identification, Prevention, and Control* (3rd ed.) New York: McGraw-Hill, 2007.
4. Saladin KS. *Anatomy and Physiology: Unity of Form and Function* (6th ed.). New York: McGraw-Hill, 2012.
5. *Understanding the Immune System: How It Works.* National Institute of Allergy and Infectious Disease, National Cancer Institute. NIH Publication No. 07-5423, September 2007. www.niaid.nih.gov/. immunesystem/documents/immune/theimmunesystem.pdf.

6. Widmaier E, Raff H, Strang K. *Vander's Human Physiology: The Mechanisms of Body Function* (12th ed.). New York: McGraw-Hill, 2011.
7. Thornley I, et al. Private cord blood banking: experiences and views of pediatric hematopoietic cell transplantation physicians. *Pediatrics,* 123(3), 1011–17, March 2009.
8. Rodriquez S, Campo-Engelsteon, Tingen C, et al. An obscure rider obstructing science: the conflation of parthenotes with embryos in the Dickey-Wicker amendment. *American Journal of Bioethics,* 11(3), 20–28, 2011.
9. Vaccine Adverse Event Reporting System (VAERS). 2011. Department of Health and Human Services, Food and Drug Administration, Centers for Disease Control and Prevention, 2011 www.vaers. hhs.gov.
10. Montgomery K, Ryan TJ, Krause A. Assessment of athletic health care facility surfaces for MRSA in the secondary school setting. *Journal of Environmental Health,* 72(6), 8–11, 2010.

11. *FDA Recommends the Over-the-Counter Cough and Cold Products Not Be Used for Infants and Children Under 2 Years of Age.* Public Health Advisory, U.S. Food and Drug Administration. Department of Health and Human Services, January 17, 2008 (updated, October 10).

12. Centers for Disease Control and Prevention. Trends in tuberculosis—United States. *Morbidity and Mortality Weekly Report,* 60(11), 333–337, 2011.

13. Centers for Disease Control and Prevention. Plan to combat extensively drug-resistant tuberculosis recommendations of the Federal Tuberculosis Task Force. *Morbidity and Mortality Weekly Report,* 58(RR-03), 1–43, 2009.

14. Extensively drug-resistant tuberculosis—United States, 1993–2006. *Morbidity and Mortality Weekly Report,* 56(11), 250–253, March 23, 2007.

15. Kariminia A, et al. Comparison of QuantiFERON TB-G to TST for detecting latent tuberculosis infection in a high-incidence area containing BCG-vaccinated population. *Journal of Evaluation in Clinical Practice,* 15(1), 148–151, February 2009.

16. Centers for Disease Control and Prevention. Updated recommendations for prevention of invasive pneumococcal disease among adults using the 23-valent pneumococcal polysaccharide vaccine (PPSV23). *Morbidity and Mortality Weekly Report,* 59(34), 1102–06, 2010.

17. *Streptococcus Pneumoniae Disease.* Division of Bacterial and Mycotic Diseases, CDC, August 11, 2005. www.cdc.gov.silibrary.org/ncidod/dbmd/diseaseinfo/streppneum_t.htm.

18. Centers for Disease Control and Prevention. Invasive pneumococcal disease in children before licensure of 13-valent pneumococcal conjugate vaccine—United States.

19. Wainberg MA, Jeang KT. XMRV as a human pathogen? *Cell Host & Microbe,* 9(4), 260–262, 2011.

20. FDANEWS. Advisory committee unanimously recommends Merck's Boceprevir. *Drug Industry Daily,* 10(84), 2010. www.fdanews.com/newsletter/article?issueId=14687&articleId=136332; FDANEWS. Committee unanimously recommends Vertex's Telaprevir. *Drug Industry Daily,* 10(85), 2010. www.fdanews.com/newsletter/article?issueId=14683&articleId=136302.

21. Centers for Disease Control. Division of vector-borne diseases. *Morbidity and Mortality Weekly Report,* 59(33), 1076–89, 2010.

22. Centers for Disease Control. Lyme disease—United States, 2003–2005. *Morbidity and Mortality Weekly Report,* 56(23), 573, 2007.

23. Rasmuson J, Andersson C, Norrman E, et al. Time to revise the paradigm of hantavirus syndromes? Hantavirus pulmonary syndrome caused by European hantavirus. *European Journal of Clinical Microbiology and Infectious Disease,* 30(5), 685–690, 2011.

24. Tabnak F, Cummings K. Center for Infectious Disease. Division of Communicable Disease Control Infectious Diseases, Epidemiologic Branch, the California Department of Public Health (CDPH). *Summary of Hantavirus Pulmonary Syndrome (HPS) in California, 2001–2008,* September 22, 2009.

25. Centers for Disease Control and Prevention. *2010 West Nile Virus Human Infections in the United States,* December 28, 2010. ww.cdc.gov/ncidod/dvbid/westnile/surv&CaseCount10_detailed.htm.

26. Centers for Disease Control and Prevention. Division of viral hepatitis. *Viral Hepatitis,* April 21, 2011. www.cdc.gov/hepatitis/.

27. FDANEWS. Advisory committee unanimously recommends Merck's Boceprevir. *Drug Industry Daily,* 10(84), 2011. www.fdanews.com/newsletter/article?issueId=14687&articleId=136332; FDANEWS. Committee unanimously recommends Vertex's Telaprevir. *Drug Industry Daily,* 10(85), 2011. www.fdanews.com/newsletter/article?issueId=14683&articleId=136302.

28. Institute of Medicine. Report. Hepatitis and liver cancer: a national strategy for prevention and control of hepatitis B and C, January 11, 2010. www.iom.edu/Reports/2010/Hepatitis-and-Liver-Cancer-A-National-Strategy-for-Pr...

29. Centers for Disease Control and Prevention, National Center for HIV/AIDS, Viral Hepatitis, STD, and TB Prevention. *HIV Surveillance Report,* 21, Tables la, 3a, 12a, 2009.

30. Eron JJ. HIV: Patients with highest CD4 counts fail to gain benefit from potent antiretroviral therapy. *Abstract THLBB201.* Presented at 18th International AIDS Conference, Vienna, July, 27, 2010.

31. Workowski KA, Berman S. Centers for Disease Control and Prevention. Sexually Transmitted Disease Guidelines. *Morbidity and Mortality Weekly Report,* 59(RR-12), 1–110, 2010.

32. Centers for Disease Control and Prevention. Discordant results from reverse sequence syphilis screening—five laboratories, United States, 2006–2011. *Morbidity and Mortality Weekly Report,* 60(05), 133–137, 2011.

33. Centers for Disease Control and Prevention. *Fact Sheet: Lice. Division of Parasitic Diseases,* May 2008. www.cdc.gov/lice.html.

34. *Fact Sheet: Bacterial Vaginosis.* Division of STD Prevention, CDC, 2007. www.cdc.gov/std/healthcomm/fact_sheets.htm.

Personal Assessment

What Is Your Risk of Contracting a Sexually Transmitted Disease?

A variety of factors interact to determine your risk of contracting a sexually transmitted disease (STD). This inventory is intended to provide you with an estimate of your level of risk.

    Circle the number of each row that best characterizes you. Enter that number on the line at the end of the row (points). After assigning yourself a number in each row, total the numbers appearing in the points column. Your total points will allow you to interpret your risk for contracting an STD.

Age

						Points
1	3	4	5	3	2	_____
0–9	10–14	15–19	20–29	30–34	35+	

Sexual Practices

0	1	2	4	6	8	_____
Never engage in sex	One sex partner	One sex partner but that person has had other partners	Two to five sex partners	Five to ten sex partners	Ten or more sex partners	

Sexual Attitudes

0	1	8	1	7	8	_____
Will not engage in nonmarital sex	Premarital sex is okay if it is with future spouse	Any kind of premarital sex is okay	Extramarital sex is not for me	Extramarital sex is okay	Believe in complete sexual freedom	

Attitudes Toward Contraception

1	1	6	5	4	8	_____
Would use condom to prevent pregnancy	Would use condom to prevent STDs	Would never use a condom	Would use the birth control pill	Would use other contraceptive measure	Would not use anything	

Attitudes Toward STD

3	3	4	6	6	6	_____
Am not sexually active so I do not worry	Would be able to talk about STDs with my partner	Would check out an infection to be sure	Would be afraid to check out an infection	Can't even talk about an infection	STDs are no problem—easily cured	

YOUR TOTAL POINTS _____

Interpretation

5–8—Your risk is well below average.
9–13—Your risk is below average.
14–17—Your risk is at or near average.
18–21—Your risk is moderately high.
22+ —Your risk is high.

TO CARRY THIS FURTHER . . .

Having taken this Personal Assessment, were you surprised at your level of risk? What is the primary reason for this level? How concerned are you and your classmates and friends about contracting an STD?

Source: Centers for Disease Control and Prevention.

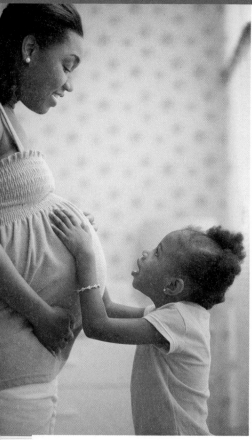

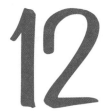

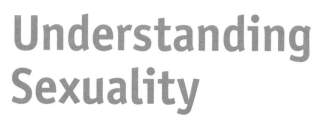

Understanding Sexuality

What Do You Know About Sexuality?

1. A fertilized ovum with the sex chromosomes XX is a biological male. True or False?

2. The release of luteinizing hormone (LH) causes ovulation to take place. True or False?

3. Hormone replacement therapy (HRT) reduces cardiovascular risks. True or False?

4. Most males are not multiorgasmic. True or False?

5. After orgasm, the length of the resolution phase is usually longer in older men. True or False?

6. Same-sex marriage is currently permitted in two U.S. states. True or False?

7. Approximately 25 percent of American adults over age 18 have not married. True or False?

Check your answers at the end of the chapter.

Early in the twenty-first century, we have reached an understanding of both the biological and psychosocial factors that contribute to the complex expression of our **sexuality.** As a society, we are now inclined to view human behavior in terms of a complex script written on the basis of both biology and conditioning. Reflecting this understanding is how we use the words *male* and *female* to refer to the biological roots of our sexuality and the words *man* and *woman* to refer to the psychosocial roots of our sexuality. This chapter explores human sexuality as it relates to the dynamic interplay of the biological and psychosocial bases that form your **masculinity** or **femininity.**

Biological Bases of Human Sexuality

Within a few seconds after the birth of a baby, someone—a doctor, nurse, or parent—emphatically labels the child: "It's a boy," or "It's a girl." For the parents and society as a whole, the child's **biological sexuality** is being displayed and identified. Another female or male enters the world.

Genetic Basis

At the moment of conception, a Y-bearing or an X-bearing sperm cell joins with the X-bearing ovum to establish the true basis of biological sexuality.[1] A fertilized ovum with sex chromosomes XX is biologically female, and a fertilized ovum bearing the XY sex chromosomes is biologically male. Genetics forms the most basic level of an individual's biological sexuality.

Gonadal Basis

The gonadal basis for biological sexuality refers to the growing embryo's development of **gonads.**[2] Male embryos develop testes about the seventh week after conception, and female embryos develop ovaries about the twelfth week after conception.

Structural Development

The development of male or female reproductive structures is initially determined by the presence or absence of hormones produced by the developing testes—androgens and the müllerian inhibiting substance (MIS). With these hormones present, the male embryo starts to develop male reproductive structures (penis, scrotum, vasa deferentia, seminal vesicles, prostate gland, and Cowper's glands).

Because the female embryo is not exposed to these male hormones, it develops the characteristic female reproductive structures: uterus, fallopian tubes, vagina, labia, and clitoris.

Biological Sexuality and the Childhood Years

The growth and development of the child in terms of reproductive organs and physiological processes has traditionally been thought to be "latent" during the childhood years. However, a gradual degree of growth occurs in both girls and boys. The reproductive organs, however, will undergo more greatly accelerated growth at the onset of **puberty** and will achieve their adult size and capabilities shortly.

Puberty

The entry into puberty is a gradual maturing process for young girls and boys. For young girls, the onset of menstruation, called **menarche,** usually occurs at about age 12 or 13 but may come somewhat earlier or later.[3] Early menstrual cycles tend to be **anovulatory.** Menarche is usually preceded by a growth spurt that includes the budding of breasts and the growth of pubic and underarm hair.[4]

Young males follow a similar pattern of maturation, including a growth spurt followed by a gradual sexual maturity. However, this process takes place about two years later than it does in young females. Genital enlargement, underarm and pubic hair growth, and a lowering of the voice commonly occur. The male's first ejaculation is generally experienced by the age of 14, most commonly through **nocturnal emission** or masturbation. For many young boys, fully mature sperm do not develop until about age 15.

Reproductive capability declines only gradually over the course of the adult years. In the woman, however, the onset of **menopause** signals a more definite turning off of the reproductive system than is the case for the male adult. By the early to mid-50s, virtually all women have entered a postmenopausal period, but for men, relatively high-level **spermatogenesis** may continue for a decade or two.[4]

The story of sexual maturation and reproductive maturity cannot, however, be solely focused on the changes that take place in the body. The psychosocial processes that accompany the biological changes are also important.

Psychosocial Bases of Human Sexuality

If the growth and development of our sexuality were to be visualized as a stepladder (see Figure 12-1), one vertical rail of the ladder would represent our biological sexuality.

> ### Key Terms
>
> **sexuality** The quality of being sexual; can be viewed from many biological and psychosocial perspectives.
>
> **masculinity** Behavioral expressions traditionally observed in males.
>
> **femininity** Behavioral expressions traditionally observed in females.
>
> **biological sexuality** Male and female aspects of sexuality.
>
> **gonads** Male or female sex glands; testes produce sperm and ovaries produce eggs.
>
> **puberty** Achievement of reproductive ability.
>
> **menarche** (muh **nar** key) Time of a female's first menstrual cycle.
>
> **anovulatory** (an **oh** vyu luh tory) Not ovulating.
>
> **nocturnal emission** Ejaculation that occurs during sleep; "wet dream."
>
> **menopause** Decline and eventual cessation of hormone production by the female reproductive system.
>
> **spermatogenesis** (sper mat oh **jen** uh sis) Process of sperm production.

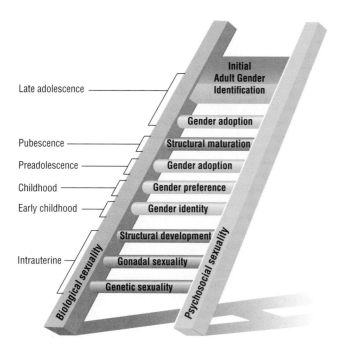

Figure 12-1 Growth and Development of Sexuality Our sexuality develops through biological and psychosocial stages.

Gender preference refers to the emotional and intellectual acceptance of one's birth gender. Reaching this rung on the psychosocial rail of the ladder takes place during the preschool years, when nearly every boy prefers being a boy and nearly every girl prefers being a girl.

(Note: The concept of gender preference is not to be confused with sexual preference. Sexual preference refers to a sexual and/or emotional attraction to sex partners. Sexual preference is discussed later in this chapter in a section titled "Sexual Orientation.")

Gender Adoption

The process of reaching an initial adult gender identification requires a considerable period of time. The specific knowledge, attitudes, and behaviors of adults must be observed, analyzed, and practiced. The process of acquiring and personalizing these "insights" about how men and women think, feel, and act is reflected by the term **gender adoption,** the first and third rungs below the initial adult gender identification rail of the ladder in Figure 12-1.

The rungs would represent the sequential unfolding of the genetic, gonadal, and structural components.

Because humans, more than any other life form, can rise above a life centered on reproduction, a second dimension (or rail) to our sexuality exists—our **psychosocial sexuality.** The reason we possess the ability to be more than reproductive beings is a question for the theologian or the philosopher. We are considerably more complex than the functions determined by biology. The process that transforms a male into a man and a female into a woman begins at birth and continues to influence us through the course of our lives.

Gender Identity

Although expectant parents may prefer to have a child of a particular **gender,** they know that this matter was determined at the moment of conception. Once the child is born, femininity or masculinity is traditionally reinforced by the parents and society in general. By age 18 months, typical children have both the language and the insight to correctly identify their gender. They have established a **gender identity.**[4] The first rung rising from the psychosocial rail of the ladder has been climbed.

Gender Preference

During the preschool years, children receive the second component of the *scripting* required for the full development of psychosocial sexuality—**gender preference.**

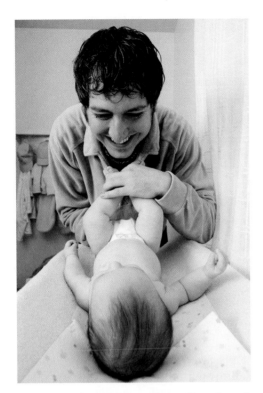

Just as women have broken into traditionally male realms, many men have taken on jobs and tasks that were once considered women's exclusive domain.

In addition to developing a personalized version of an adult sexual identity, the child—and particularly the adolescent—must construct a *gender schema* for a member of the opposite gender. The world of adulthood, involving intimacy, parenting, and employment, requires that men know women and women know men. Gender adoption provides an opportunity to begin constructing the equally valuable "pictures" of what both genders are like.

Initial Adult Gender Identification

By the time young people have climbed all of the rungs of the sexuality ladder, they have arrived at the chronological point in the life cycle when they need to construct their own initial adult **gender identification.** You might notice that this label seems remarkably similar to the terminology used to describe one of the developmental tasks discussed in this textbook. In fact, the task of forming an initial adult identity is closely related to developing an initial adult image of oneself as a man or a woman. Although most of us currently support the concept of "person" in many gender-neutral contexts (for some very valid reasons), we still must identify ourselves as either a man or a woman. This process includes having a good understanding of the **gender roles** common to our society.

Reproductive Systems

The most familiar aspects of biological sexuality are the structures comprised in the reproductive systems. Each structure contributes to the reproductive process in unique ways. Thus, with these structures, males have the ability to impregnate. Females have the ability to become pregnant, give birth, and nourish infants through breast-feeding. Many of these structures are also associated with nonreproductive sexual behavior.

Male Reproductive System

The male reproductive system consists of external structures of genitals (the penis and scrotum) and internal structures (the testes, various passageways or ducts, seminal vesicles, the prostate gland, and the Cowper's glands) (see Figure 12-2).

Testes The *testes* (also called *gonads* or *testicles*) are two egg-shaped bodies that lie within a saclike structure called the *scrotum*. During most of fetal development, the testes lie within the abdominal cavity. They descend into the scrotum during the last two months of fetal life.

The testes are housed in the scrotum because a temperature lower than the body core temperature is required for adequate sperm development. The walls of the scrotum are composed of contractile tissue and, with the help of the **cremasteric muscles,** can draw the testes closer to the body during cold temperatures (and sexual arousal) and relax during warm temperatures. Scrotal movements allow a constant, productive temperature to be maintained in the testes.

Each testis contains an intricate network of structures called *seminiferous tubules*. Within these 300 or so seminiferous tubules, the process of sperm production (*spermatogenesis*) takes place. Sperm cell development starts at about age 11 in boys and is influenced by the release of the hormone **interstitial cell-stimulating hormone (ICSH)** from the pituitary gland. ICSH does primarily what its name suggests: It stimulates specific cells (called *interstitial cells*) within the testes to begin producing the male sex hormone *testosterone*. Testosterone in turn is primarily responsible for the gradual development of the male secondary sex characteristics at the onset of puberty. By the time a boy is approximately 15 years old, sufficient levels of testosterone exist that the testes become capable of full spermatogenesis.

Before the age of about 15, most of the sperm cells produced in the testes are incapable of fertilization. The production of fully mature sperm (*spermatozoa*) is triggered by another hormone secreted by the brain's pituitary gland—**follicle-stimulating hormone (FSH).** FSH influences the seminiferous tubules to begin producing spermatozoa that are capable of fertilization.

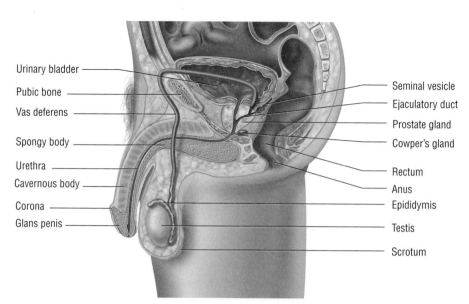

Figure 12-2 The Male Reproductive System

Urinary bladder
Pubic bone
Vas deferens
Spongy body
Urethra
Cavernous body
Corona
Glans penis

Seminal vesicle
Ejaculatory duct
Prostate gland
Cowper's gland
Rectum
Anus
Epididymis
Testis
Scrotum

Ducts   Spermatogenesis takes place around the clock, with hundreds of millions of sperm cells produced daily. The sperm cells do not stay in the seminiferous tubules but rather are transferred through a system of *ducts* that lead into the *epididymis*. The epididymis is a tubular coil that attaches to the back side of each testicle. These collecting structures house the maturing sperm cells for two to three weeks. During this period, the sperm finally become capable of motion, but they remain inactive until they mix with the secretions from the accessory glands (the seminal vesicles, prostate gland, and Cowper's glands).

Each epididymis leads into an 18-inch passageway known as the *vas deferens*. Sperm, moved along by the action of hairlike projections called *cilia,* can also remain in the vas deferens for an extended time without losing their ability to fertilize an egg.

Seminal Vesicles   The two vasa deferentia extend into the abdominal cavity, where each meets with a *seminal vesicle*—the first of the three accessory structures or glands. Each seminal vesicle contributes a clear, alkaline fluid that nourishes the sperm cells with fructose and permits the sperm cells to be suspended in a movable medium. The fusion of a vas deferens with the seminal vesicle results in the formation of a passageway called the *ejaculatory duct*. Each ejaculatory duct is only about 1 inch long and empties into the final passageway for the sperm—the urethra.

Prostate Gland   The ejaculatory duct is located within the second accessory gland—the *prostate gland.* The prostate gland secretes a milky fluid containing a variety of substances, including proteins, cholesterol, citric acid, calcium, buffering salts, and various enzymes. The prostate secretions further nourish the sperm cells and also

raise the pH level, making the mixture quite alkaline. This alkalinity permits the sperm to have greater longevity as they are transported during ejaculation through the urethra, out of the penis, and into the highly acidic vagina.

Cowper's Glands   The third accessory glands, the *Cowper's glands,* serve primarily to lubricate the urethra with a clear, viscous mucus. These paired glands empty their small amounts of preejaculatory fluid during the plateau stage of the sexual response cycle. Alkaline in nature, this fluid also neutralizes the acidic level of the urethra. Viable sperm cells can be suspended in this fluid and can enter the female reproductive tract before full ejaculation by the male.[5] This may account for many of the failures of the "withdrawal" method of contraception.

Semen   The sperm cells, when combined with secretions from the seminal vesicles, the prostate gland, and the Cowper's glands, form a sticky substance called **semen.**[6] Interestingly, the microscopic sperm actually makes up less than 5 percent of the seminal fluid discharged at ejaculation. Contrary to popular belief, the paired seminal vesicles contribute about 60 percent of the semen volume, and the prostate gland adds about 30 percent.[6] Thus, the fear of some men that a **vasectomy** will destroy their ability to ejaculate is completely unfounded (see Chapter 13).

During *emission* (the gathering of semen in the upper part of the urethra), a sphincter muscle at the base of the bladder contracts and inhibits semen from being pushed into the bladder and urine from being deposited into the urethra.[7] Thus, semen and urine rarely intermingle, even though they leave the body through the same passageway.

Figure 12-3 The Female Reproductive System

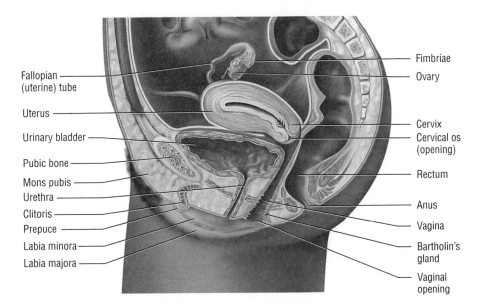

Fallopian (uterine) tube

Uterus

Urinary bladder

Pubic bone

Mons pubis

Urethra

Clitoris

Prepuce

Labia minora

Labia majora

Fimbriae

Ovary

Cervix

Cervical os (opening)

Rectum

Anus

Vagina

Bartholin's gland

Vaginal opening

Penis   Ejaculation takes place when the semen is forced out of the *penis* through the urethral opening. The involuntary, rhythmic muscle contractions that control ejaculation result in a series of pleasurable sensations known as *orgasm.*

The urethra lies on the underside of the penis and extends through one of three cylindrical chambers of erectile tissue (two *cavernous bodies* and one *spongy body*). Each of these three chambers provides the vascular space required for sufficient erection of the penis. When a male becomes sexually aroused, these areas become congested with blood (*vasocongestion*). After ejaculation or when a male is no longer sexually stimulated, these chambers release the blood into the general circulation and the penis returns to a **flaccid** state.

The *shaft* of the penis is covered by a thin layer of skin that is an extension of the skin that covers the scrotum. This loose layer of skin is sensitive to sexual stimulation and extends over the head of the penis, except in males who have been circumcised. The *glans* (or head) of the penis is the most sexually sensitive (to tactile stimulation) part of the male body. Nerve receptor sites are especially prominent along the *corona* (the ridge of the glans) and the *frenulum* (the thin tissue at the base of the glans).

Female Reproductive System

The external structures (genitals) of the female reproductive system consist of the mons pubis, labia majora, labia minora, clitoris, and vestibule (see Figure 12-3). Collectively, these structures form the *vulva* or vulval area.

Mons Pubis   The *mons pubis* is the fatty covering over the pubic bone. The mons pubis (or *mons veneris,* "mound of Venus") is covered by pubic hair and is quite sensitive to sexual stimulation.

Labia Majora and Labia Minora   The *labia majora* are large longitudinal folds of skin that cover the entrance to the vagina, whereas the *labia minora* are the smaller longitudinal skin folds that lie within the labia majora. These hairless skin folds of the labia minora join at the top to form the *prepuce* or *clitoral hood.*

Clitoris   The prepuce covers the glans (or head) of the *clitoris,* which is the most sexually sensitive part of the female body. A rather direct analogy can be made between the penis and the clitoris. In terms of the tactile sensitivity, both structures are the most sensitive parts of the male and female genitals. Both contain a glans and a shaft (although the clitoral shaft is beneath the skin surface). Both organs are composed of erectile tissue that can become engorged with blood. Both are covered by skin folds (the clitoral prepuce of the female and the foreskin of the male), and both structures can collect **smegma** beneath these tissue folds.[4]

> ### Key Terms
>
> **semen**   Secretion containing sperm and nutrients discharged from the urethra at ejaculation.
>
> **vasectomy**   Surgical procedure in which the vasa deferentia are cut to prevent the passage of sperm from the testicles; the most common form of male sterilization.
>
> **flaccid** (**fla** sid)   Nonerect; the state of erectile tissue when vasocongestion is not occurring.
>
> **smegma**   Cellular discharge that can accumulate beneath the clitoral hood and the foreskin of an uncircumcised penis.

Vestibule   The *vestibule* is the region enclosed by the labia minora. Evident here are the urethral opening and the entrance to the vagina (or vaginal orifice). Also located at the vaginal opening are the *Bartholin's glands,* which secrete a minute amount of lubricating fluid during sexual excitement.

The *hymen* is a thin layer of tissue that stretches across the opening of the vagina. Once thought to be the only indication of virginity, the intact hymen rarely covers the vaginal opening entirely. Openings in the hymen are necessary for the discharge of menstrual fluid and vaginal secretions. Many hymens are stretched or torn to full opening by adolescent physical activity or by the insertion of tampons. In women whose hymens are not fully ruptured, the first act of sexual intercourse will generally accomplish this. Pain may accompany first intercourse in females with relatively intact hymens.

The internal reproductive structures of the female include the vagina, uterus, fallopian tubes, and ovaries.

Vagina   The *vagina* is the structure that accepts the penis during sexual intercourse. Normally, the walls of the vagina are collapsed, except during sexual stimulation, when the vaginal walls widen and elongate to accommodate the erect penis. Only the outer third of the vagina is especially sensitive to sexual stimulation. In this location, vaginal tissues swell considerably to form the **orgasmic platform.** [7] This platform constricts the vaginal opening and in effect "grips" the penis (or other inserted object)—regardless of its size. So the belief that a woman receives considerably more sexual pleasure from men with large penises is not supported from an anatomical standpoint.

Uterus   The *uterus* (or *womb*) is approximately the size and shape of a small pear. This highly muscular organ is capable of undergoing a wide range of physical changes, as evidenced by its enlargement during pregnancy, its contraction during menstruation and labor, and its movement during the orgasmic phase of the female sexual response cycle. The primary function of the uterus is to provide a suitable environment for the possible implantation of a fertilized ovum, or egg. This implantation, should it occur, takes place in the innermost lining of the uterus—the *endometrium.* In the mature female, the endometrium undergoes cyclic changes as it prepares a new lining on a near-monthly basis.

The lower third of the uterus is called the *cervix.* The cervix extends slightly into the vagina. Sperm enter the uterus through the cervical opening, or *cervical os.* Mucous glands in the cervix secrete a fluid that is thin and watery near the time of ovulation. Mucus of this consistency apparently facilitates sperm passage into the uterus and deeper structures. However, cervical mucus is much thicker during certain points in the menstrual cycle when pregnancy is improbable and during pregnancy, to protect against bacterial agents and other substances that are especially dangerous to the developing fetus.

The upper two-thirds of the uterus is called the *corpus,* or *body.* This is where implantation of the fertilized ovum generally takes place.

Fallopian Tubes   The upper portion of the uterus opens into two *fallopian tubes,* or *oviducts,* each about 4 inches long. The fallopian tubes are each directed toward an *ovary.* They serve as a passageway for the ovum in its weeklong voyage toward the uterus. Usually, conception (the joining of an ovum and a sperm) takes place in the upper third of the fallopian tubes.

Ovaries   The ovaries are analogous to the testes in the male. Their function is to produce the ovum, or egg. Usually, one ovary produces and releases just one egg each month. Approximately the size and shape of an unshelled almond, an ovary produces viable ova in the process known as *oogenesis.* The ovaries also produce the female sex hormones through the efforts of specific structures within the ovaries. These hormones play multiple roles in the development of female secondary sex characteristics, but their primary function is to prepare the endometrium of the uterus for possible implantation of a fertilized ovum. In the average healthy female, this preparation takes place about 13 times a year for a period of about 35 years. At menopause, the ovaries shrink considerably and stop nearly all hormonal production.

Menstrual Cycle

Each month or so, the inner wall of the uterus prepares for a possible pregnancy. When a pregnancy does not occur (as is the case throughout most months of a woman's fertile years), this lining must be released and a new one prepared. The breakdown of this endometrial wall and the resultant discharge of blood and endometrial tissue is known as *menstruation* (or *menses*) (see Figure 12-4). The cyclic timing of menstruation is governed by hormones released from two sources: the pituitary gland and the ovaries.

Girls generally have their first menstrual cycle, the onset of which is called *menarche,* sometime around age 12 or 13. Over the past few decades, the age of menarche has been dropping gradually. This drop appears to be related to heredity, improved overall health, better childhood nutrition, and increased caloric intake. These factors in combination produce the increased body weight evident today in many young adolescent girls that seems to trigger an earlier menarche.

After a girl first menstruates, she may be anovulatory for a year or longer before a viable ovum is released during her cycle. This cyclic activity will continue until about ages 45–55.

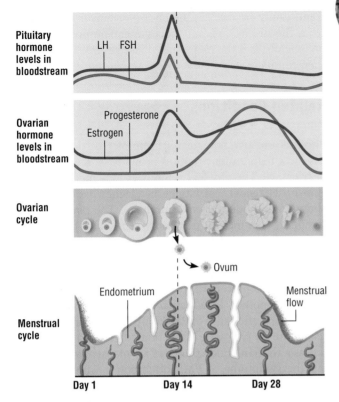

Pituitary hormone levels in bloodstream

LH   FSH

Ovarian hormone levels in bloodstream

Progesterone
Estrogen

Ovarian cycle

Ovum

Endometrium

Menstrual flow

Menstrual cycle

Day 1   Day 14   Day 28

Figure 12-4 Menstrual Cycle   The menstrual cycle involves the development and release of an ovum, supported by hormones from the pituitary gland, and the buildup of the endometrium, supported by hormones from the ovaries, for the purpose of establishing a pregnancy.

This text refers to a menstrual cycle that lasts 28 days. However, few women display perfect 28-day cycles. Most women fluctuate by a few days to a week around this 28-day pattern, and some women vary greatly from this cycle.

It is not uncommon for some women to experience irregular cycles (cycles that differ in length) and even occasional midcycle spotting (with small amounts of reddish discharge). These events are most likely to occur in young women who are just establishing their cycles, women who are approaching or moving through menopause, and women who are just starting to use hormone-based contraceptives. Major life changes, certain illnesses and medications, and unresolved stress can also affect the length of a woman's cycle. Any woman who experiences a significant, dramatic change from her usual pattern should contact her physician or health care practitioner.[4]

Your knowledge about the menstrual cycle is critical for your understanding of pregnancy, contraception, menopause, and issues related to the overall health and comfort of women (see the box "Endometriosis"). Although at first this cycle may sound like a complicated process, each segment of the cycle can be studied separately for better understanding.

Endometriosis

Endometriosis is a condition in which endometrial tissue that normally lines the uterus is found growing within the pelvic cavity. Because the tissue remains sensitive to circulating hormones, it is the source of pain and discomfort during the latter half of the menstrual cycle. Endometriosis is most commonly found in younger women and is sometimes related to infertility in women with severe cases.

In addition to painful cramping before and during menstruation, the symptoms of endometriosis include low back pain, pain during intercourse, painful bowel movements, heavy menstrual flow, and difficulty becoming pregnant. Many women with endometriosis, however, experience no symptoms.*

Treatment of endometriosis largely depends on its extent. For some women, over-the-counter anti-inflammatory drugs can relieve pain and reduce bleeding. Drugs to suppress ovulation, including birth control pills, may be helpful in mild cases. For more severe cases, surgical removal of the tissue or a hysterectomy may be necessary. For some women, endometriosis is suppressed during pregnancy and does not return after pregnancy.

*WebMd, Endometriosis: topic overview, February 22, 2011. http://women.webmd.com/endometriosis/endometriosis-topic-overview?page2.

The menstrual cycle can be thought of as occurring in three segments or phases: the menstrual phase (lasting about one week), the preovulation phase (also lasting about one week), and the postovulation phase (lasting about two weeks). Day 1 of this cycle starts with the first day of bleeding, or menstrual flow.

Menstrual Phase   The *menstrual phase* signals the woman that a pregnancy has not taken place and that her uterine lining is being sloughed off. During a five- to seven-day period, a woman will discharge about one-quarter to one-half cup of blood and tissue. (Only about one ounce of the menstrual flow is blood.) The menstrual flow is heaviest during the first days of this phase. Since the muscular uterus must contract to accomplish this tissue removal, some women have uncomfortable cramping during menstruation. Most women, however, report more pain and discomfort during the few days before the first day of menstrual flow. (See the following discussion of premenstrual syndrome [PMS].)

Today's methods of absorbing menstrual flow include the use of internal tampons and external pads. Caution must be exercised by the users of tampons to prevent the possibility of toxic shock syndrome (TSS) (see Chapter 11). Since menstrual flow is a positive sign of good health, women are encouraged to be normally active during menstruation.

Preovulation Phase The *preovulation phase* of the menstrual cycle starts about the time menstruation stops. Lasting about one week, this phase is first influenced by the release of follicle-stimulating hormone (FSH) from the pituitary gland. FSH circulates in the bloodstream and directs the ovaries to start the process of maturing approximately 20 primary ovarian *follicles*. Thousands of primary egg follicles are present in each ovary at birth. These follicles resemble shells that house immature ova. As these follicles ripen under FSH influence, they release the hormone *estrogen*. Estrogen's primary function is to direct the endometrium to start the development of a thick, highly vascular wall. As the estrogen levels increase, the pituitary gland's secretion of FSH is reduced. Now the pituitary gland prepares for the surge of the **luteinizing hormone (LH)** required to accomplish ovulation.[8]

In the days immediately preceding ovulation, one of the primary follicles (called the *graafian follicle*) matures fully. The other primary follicles degenerate and are absorbed by the body. The graafian follicle moves toward the surface of the ovary. When LH is released in massive quantities on about day 14, the graafian follicle bursts to release the fully mature ovum. The release of the ovum is called **ovulation.** Regardless of the overall length of a woman's cycle, ovulation occurs 14 days before her first day of menstrual flow.

The ovum is quickly captured by the fingerlike projections (*fimbriae*) of the fallopian tubes. In the upper third of the fallopian tubes, the ovum is capable of being fertilized in a 24- to 36-hour period. If the ovum is not fertilized by a sperm cell, it will begin to degenerate and eventually will be absorbed by the body. (See Figure 13-1 for information about the days in which a woman is most likely to conceive.)

Postovulation Phase After ovulation, the *postovulation phase* of the menstrual cycle starts when the remnants of the graafian follicle restructure themselves into a **corpus luteum.** The corpus luteum remains inside the ovary, secreting estrogen and a fourth hormone called *progesterone*. Progesterone, which literally means "for pregnancy," continues to direct the endometrial buildup. If pregnancy occurs, the corpus luteum monitors progesterone and estrogen levels throughout the pregnancy. If pregnancy does not occur, high levels of progesterone signal the pituitary gland to stop the release of LH and the corpus luteum starts to degenerate on about day 24. When estrogen and progesterone levels diminish significantly by day 28, the endometrium is discharged from the uterus and out the vagina. The postovulation phase ends, and the menstrual phase begins. The cycle is then complete.

Related Conditions

Premenstrual Syndrome (PMS) PMS is a collection of physical and psychological symptoms that occur in the days just before menstruation in many women of childbearing age. The physical symptoms may include weight gain, breast tenderness, fatigue, headaches, backaches, and abdominal cramps (**dysmenorrhea**). The psychological symptoms can include irritability, tension, anxiety, mood swings, depression, difficulty concentrating, and aggressiveness. These symptoms vary from woman to woman and from one menstrual cycle to the next. It has been estimated that 85 percent of women experience at least some of these symptoms on a regular basis.[9]

The specific cause of PMS is unknown, but it is likely related to the changing levels of estrogen and progesterone as a woman's body prepares for menstruation. Treating the symptoms of PMS often starts with a healthy diet—reducing one's intake of caffeine, salt, and simple sugar, and increasing one's intake of complex carbohydrates by eating more fresh fruits and vegetables. A simple, daily vitamin/mineral combination pill might also be helpful. Physical exercise is highly recommended to reduce PMS symptoms and elevate one's mood.

Over-the-counter nonsteroidal anti-inflammatory drugs (NSAIDs), such as ibuprofen and naproxen, and over-the-counter diuretics can help alleviate uncomfortable physical symptoms. A physician can prescribe medications for severe cases of PMS. These might include certain antidepressants and prescription diuretics. Although in the past progesterone therapy or birth control pills were prescribed for relief from PMS, there is little research data to support their effectiveness. Also found to be ineffective or of little benefit is the use of primrose oil, black cohosh, wild yam root, chaste tree fruit, dong quai, and vitamin B$_6$.[9]

Premenstrual Dysphoric Disorder (PMDD) Premenstrual dysphoric disorder (PMDD) is a severe form of PMS that occurs in about 2–10 percent of menstruating women.[10] As with PMS, PMDD expresses itself in the latter half of the menstrual cycle, in the days before menstruation begins. The symptoms of PMDD are similar to those of PMS, but they are so severe that they cause major disruptions in a woman's personal relationships, social activities, and employment. With PMDD, the mood swings, tension, irritability, depression, anger, appetite changes, sleep problems, loss of control, difficulties concentrating, and physical symptoms are magnified far beyond the symptoms seen in women with PMS.

Methods of treatment for PMDD focus on many of the same strategies used to manage PMS. Additionally, the U.S.

Food and Drug Administration (FDA) has approved the use of three prescription antidepressants and some newer types of birth control pills to help relieve the symptoms of PMDD. Some physicians prescribe regular birth control pills or other hormonal drugs to women coping with PMDD, although their effectiveness remains uncertain.[10]

Fibrocystic Breast Condition   In some women, particularly those who have never been pregnant, stimulation of the breast tissues by estrogen and progesterone during the menstrual cycle results in an unusually high degree of secretory activity by the cells lining the ducts. The fluid released by the secretory lining finds its way into the fibrous connective tissue areas in the lower half of the breast, where in pocketlike cysts the fluid presses against neighboring tissues. This activity produces a benign fibrocystic breast condition characterized by swollen, firm or hardened, tender breast tissue before menstruation.

Researchers have begun to describe the importance of a healthy diet in preventing fibrocystic breast condition, in particular a low-fat, low-salt, low-red-meat diet that is rich in whole grains, fish, and poultry. The reduction or elimination of caffeine found in coffee, tea, soft drinks, and chocolate might also help reduce these benign breast changes. In some cases, vitamin E and vitamin B-complex supplementation have helped.[4]

Women who experience more extensive fibrocystic conditions can be treated with drugs that have a "calming" effect on progesterone production. Occasional draining of cysts can bring relief.

Menopause   For the vast majority of women in their late 40s through their mid-50s, a gradual decline in reproductive system function, called *menopause*, occurs. Menopause is a normal physiological process, not a disease process. It can, however, become a health concern for some middle-aged women who have unpleasant side effects resulting from this natural stoppage of ovum production and menstruation.

As ovarian function and hormone production diminish, adjustments must be made by the hypothalamus, ovaries, uterus, and other estrogen-sensitive tissues. The extent of menopause as a health problem is determined by the degree to which **hot flashes**, night sweats, insomnia, vaginal wall dryness, depression and melancholy, breast changes, and the uncertainty of fertility are seen as problems.

In comparison with past generations, today's midlife women are much less likely to find menopause to be a negative experience. The end of fertility, perhaps combined with children leaving the home, makes the middle years a period of personal rediscovery for many women.

For women who are troubled by the changes brought about by menopause, physicians may prescribe **hormone replacement therapy (HRT).** This can relieve many symptoms and help reduce the incidence of osteoporosis (see Chapter 4). However, some forms of HRT have also been found to increase the risk of breast cancer and cardiovascular problems[11,12] (see Chapters 9 and 10).

There are alternate approaches to HRT that women can try to ease the symptoms of menopause. Reducing the intake of spicy foods, caffeine, and alcohol may help with hot flashes and night sweats. Vitamin E and soy products provide relief for some women, and the potential benefits of certain herbs (especially black cohosh) are being studied. Prescription antidepressants may reduce hot flashes in some women.

Vaginal dryness can be treated with over-the-counter lubricants and moisturizers, and vaginal estrogen creams, and regular sexual activity may help as well. Insomnia can be countered with good sleeping patterns (consistent bedtime hour, a glass of warm milk, and reduced caffeine, alcohol, and food intake before bed).

Interestingly, physical activity cuts across most of the issues related to menopause. Physical activity has been demonstrated to benefit sleep patterns, provide emotional balance, encourage mental acuity, and bolster cardiovascular function. Physical activity also makes people feel better about their bodies and, thus, become potentially more interested in sexual activity, which can help maintain vaginal lubrication.

Human Sexual Response Pattern

Although history has many written and visual accounts of the human ability to be sexually aroused, it was not until the pioneering work of Masters and Johnson[13] that the events associated with arousal were clinically documented. Five questions posed by these researchers gave direction to a series of studies involving the scientific evaluation of human sexual response.

> **Key Terms**
>
> **luteinizing hormone (LH)** (**loo** ten eye zing) A gonadotropic hormone of the female required for fullest development and release of ova; ovulating hormone.
>
> **ovulation** The release of a mature egg from the ovary.
>
> **corpus luteum** (**kore** pus **loo** tee um) Cellular remnant of the graafian follicle after the release of an ovum.
>
> **dysmenorrhea** Abdominal pain caused by muscular cramping during the menstrual cycle.
>
> **hot flashes** Unpleasant, temporary feelings of warmth experienced by women during and after menopause, caused by blood vessel dilation.
>
> **hormone replacement therapy (HRT)** Medically administered estrogen and progestin to replace hormones lost as the result of menopause.

Do the Sexual Responses of Males and Females Have a Predictable Pattern?

The answer to the first question posed by the researchers was an emphatic yes. A predictable sexual response pattern was identified;[13] it consists of an initial **excitement stage,** a **plateau stage,** an **orgasmic stage,** and a **resolution stage.** Each stage involves predictable changes in the structural characteristics and physiological function of reproductive and nonreproductive organs in both the male and the female. These changes are shown in Figure 12-5.

Is the Sexual Response Pattern Stimuli-Specific?

The research of Masters and Johnson clearly established a *no* answer to the second question concerning stimuli specificity. Their findings demonstrated that numerous senses can supply the stimuli necessary for initiating the sexual response pattern. Although touching activities might initiate arousal in most people and maximize it for the vast majority of people, in both males and females, sight, smell, sound, and *vicariously formed stimuli* can also stimulate the same sexual arousal patterns.

What Differences Occur in the Sexual Response Pattern?

Several differences are observable when the sexual response patterns of males and females are compared:

- With the exception of some later adolescent males, the vast majority of males are not multiorgasmic. The **refractory phase** of the resolution stage prevents most males from experiencing more than one orgasm in a short period, even when sufficient stimulation is available.

- Females possess a **multiorgasmic capacity.** Masters and Johnson found that as many as 10–30 percent of female adults routinely experience multiple orgasms.

- Although they possess multiorgasmic potential, about 10 percent of all female adults are *anorgasmic*—that is, they never experience an orgasm through **coitus.**[13] For many of these women, orgasms can be experienced when masturbation provides the stimulation.

- When measured during coitus, males reach orgasm far more quickly than do females. However, when masturbation is the source of stimulation, females reach orgasm as quickly as do males.

More important than any of the differences pointed out is the finding that the sexual response patterns of males and females are far more alike than they are different.

Not only do males and females experience the four basic stages of the response pattern, but they also have similar responses in specific areas, including the **erection** and *tumescence* of sexual structures; the appearance of a **sex flush;** the increase in cardiac output, blood pressure, and respiratory rate; and the occurrence of *rhythmic pelvic thrusting.*[13]

Not all women and men move through the sexual response pattern in a similar way. There is great variation among women and great variation among men. Also, for a given man or woman, movement through the response pattern can vary greatly from one day to the next. Factors such as the aging process, changes in general health status, alcohol or other drug use, and changes in a sex partner can cause one's own sexual response to change from one sexual experience to another.

What Are the Basic Physiological Mechanisms Underlying the Sexual Response Pattern?

The basic mechanisms in the fourth question posed by Masters and Johnson are now well recognized. One factor, *vasocongestion,* or the retention of blood or fluid within a particular tissue, is critically important in the development of physiological changes that promote the

---

Key Terms

excitement stage Initial arousal stage of the sexual response pattern.

plateau stage Second stage of the sexual response pattern; a leveling off of arousal immediately before orgasm.

orgasmic stage Third stage of the sexual response pattern; the stage during which neuromuscular tension is released.

resolution stage Fourth stage of the sexual response pattern; the return of the body to a preexcitement state.

refractory phase That portion of the male's resolution stage during which sexual arousal cannot occur.

multiorgasmic capacity Potential to have several orgasms within a single period of sexual arousal.

coitus (co ih tus) Penile-vaginal intercourse.

erection The engorgement of erectile tissue with blood; characteristic of the penis, clitoris, nipples, labia minora, and scrotum.

sex flush The reddish skin response that results from increasing sexual arousal.

sexual response pattern.[13] The presence of erectile tissue underlies the changes that can be noted in the penis, breasts, and scrotum of the male and the clitoris, breasts, and labia minora of the female.

A second factor now recognized as necessary for the development of the sexual response pattern is that of *myotonia,* or the buildup of *neuromuscular tonus* within a variety of body structures.[7] At the end of the plateau stage of the response pattern, a sudden release of the accumulated neuromuscular tension gives rise to the rhythmic muscular contractions and pleasurable muscular spasms that constitute orgasm, as well as ejaculation in the male.[3]

What Role Is Played by Specific Organs and Organ Systems in the Sexual Response Pattern?

The fifth question posed by Masters and Johnson, which concerns the role played by specific organs and organ systems during each stage of the response pattern, can be readily answered by referring to the material presented in Figure 12-5. As you study this figure, remember that direct stimulation of the penis and either direct or indirect stimulation of the clitoris are the principal avenues toward orgasm. Also, intercourse represents only one activity that can lead to orgasmic pleasure.[14]

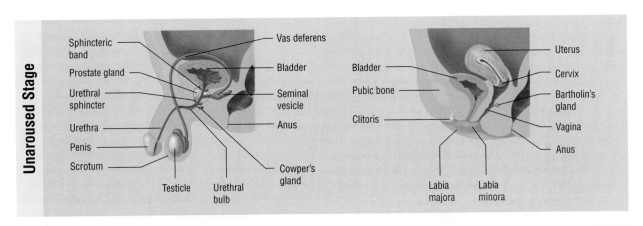

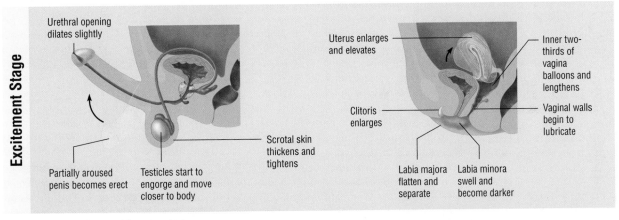

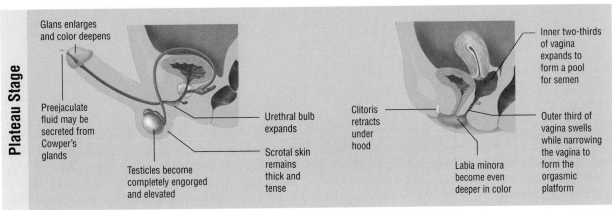

Figure 12-5 The Sexual Response Pattern in Men and Women

Continued on next page

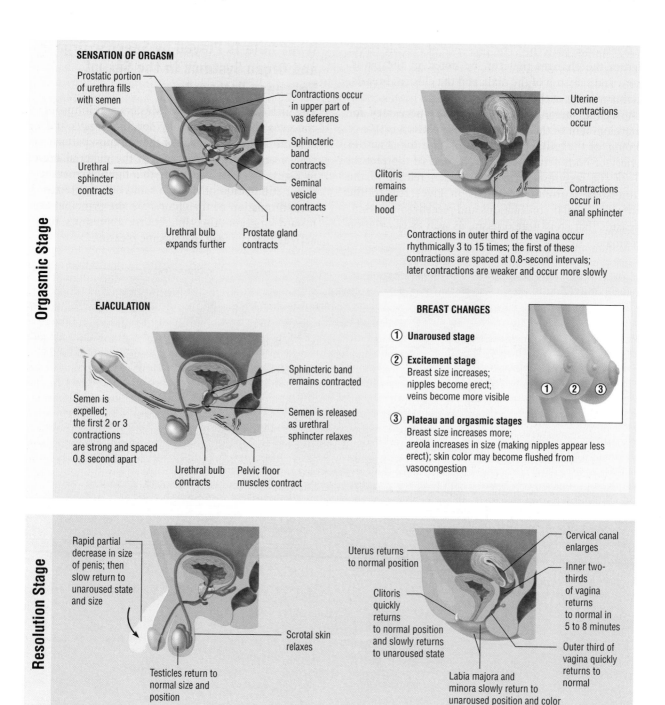

Figure 12-5 *Continued*

Patterns of Sexual Behavior

Although sex researchers may see sexual behavior in terms of the human sexual response pattern just described, most people are more interested in the observable dimensions of sexual behavior. Also consider that sexual behavior can involve profound emotional experiences (see the box "Sexuality as a Means of Spiritual Discovery" on page 316).

Celibacy

Celibacy can be defined as the self-imposed avoidance of sexual intimacy. It is synonymous with sexual abstinence. There are many reasons people could choose not to have a sexually intimate relationship. For some, celibacy is part of a religious doctrine. Others might be afraid of sexually transmitted diseases (STDs). For most, however, celibacy is preferred simply because it seems appropriate for them. Celibate people can certainly have deep, intimate relationships with other people—just not sexual relationships. Celibacy may be short-term or last a lifetime. In any case, no identified physical or psychological complications appear to result from a celibate lifestyle.

Masturbation

Throughout recorded history, **masturbation** has been a primary method of achieving sexual pleasure. Through masturbation, people can explore their sexual response patterns. Traditionally, some societies and religious groups have condemned this behavior based on the belief that intercourse is the only "right" sexual behavior. With sufficient lubrication, masturbation cannot do physical harm. Today masturbation is considered by most sex therapists and researchers to be a normal source of self-pleasure.

Fantasy and Erotic Dreams

The brain is the most sensual organ in the body. In fact, many sexuality experts classify **sexual fantasies** and **erotic dreams** as forms of sexual behavior. Particularly for people whose verbal ability is highly developed, the ability to create imaginary scenes enriches other forms of sexual behavior.

When fantasies occur in conjunction with another form of sexual behavior, the second behavior may be greatly enhanced by the supportive fantasy. Both women and men fantasize during foreplay and intercourse. Masturbation and fantasizing are inseparable activities.

Erotic dreams occur during sleep in both men and women. The association between these dreams and ejaculation resulting in a nocturnal emission (wet dream) is readily recognized in males. In females, erotic dreams can lead not only to vaginal lubrication but to orgasm as well.

Shared Touching

Virtually the entire body can be an erogenous (sexually sensitive) zone when shared touching is involved. A light touch, a slight application of pressure, the brushing back of a partner's hair, and gentle massage are all forms of communication that heighten sexual arousal.

Sexting

Within the past five years, a new pattern of sexually related behavior has emerged that is intrinsically connected to the digital world. This behavior is called **sexting.** Typically, sexting refers to the sharing of nude or seminude photos by cell phone or some other digital media device. While a definition of sexting can also include the sending of sexy or suggestive e-mail messages (and not photos), transmitting nude photographs has very significant legal and psychological consequences.[15]

Laws vary from state to state, but generally, the transmission of nude of seminude photos of minors amounts to producing, possessing, or distributing child pornography. It is illegal to send photos of yourself to someone else if you, the person in the photo, or the recipient is a minor. If the photos are sent to someone in another state, the crime becomes a federal felony. Some college students may think that these laws do not apply to them because most are older than 18 years. However, think of instances in which an 18-year-old freshman has a boyfriend or girlfriend still in high school. If these two send each other naked photos, they could be setting themselves up for some really serious legal charges in many states.

While it is true that the present child pornography laws in many states were developed years ago (well before personal digital photo transmission was possible), until these laws are reconsidered and perhaps changed, the harsh penalties will remain. Beyond the legal consequences are the psychological consequences of having intimate photos of yourself distributed online.[15] Lovers and friends can become ex-lovers and ex-friends, and some jilted lovers can work very hard to destroy your reputation and embarrass you. So, it is critically important that you think carefully and stay alert when using digital media. Are you aware of the laws in your state that pertain to sexting? You could probably locate these laws if you consult the web page for the office of your state's attorney general.

Genital Contact

Two important uses can be identified for the practice of stimulating a partner's genitals. The first is that of being the tactile component of **foreplay.** Genital contact, in the form of holding, rubbing, stroking, or caressing, heightens arousal to a level that allows for progression to intercourse.

Key Terms

masturbation Self-stimulation of the genitals.

sexual fantasies Fantasies with sexual themes; sexual daydreams or imaginary events.

erotic dreams Dreams whose content elicits a sexual response.

sexting The sharing of sexually explicit photos or messages by cell phone or other digital media device.

foreplay Activities, often involving touching and caressing, that prepare individuals for sexual intercourse.

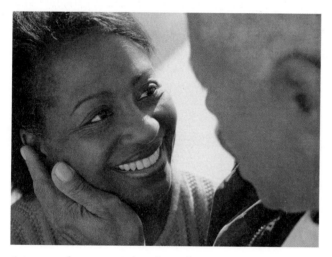

Any sensual contact can be a form of communication and sexual expression between partners.

The second role of genital contact is that of *mutual masturbation to orgasm.* Stimulation of the genitals so that both partners have orgasm is a form of sexual behavior practiced by many people, as well as couples during the late stage of a pregnancy. For couples not desiring pregnancy, the risk of conception is virtually eliminated when this becomes the form of sexual intimacy practiced.

As is the case of other aspects of intimacy, genital stimulation is best enhanced when partners can talk about their needs, expectations, and reservations. Practice and communication can shape this form of contact into a pleasure-giving approach to sexual intimacy.

Oral-Genital Stimulation

Oral-genital stimulation brings together two of the body's most erogenous areas: the genitals and the mouth. Because oral-genital stimulation can involve an exchange of body fluids, the risk of disease transmission is real. Small tears in the mouth or genital tissue may allow transmission of disease-causing pathogens. Only couples who are absolutely certain that they are free from all sexually transmitted diseases (including HIV infection) can practice unprotected oral sex. Couples in doubt should refrain from oral-genital sex or carefully use a condom (on the male) or a latex square to cover the female's vulval area. Increasingly, latex squares (dental dams) can be obtained from drugstores or pharmacies or purchased online.

Three basic forms of oral-genital stimulation are practiced.[4] **Fellatio,** in which the penis is sucked, licked, or kissed by the partner, is the most common of the three. **Cunnilingus,** in which the vulva of the female is kissed, licked, or penetrated by the partner's tongue, is only slightly less frequently practiced.

Mutual oral-genital stimulation, the third form of oral-genital stimulation, combines both fellatio and cunnilingus. When practiced by a heterosexual couple, the female partner performs fellatio on her partner while her male partner performs cunnilingus on her. Gay couples can practice mutual fellatio or cunnilingus.

Intercourse

Sexual intercourse (coitus) refers to the act of inserting the penis into the vagina. Intercourse is the sexual behavior that is most directly associated with **procreation.** For some, intercourse is the only natural and appropriate form of sexual intimacy.

The incidence and frequency of sexual intercourse is a much-studied topic. Information concerning the percentages of people who have engaged in intercourse is readily available in textbooks used in sexuality courses. Data concerning sexual intercourse among college students may be changing somewhat because of concerns about HIV infection and other STDs, but a reasonable estimate of college students reporting having had sexual intercourse is 60–75 percent.

These percentages reflect two important concepts about the sexual activity of college students. The first is that most college students are having (or have had) intercourse. The second concept is that a sizable percentage (25–40 percent) of students are choosing to refrain from intercourse. Indeed, the belief that "everyone is doing it" may be a bit shortsighted. From a public health standpoint, we believe it is important to provide accurate health information to protect those who choose to have intercourse and to actively support a person's right to choose not to have intercourse.

Couples need to share their expectations concerning sexual techniques and frequency of intercourse. Even the "performance" factors, such as depth of penetration, nature of body movements, tempo of activity, and timing of orgasm, are of increasing importance to many couples. Issues concerning sexually transmitted diseases (including HIV infection) are also critically important for couples who are contemplating intercourse. These factors need to be explored through open communication.

There are a variety of books (including textbooks) that provide written and visually explicit information on intercourse positions. Four basic positions for intercourse—*male above, female above, side by side,* and *rear entry*—each offer relative advantages and disadvantages.

Anal Sexual Activity

Some couples practice **anal intercourse,** in which the penis is inserted into the rectum of a partner. Anal intercourse can be performed by both heterosexual couples and gay men. According to a report in the journal *Archives of Sexual Behavior,* about 20–25 percent of college students have experienced anal intercourse.[16] The anal sphincter muscles contract tightly and tend to resist entry. Thus, couples who engage in anal intercourse must do so slowly and gently, and with adequate amounts of water-based lubricants. Because of the danger of tearing tissues in the rectal area, HIV transmission risk is increased if the inserting male is infected.[3] Unless it is absolutely certain that both partners are uninfected, the inserting male should always wear a condom. Even with a condom, disease transmission is possible, because during anal intercourse condoms are more likely to tear

than during penis-vaginal intercourse. Couples practicing anal sex must not follow anal insertion with insertion into the mouth or vagina because of the likelihood of transmitting infectious agents.

Sexuality and Aging

Students are often curious about how aging affects sexuality. This is understandable because we live in a society that idolizes youth and demands performance. Many younger people become anxious about growing older because of what they think will happen to their ability to express their sexuality. Interestingly, young adults are willing to accept other physical changes of aging (such as the slowing down of basal metabolism, reduced lung capacity, and even wrinkles) but not those changes related to sexuality.

Most of the research in this area suggests that older people are quite capable of performing sexually. As with other aspects of aging, certain anatomical and physiological changes will be evident, but these changes do not necessarily reduce the ability to enjoy sexual activity.[4] Most experts in sexuality report that many older people remain interested in sexual activity. Furthermore, those who are exposed to regular sexual activity throughout a lifetime report being most satisfied with their sex lives as older adults.

As people age, the likelihood of alterations in the male and female sexual response patterns increases. In postmenopausal women, vaginal lubrication commonly begins more slowly, and the amount of lubrication usually diminishes. However, clitoral sensitivity and nipple erection remain the same as in earlier years. The female capacity for multiple orgasms remains the same, although the number of contractions that occur at orgasm typically is reduced.

In the older man, physical changes are also evident. This is thought to be caused by the decrease in the production of testosterone between the ages of 20 and 60. After age 60 or so, testosterone levels remain relatively steady. Thus, many men, despite a decrease in sperm production, remain fertile into their 80s.[4] Older men typically take longer to achieve an erection (however, they are able

---

Key Terms

fellatio (feh **lay** she oh) Oral stimulation of the penis.

cunnilingus (cun uh **ling** gus) Oral stimulation of the vulva or clitoris.

procreation Reproduction.

anal intercourse A sexual act in which the erect penis is inserted into the rectum of a partner.

Chapter Twelve Understanding Sexuality

to maintain their erection longer before ejaculation), have fewer muscular contractions at orgasm, and ejaculate less forcefully than they once did. The volume of seminal fluid ejaculated is typically less than in earlier years, and its consistency is somewhat thinner. The resolution phase is usually longer in older men. In spite of these gradual changes, some elderly men engage in sexual intercourse with the same frequency as do much younger men.

Sexual Orientation

Sexual orientation refers to the direction in which people focus their sexual interests. People can be attracted to opposite-gender partners (heterosexuality), same-gender partners (homosexuality), or partners of both genders (bisexuality).

The distinctions among the three categories of sexual orientation are much less clear than their definitions might suggest. Most people probably fall somewhere along a continuum between exclusive heterosexuality and exclusive homosexuality. As far back as 1948, Kinsey presented just such a continuum.[17]

Heterosexuality

Heterosexuality (or heterosexual orientation) refers to an attraction to opposite-gender partners. (*Heteros* is a Greek word that means "the other.") A heterosexual person is sometimes called *straight*. Throughout the world, this is the most common sexual orientation. For reasons related to species survival, heterosexuality has its most basic roots in the biological dimension of human sexuality. Beyond its biological roots, heterosexuality has significant cultural and religious support in virtually every country in the world. Worldwide, laws related to marriage, living arrangements, health benefits, child rearing, financial matters, sexual behavior, and inheritance generally support relationships that are heterosexual in nature. However, this may be gradually changing. (See page 323 for an update on same-sex marriage.)

Homosexuality

Homosexuality (or homosexual orientation) refers to an attraction to same-gender partners. (*Homos* is a Greek word that means "the same.") The term *gay* refers to either males or females, whereas the word *lesbian* is used only in reference to females.

What percentage of the population is gay? This is difficult to determine accurately, because many people refuse to reveal their orientations and prefer to remain "in the closet." However, it is safe to say that the number of gay people in our society is probably much greater than most people realize. Kinsey estimated that about 2 percent of American females and 4 percent of American males were

exclusively homosexual.[17,18] More recent estimates place the overall figure at about 10 percent of the population. The expression of same-gender attraction is widespread. (See the box "'Don't Ask, Don't Tell' Policy Repealed" for discussion of a current issue affecting United States military personnel.)

Bisexuality

People who are attracted to either gender are referred to as *bisexual*. Bisexuals generally are in one of several groups: those who are (1) genuinely attracted emotionally and physically to both genders, (2) those who are gay but feel the need to behave heterosexually, (3) those who are aroused physically by the same gender but attracted emotionally to the opposite gender, or (4) those who are aroused physically by the opposite gender but attracted emotionally to the same gender. Some participate in a bisexual lifestyle for an extended period of time, while others move on more quickly to a more exclusive orientation. The size of the bisexual population is unknown.

Origins of Sexual Orientation

Students often wonder, What makes a person gay? This question has no simple answer. (College sexuality textbooks devote entire chapters to this topic.) Some research has pointed to differences in the sizes of certain brain structures as a possible biological or anatomical basis for homosexuality.[19] Other research proposes possible genetic, environmental, hormonal, or other foundations.

No single theory has emerged that fully explains this complex developmental process. The consensus of scientific opinion is that people do not choose their sexual orientation. Thus, being straight or being gay is something that "just happens." Indeed, most gays and lesbians report that no specific event "triggered" them into becoming gay. Many gays also indicate that their orientations seemed different from those of other children as far back as their prepuberty years.

Given the many challenges of being gay in a mostly straight world, it would seem logical that gays and lesbians do not make conscious efforts to choose to become gay. (Who would want to be a magnet for taunts, discrimination, and violence?) In a similar manner, it is highly likely that heterosexual persons do not actually choose to become straight. Sexual orientation is something that just unfolds in a person's life. (See the box "Coming Out—Then What?" on page 320 for insight into some of the issues that gay men and women need to face.)

Bonds Between People

As people develop relationships, they form bonds that can develop into intimacy and love.

"Don't Ask, Don't Tell" Policy Repealed

In late December 2010, President Barack Obama followed up on a 2008 campaign promise by signing a landmark congressional law that repealed the 1993 "Don't Ask, Don't Tell" military policy.* The 17-year-old policy required gay soldiers to hide their sexual orientation or face dismissal. Under the existing policy, over 14,000 troops had been dismissed.[†] However, the provisions of the repeal were not to be implemented until the military could certify that the new policy would not diminish combat readiness. Defense Secretary Robert Gates and Joint Chiefs of Staff Admiral Mike Mullen were advocates for this change in policy.

The Pentagon was expected to produce the implementation guidelines that would determine, among other things, how to educate troops about sexual orientation and how to readmit soldiers who were ousted under the old policy. This process was expected to take up to a year. However on September 20, 2011, the new guidelines were certified and the "Don't Ask, Don't Tell" policy came to an end. Gay soldiers now can openly serve in the U.S. military.

*MSNBC.com, Obama signs repeal of don't ask, don't tell, December 22, 2010. http://www.msnbc.msn.com/id/40777922/ns/politics-white house.

[†]Shane III, L, GAO: Ban cost military $53,000 per dismissal. *Stars and Stripes online,* January 20, 2011.

Love

Love may be one of the most elusive yet widely recognized concepts that describe some level of emotional attachment to another. Forms of love include friendly, erotic, devotional, parental, and altruistic love. Two types of love are most closely associated with dating and mate selection: *passionate love* and *companionate love.*[4]

Passionate love, also described as romantic love or **infatuation,** is a state of extreme absorption in another person. It is characterized by intense feelings of tenderness, elation, anxiety, sexual desire, and ecstasy. Often appearing early in a relationship, passionate love typically does not last very long. Passionate love is driven by the excitement of being closely involved with a person whose character is not fully known.

If a relationship progresses, passionate love is gradually replaced by companionate love. This type of love is less emotionally intense than passionate love. It is characterized by friendly affection and a deep attachment that is based on extensive familiarity with the partner. This love is enduring and capable of sustaining long-term mutual growth. Central to companionate love are feelings of empathy for, support of, and tolerance of the partner. Complete the Personal Assessment at the end of this chapter to determine whether you and your partner are truly compatible.

Intimacy

When most people hear the word **intimacy,** they immediately think about physical intimacy. They think about shared touching, kissing, and even intercourse. However, sexuality experts and family therapists prefer to view intimacy more broadly, as any close, mutual, verbal or nonverbal behavior within a relationship. In this sense, intimate behavior can range from sharing deep feelings and experiences with a partner to sharing profound physical pleasures with a partner.

Intimacy is present in both love and friendship. You have likely shared intimate feelings with your closest friends, as well as with those you love. Intimacy helps us feel connected to others and allows us to feel the full measure of our own self-worth.

 TALKING POINTS Your teenage son equates intimacy with sex. How would you explain the emotional intimacy involved in marriage?

Qualities of a Healthy Relationship

Perhaps the best thing a person could have is a truly fantastic relationship with someone. Such a relationship might be better than getting straight A's, better than looking like a movie star, and better than winning the lottery. But how do you know if what you have is a great relationship? Put another way, what are the qualities that reflect a healthy relationship?

Although bookstore shelves are filled with books that try to pinpoint the answer to this question, here are some basic qualities that reflect a healthy relationship. In a healthy relationship, partners should feel safe and treat each other with respect. Partners should enjoy spending time with each other, yet still feel good about having some personal, private time. In a healthy relationship, partners trust each other and openly communicate

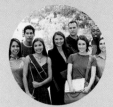

Learning from Our Diversity

Coming Out—Then What?

If you are openly gay, when you finally told your family and friends about your sexual orientation, a lot of things changed. But one thing probably stayed the same—you still feel like an outsider. Most of the couples holding hands on campus are young men and women. TV sit-coms are centered on heterosexual couples. They may include a gay character, but usually in a minor role. Popular magazines—through their ads, their features, their entire focus—are telling you how to be attractive to the opposite sex.

Being openly gay has probably made you wonder about some of the mixed messages you receive. The person who says it's okay that you're gay also seems to feel sorry for you, because you can't have a "normal" life and enjoy some of the things she does. Your mother makes remarks that suggest she still has hopes that someday you'll marry her best friend's son.

Feeling good about being gay in a straight world doesn't come easily. You've got to work at it. Start by finding support among your gay friends. Knowing that you're not alone is important—especially right after coming out. Realizing that other good, whole people are gay helps to reinforce your self esteem. Joining a campus gay organization is good for ongoing support, but don't limit yourself to that group. To grow as an individual, you also need to interact with and be part of heterosexual society.

Focus on what you value about yourself. Are you creative? Someone who gets things accomplished? A dependable friend? Think about the contributions you make—to your family, school, friends, church, and community. Remind yourself that you're a worthy person.

What do your friends appreciate about you? Do they value your advice? Like your sense of humor? Admire your courage? Think you're a strong leader?

Reinforcing the fact that you're a whole, worthy person is up to you. Listen to the "tapes" that are constantly playing in your head—both positive and negative. Edit out the negative thoughts, and turn up the volume on the positive ones. Take charge of what you think about yourself, rather than accepting what others think you are or should be.

their needs, concerns, and feelings. Partners in a good relationship are interested in each other's lives, including their families, work activities, and recreational needs. If the relationship is sexually intimate, partners are honest and open about their past and current sexual activity. There also should be no sexual coercion in a healthy relationship.[20]

Even great relationships have their ups and downs (see the box "How 'Real' Are the Relationships Seen on Television?"). For the long run, partners need to have some healthy optimism, a measure of flexibility, and a willingness to compromise during the tough times. Perhaps the simplest sign of a healthy relationship is that it has a lot more positive aspects to it than negative ones.

Communication in Relationships

As you read this chapter, you might notice that one of the recurring messages is the importance of effective communication between partners in a relationship. When you think about it, effective communication is the basis for *all healthy relationships,* not just ones related to love and intimacy.

For this reason, we encourage all readers to take advantage of available opportunities to learn effective communication skills. You might find these opportunities in college courses. Most speech and communication departments have courses that teach personal communication skills. Look for pertinent courses in psychology and counseling psychology departments. Most colleges

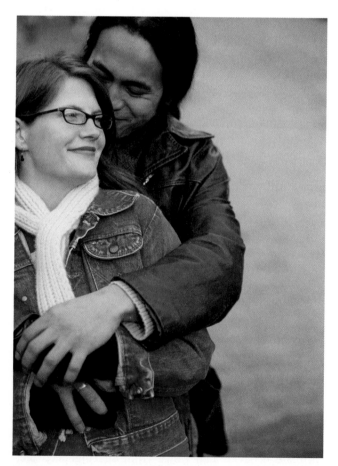

Healthy relationships are characterized by trust, respect, and open communication.

and universities also offer one or more human sexuality courses in their biology, psychology, sociology, consumer sciences, or health sciences departments. The counseling center on your campus may offer programs that can improve your communication skills. Your campus library or bookstore will certainly have popular books that may be very useful.

Recognizing Unhealthy Relationships

Sadly, sometimes people do not recognize or heed the warning signs of an unstable relationship, so they stay involved long after the risks outweigh the benefits. These warning signs include abusive behavior, whether emotional or physical, or both (see Chapter 15). Another red flag is excessive jealousy about a partner's interactions with others. Sometimes excessive jealousy evolves into controlling behavior, and one partner attempts to manage the daily activities of the other partner. By definition, controlling behavior limits your creativity and freedom.

Other warning signs are dishonesty, irresponsibility, lack of patience, and any kind of drug abuse. We certainly do not want to see these qualities in those we have initially judged to be "nice people," even though these unappealing characteristics may be obvious to others. If you suspect that any of these problems may be undermining your relationship, talk about your concerns with one or two trusted friends, and seek the advice of a professional counselor at your college or university. Try to realize that ending your relationship might be the best thing you could do for yourself.

Ending a Relationship

One of life's real challenges is dealing with the breakup of a relationship. Generally, the longer the relationship lasts, the more difficult it is to end it. While a bad first date can halt a potential relationship quickly, a partnership that has gone on for a few weeks, months, or years can be much more complicated. However, it is best to act quickly after making the firm judgment that the relationship is over. This allows you both not to waste time on a relationship that just isn't working out.

Each breakup situation is different, but there are some common threads to keep in mind. Unless you have been treated poorly (by a partner who cheated, lied, abused, manipulated, or disrespected you), try to show some personal *respect and courtesy* to the other person. Whether it is in a face-to-face meeting, a phone call, a text message, or an e-mail, try also to keep the message *clear and simple*. You can state that you just don't think the relationship is working and that you want to move on. Don't feel that you have to identify a specific event that caused you to want to break up, and don't place blame on the other person. Don't feel that you have to justify yourself or explain your reasons, either. Keep the message *short*.[21]

Hopefully, the ending of a relationship will be emotionally beneficial for both of you. If not, and you have lingering concerns over the breakup, you should seek help from your college's counseling center or a trusted friend or professor. If your former partner becomes abusive or threatening in some way (perhaps by harassing you through stalking, constant e-mailing, or incessant phoning), you should contact your campus security department or local police. (See Chapter 15 for additional information about stalking and protecting yourself on campus. Also, if you or someone you know is being stalked, refer to valuable information from the Stalking Resource Center at the National Center for the Victims of Crime website, www.ncvc.org.)

Lifestyles and Relationships

A variety of informal and formal lifestyles and relationships exist in our society. Here are a few of the most common ones.

Singlehood

One lifestyle option for adults is *singlehood*. For many people, being single is a lifestyle that affords the potential for pursuing intimacy, if desired, and provides an uncluttered path for independence and self-directedness. Other people, however, are single because of divorce, separation, death, or the absence of an opportunity to establish a partnership. The U.S. Census Bureau indicates that 44 percent of women and 41 percent of men over the age of 18 are currently single.[22]

Many different living arrangements are seen among singles. Some single people live alone and choose not to share a household. Other arrangements for singles include cohabitation, periodic cohabitation, singlehood during the week and cohabitation on the weekends or during vacations, or the *platonic* sharing of a household with others. Among young adults, large percentages of single men and women live with their parents.

Like habitation arrangements, the sexual intimacy patterns of singles are individually tailored. Some singles practice celibacy, others pursue intimate relationships in a **monogamous** pattern, and still others may have multiple partners. As in all interpersonal relationships, including marriage, the levels of commitment are as variable as the people involved.

Cohabitation

Cohabitation, or the sharing of living quarters by unmarried people, represents another alternative to marriage. According to the U.S. Census Bureau, the number of unmarried, opposite-gender couples living together totals over 5.6 million. The number of reported same-gender couples totaled 565,000 in the year 2008.[22]

Although cohabitation may seem to imply a vision of sexual intimacy between roommates, several forms of shared living arrangements can be viewed as cohabitation. For some couples, cohabitation is only a part-time arrangement for weekends, during summer vacation, or on a variable schedule. In addition, **platonic** cohabitation can exist when a couple shares living quarters but does so without establishing an intimate relationship. Close friends and people of retirement age might be included in a group called *cohabitants*.

How well do cohabitation arrangements fare against marriage partnerships in terms of long-term stability? A report prepared by the CDC's National Center for Health Statistics[23] indicated that unmarried cohabitations are generally less stable than marriages are. The probability of a first marriage ending in separation or divorce within 5 years was found to be 20 percent, but the probability of a premarital cohabitation breaking up within 5 years was 49 percent. After 10 years, the probability of a first marriage ending was 33 percent, compared to 62 percent for cohabitations.

Gay and Lesbian Partnerships

To believe that adult partnerships are reserved only for heterosexual couples is to avoid reality. In the United States and in many parts of the world, gays and lesbians are forming partnerships that in many ways are similar to those of heterosexuals. It no longer is unusual to see same-sex men and women openly living together in one household. Gay and lesbian couples buy houses together and share property rights. As businesses restructure their employee benefits packages, gays and lesbians are covering their partners on health care plans and making them beneficiaries on their insurance policies and retirement plans.

A search of the literature indicates that gay and lesbian partnerships have many of the same characteristics and problems as heterosexual couples.[3] Like straight couples, they struggle with interpersonal issues related to their relationship and their lifestyle. They work to decide how best to juggle their financial resources, their leisure time, and their friends and extended families. If they live

> **Key Terms**
>
> **monogamous** (mo **nog** a mus) Paired relationship with one partner.
>
> **cohabitation** Sharing of a residence by two unrelated, unmarried people; living together.
>
> **platonic** (pluh **ton** ick) Close association between two people that does not include a sexual relationship.

together in an apartment or house, they must decide how to divide the household tasks.

If children are present in the household, they must be cared for and nurtured. These children could have come from an adoption, a previous heterosexual relationship, or, in the case of a lesbian couple, from artificial insemination. Research indicates that children raised in lesbian or gay families overwhelmingly grow up with a heterosexual orientation, and are like other children from heterosexual families in terms of their adjustment, mental health, social skills, and peer acceptance.[3]

Same-Sex Marriage

One area in which gay and lesbian couples differ from heterosexual couples is in their ability to obtain a legal marriage. In the last few years, this inequity has been the focus of an intense national debate over same-sex marriage. The issues are complex, primarily because of the differences in state laws and the various courts' interpretations of those laws. At this point in the debate, here is where same-sex marriage stands.

If enacted, same-sex marriages would grant gay couples a legal marriage document that allows for an array of legal and economic benefits, including joint parental custody, insurance and health benefits, joint tax returns, alimony and child support, inheritance of property, hospital visitation rights, family leave, and a spouse's retirement benefits. (Social Security benefits come from a federal program and are not influenced by state laws.)

As of July 2011, the states of Massachusetts, Connecticut, Iowa, Vermont, New Hampshire, New York, and the District of Columbia issue marriage licenses to same-sex couples.[24] (California, which once permitted same-sex marriages, currently does not do so because the law is mired in a complicated "legal limbo.") With the exceptions of New York and Maryland, states do not recognize same-sex marriages performed in other jurisdictions.

In 2000, the Vermont legislature passed the nation's first "civil union" law, which granted legal status to gay and lesbian couples. Vermont's law conferred on same-sex couples all the benefits that the state allowed for heterosexual married couples. Since then, Delaware, Hawaii, Illinois, Rhode Island, and New Jersey have also passed civil union statutes while Vermont, Connecticut, and New Hampshire have replaced their civil union laws with same-sex marriage laws.

A number of states, including California, Oregon, Nevada, and Washington, have elected to provide nearly all state-level spousal rights to unmarried couples in "domestic partnership" relationships. Hawaii, Maine, Wisconsin, and the District of Columbia provide more limited state-level spousal rights to unmarried couples in domestic partnerships. States generally do not recognize domestic partnerships or civil unions from other states.

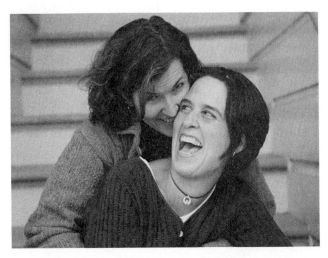

Legalization of same-sex marriage would grant gay and lesbian couples a wide range of legal and economic rights.

In 1996, the U.S. Congress passed the Defense of Marriage Act (DOMA), which prohibited federal recognition of same-sex marriages and allowed states to enact their own laws to prohibit the recognition of same-sex marriages. At the time of this writing, 39 states have laws that define marriage as between a man and a woman, and 30 states have state constitutions that define marriage as between a man and a woman.[24]

In February 2011, President Barack Obama made headlines when he instructed the Department of Justice to stop enforcing the Defense of Marriage Act because of the administration's belief that part of that federal law (Section 3) is unconstitutional.[25] In the 15 years since DOMA was enacted, the American political landscape has clearly changed, with the Supreme Court ruling that laws criminalizing homosexual conduct are unconstitutional, the repeal of the military's "Don't Ask, Don't Tell" policy, and several lower courts' rulings that DOMA is unconstitutional. These recent legal changes called into question the constitutionality of DOMA.

Despite not defending the constitutionality of DOMA in court, the Obama administration continues to support the enforcement of the law, until the time that either Congress repeals DOMA or there is a final judicial finding that the law is unconstitutional. Many observers believe that, within a few years, the U.S. Supreme Court will rule on the constitutionality of DOMA and the legality of same-sex marriage throughout the country.

Single Parenthood

Unmarried young women continue to become pregnant and then become single parents in this country. In 2007, unmarried mothers accounted for 40 percent of all newborns in the United States.[22] There is also a significantly different form of single parenthood: the planned entry into single parenthood by older, better-educated, financially stable people, the vast majority of whom are women.

In contrast to the teenaged girl who becomes a single parent through an unwed pregnancy, the more mature woman who desires single parenting has usually planned carefully for the experience. She has explored several important concerns, including the way she will become pregnant (with or without the knowledge of a male partner or through artificial insemination), the need for a father figure for the child, the effect of single parenting on her social life, and its effect on her career development. Once these questions have been resolved, no legal barriers stand in the way of her becoming a single parent.

A very large number of women and a growing number of men are becoming single parents through a divorce settlement or separation agreement. Additionally, increasing numbers of single persons are adopting children. In 2009, single women headed up 9.9 million households with children under age 18. In contrast, single men headed up 1.7 million households in 2009 with children under age 18.[22]

A few single parents have been awarded children through adoption. The likelihood of a single person's receiving a child this way is small, but more people have been successful recently in single-parent adoptions.

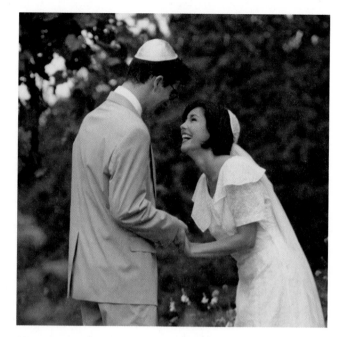

Marriage is a form of emotional and legal bonding.

Marriage

Just as there is no single best way for two people to move through dating and mate selection, marriage is also a variable undertaking. In marriage, two people join their lives in a way that affirms each as an individual and both as a legal pair. Some are able to resolve conflicts constructively (see the box "Resolving Conflict Through Better Communication"). However, for a large percentage of couples, the demands of marriage are too rigorous, confining, and demanding. They will find resolution for their dissatisfaction through divorce or extramarital affairs. For most, though, marriage will be an experience that alternates periods of happiness, productivity, and admiration with periods of frustration, unhappiness, and disillusionment with the partner. Each of you who marries will find the experience unique in every regard.

Currently, certain trends regarding marriage are evident. The most obvious of these is the age at first marriage. Today men are waiting longer than ever to marry. In 2010, the median age at first marriage for men is 28.2 years.[26] In addition, these new husbands are better educated than in the past and are more likely to be established in their careers. Women are also waiting longer to get married and tend to be more educated and career oriented than they were in the past. Recent statistics indicate that the median age at first marriage for women is 26.1 years.[26]

Marriage still appeals to most adults. Currently, 74 percent of adults age 18 and older are either married, widowed, or divorced.[22] Thus, about one-quarter of today's adults have not married.

Divorce

Marriages, like many other kinds of interpersonal relationships, can end. Today, marriages—relationships begun with the intent of permanence, "until death do us part"—end through divorce nearly as frequently as they continue.

Why should approximately half of marital relationships be so likely to end? Unfortunately, marriage experts cannot provide one clear answer. Rather, they suggest that divorce is a reflection of unfulfilled expectations for marriage on the part of one or both partners, including the following:

- The belief that marriage will ease your need to deal with your own faults and that your failures can be shared by your partner

- The belief that marriage will change faults that you know exist in your partner

- The belief that the high level of romance of your dating and courtship period will continue through marriage

- The belief that marriage can provide you with an arena for the development of your personal power and that, once married, you will not need to compromise with your partner

- The belief that your marital partner will be successful in meeting all of your needs

If these expectations seem to be ones you anticipate through marriage, then you may find that disappointments will abound. To varying degrees, marriage is a partnership that requires much cooperation and compromise. Marriage can be complicated. Because of the high expectations that many people hold for marriage, the termination of marriage can be an emotionally difficult process to undertake.

Concern is frequently voiced over the well-being of children whose parents divorce. Different factors, however, influence the extent to which divorce affects children. Included among these factors are the gender and age of the children, custody arrangements, financial support, and the remarriage of one or both parents. For many children, adjustments must be made to accept their new status as a member of a blended family.

 TALKING POINTS A couple you know well is going through a divorce. How could you show support for each person without taking sides?

Taking Charge of Your Health

- Take the Personal Assessment at the end of this chapter to find out how compatible you and your partner are.

- If being around someone whose sexual orientation is different from yours makes you feel uncomfortable, focus on getting to know that person better as an individual.

- If you are in an unhealthy relationship, take the first step toward getting out of it through professional counseling or group support.

- If you are in a sexual relationship, communicate your sexual needs to your partner clearly. Encourage him or her to do the same so that you will both have a satisfying sex life.

- Consider whether your lifetime plan will involve marriage, singlehood, or cohabitation. Evaluate your current situation in relation to that plan.

SUMMARY

- Biological and psychosocial factors contribute to the complex expression of our sexuality.
- The structural basis of sexuality begins in the growing embryo and fetus. Structural sexuality changes as one moves through adolescence and later life.
- The psychosocial processes of gender identity, gender preference, and gender adoption form the basis for an initial adult gender identification.
- The complex functioning of the male and female reproductive structures is controlled by hormones.
- The menstrual cycle's primary functions are to produce mature ova and to develop a supportive environment for the fetus in the uterus.

- The sexual response pattern consists of four stages: excitement, plateau, orgasmic, and resolution.
- Three sexual orientations are heterosexuality, homosexuality, and bisexuality.
- Many older people remain interested in sexual activity and are sexually active. Physiological changes may alter the way in which some older people perform sexually.
- Abusive behavior, extreme jealousy, controlling behaviors, dishonesty, and drug abuse are warning signs of an unhealthy relationship.
- A variety of lifestyles and relationships exist in our society.

REVIEW QUESTIONS

1. Describe the following foundations of our biological sexuality: the genetic basis, the gonadal basis, and structural development.
2. Define and explain the following terms: *gender identity, gender preference, gender adoption,* and *initial adult gender identification.*
3. Identify the major components of the male and female reproductive systems. Trace the passageways for sperm and ova.
4. Explain the menstrual cycle. Identify and describe the four main hormones that control the menstrual cycle.
5. What similarities and differences exist between the sexual response patterns of males and females?
6. What is the refractory period?
7. How do myotonia and vasocongestion differ?
8. Approximately what percentage of today's college students report having had sexual intercourse?
9. Explain the differences between heterosexuality, homosexuality, and bisexuality. How common are each of these sexual orientations in our society?
10. What are some key strategies to keep in mind when ending a relationship?

ANSWERS TO THE "WHAT DO YOU KNOW?" QUIZ

1. False   2. True   3. False   4. True   5. True   6. False   7. True

Visit the Online Learning Center (**www.mhhe.com/hahn11e**), where you will find tools to help you improve your grade including practice quizzes, key terms flashcards, audio chapter summaries for your MP3 player, and many other study aids.

SOURCE NOTES

1. Patten KT, Thibodeau GA. *Anatomy and Physiology* (7th ed.). St. Louis, MO: Mosby, 2010.
2. Sherwood L. *Human Physiology: From Cells to Systems* (7th ed.). Belmont, CA: Brooks/Cole, Cengage Learning, 2010.
3. Hyde JS, DeLamater JD. *Understanding Human Sexuality* (11th ed.). New York: McGraw-Hill, 2011.
4. Crooks R, Baur K. *Our Sexuality* (11th ed.). Belmont, CA: Wadsworth, Cengage Learning, 2011.
5. Kelly GF. *Sexuality Today* (10th ed.). New York: McGraw-Hill, 2011.
6. Saladin KS. *Human Anatomy* (3rd ed.). New York: McGraw-Hill, 2011.
7. Yarber WL, Sayad BW, Strong B. *Human Sexuality: Diversity in Contemporary America* (7th ed.). New York: McGraw-Hill, 2010.
8. Hatcher RA, et al. *Contraceptive Technology* (19th ed.). New York: Ardent Media, 2007.
9. WebMd. Your guide to premenstrual syndrome, or PMS, February 17, 2011. http://women.webmd.com/mental-health/premenstrual-syndrome.
10. WebMd. Your guide to premenstrual dysphoric disorder, February 17, 2011. http://www.webmd.com/mental-health/premenstrual-dysphoric-disorder.
11. Writing Group for the Women's Health Initiative Investigation. Risks and benefits of estrogen plus progestin in healthy postmenopausal women: principal results from the Women's Health Initiative Randomized Controlled Trial. *Journal of the American Medical Association,* 288(3), 321–333, 2002.
12. Mayo Clinic. Hormone therapy: Is it right for you? February 22, 2011. http://www.mayoclinic.com/health/hormone-therapy/WO00046.
13. Masters WH, Johnson VE. *Human Sexual Response.* Philadelphia: Lippincott, Williams & Wilkins, 1966.
14. Carroll JL. *Sexuality Now: Embracing Diversity* (3rd ed.). Belmont, CA: Wadsworth, Cengage Learning, 2010.
15. Connect Safely. *Tips to Prevent Sexting,* accessed February 28, 2011. www.connectsafely.org/Safety-Tips/tips-to-prevent-sexting.html.
16. Baldwin JI, Baldwin JD. Heterosexual anal intercourse: an understudied, high-risk sexual behavior. *Archives of Sexual Behavior,* 29(4), 357–373, 2000.
17. Kinsey AC, Pomeroy WB, Martin CE. *Sexual Behavior in the Human Male* (reprint ed.). Bloomington: Indiana University Press, 1998.
18. Kinsey AC, et al. *Sexual Behavior in the Human Female* (reprint ed.). Bloomington: Indiana University Press, 1998.
19. Allen LS, Gorski RA. Sexual orientation and the size of the anterior commissure in the human brain. *Proceedings of the National Academy of Sciences,* 89(15), 7199–7202, 1992.
20. Health Services at Columbia University. Healthy vs. unhealthy relationships, accessed February 27, 2011. www goaskalice .columbia.edu.
21. Health Services at Columbia University. Breaking up can be hard to do, accessed February 25, 2011. www.goaskalice.columbia.edu.
22. U.S. Census Bureau. *Statistical Abstract of the United States: 2011* (130th ed.). Washington, DC: U.S. Department of Commerce, 2010.
23. Bramlett MD, Mosher WD. Cohabitation, marriage, divorce, and remarriage in the United States. U.S. Centers for Disease Control and Prevention, National Center for Health Statistics. *Vital Health Statistics,* 23(22), 2002.
24. National Conference of State Legislatures. *Same Sex Marriage, Civil Unions and Domestic Partnerships,* July 14, 2011. www.ncsl.org.
25. U.S. Department of Justice, Office of Public Affairs. *Statement of the Attorney General on Litigation Involving the Defense of Marriage Act,* February 23, 2011 (press release). www.justice.gov.
26. U.S. Census Bureau. Current Population Survey, *Estimated Median Age at First Marriage, by Sex: 1890–the Present* (Table MS-2), accessed March 1, 2011. www.census.gov.

Personal Assessment

How Compatible Are You?

This quiz will help test how compatible you and your partner's personalities are. You should each rate the truth of these 20 statements based on the following scale. Circle the number that reflects your feelings. Total your scores and check the interpretation following the quiz.

1 = Never true
2 = Sometimes true
3 = Frequently true
4 = Always true

1. We can communicate our innermost thoughts effectively. 1 2 3 4
2. We trust each other. 1 2 3 4
3. We agree on whose needs come first. 1 2 3 4
4. We have realistic expectations of each other and of ourselves. 1 2 3 4
5. Individual growth is important within our relationship. 1 2 3 4
6. We will go on as a couple even if our partner doesn't change. 1 2 3 4
7. Our personal problems are discussed with each other first. 1 2 3 4
8. We both do our best to compromise. 1 2 3 4
9. We usually fight fairly. 1 2 3 4
10. We try not to be rigid or unyielding. 1 2 3 4
11. We keep any needs to be "perfect" in proper perspective. 1 2 3 4
12. We can balance desires to be sociable and the need to be alone. 1 2 3 4
13. We both make friends and keep them. 1 2 3 4
14. Neither of us stays down or up for long periods. 1 2 3 4
15. We can tolerate the other's mood without being affected by it. 1 2 3 4
16. We can deal with disappointment and disillusionment. 1 2 3 4
17. Both of us can tolerate failure. 1 2 3 4
18. We can both express anger appropriately. 1 2 3 4
19. We are both assertive when necessary. 1 2 3 4
20. We agree on how our personal surroundings are kept. 1 2 3 4

YOUR TOTAL POINTS _____

Interpretation

20–35 points—You and your partner seem quite incompatible. Professional help may open your lines of communication.

36–55 points—You probably need more awareness and compromise.

56–70 points—You are highly compatible. However, be aware of the areas where you can improve.

71–80 points—Your relationship is very fulfilling.

TO CARRY THIS FURTHER . . .

Ask your partner to take this test too. You may have a one-sided view of a "perfect" relationship. Even if you scored high on this assessment, be aware of areas where you can still improve.

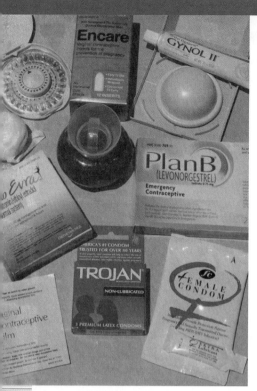

Managing Your Fertility

What Do You Know About Managing Your Fertility?

1. Birth control and contraception mean the same thing. True or False?

2. In the United States, condoms are available in one size only. True or False?

3. Intrauterine devices (IUDs) are safe and effective for most women. True or False?

4. Emergency contraception produces a medication abortion. True or False?

5. The acid in the vagina is destructive to sperm. True or False?

6. Typically, the first stage of labor is the longest stage. True or False?

7. IVF-ET is the most frequently used assisted reproductive technology. True or False?

Check your answers at the end of the chapter.

How you decide to control your **fertility** will have an important effect on your future. Your understanding of information and issues related to fertility control will help you make responsible decisions in this complex area.

For traditional-age students, these decisions may be fast approaching. (See the box "There's More to Sex Than You Thought" for a discussion of decision making about sex and the spiritual dimension of sexuality.) Frequently, nontraditional students are parents who have had experiences that make them useful resources for other students in the class.

Basic Concepts of Fertility Control

This chapter begins with some basic concepts related to fertility control. After reading the material in the next three subsections, you should be better prepared to examine closely the many birth control methods available today. We start with a terminology distinction.

Are you ready for sex? If you're not sure, take time to think it over. If you start having sex before you're ready, you might feel guilty. Or you might feel bad because you realize this step isn't right for you now. Or your religious upbringing may make you feel as though you're doing something wrong. You also may not be ready for the emotional aspects of a sexual relationship. Most important, you will probably have difficulty handling the complexities of an unplanned pregnancy or a sexually transmitted disease.

If you do feel ready for sex, you still have a choice. Sex may be okay for you now. It may be personally fulfilling, something that enhances your self-esteem. Alternatively, you can choose to abstain from sex until later—another way of enhancing your self-esteem. You'll feel empowered by making the decision for yourself, rather than doing what is expected. Being strong enough to say "no" can also make you feel good about yourself. For some, making this decision may reflect a renewed commitment to spiritual or religious concerns.

If you're in a committed relationship, sex is a good way of connecting as a couple. It's something that the two of you alone share. It's a time to give special attention to each other—taking a break from the kids, your jobs, and your other responsibilities. It's a way of saying "This relationship is important—it's something I value."

Going through a pregnancy together is another opportunity for closeness. From the moment you know that you're going to be parents, you're connected in a new way. Your focus becomes the expected child. You'll watch the fetus grow on ultrasound, go to parenting and Lamaze classes together, visit the doctor together, mark the various milestones, and share new emotions. When your child is born, you'll be connected as never before.

Whether you're thinking about starting to have sex, making the decision to wait, or examining the sexual life you have now, you can't ignore the possibilities and the consequences. Is the time right for you? Are you doing this for yourself or for someone else? What do you think you will gain from waiting? Do you expect your future partner to also have made the decision to wait? What do you expect to get from a sexual relationship—pleasure, intimacy, love? What do you expect to give? Do you want an emotional commitment? Do you view sex and love as inseparable? Do you understand how sex can enhance your spirituality? Taking time to consider these questions can make you feel good about yourself—no matter what you decide.

Birth Control Versus Contraception

Any discussion about the control of your fertility should start with an explanation of the subtle differences between the terms **birth control** and **contraception.** Although many people use the words interchangeably, they reflect different perspectives about fertility control. *Birth control* is an umbrella term that refers to all the procedures you might use to prevent the birth of a child. Birth control includes all available contraceptive measures, as well as all sterilization and abortion procedures.

Contraception is a much more specific term for any procedure used to prevent the fertilization of an ovum. Contraceptive measures vary widely in the mechanisms they use to accomplish this task. They also vary considerably in their method of use and their rate of success in preventing conception. A few examples of contraceptives are condoms, hormonal contraceptives, spermicides, and diaphragms.

Beyond the numerous methods mentioned, certain forms of sexual behavior not involving intercourse could be considered forms of contraception. For example, mutual masturbation by couples virtually eliminates the possibility of pregnancy. This practice, as well as additional forms of sexual expression other than intercourse (such as kissing, touching, and massage), has been given the generic term **outercourse.** Not only does outercourse protect against unplanned pregnancy, it may also significantly reduce the transmission of sexually transmitted diseases (STDs), including HIV infection.

Theoretical Effectiveness Versus Use Effectiveness

People considering the use of a contraceptive method need to understand the difference between the two effectiveness rates given for each form of contraception. *Theoretical effectiveness* is a measure of a contraceptive method's ability to prevent a pregnancy when the method is used precisely as directed during every act of intercourse. *Use effectiveness,* however, refers to the effectiveness of a method in preventing conception when used by the

---

> **Key Terms**
>
> **fertility** The ability to reproduce.
>
> **birth control** All the methods and procedures that can prevent the birth of a child.
>
> **contraception** Any method or procedure that prevents fertilization.
>
> **outercourse** Sexual activity that does not involve intercourse.

general public. Use-effectiveness rates take into account factors that lower effectiveness below that based on "perfect" use. Failure to follow proper instructions, illness of the user, forgetfulness, physician (or pharmacist) error, and a subconscious desire to experience risk or even pregnancy are a few of the factors that can lower the effectiveness of even the most theoretically effective contraceptive technique.

Effectiveness rates are often expressed in terms of the percentage of women users of childbearing age who do not become pregnant while using the method for one year. For some methods, the theoretical-effectiveness and use-effectiveness rates are vastly different; the theoretical rate is always higher than the use rate. Table 13.1 presents data concerning effectiveness rates, advantages, and disadvantages of many birth control methods.

Table 13.1 Effectiveness Rates of Birth Control for 100 Women During the First Year of Use

Method	Estimated Effectiveness		Advantages	Disadvantages
	Theoretical	Use		
No method (chance)	15%	15%	Inexpensive	Totally ineffective
Withdrawal	96%	73%	No supplies or advance preparation needed; no side effects; men share responsibility for family planning	Interferes with coitus; very difficult to use effectively; women must trust men to withdraw as orgasm approaches
Periodic abstinence	91–99%	75%	No supplies needed; no side effects; men share responsibility for family planning; women learn about their bodies	Difficult to use, especially if menstrual cycles are irregular, as is common in young women; abstinence may be necessary for long periods; lengthy instruction and ongoing counseling may be needed
Spermicide (gel, foam, suppository, film)		71%	No health risks; can be used with condoms to increase effectiveness considerably	Must be inserted 5–30 minutes before coitus; effective for only 30–60 minutes; some concern about nonoxynol-9
Diaphragm	94%	84%	No major health risks; easily carried in purse, can be used during breast-feeding; no impact on woman's hormones; usually cannot be felt by either partner	Cannot be used during menstruation; must be left in place for at least 6 hours after coitus; must be fitted by health care personnel; some women may find it awkward or embarrassing to use; some concern about nonoxynol-9
FemCap (no previous births) (previous births)	? ?	86% 71%	No major health risks; easily carried in purse; can be used during breast-feeding; no impact on woman's hormones; usually cannot be felt by either partner	Similar to diaphragm disadvantages above; must not be left in place more than 48 hours
Sponge (no previous births) (previous births)	91% 80%	84% 68%	Easy to use; not messy; protection is good for 24 hours and multiple acts of intercourse; no prescription required	Not reusable; contraceptive protection is reduced for women with previous births; some concern about nonoxynol-9
Male condom Male condom with spermicide	98% 99%	85% 95%	Easy to use; inexpensive and easy to obtain; no health risks; very effective protection against some STDs; men share responsibility for family planning	Must be put on just before coitus; some men and women complain of decreased sensation; some concern about nonoxynol-9
Female condom	95%	79%	Relatively easy to use; no prescription required; polyurethane is stronger than latex; provides some STD protection; silicone-based lubrication provided; useful when male will not use condom	Contraceptive effectiveness not as high as with male condom; couples may be unfamiliar with device that extends outside the vagina; more expensive than male condoms
IUD ParaGard (Copper T) Mirena (progestin)	99%+ 99%+	99%+ 99%+	Easy to use; highly effective in preventing pregnancy; does not interfere with coitus; repeated action not needed; with Mirena, may result in reduced menstrual flow or the absence of periods	May increase risk of pelvic infection and infertility in very small percentage of women; not usually recommended for women who have never had child; must be inserted by health care personnel; may cause heavy bleeding and pain in some women
Combined pill (estrogen + progestin) Minipill (progestin only)	99%+ 99%+	92% 92%	Easy to use; highly effective in preventing pregnancy; does not interfere with coitus; regulates menstrual cycle; reduces heavy bleeding and menstrual pain; helps protect against ovarian and endometrial cancer	Must be taken every day; requires medical examination and prescription; minor side effects such as nausea or menstrual spotting; possibility of cardiovascular problems in small percentage of users

(continued)

Table 13.1 Continued

| Method | Estimated Effectiveness | | Advantages | Disadvantages |
	Theoretical	Use		
Contraceptive ring (estrogen + progestin)	99%+	92%	Easy to use after learning how to insert; remains in place 3 weeks	Like other hormonal methods, does not protect against STDs; requires physician prescription; possibility of cardiovascular problems in small percentage of users
Contraceptive patch (estrogen + progestin)	99%+	92%	Easy to apply; must be changed weekly for 3 weeks	No STD protection; requires physician prescription; possibility of cardiovascular problems in small percentage of users
Depo-Provera	99%+	97%	Easy to use; highly effective for 3-month period; continued use prevents menstruation	Requires supervision by physician; administered by injection; some women experience irregular menstrual spotting in early months of use
Contraceptive implant	99%+	99%+	Easy to use; protection is good for 3 years; progestin only; can be used while breast-feeding; no medicine to take daily	No STD protection; requires physician to insert or remove; may cause temporary irregular bleeding; possibility of cardiovascular problems in small percentage of users
Tubal ligation	99%+	99%+	Permanent; removes fear of pregnancy	Surgery-related risks; generally considered irreversible
Vasectomy	99%+	99%+	Permanent; removes fear of pregnancy	Generally considered irreversible

Sources: Adapted from Hatcher RA, et al., *Contraceptive Technology* (19th ed.). New York: Ardent Media, 2007; and Planned Parenthood Federation of America, *Birth Control.* www.plannedparenthood.org.

Selecting Your Contraceptive Method

In this section, we discuss some of the many factors that should be important to you as you consider selecting a contraceptive method. Remember that no method possesses equally high marks in all of the following areas. You and your partner should select a contraceptive method that is both acceptable and effective, as determined by your unique needs and expectations. Completing the Personal Assessment at the end of this chapter will help you make this decision.

For a contraceptive method to be acceptable to those who wish to exercise a large measure of control over their fertility, the following should be given careful consideration:

- *It should be safe.* The contraceptive approach you select should not pose a significant health risk for you or your partner.
- *It should be effective.* Your approach must have a high success rate in preventing pregnancy.
- *It should be reliable.* The form you select must be able to be used over and over again with consistent success.
- *It should be reversible.* Couples who eventually want to have a family should select a method that can be reversed.
- *It should be affordable.* The cost of a particular method must fit comfortably into a couple's budget.

- *It should be easy to use.* Complicated instructions or procedures can make a method difficult to use effectively.
- *It should not interfere with sexual expression.* An ideal contraceptive fits in comfortably with a couple's intimate sexual behavior.

Behavioral Contraceptive Methods

The first contraceptives we'll discuss are those that are based on the sexual behavior of a couple. As with all approaches to contraception, a clear understanding of each method can help you make decisions about sexual activity and birth control that are right for you. For guidelines on locating accurate information on the Web, see the box "Information Online—Birth Control and Sexuality."

Abstinence

Abstinence as a form of birth control has gained attention recently on college campuses. This method is as close to 100 percent effective as possible. There have been isolated reports in the medical literature of pregnancy without sexual intercourse, usually involving ejaculation by the male near the woman's vagina. Avoiding this situation should raise the effectiveness of abstinence to 100 percent.

Information Online—Birth Control and Sexuality

The Internet offers a number of resources for locating information about birth control, sexuality, and related topics. The Planned Parenthood Federation of America provides one of the most comprehensive sites at www.plannedparenthood.org. At this site you will learn about women's health issues, birth control, pregnancy, sexually transmitted infections and diseases, gynecological exams, sexuality and relationships, health centers in your area, and teen sexuality. A number of new podcasts are available on different topics. Planned Parenthood believes that when people are empowered with knowledge, they are better able to make sound decisions about their health and sexuality.

Three other sites offer information about sexuality and reproductive choices. The Guttmacher Institute (www.guttmacher.org) is a nonprofit organization focused on "sexual and reproductive health research, policy analysis, and public education." Its mission is to protect reproductive choices for all men and women. The Guttmacher Institute publishes scientific research papers in the areas of contraception, HIV/AIDS and STDs, sexual and reproductive health, abortion, technology, and bioethics.

The Sexuality Information and Education Council of the United States (SIECUS) is a nonprofit organization dedicated to developing, collecting, and disseminating information about sexuality. This group (www.siecus.org) promotes comprehensive sexuality education and distributes thousands of pamphlets, booklets, and bibliographies each year to professionals and the general public.

If you want to search for information about certain sexuality topics from a pro-life perspective, you might wish to examine the website for the National Right to Life Committee (NRLC) at www.nrlc.org. This group, founded shortly after the January 22, 1973, *Roe v. Wade* decision, has as its goal to "restore legal protection to innocent human life." The main focus is on the abortion controversy, but the NRLC is also concerned about matters of medical ethics that are related to euthanasia or infanticide. The NRLC closely monitors current issues in the courts and legislative bodies.

When searching websites for accurate sexuality information, here are some good strategies you can use: (1) *Don't settle for just one site.* Look at a number of sites to see if the information is substantiated in more than one place. (2) *Check for references* to high-quality professional publications or government reports. (3) *Locate the "About Us" link* that the website provides—this can tell you why the site exists, who funds the site, and what the mission of the site is. Finally, (4) *check to see if the topic you are searching for is covered in your textbook.* Since most textbooks are reviewed by top professionals in their field, your book should be a confirmatory source of information. By thinking critically about the quality of an online site, you can be more certain that the information is valid and useful.

Abstinence as a form of birth control has additional advantages in that it provides nearly 100 percent protection from sexually transmitted diseases, it is free, and it does not require a visit to a physician or a health clinic.

However, significant concerns exist about the effectiveness of educational programs that encourage abstinence. A large, five-year study published in the journal *Pediatrics* supported earlier studies that found that teens who "pledged virginity until marriage" were just as likely to have sex as nonpledgers, were less likely to use contraceptives when they had sex, had similar rates of oral and anal sex, and had similar rates of sexually transmitted diseases as nonpledgers. Also, pledgers did not differ in lifetime number of sexual partners and age at time of first sex.[1]

Abstinence works effectively only when it is broadly defined (to include many sexual behaviors) and used correctly and consistently. Abstinence is a challenging proposition for many adolescents and young adults.

Withdrawal

Withdrawal, or **coitus interruptus,** is the contraceptive practice in which the erect penis is removed from the vagina just before ejaculation of semen. Theoretically this procedure prevents sperm from entering the deeper structures of the female reproductive system. The use effectiveness of this method, however, reflects how unsuccessful this method is in practice.

There is strong evidence to suggest that the clear preejaculate fluid that helps neutralize and lubricate the male urethra can contain *viable* (capable of fertilization) sperm.[2] This sperm can be deposited near the cervical opening before withdrawal of the penis. This phenomenon may in part explain the relatively low effectiveness of this method. Furthermore, withdrawal does not protect users from the transmission of STDs.

Periodic Abstinence

Five approaches are included in the birth control strategy called **periodic abstinence:** (1) the calendar method, (2) the temperature method, (3) the cervical mucus method, (4) the symptothermal method, and (5) the standard days method.[3] All five methods attempt to determine the time a woman ovulates. Figure 13-1 shows a day-to-day fertility calendar that reflects a woman's fertile periods. Most research indicates that an ovum is viable for only about 24–36 hours after its release from the ovary. (Once inside the female reproductive tract, some sperm can survive up to a week.)

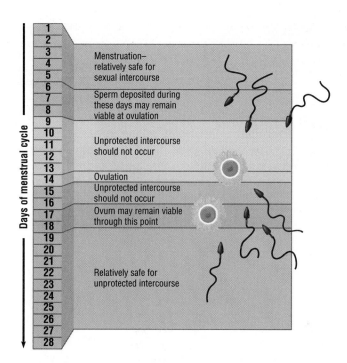

Figure 13-1 Periodic Abstinence   These methods try to pinpoint when a woman is most likely to ovulate. Remember that most women's cycles are not consistently perfect 28-day cycles, as shown in most illustrations. This figure is only an approximation of a woman's cycle.

Within the figure:

Days of menstrual cycle (1–28)

Menstruation— relatively safe for sexual intercourse

Sperm deposited during these days may remain viable at ovulation

Unprotected intercourse should not occur

Ovulation

Unprotected intercourse should not occur

Ovum may remain viable through this point

Relatively safe for unprotected intercourse

When a woman can accurately determine when she ovulates, she must refrain from intercourse long enough for the ovum to begin to disintegrate. *Fertility awareness, rhythm, natural birth control,* and *natural family planning* are terms interchangeable with periodic abstinence. Remember that periodic abstinence methods do *not* provide protection against the spread of STDs.[2]

Periodic abstinence is the only acceptable method endorsed by the Roman Catholic Church. For some people who have deep concerns for the spiritual dimensions of their health, the selection of a contraceptive method other than periodic abstinence may indicate a serious compromise of beliefs.

The **calendar method** requires close examination of a woman's menstrual cycle for the last 6–12 cycles. Records are kept of the length (in days) of each cycle. A *cycle* is defined as the number of days from the first day of menstrual flow in one cycle to the first day of menstrual flow in the next cycle.

To determine the days she should abstain from intercourse, a woman should subtract 18 from her shortest cycle; this is the first day she should abstain from intercourse in an upcoming cycle. Then she should subtract 11 from her longest cycle; this is the last day she must abstain from intercourse in an upcoming cycle.[4]

The *temperature method* requires a woman (for about three or four successive months) to take her body temperature every morning before she gets out of bed.

A finely calibrated, basal thermometer, available in many drugstores, is used for this purpose. The theory behind this method is that a distinct correlation exists between body temperature and the process of ovulation. Around the time of ovulation, the body temperature rises at least 0.4°F and remains elevated until the start of menstruation. The woman is instructed to refrain from intercourse during the interval when the temperature change takes place.

Drawbacks of this procedure include the need for consistent, accurate readings and the realization that all women's bodies are different. Some women may not fit the temperature pattern projection because of biochemical differences in their bodies. Also, body temperatures can fluctuate because of a wide variety of illnesses and physical stressors. A basal thermometer costs about $10.[5]

The *cervical mucus method* is another periodic abstinence technique. Generally used with other periodic abstinence techniques, this method requires a woman to evaluate the daily mucus discharge from her cervix. Users of this method become familiar with the changes in both appearance (from clear to cloudy) and consistency (from watery to thick) of their cervical mucus throughout their cycles. Women are taught that the unsafe days are when the mucus becomes clear and is the consistency of raw egg whites. Such a technique of ovulation determination must be learned from a physician or family planning professional.

The *symptothermal method* of periodic abstinence combines the use of the calendar, temperature, and cervical mucus methods. Couples using the symptothermal method are already using a calendar to chart the woman's body changes. Family planning professionals consider the symptothermal method preferable to a single periodic abstinence approach.

The newest periodic abstinence approach is called the *standard days method.* This method is appropriate only for women who have menstrual cycles that are consistently between 26 and 32 days long. It is not to be used by women who have variable cycles that are shorter than 26 days or longer than 32 days. Having had just one cycle in the past year shorter than 26 days or longer than 32 days should encourage a woman *not* to use the standard days method. She should meet with her health care provider and discuss an alternative method.

To use this method, women must count the days of their menstrual cycle, with day 1 as the first day of menstrual bleeding. Women can have intercourse on days 1 to 7. On days 8–19, women should refrain from penis-vaginal intercourse or use a barrier method of contraception. Days 8–19 are the fertile days. From day 20 until the end of the cycle, unprotected intercourse can take place.[4] Keep in mind that the standard days method does not protect against the transmission of STDs.

Over-the-Counter Contraceptive Methods

These are methods that couples can choose easily because they do not require a physician's prescription, they are readily available in supermarkets or drugstores, and they are approved by the U.S. Food and Drug Administration (FDA). They all work by providing some kind of obstacle or mechanism that prevents the sperm from joining an ovum.

Spermicides

Spermicides are agents that are capable of killing sperm. When used alone, they offer a moderately effective form of contraception for the woman who is sexually active on an infrequent basis. Modern spermicides are generally safe (but see the following precaution), reversible forms of contraception that can be obtained without a physician's prescription in most drugstores and supermarkets. They are available in foams, creams, gels, film, or suppositories. Spermicides are relatively inexpensive. Applicator kits cost about $8, and refills cost around $4–8 (see Figure 13-2). Suppositories and film are also priced in this range.[5]

Spermicides have water-soluble bases with a sperm-killing agent in the base. Frequently, spermicides are used with other contraceptives, such as diaphragms, caps, and condoms, to increase contraceptive effectiveness. Spermicides do not protect users from contracting pathogens that cause various STDs. In fact, people who use nonoxynol-9 many times each day or people who are at risk for HIV are more likely to transmit infections. This is due to an increase in skin irritations and abrasions, which provides the avenue for passage into the bloodstream.[6]

Couples should realize that condoms, when used consistently and correctly, provide much better disease protection and contraceptive effect than spermicides used alone. However, the small amount of nonoxynol-9

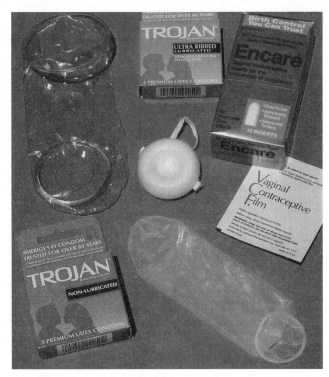

Over-the-counter methods of contraception are widely available in drugstores and supermarkets. They include male and female condoms, spermicides, and the contraceptive sponge.

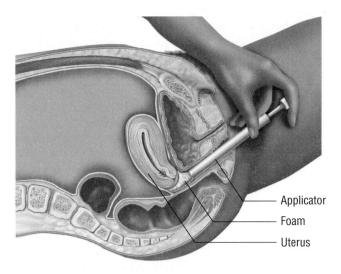

Figure 13-2 Use of Spermicide Spermicidal foams, gels, and suppositories are placed deep into the vagina in the region of the cervix no longer than 30 minutes before intercourse.

that is added to the lubricant with some condoms is not a sufficient backup contraceptive if the condom breaks. Thus, some health centers and family planning agencies have stopped distributing condoms coated with a spermicide. If you and/or your partner have concerns about your use of spermicides, you should seek advice from your health care provider.

Putting on a condom seems so easy. Is there anything else I need to know about condom use?

These simple directions for using condoms correctly, in combination with your motivation and commitment to regular use, should provide you with reasonable protection:

- *Keep a supply of condoms at hand.* Condoms should be stored in a cool, dry place so that they are readily available at the time of intercourse. Condoms that are stored in wallets or glove compartments may not be in satisfactory condition when they are used. Temperature extremes are to be avoided. Check the condom package for the expiration date.
- *Do not test a condom by inflating or stretching it.* Handle it gently and keep it away from sharp fingernails.
- *For maximum effectiveness, put the condom on before genital contact.* Either the man or the woman can put the condom in place. Early application is particularly important in the prevention of STDs. Early application also lessens the possibility of the release of preejaculate fluid into the vagina.
- *Unroll the condom on the erect penis.* For those using a condom without a reservoir tip, a ½-inch space should be left to catch the ejaculate. To leave this space, pinch the tip of the condom as you roll it on the erect penis. Do not leave any air in the tip of the condom.
- *Lubricate the condom if this has not already been done by the manufacturer.* When doing this, be certain to use a water-soluble lubricant and not a petroleum-based product such as petroleum jelly. Petroleum can deteriorate the latex material. Other oil-based lubricants, such as mineral oil, baby oil, vegetable oil, shortening, and certain hand lotions, can quickly damage a latex condom. Use water-based lubricants only!
- *After ejaculation, be certain that the condom does not become dislodged from the penis.* Hold the rim of the condom firmly against

the base of the penis during withdrawal. Do not allow the penis to become flaccid (soft) while still in the vagina.

- *Inspect the condom for tears before throwing it away.* If the condom is damaged in some way, immediately insert a spermicidal agent into the vagina or consider using emergency contraception (see page 341).

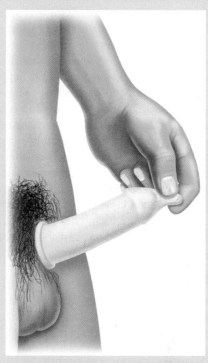

Pinch the end of the condom to leave ½ inch of space at the tip.

Condoms

Colored or natural, smooth or textured, straight or shaped, plain or reservoir-tipped, dry or lubricated—the latex condom is approaching an art form. Still, the familiar **condom** remains a safe, effective, reversible contraceptive device. All condoms manufactured in the United States must be approved by the FDA.

For couples who are highly motivated to prevent a pregnancy, the effectiveness of a male condom can approach that of an oral contraceptive—especially if condom use is combined with a spermicide. For couples who are less motivated, the condom can be considerably less effective. Condoms cost from 50¢ to $2.50 each but are often free at college health centers or local health departments or clinics.

The male latex condom offers substantial protection against STDs. For both the man and the woman, chlamydial infections, gonorrhea, HIV infection, and other STDs are less likely to be acquired when the condom is used correctly (see the box "Maximizing the Effectiveness

> **Key Terms**
>
> **spermicides** Chemicals capable of killing sperm.
>
> **condom** A shield designed to cover the erect penis and retain semen on ejaculation; "rubber." Various types of condoms are available, including latex, polyurethane, lambskin, and female condoms.

of Condoms"). However, "natural" or lambskin condoms, made from animal membranes, have tiny pores that can permit viruses (such as herpes, hepatitis B, and HIV) to pass through and cause serious infections.

Some lubricated condoms also contain a spermicide, yet the small amount of spermicide present in the condom's lubricant is not enough to consistently prevent conception if the condom should break. Current recommendations are to use lubricated condoms without spermicide or to use dry condoms and add lubrication and/or contraceptive gel or foam for comfort and contraceptive protection. Any lubricants used should be water-based. Nonlubricated condoms can be used for oral sex.

The FDA has approved both male and female types of polyurethane condoms. These are available as one-time-use condoms. These condoms are good alternatives for people who have an allergic sensitivity to latex, estimated to be up to 7 percent of the population.[7] Also, they are thinner and stronger than latex condoms and can be used with oil-based or water-based lubricants. Currently, these condoms are believed to provide protection against STDs that is close to that of latex condoms. The contraceptive effectiveness of polyurethane condoms remains somewhat less than that of the male latex condom.[8]

Female and male condoms should not be used together since they might adhere to each other and cause slippage or displacement. Female condoms cost about $4 each.

Contraceptive Sponge

The contraceptive sponge is a small, pillow-shaped polyurethane device containing nonoxynol-9 spermicide. The sponge is dampened with water and inserted deep in the vagina to cover the cervical opening. The device provides contraceptive protection for up to 24 hours, regardless of the number of times intercourse occurs. After the last act of intercourse, the sponge must be left in place for at least 6 hours. Once removed, the sponge must be discarded. The sponge must not be left in place for more than 30 hours because of the risk of toxic shock syndrome.[4] (Consult your physician if you are concerned about the use of nonoxynol-9.)

It is important to remember that the sponge does not protect users from contracting STDs. In women who have not given birth, the contraceptive effectiveness of the sponge is similar to that of the diaphragm. The sponge is less effective in women who have already given birth.[4] A package of three sponges costs $9–15.[5]

Prescription Contraceptive Methods

There are many approaches to contraception that require a physician's prescription. Generally, these methods have higher effectiveness rates, but they also come with possible risks and side effects to the user. Some devices require careful fitting or placement. Some prescription methods use devices that require the user to follow careful instructions. Some approaches use hormones that can have dangerous consequences for a very small percentage of users. For these reasons, these products or approaches are not available over-the-counter.

Diaphragm

The **diaphragm** is a soft rubber cup with a springlike metal rim that, when properly fitted and correctly inserted by the user, rests in the top of the vagina. The diaphragm covers the cervical opening (see Figure 13-3). During intercourse, the diaphragm stays in place quite well and usually cannot be felt by either partner.

The diaphragm is always used with a spermicidal cream or gel. The diaphragm should be covered with an adequate amount of spermicide inside the cup and around the rim. When used properly with a spermicide, the diaphragm is a relatively effective contraceptive, and when combined with the man's use of a condom, its effectiveness is even greater.

The diaphragm must be inserted before intercourse. It should provide effective protection for 6 hours. If this time interval extends beyond 6 hours, some clinicians recommend that additional spermicide be placed in the vagina. Use of additional spermicide with multiple acts of intercourse is optional. After intercourse, the diaphragm must be left in place for at least 6 hours before it is removed. Because of the risk of toxic shock syndrome (TSS), the diaphragm must not remain in the vagina longer than 24 hours.[4] Women should avoid using

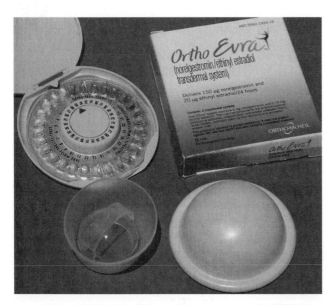

Prescription methods of contraception are those that include hormones, such as combined oral contraceptives and the contraceptive patch, and those that require expert fitting, such as the diaphragm and FemCap.

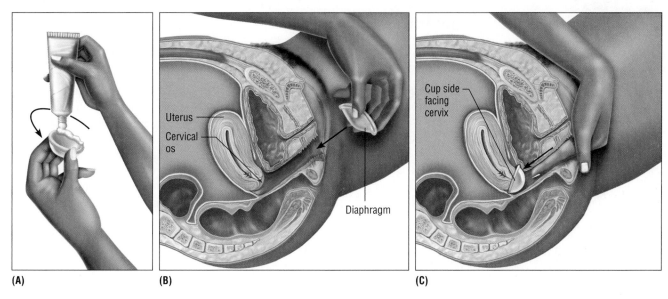

(A)   **(B)**   **(C)**

Figure 13-3 Use of a Diaphragm   A: Spermicidal cream or gel is placed around the rim and inside the cup of the diaphragm. **B:** The diaphragm is folded lengthwise and inserted into the vagina. **C:** The diaphragm is then placed against the cervix so that the cup portion with the spermicide is facing the cervix. The outline of the cervix should be felt through the central part of the diaphragm.

diaphragms or cervical caps during any kind of vaginal bleeding, including menstruation.[5] It is always best to ask a health care provider for specific instructions.

Diaphragms must always be fitted and prescribed by a physician.[9] Typically, it costs $15–75 for a diaphragm and $8–17 for the spermicide. An examination may cost $50–200, but it will be less at a family planning clinic.[5] Also, a high level of motivation to follow the instructions *exactly* is important.

Diaphragms and cervical caps do not provide reliable protection against STDs and HIV infection. Concerns about the spermicide nonoxynol-9 should prompt users to ask their physicians to recommend a cream or gel to use with a diaphragm. If you are concerned about possible infection, either avoid sexual activity or have the man use a latex condom.

FemCap

Approved by the FDA in 2002, the *FemCap* is a reusable (up to two years), hat-shaped cervical cap. The FemCap is the only cervical cap available in the United States today. Made of silicone rubber, the FemCap completely covers the cervix. Coated with spermicide, the Fem-Cap's brim fits snugly against the deep vaginal walls. The attached strap helps in the removal of this device. The FemCap must be prescribed by a physician and comes in three sizes. Among women who have never been pregnant or given birth vaginally, the use-effectiveness rate of this device is 86 percent. For women who have given birth vaginally, the effectiveness rate drops to 71 percent. The cost of the FemCap is about the same as for the diaphragm.[5]

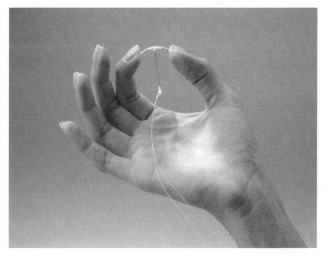

The T-shaped ParaGard IUD works by releasing copper ions that impair sperm function and prevent fertilization.

Intrauterine Device (IUD)

The **intrauterine device (IUD)** is the most popular reversible contraceptive method in the world, although the number of users in the United States is relatively small.

> **Key Terms**
>
> **diaphragm** A soft rubber cup designed to cover the cervix.
>
> **intrauterine device (IUD)** A small, plastic, medicated or unmedicated contraceptive device that prevents pregnancy when inserted into the uterus.

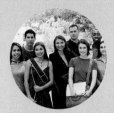
This can be an excellent choice for women who desire a long-term, hassle-free, reversible, highly effective method of contraception. The IUD is especially advantageous for women who have already had at least one child; are in a stable, monogamous relationship; and perhaps are unable to take daily birth control pills.

Two types of IUDs are available in the United States: a T-shaped one containing the hormone progestin (Mirena) and a T-shaped one wrapped with copper wire (ParaGard). The Mirena IUD works by thickening cervical mucus, inhibiting sperm survival, and producing a thin endometrial lining that will not support a fertilized ovum. In some women, Mirena inhibits ovulation. The ParaGard works by releasing copper ions that impair sperm function and prevent fertilization.[4] The Mirena IUD substantially reduces menstrual flow, but the ParaGard may increase menstrual flow. About 20 percent of women who use the Mirena IUD stop having their periods altogether.[10]

The Mirena provides highly effective contraceptive protection for 5 years, and the ParaGard for 12 years. Only a skilled clinician can prescribe and insert an IUD. As with many other forms of contraception, IUDs do not offer protection against STDs, including the AIDS virus.[9]

For many years, the public has been concerned about two potentially serious side effects: *uterine perforation* (in which the IUD embeds itself in the uterine wall) and pelvic inflammatory disease (PID, a widespread infection of the abdominal cavity). However, these events rarely happen, especially when the IUD is inserted by a skilled clinician. Between 2 percent and 10 percent of IUD users experience *expulsion* (muscular contractions that force the IUD out of the uterus) within the first year of use.[4] As Table 13.1 indicates, IUDs are highly effective birth control devices. The cost for an IUD ranges from $500 to $1,000, which includes an exam, insertion, and a follow-up visit. The Mirena tends to cost more than the ParaGard.[5]

Oral Contraceptives

First introduced in the United States in 1960, today's **oral contraceptive pill** provides one of the highest effectiveness rates of any of the reversible contraceptive methods. Only the IUD, the implant, and the injection provide higher effectiveness rates. Worldwide, more than 75 million women are currently using oral contraceptives.[4] A successful male version has not yet been developed (see the box "The Male Contraceptive Pill" for more information).

Use of the pill requires a physical examination by a physician and a prescription. Since oral contraceptives are available in a wide range of formulas, follow-up examinations are important to ensure that a woman is receiving an effective dosage with as few side effects as possible. Determining the right prescription for a particular woman may require a few consultations.

Combined Pills All oral contraceptives contain synthetic (laboratory-made) hormones. The typical *combined pill* uses both synthetic estrogen and synthetic progesterone in each of 21 pills. With *triphasic pills,* the level of estrogen remains constant, but the level of progestin varies every seven days.

The FDA has approved three *extended-cycle oral contraceptives.* Seasonale contains synthetic estrogen and progesterone and is taken for 81 straight days and then followed by 7 days of inactive pills. Seasonique also contains synthetic estrogen and progesterone and is taken for 84 days, but is then followed by 7 days of low-estrogen pills. Women who use either of these contraceptives have only four periods each year. In 2007, the FDA approved the newest extended-cycle pill, called Lybrel. Women take this combined pill each day for a full year and have no periods for 365 days. Although it might seem unnatural to reduce (or eliminate) the frequency of one's period, extended-cycle pills are reported to be as safe as traditional pills. Some women report irregular breakthrough bleeding or spotting when using extended-cycle contraceptives.[11]

The contraceptive effect of the pill can be compromised in women who are also taking certain medicines or supplements. The antibiotic rifampin reduces the pill's effectiveness. Interestingly, other antibiotics do not make the pill less effective. Certain antifungal drugs taken orally for yeast infections, certain anti-HIV protease inhibitors, some antiseizure medications, and the over-the-counter herbal supplement St. John's wort (sometimes used for mild depression) all have the ability to make the pill less effective. Thus, it is very important for a woman to talk with her clinician about the medicines she is taking before she is given any prescription method of birth control.[5]

Oral contraceptives function in several ways. The estrogen in the pill tends to reduce ova development. The progesterone in the pill helps reduce the likelihood of ovulation (by lowering the release of luteinizing hormone). The progesterone in the pill also causes the uterine wall to develop inadequately and helps thicken cervical mucus, thus making it difficult for sperm to enter the uterus. As with many forms of contraception, *oral contraceptives do not provide protection from the transmission of STDs or HIV infection.*

The physical changes produced by the oral contraceptive provide some beneficial side effects in women. Since the synthetic hormones are taken for 21 days and then are followed by **placebo pills** or no pills for 7 days, the menstrual cycle becomes regulated. Even women who have irregular cycles immediately become "regular." Since the uterine lining is not developed to the extent seen in a nonuser, the uterus is not forced to contract with the same amount of vigor. Thus, menstrual cramping is reduced, and the resultant menstrual flow is diminished. Research indicates that the combined pill can provide protection against anemia, PID, noncancerous breast tumors, acne, breast and ovarian cysts, ectopic pregnancy, endometrial cancer, ovarian cancer, and endometriosis.[4]

The negative side effects of the oral contraceptive pill can be divided into two general categories: (1) unpleasant and (2) potentially dangerous. The unpleasant side effects generally subside within two or three months for most women. A number of women report some or many of the following symptoms:

- Tenderness in breast tissue
- Nausea
- Mild headaches
- Slight, irregular spotting
- Weight gain
- Fluctuations in sex drive
- Mild depression
- More frequent vaginal infections

The potentially dangerous side effects of the oral contraceptive pill are most often seen in the cardiovascular system. Blood clots, strokes, hypertension, and heart attack seem to be associated with the estrogen component of the combined pill. However, when compared with the risk to nonusers, the risk of dying from cardiovascular complications is only slightly increased among healthy young oral contraceptive users. Additionally, multiple scientific studies have determined that oral contraceptive use has little, if any, effect on the development of breast cancer, even among women with a family history of breast cancer. This is especially true in women who started taking the pill after 1978, when lower dose formulations began.[4]

Most health professionals agree that the risks related to pregnancy and childbirth are much greater than those associated with oral contraceptive use. Certainly, a woman who is contemplating the use of the pill must discuss all of the risks and benefits with her physician.

There are some **contraindications** for the use of oral contraceptives. If you think you might be pregnant; have a history of blood clots, migraine headaches, liver

---

Key Terms

oral contraceptive pill A pill taken orally, composed of synthetic female hormones that prevent ovulation or implantation; "the pill."

placebo pills Pills that contain no active ingredients.

contraindications Factors that make the use of a drug inappropriate or dangerous for a particular person.

disease, a heart condition, high blood pressure, obesity, diabetes, breast or uterine cancer, hepatitis, or cirrhosis; or have not established regular menstrual cycles, the pill probably should not be your contraceptive choice. Providing a physician with a complete and accurate health history is critically important before a woman starts to take the pill.

Two additional contraindications are well understood by the medical community. Cigarette smoking and advancing age are highly associated with an increased risk of potentially serious side effects. Increasing numbers of physicians are not prescribing oral contraceptives for their patients who smoke. The risk of cardiovascular-related deaths is enhanced for women over age 35. The risk is even higher for female smokers over age 35.[4]

For the vast majority of women, however, the pill, when properly prescribed, is safe and effective. Careful scrutiny of a woman's health history and careful follow-up examinations when a problem is suspected are essential elements that can provide a good margin of safety. Monthly pill packs cost $15–50. An exam may cost $35–250.[5]

Minipills Some women prefer not to use the combined oral contraceptive pill. To avoid some of the potentially serious side effects of the combined pill, some physicians are prescribing **minipills.** These oral contraceptives contain no estrogen—only low-dose progesterone in all pills in a 28-day pill pack. The minipill seems to work by thickening cervical mucus, preventing ovulation, and producing a thin endometrial lining.[4]

The effectiveness of the minipill is slightly lower than that of the combined pill. *Breakthrough bleeding* and **ectopic pregnancy** are more common in minipill users than in combined-pill users. Yet some women using minipills have no periods, some get a period in the fourth week, and some have irregular bleeding throughout the 28-day month. The cost of minipills is similar to that of combined pills.

Injectable Contraceptive

Depo-Provera is a highly effective (99 percent+) injectable progesterone contraceptive that provides protection for three months. This hormone shot works primarily by preventing ovulation and thickening the cervical mucus to keep sperm from joining with the egg.

The most common side effects of Depo-Provera are irregular bleeding and spotting followed by *amenorrhea* (the absence of periods).[4] When the woman's body adjusts to the presence of this drug, breakthrough bleeding diminishes, and the most common side effect is amenorrhea. Many women see this as a desirable effect. Women who stop using Depo-Provera may experience infertility for a period of up to one year.[4] The cost of Depo-Provera

ranges from $35 to $75 per injection. The initial exam could cost $35–250.[12]

Contraceptive Implant

In July 2006, the FDA approved the use of a progestin-based contraceptive implant called Implanon. This thin, flexible plastic device, about the size of a matchstick, is inserted just under the skin of the upper arm. Implanon works by slowly releasing progestin for up to three years.[12] The progestin inhibits ovulation and also thickens the cervical mucus to prevent the sperm from joining with an egg. Studies indicate that this contraceptive implant is nearly as effective as sterilization.[4]

Many of the health concerns that apply to other hormone-based contraceptives (including drug interactions that can lower its effectiveness) apply to the implant as well. The cost of this device and its insertion ranges from $400 to $800. Removal of the implant costs $75–150.[5]

Contraceptive Ring

One of the newest contraceptives on the market is the vaginal **contraceptive ring** (NuvaRing). Available by prescription, NuvaRing is a thin polymer ring (2⅛ inches in diameter and ⅛ inch thick) that contains synthetic estrogen and progestin. Users insert this device deep into the vagina where it remains for three weeks. At the end of the third week, the device is removed for a week and the woman has her period.[13] The NuvaRing provides effective contraception (99 percent+ effective when used perfectly) for the entire four-week time frame.

The ring functions in a manner similar to the oral contraceptive pill: It reduces the chances of ovulation and thickens cervical mucus. Women who use the ring cannot at the same time use caps or diaphragms as a backup method. The contraceptive ring does not protect against sexually transmitted diseases. As with all prescribed forms of contraception, women should discuss all the benefits, risks, and possible side effects with their health care providers. The costs of the contraceptive ring are about $15–70 per month for the device and $35–250 for the initial exam.[5]

Contraceptive Patch

In 2002, the Ortho Evra **contraceptive patch** became available to women. This patch contains continuous levels of estrogen and progestin delivered from a 1¾-inch square patch that is applied weekly to one of four areas on the woman's body: the buttocks, abdomen, upper chest (front and back, excluding the breasts), or upper outer arm.[14] The patch remains attached even while a woman bathes, swims, or exercises. After three weeks of

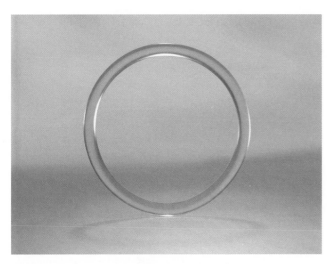

The NuvaRing contraceptive ring is a flexible ring about 2⅛ inches in diameter. When inserted into the vagina, it delivers a low dose of hormones similar to those found in oral contraceptives.

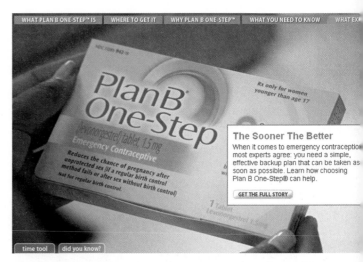

Plan B One-Step emergency contraception consists of one pill taken within 72 hours of unprotected sex. Nonprescription behind-the-counter access to Plan B One-Step (or Next Choice) has been approved for persons age 17 and older.

patches, the woman uses no patch for the fourth week, during which time she has her period. The patch functions in a manner similar to the oral contraceptive pill. Like all hormonal methods of contraception, the patch does not protect against sexually transmitted diseases. The patch costs about $15–70 per month and $35–250 for the initial exam.[5]

Many women have used the patch successfully, but some concerns have arisen over possible increased cardiovascular risks (blood clots, strokes, heart attacks) due to the way the hormones are delivered to the user. On the home page of the Ortho Evra website, the manufacturer clearly states that patch users will be exposed to about 60 percent more estrogen than that coming from a typical birth control pill taken by mouth that contains 35 micrograms (μg) of estrogen.[14] For this reason, it is especially important that potential users discuss with their health care provider whether this is a good contraceptive choice. This precaution is even more important for women who are smokers and women over the age of 35.

Emergency Contraception

Emergency contraception is designed to prevent pregnancy after unprotected vaginal intercourse, such as when a condom breaks, when a couple uses no method of contraception, or when someone forces another to have intercourse. This method is also called *postcoital* or *"morning after"* contraception. (Emergency contraception is not the "abortion pill" or RU-486.) Emergency contraception is available in two forms: emergency hormonal contraception and the insertion of an IUD.

Emergency contraception works by preventing ovulation or fertilization, thickening cervical mucus, and thinning the lining of the uterus. It won't work if you are already pregnant, and it won't terminate an existing pregnancy. Emergency contraception will not prevent STDs or infections.[5]

Currently, the FDA has approved three drugs for emergency contraception. All three use oral pills. Plan B One-Step is a single progesterone pill taken in one dose. Next Choice is a two-progesterone-pill approach. Women using either plan are instructed to start their emergency contraception as soon as possible but no later than 72 hours (three days) after contraceptive failure or unprotected sex. (Women using Next Choice would take their second pill 12 hours after their first one.) If taken correctly, these drugs reduce the risk of pregnancy by 89 percent.[5]

Key Terms

minipills Low-dose progesterone oral contraceptives.

ectopic pregnancy A pregnancy in which the fertilized ovum implants at a site other than the uterus, typically in the fallopian tubes.

contraceptive ring A thin, polymer contraceptive device containing estrogen and progestin; placed deep within the vagina for a three-week period.

contraceptive patch Contraceptive skin patch containing estrogen and progestin; replaced each week for a three-week period.

emergency contraception Contraceptive measures used to prevent pregnancy within five days of unprotected intercourse; also called *postcoital* or *morning-after contraception*.

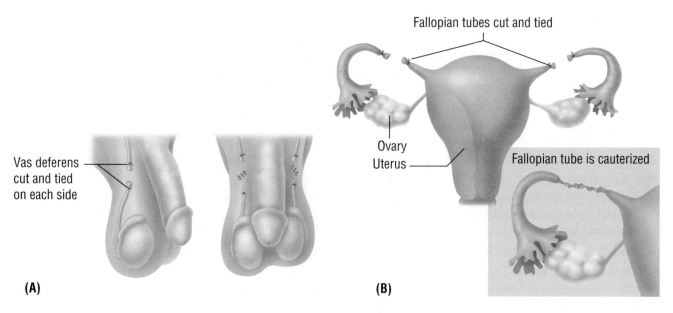

Figure 13-4 The Most Frequently Used Forms of Male and Female Sterilization   A: Vasectomy. B: Tubal ligation.

Plan B One-Step and Next Choice are available at drugstores as over-the-counter products to women and men age 17 and older. However, they are not available on aisle shelves. Like nicotine-replacement medications, these drugs are located behind the pharmacist's counter. Some pharmacists may ask for identification to verify a young person's age.

The third form of emergency contraception is the latest approach. Approved in 2010, *ella* is a pill that uses not progesterone, but rather a nonhormonal drug that blocks the likelihood of ovulation and, possibly, implantation. *Ella*'s key difference from the other approved emergency contraceptives is that it does not lose its effectiveness for 120 hours (or five days) after unprotected intercourse.[15] However, *ella* is not available over-the-counter. Users will need a physician's prescription to purchase *ella*.

The most commonly reported side effects of emergency hormonal contraception are nausea and vomiting. Less than 25 percent of users experience nausea. The use of antinausea medication can help offset the nausea and vomiting. Some women also report fatigue, breast tenderness, abdominal pain, headaches, and dizziness. These side effects subside within a day or two after treatment. Costs for emergency contraception range from $10 to $70.[5]

The copper-wrapped IUD is a less commonly used, but highly effective, form of emergency contraception. To function as a contraceptive, however, the ParaGard IUD must be inserted within 5 days after unprotected intercourse.

Permanent Contraceptive Methods

All the contraceptive mechanisms or methods already discussed have one quality in common: They are reversible.

Although microsurgical techniques are providing medical breakthroughs, **sterilization** should generally be considered an irreversible procedure. Attempts to reverse sterilization are quite difficult and very expensive.

Therefore, couples considering sterilization procedures usually must undergo extensive discussions with a physician or family planning counselor to identify their true feelings about this finality. Sterilization does not protect one against sexually transmitted diseases, including HIV infection.

Male Sterilization

The male sterilization procedure is called a *vasectomy*. Accomplished with a local anesthetic in a physician's office, this 20- to 30-minute procedure consists of the surgical removal of a section of each vas deferens. After a small incision is made through the scrotum, the vasa deferentia are located and a small section from each removed. The remaining ends are either tied, clamped, or *cauterized* (see Figure 13-4A). A nonincision (no-scalpel, no-sutures) vasectomy method uses a tiny puncture tool to reach both tubes. This procedure is gaining in popularity because of its simplicity, effectiveness, and quick recovery time.

After a vasectomy, sperm may still be present in the vasa deferentia. A backup contraceptive is recommended until a physician microscopically examines a semen specimen. This examination usually occurs about three months after the surgery. After a vasectomy, men can still produce male sex hormones, get erections, have orgasms, and ejaculate. (Recall that sperm account for only a small portion of the semen.) Some men even report increased interest in sexual activity, since their chances of impregnating a woman are virtually eliminated. Most men wait about a week before resuming sexual activity.

What happens to the process of spermatogenesis within each testicle? Sperm cells are still being produced, but they are destroyed by specialized white blood cells called *phagocytic leukocytes*. The cost of a vasectomy ranges from $350 to $1,000.[5]

Female Sterilization

Female sterilization can be accomplished in a number of ways.

Tubal Ligation   The most common method of female sterilization is *tubal ligation*. During this procedure, the fallopian tubes are cut and the ends are tied back. Some physicians cauterize the tube ends to ensure complete sealing (see Figure 13-4B). The fallopian tubes are usually reached through the abdominal wall. In a *minilaparotomy*, a small incision is made in the abdominal wall just below the navel. The resultant scar is quite small and is the basis for the term *Band-Aid surgery*.

Female sterilization requires about 20–30 minutes, with the patient under local or general anesthesia. The use of a *laparoscope* has made female sterilization much simpler than in the past. The laparoscope is a small tube equipped with mirrors and lights. Inserted through a single incision, the laparoscope locates the fallopian tubes before they are cut, tied, or cauterized. When a laparoscope is used through an abdominal incision, the procedure is called a *laparoscopy*.

Nonincision Sterilization   Two new nonincision methods of female sterilization, Essure and Adiana, have been approved by the FDA. In the Essure approach, a physician inserts a small, soft metallic coil into the vagina, through the cervix, and directly into each fallopian tube. This procedure is done under local anesthetic and takes about a half-hour. Once inserted, the coils encourage scar tissue growth that eventually blocks the fallopian tubes. If the tubes are obstructed, sperm are blocked from meeting the ovum. After three months, a woman returns to her physician for an x-ray test to determine whether the tubes are fully obstructed. During these first three months, couples must use another form of birth control. Cramping is the most common side effect. Reports indicate that Essure has a near 100 percent effectiveness rate.[4]

Adiana is the most recent nonincision sterilization procedure. Similar to the Essure coil, this procedure involves placing an insert into each fallopian tube to encourage scar tissue growth. Adiana differs from Essure in two main ways: (1) Adiana uses a low level of radiofrequency waves to create a small, superficial lesion in each fallopian tube where the insert will be placed, and (2) the Adiana insert is a silicone matrix (not a metallic coil) about the size of a grain of rice.

After the 12-minute procedure to insert the matrix, women recover quickly and can resume normal activities within a day. They must use a backup method of birth control for three months, until a special test determines whether the tubes are fully blocked. Adiana's website reports that, after three years of clinical data, Adiana is 98.4 percent effective in preventing pregnancy.[16]

Women who are sterilized still produce female hormones, ovulate, and menstruate. However, the ovum cannot move down the fallopian tube. Within a day of its release, the ovum will start to disintegrate and be absorbed by the body. Freed of the possibility of becoming pregnant, many sterilized women report an increase in sex drive and activity. Sterilization does not initiate signs or symptoms of menopause or cause menopause to occur earlier. Tubal ligation costs range from $1,500 to $6,000.[5]

Other Approaches   Two other procedures produce sterilization in women: *ovariectomy* (the surgical removal of the ovaries) and *hysterectomy* (the surgical removal of the uterus). However, these procedures are used to remove diseased (cancerous, cystic, or hemorrhaging) organs and are not considered primary sterilization techniques.

Abortion

Regardless of the circumstances under which pregnancy occurs, women may now choose to terminate their pregnancies. No longer must women who do not want to be pregnant seek potentially dangerous, illegal abortions. On the basis of current technology and legality, women need never experience childbirth. The decision is theirs to make.

Abortion should never be considered a first-line, preferred form of fertility control. Rather, abortion is a final, last-chance undertaking. It should be used only when responsible control of one's fertility could not be achieved. The decision to abort a fetus is a highly controversial, personal one—one that needs serious consideration by each woman.

On the basis of the landmark 1973 U.S. Supreme Court case *Roe v. Wade*, the United States joined many of the world's most populated countries in legalizing abortions. Abortions are quite common. Among women in the United States, more than one out of three have had an abortion by age 45.[5] In 2008, 1.21 million women in the United States made the decision to terminate a pregnancy.[17]

Key Terms

sterilization   Generally permanent birth control techniques that surgically disrupt the normal passage of ova or sperm.

abortion   Induced premature termination of a pregnancy.

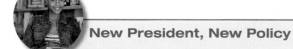
Thousands of additional women probably considered abortion but elected to continue their pregnancies.

Abortion is a political issue (see the box "New President, New Policy"). The rhetoric from both sides of the debate can be intense. For example, anti-abortion (pro-life) supporters often claim that women who have abortions increase their risk of developing breast cancer. However, the National Cancer Institute (NCI), the American Cancer Society (ACI), and the American College of Obstetricians and Gynecologists continue to report that abortion, whether induced or spontaneous, is not linked to an increase in breast cancer risk.[18,19] The heated arguments will undoubtedly continue.

Regardless of the eventual outcomes of this multi-faceted debate, here are the present abortion procedures available in the United States.

First-Trimester Abortion Procedures

The first trimester consists of the first 13 weeks (91 days) of pregnancy. During the first 49 days after a woman's last menstrual period, a woman has two options for terminating a pregnancy: *vacuum aspiration* or *medication abortion*. Once 63 days have passed, only vacuum aspiration is an abortion option.[4] Eighty-eight percent of all abortions are performed during the first trimester.[17]

Vacuum Aspiration There are two common methods of performing vacuum aspiration abortions. Both procedures can be performed in a physician's office or in a hospital. Both procedures require **dilation** of the cervix. The method used depends on how long the woman has been pregnant. Together, these methods represent the most widely used abortion procedures in the United States.

The **manual vacuum aspiration (MVA)** procedure can be performed in the earliest part of the first trimester, from the time a woman knows she is pregnant and up to 10 weeks after her last period. After a physician injects a local anesthetic into the cervix, dilators can be used to enlarge the cervical opening. The physician then inserts a small tube into the uterus and applies suction with a handheld instrument. By rotating and moving this small tube across the uterine wall, the physician can empty the uterus. A return visit to the physician is an important follow-up procedure.[4]

After the first month of pregnancy and throughout the first trimester, physicians typically select **dilation and suction curettage (D&C)** (frequently called *vacuum aspiration*) as the abortion procedure of choice. D&C is similar to MVA, but the clinician uses a vacuum machine rather than a manually operated suction instrument. The clinician tends to use more sedation for the woman, in addition to the local cervical anesthetic. The cervix is stretched open with dilators that gradually enlarge the opening to permit the insertion of a tube. This tube is attached to a vacuum machine that empties the uterus with gentle suction. If the physician believes that additional endometrial tissue remains in the uterus, he or she can use a **curette** to scrape the wall of the uterus. A subsequent visit to the clinician is an important follow-up procedure. Costs range from $350 to $950.[5]

Medication Abortion Mifepristone is an oral pill that a woman can use under medical supervision to induce a **medication abortion** during the first trimester. Formerly known as RU-486, mifepristone blocks the action of progesterone and causes the uterine lining and any fertilized egg to shed. The pill is marketed as Mifeprex and is available only through physicians and clinics.[20] The cost of a medication abortion is about the same as the cost of first-trimester surgical procedures, or about $350–650.[5]

Under FDA guidelines, women must use mifepristone within 49 days of the start of their last menstrual period. Women take three pills at the first doctor visit and then return 48 hours later to take a second drug, misoprostol, which causes menstruation to occur, usually within about 5 hours. A third visit to a physician is necessary to ensure that the abortion was successful and the woman is recovering well from the procedure. With a success rate of 92–95 percent, the abortion pill is a highly effective approach.[5] In 2008, 17 percent of all abortions in the United States were medication abortions.[17]

Second-Trimester Abortion Procedures

When a woman's pregnancy continues beyond the thirteenth week of gestation, termination becomes a more difficult matter. The procedures at this stage are more complicated and take longer to complete. Generally, they cost more than first-trimester abortions.

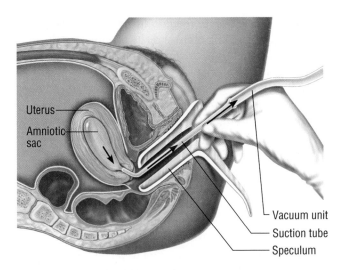

Uterus
Amniotic sac

Vacuum unit
Suction tube
Speculum

Figure 13-5 Dilation and Evacuation The cervix is dilated and the contents of the uterus are aspirated (removed by suction). This procedure is used to perform abortions during the second trimester.

Dilation and Evacuation Between 13 and 16 weeks of pregnancy, the abortion method of choice is **dilation and evacuation (D&E).** In the United States, almost all second-trimester abortions use the D&E procedure. Some physicians use this method up through 24 weeks or more of pregnancy.[4] The D&E is a more involved surgical procedure than is a D&C and generally requires greater dilation of the cervix, larger medical instruments (including forceps), suction, and curettage (see Figure 13-5). Some women may be given a general anesthetic during D&E procedures. After a D&E, a return visit to the clinician is an important follow-up procedure.

The cost of a second-trimester abortion is greater than that for a first-trimester abortion. The cost will vary depending on the length of the pregnancy and the facility one selects. Hospitals are usually more expensive than clinics.[5]

Note: Procedures that once used drugs or salt solutions to produce a second-trimester abortion are rarely used today.

Third-Trimester Abortion Procedures

If termination of a pregnancy is required in the latter weeks of the gestational period, a surgical procedure in which the fetus is removed (*hysterotomy*) or in which the entire uterus is removed (*hysterectomy*) can be undertaken. These procedures are more complicated and involve longer hospitalization, major abdominal surgery, and an extended period of recovery.

A Final Word About Birth Control

In the heat of passion, people often fail to think rationally about the potential outcomes of unprotected sex. Therefore,

the time to prepare for the romantic moment is *before* you are in a position where you don't want to think about the possibility of an unintended result. If you choose to be sexually active, find a form of protection that works well for you and use it consistently. If you choose not to be sexually active, realize that this is a viable choice that can be 100 percent effective.

Pregnancy

Pregnancy is a condition that requires a series of complex yet coordinated changes to occur in the female body. This discussion follows pregnancy from its beginning, at fertilization, to its conclusion, with labor and childbirth.

Physiological Obstacles and Aids to Fertilization

Many sexually active young people believe that they will become pregnant (or impregnate someone) only when they want to, despite their haphazard contraceptive practices. Because of this mistaken belief, many young people are not sold on the use of contraceptives. It is important for young adults to remember that from a species survival standpoint, our bodies were designed to promote pregnancy. It is estimated that about 85 percent of sexually active women of childbearing age will become pregnant within one year if they do not use some form of contraception.[4]

With regard to pregnancy, each act of intercourse can be considered a game of physiological odds. There are obstacles that may reduce a couple's chance of pregnancy, including the following.

> **Key Terms**
>
> **dilation** Gradual expansion of an opening or passageway, such as the cervix.
>
> **manual vacuum aspiration (MVA)** The abortion procedure performed in the earliest weeks after a pregnancy is established.
>
> **dilation and suction curettage (D&C)** A surgical procedure in which the cervical canal is dilated to allow the uterine wall to be scraped; vacuum aspiration.
>
> **curette** A metal scraping instrument that resembles a spoon with a cup-shaped cutting surface on its end.
>
> **medication abortion** An abortion caused by the use of prescribed drugs.
>
> **dilation and evacuation (D&E)** A second-trimester abortion procedure that requires greater dilation, suction, and curettage than first-trimester vacuum aspiration procedures.

Obstacles to Fertilization

- *The acid in the vagina is destructive to sperm.* The low pH of the vagina kills sperm that fail to enter the uterus quickly.

- *The cervical mucus is thick during most of the menstrual cycle.* Sperm movement into the uterus is more difficult, except during the few days surrounding ovulation.

- *The sperm must locate the cervical opening.* The cervical opening is small compared with the rest of the surface area where sperm are deposited.

- *Half of the sperm travel through the wrong fallopian tube.* Most commonly, only one ovum is released at ovulation. The two ovaries generally "take turns" each month. The sperm have no way of "knowing" which tube they should enter. Thus, it is probable that half will travel through the wrong tube.

- *The distance sperm must travel is relatively long compared with the tiny size of the sperm cells.* Microscopic sperm must travel about 7 or 8 inches once they are inside the female.

- *The sperm's travel is relatively "upstream."* The anatomical positioning of the female reproductive structures necessitates an "uphill" movement by the sperm.

- *The contoured folds of the tubal walls trap many sperm.* These folds make it difficult for sperm to locate the egg. Many sperm are trapped in this maze.

There are also a variety of aids that tend to help sperm and egg cells join. Some of these are listed here.

Aids to Fertilization

- *An astounding number of sperm are deposited during ejaculation.* Each ejaculation contains about a teaspoon of semen.[2] Within this quantity are 200–500 million sperm cells. Even with large numbers of sperm killed in the vagina, millions are able to move to the deeper structures.

- *Sperm are deposited near the cervical opening.* Penetration into the vagina by the penis allows for the sperm to be placed near the cervical opening.

- *The male accessory glands help make the semen nonacidic.* The seminal vesicles, prostate gland, and Cowper's glands secrete fluids that provide an alkaline environment for the sperm. This environment helps sperm be better protected in the vagina until they can move into the deeper, more alkaline uterus and fallopian tubes.[3]

- *Uterine contractions aid sperm movement.* The rhythmic muscular contractions of the uterus tend to cause the sperm to move in the direction of the fallopian tubes.

- *Sperm cells move rather quickly.* Despite their tiny size, sperm cells can move relatively quickly—just about 1 inch per hour. Powered by sugar solutions from the male accessory glands and the whiplike movements of their tails, sperm can reach the distant third of the fallopian tubes in less than eight hours as they swim in the direction of the descending ovum.

- *Once inside the fallopian tubes, sperm can live for days.* Most sperm will survive an average of 48–72 hours. However, some sperm may be viable for up to a week after reaching the comfortable, nonacidic environment of the fallopian tubes. Thus, they can "wait in the wings" for the moment an ovum is released from the ovary (see Figure 13-6).

- *The cervical mucus is thin and watery at the time of ovulation.* This mucus allows for better passage of sperm through the cervical opening when the ovum is most capable of being fertilized.

Signs of Pregnancy

Aside from pregnancy tests done in a professional laboratory, a woman can sometimes recognize early signs and symptoms. The signs of pregnancy have been divided into three categories.

Presumptive Signs of Pregnancy

- Missed period after unprotected intercourse the previous month
- Nausea on awakening (morning sickness)
- Increase in the size and tenderness of breasts
- Darkening of the areolar tissue surrounding the nipples

Probable Signs of Pregnancy

- Increase in the frequency of urination (the growing uterus presses against the bladder)
- Increase in the size of the abdomen
- Cervix becomes softer by the sixth week (detected by a pelvic examination by clinician)
- Positive pregnancy test

Positive Signs of Pregnancy

- Determination of a fetal heartbeat
- Feeling of the fetus moving (*quickening*)
- Observation of the fetus by ultrasound or optical viewers

Home Pregnancy Tests   Using a woman's urine, home pregnancy tests detect the presence of human chorionic gonadotropin (hCG), a hormone produced during pregnancy by the woman's placenta.[21] These tests contain

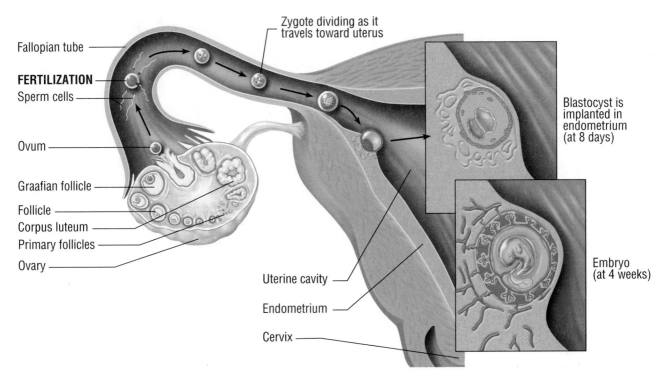

Figure 13-6 Fertilization and Implantation After its release from the follicle, the ovum begins its weeklong journey down the fallopian tube. Fertilization generally occurs in the outermost third of the tube. After conception, the zygote progresses toward the uterus, where it embeds itself in the endometrium. A pregnancy is established.

The labels in the figure are:
- Fallopian tube
- **FERTILIZATION**
- Sperm cells
- Ovum
- Graafian follicle
- Follicle
- Corpus luteum
- Primary follicles
- Ovary
- Zygote dividing as it travels toward uterus
- Blastocyst is implanted in endometrium (at 8 days)
- Embryo (at 4 weeks)
- Uterine cavity
- Endometrium
- Cervix

monoclonal antibodies, which are molecules coated with a substance that bonds to the hCG hormone. If hCG is present, a colored stripe, dot, or other symbol appears in the test windows. Improved technology has made these home test kits highly accurate.

Although the makers of today's tests say their products can detect hCG as soon as the very day a missed period was supposed to begin, they also advise taking the test again a few days later to confirm the result. If the result is positive, one should see a doctor as soon as possible.

Agents That Can Damage a Fetus

A large number of agents that come into contact with a pregnant woman can affect fetal development. Many of these (rubella and herpes viruses, tobacco smoke, alcohol, and virtually all other drugs) are discussed in other chapters of this text. The best advice for a pregnant woman is to maintain close contact with her obstetrician during pregnancy and to consider carefully the ingestion of any OTC drug (including aspirin, caffeine, and antacids) that could possibly harm the fetus.

All pregnant women should also avoid exposure to radiation during pregnancy. Such exposure, most commonly through excessive x-rays or radiation fallout from nuclear testing, can irreversibly damage fetal genetic structures. In addition, pregnant women should avoid

taking Accutane, a drug prescribed for the treatment of cystic acne, because it can severely damage a fetus.[9]

Maintaining a Healthy Pregnancy

The process of having a healthy pregnancy and delivering a healthy child actually should begin in the months before conception. During these preconception months, obstetricians advise women to stop smoking, stop drinking alcoholic beverages, eat well, get physical exercise, avoid or treat infections, avoid unnecessary exposure to toxic chemicals, and ask a physician before consuming any drug (prescription or over-the-counter).

Once the pregnancy is established, it is important to follow additional guidelines:

- Arrange for prenatal care.
- Consume a well-balanced diet.
- Take a vitamin supplement that contains folic acid.
- Exercise according to a physician's recommendation.
- Avoid and treat infections.
- Avoid alcohol, tobacco, and other drugs.
- Limit caffeine intake.
- Stay away from x-rays, hot tubs, and saunas.
- Stay away from toxic chemicals.

An expectant father can also participate in this healthy regimen by matching the woman's lifestyle changes. This provides sound emotional support for the pregnancy and, as an added bonus, improves the overall health of the dad. (See the box "Keepsake Ultrasounds" for an additional concern for expectant parents.)

Intrauterine Development

Intrauterine development takes place over the course of three **trimesters.** Most pregnancies last 38–42 weeks. For purposes of illustration, we will consider each trimester to be 13 weeks. The growth and development during these trimesters occurs in a typical pattern for most pregnancies.

First Trimester   The first 13-week trimester starts at conception, when the egg and sperm unite to form a structure called a **zygote.** The zygote, or fertilized egg, undergoes a series of cellular changes as it grows and makes its weeklong journey down the fallopian tube to the uterus. On about the tenth day after conception, the zygote, now called a **blastocyst,** embeds itself in the endometrial lining of the uterus. From the end of the second week after conception until the end of the eighth week, the growing structure is called an **embryo.** After eight weeks and until the birth, it is called a **fetus.**

The first trimester is characterized by rapid cellular growth. By the end of the first trimester, the fetus weighs only about 1 ounce, yet most body organs are formed and the fetus can move.[22] It is currently thought that about half of all pregnancies end in **spontaneous abortion** during the early weeks of the first trimester, usually before the woman realizes she is pregnant. These miscarriages usually result from a genetic defect or a fatal error in fetal development.

Second Trimester   The second trimester is characterized by continued growth and maturation. During this time, the organs continue to grow and physicians can easily hear the fetal heartbeat with a stethoscope. The bone structures are fully evident during the second trimester. The fetus starts to look more like an infant.

Additionally, the mother's breast weight increases by about 30 percent because of the deposition of 2–4 pounds of fat. This fat serves as a reserve energy source for the mother should she decide to nurse her baby. For this reason, good maternal nutrition is essential during the second trimester.[22]

Third Trimester   The third trimester is another critical time for the developing fetus. At the beginning of this trimester, the fetus generally weighs about 2–3 pounds. Over the final 13 weeks of gestation, the fetus will double in length and multiply its weight by three to four times.

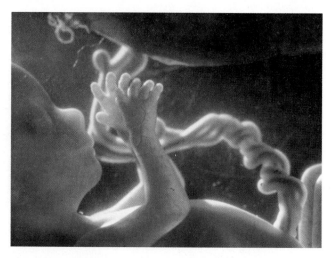

The fetus at 16 weeks' gestation within the amniotic sac.

This is also the time when the fetus absorbs considerable amounts of the minerals iron and calcium from the mother. For this reason, the mother must maintain sound eating patterns and avoid depleting her body's mineral stores, perhaps by taking a vitamin and mineral supplement containing iron, which would reduce her risk of developing anemia during the final trimester.[22]

Childbirth: The Labor of Delivery

Childbirth, or *parturition,* is one of the true peak life experiences for both men and women. Most of the time, childbirth is a wonderfully exciting venture into the unknown. For the parents, this intriguing experience

> **Key Terms**
>
> **trimester** A three-month period of time; human pregnancies encompass three trimesters.
>
> **zygote** A fertilized ovum.
>
> **blastocyst** Early stage of the developing life form that embeds itself in the endometrial lining of the uterus.
>
> **embryo** Developmental stage from the end of the second week after conception until the end of the eighth week.
>
> **fetus** Developmental stage from the beginning of the ninth week after conception until birth.
>
> **spontaneous abortion** Any cessation of pregnancy resulting from natural causes; also called a *miscarriage.*
>
> **false labor** Conditions that resemble the start of true labor; may include irregular uterine contractions, pressure, and discomfort in the lower abdomen.

Keepsake Ultrasounds

The March of Dimes, the FDA, and many health experts believe that ultrasound screening procedures, when properly used by medical personnel, are safe and will not cause harmful side effects to the mother or her baby.* Unlike x-ray tests that use radiation, ultrasound uses high-frequency sound waves, inaudible to the human ear. Typical ultrasounds produce somewhat "fuzzy photographs" of the baby that trained personnel can use to detect various health indicators and possible health complications. Parents often like to keep these as mementos.

Newer types of ultrasound have the ability to show three-dimensional views of the fetus. These are called *3-D* (for three-dimensional pictures) and *4-D* (for moving picture) *ultrasounds*. Since they produce a clarity that exceeds that seen in regular ultrasounds, they can be especially helpful in detecting birth defects when performed in a medical center.

However, there has been an increase in the number of parents who are going to commercial facilities and requesting ultrasounds (including 3-D and 4-D) to keep as family mementos or keepsakes. This has drawn the ire of the FDA, the March of Dimes, and medical experts. Their concern is that nonmedical ultrasounds could be given by untrained and unsupervised personnel who could then provide inaccurate or harmful information to the parents. The consensus recommendation is to avoid nonmedical ultrasounds.[†]

*WebMd, Prenatal ultrasound. www.webmd.com/baby/ultrasound, accessed March 26, 2011.
[†]March of Dimes, Prenatal care: ultrasound. www.marchofdimes.com/pregnancy/prenatalcare_ultrasound, accessed March 26, 2011.

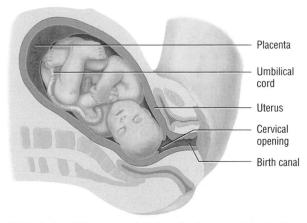

(A) First stage: Effacement and dilation. Uterine contractions thin the cervix and enlarge the cervical opening.

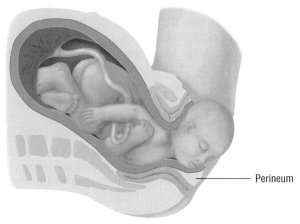

(B) Second stage: Delivery of the fetus. Uterine contractions are aided by mother's voluntary contractions of abdominal muscles. The fetus moves through dilated cervical opening and birth canal.

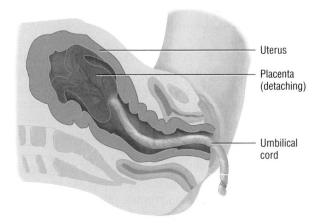

(C) Third stage: Delivery of the placenta. Placenta detaches from uterine wall and is delivered through the birth canal.

Figure 13-7 Labor and Delivery

can provide a stage for personal growth, maturity, and insight into a dynamic, complex world.

During the last few weeks of the third *trimester,* most fetuses move deeper into the pelvic cavity in a process called *lightening.* During this movement, the fetus's body rotates and the head begins to engage more deeply in the mother's pelvic girdle. Many women will report that the baby has "dropped."

Another indication that parturition may be relatively near is the increased reporting of *Braxton Hicks contractions.*[6] These uterine contractions, which are of mild intensity and often occur at irregular intervals, may be felt throughout a pregnancy. During the last few weeks of pregnancy (*gestation*), these mild contractions can occur more frequently and may cause a woman to feel as if she is going into labor (**false labor**).

Labor begins when uterine contractions become more intense and occur at regular intervals. The birth of a child can be divided into three stages: (1) *effacement* and dilation of the cervix, (2) delivery of the fetus, and (3) delivery of the placenta (see Figure 13-7). For a woman having her first child, the birth process lasts an average of 12–16 hours. The average length of labor for subsequent births is much shorter—from 4 to 10 hours on average. Labor is very unpredictable: labors that last between 1 and 24 hours occur daily at most hospitals.

Stage One: Effacement and Dilation of the Cervix

In the first stage of labor, the uterine contractions attempt to thin (*efface*) the normally thick cervical walls and to enlarge (*dilate*) the cervical opening.[2] These contractions are directed by the release of prostaglandins and the hormone oxytocin into the circulating bloodstream.

The first stage of labor is often the longest. The cervical opening must thin and dilate to a diameter of 10 cm before the first stage of labor is considered complete.[3] Often this stage begins with the dislodging of the cervical mucus plug. The subsequent *bloody show* (mucus plug and a small amount of blood) at the vaginal opening may indicate that effacement and dilation have begun. Another indication of labor's onset may be the bursting or tearing of the fetal amniotic sac. "Breaking the bag of waters" refers to this phenomenon, which happens in various measures in expectant women.

The uterine contractions become more intense as the woman moves through this first stage of labor. As the cervical opening effaces and dilates 0–3 cm, many women report feeling happy, exhilarated, and confident. In the *early phase of the first stage* of labor, the contractions are relatively short (lasting 15–60 seconds), and the intervals between contractions range from 20 minutes to 5 minutes as labor progresses. However, these rest intervals will become shorter and the contractions more forceful when the woman's uterus contracts to dilate 4–7 cm.

In this *second phase of the first stage* of labor, the contractions usually last about 1 minute each, and the rest intervals drop from about 5 minutes to 1 minute over a period of 5–9 hours.

The *third phase of the first stage* of labor is called *transition*. During transition, the uterus contracts to dilate the cervical opening to the full 10 cm required for safe passage of the fetus out of the uterus and into the birth canal (vagina).[9] This period of labor is often the most painful part of the entire birth process. Fortunately, it is also the shortest phase of most labors. Lasting 15–30 minutes, transition contractions often last 60–90 seconds each. The rest intervals between contractions are short and vary from 30 to 60 seconds.

An examination of the cervix by a nurse or physician will reveal whether full dilation of 10 cm has occurred. Until the full 10-cm dilation, women are cautioned not to "push" the fetus during the contractions. Special breathing and concentration techniques help many women cope with the first stage of labor.

Stage Two: Delivery of the Fetus

Once the mother's cervix is fully dilated, she enters the second stage of labor, the delivery of the fetus through the birth canal. Now the mother is encouraged to help push the fetus out (with her abdominal muscles) during each contraction. In this second stage, the uterine contractions are less forceful than during the transition phase of the first stage and may last 60 seconds each, with a 1- to 3-minute rest interval.

This second stage may last up to 2 hours in first births.[2] For subsequent births, this stage will usually be much shorter. When the baby's head is first seen at the vaginal opening, *crowning* is said to have taken place. Generally, the back of the baby's head appears first. (Infants whose feet or buttocks are presented first are said to be delivered in a *breech position*.) Once the head is delivered, the baby's body rotates upward to let the shoulders come through. The rest of the body follows quite quickly. The second stage of labor ends when the fetus is fully expelled from the birth canal.

Stage Three: Delivery of the Placenta

Usually within 30 minutes after the fetus is delivered, the uterus again initiates a series of contractions to expel the placenta (or *afterbirth*). The placenta is examined by the attending physician to ensure that it was completely expelled. Torn remnants of the placenta could lead to dangerous *hemorrhaging* by the mother. Often the physician will perform a manual examination of the uterus after the placenta has been delivered.

Once the placenta has been delivered, the uterus will continue with mild contractions to help control bleeding and start the gradual reduction of the uterus to its normal, nonpregnant size. This final aspect of the birth process is called **postpartum.** External abdominal massage of the lower abdomen seems to help the uterus contract, as does an infant's nursing at the mother's breast (see the box "Benefits of Successful Breast-Feeding").

Cesarean Deliveries

A **cesarean delivery** (cesarean birth, C-section) is a procedure in which the fetus is surgically removed from the mother's uterus through the abdominal wall. This type of delivery, which is completed in up to an hour, can be performed with the mother having a regional or a general anesthetic. A cesarean delivery is necessary when the health of either the baby or the mother is at risk.

Although a cesarean delivery is considered major surgery, most mothers cope well with the delivery and

---

Key Terms

postpartum The period after the birth of a baby, during which the mother's body returns to its prepregnancy state.

cesarean delivery Surgical removal of a fetus through the abdominal wall.

postsurgical and postpartum discomfort. The hospital stay is usually a few days longer than for a vaginal delivery. In 2008, the percentage of cesarean deliveries reached an all-time high of 32.3 percent of all births in the United States.[23]

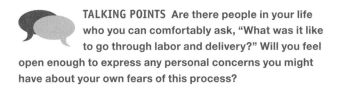

TALKING POINTS Are there people in your life who you can comfortably ask, "What was it like to go through labor and delivery?" Will you feel open enough to express any personal concerns you might have about your own fears of this process?

Infertility

Most traditional-age college students are interested in preventing pregnancy. However, other people are trying to do just the opposite: They are trying to become pregnant. It is estimated that about 10–15 percent of the U.S. population has a problem with *infertility*. These couples wish to become pregnant but are unsuccessful. The general criterion for infertility is the inability to conceive after a year of frequent unprotected intercourse.

Causes of Infertility

What causes infertility? About 40 percent of infertility problems are attributed to male factors, and about 40 percent are explained by female factors. Approximately 10 percent of the problems stem from a combination of male and female factors, while the remaining 10 percent come from unknown origins.

Factors in infertility in males include low sperm count, inability of the sperm to move properly, and structural abnormalities of the sperm. Female factors center on lack of ovulation and obstructions in the fallopian tubes.

Preventing Infertility

Can you do anything to prevent being infertile? There are many ways you can increase your chances of remaining fertile. Avoiding sexually transmitted diseases is one crucial factor. (See the guidelines for safer sex in Chapter 11.) The risk from multiple partners should encourage responsible sexual activity. Men and women should avoid working around hazardous chemicals or using psychoactive drugs. Being overweight or underweight, endometriosis, smoking, and heavy alcohol consumption are risk factors that reduce fertility.[24] Maintaining overall good health and having regular medical (and, for women, gynecological) checkups are excellent ideas. Because infertility is directly linked with advancing age, couples may not want to indefinitely delay having children.

Enhancing a Couple's Fertility

A number of approaches can be used to increase sperm counts. Among the simple approaches are the application of periodic cold packs on the scrotum and the replacement of tight underwear with boxer shorts. When a structural problem or obstruction reduces sperm production, surgery

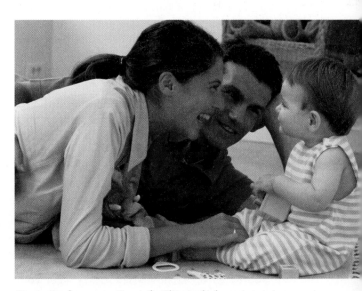

Strategies for preventing infertility include maintaining a healthy lifestyle, protecting yourself from sexually transmitted diseases, and avoiding use of tobacco, alcohol, and other drugs.

can be helpful. Most experts (reproductive endocrinologists) suggest that couples have frequent intercourse starting three days before ovulation and continuing for two or three days after the woman thinks she has ovulated. This helps increase the odds of becoming pregnant.[25]

Treatments for Infertility

A variety of approaches can be used with couples who are having fertility problems. These include artificial insemination, surgical remedies, fertility drugs, and assisted reproductive technologies (ARTs).

Artificial Insemination Men can also collect (through masturbation) and save samples of their sperm to use in a procedure called *artificial insemination by partner*. Near the time of ovulation, the collected samples of sperm are then deposited near the woman's cervical opening. In the related procedure called *artificial insemination by donor*, the sperm of a donor are used. Donor semen is screened for the presence of pathogens, including the AIDS virus.

Surgical Remedies Causes of infertility in women center mostly on obstructions in the reproductive tract and the inability to ovulate. The obstructions sometimes result from tissue damage (scarring) caused by infections. Chlamydial and gonorrheal infections often produce fertility problems. Other possible causes of structural abnormalities include scar tissue from previous surgery, fibroid tumors, polyps, and endometriosis. A variety of microsurgical techniques may correct some of these complications.

One of the more recent innovative procedures involves the use of **transcervical balloon tuboplasty.** In this procedure, a series of balloon-tipped catheters are inserted through the uterus into the blocked fallopian tubes. Once inflated, these balloon catheters help open the scarred passageways.

Fertility Drugs When a woman has ovulation difficulties, pinpointing the specific cause can be very difficult. In women of normal weight who are not approaching menopause, it appears that ovulation difficulties are caused by lack of synchronization between the hormones governing the menstrual cycle. Fertility drugs can help alter the menstrual cycle to produce ovulation. Clomiphene citrate (Clomid), in oral pill form, or injections of human menopausal gonadotropin (Pergonal) are two of the most common fertility drugs available. Both are capable of producing multiple ova at ovulation.[26]

Assisted Reproductive Technologies (ART) For couples who are unable to conceive after drug therapy, surgery, and artificial insemination, the use of one of four assisted reproductive technologies (ART) can be helpful. One option is *in vitro fertilization and embryo transfer*

(IVF-ET). This method is sometimes referred to as the "test tube" procedure. Costing over $12,000 per attempt, IVF-ET consists of surgically retrieving fertilizable ova from the woman and combining them in a glass dish with sperm. After several days, the fertilized ova are transferred into the uterus. IVF-ET accounts for 99 percent of all ART procedures.[27]

A second test tube procedure is called *gamete intrafallopian transfer (GIFT)*. Similar to IVF-ET, this procedure involves depositing a mixture of retrieved eggs and sperm directly into the fallopian tubes.

Fertilized ova (zygotes) can also be transferred from a laboratory dish into the fallopian tubes in a third procedure called *zygote intrafallopian transfer (ZIFT)*. One advantage of this procedure is that the clinicians are certain that ova have been fertilized before the transfer to the fallopian tubes. GIFT and ZIFT combined account for just 1 percent of ART procedures.[27]

The fourth (and newest) procedure is *intracytoplasmic sperm injection (ICSI)*. This is a laboratory procedure in which a single sperm cell is injected into a woman's retrieved egg. The fertilized egg is then transplanted into the woman's uterus. The cost and technical expertise involved in ICSI make it a seldom-used procedure for infertile couples.

Ethical Questions Remain The January 2009 births of eight babies to a California woman (who already had six children through IVF-ET procedures) raised the eyebrows of many who struggle with the ethical issues surrounding high-tech infertility treatments. This was the second set of octuplets ever recorded in the United States.[28] The biggest challenge with extreme multiple births is the overall health of the babies and the mother. The risks to the infants include bleeding in the brain, intestinal problems, developmental delays, and learning disabilities that last a lifetime. (At the time of this writing, however, all eight toddlers and the mother appeared to be in good physical health.)

The general consensus among medical ethicists seems to be that the decision to implant such a large number of embryos into the woman was irresponsible. European countries limit the number of embryos to be implanted at one to three. In the so-called octomom's case, she was apparently offered "selective reduction" to lower the number of implanted embryos, but she declined. A representative of the American Society for Reproductive Medicine indicated that the organization's guidelines

> **Key Terms**
>
> **transcervical balloon tuboplasty** The use of inflatable balloon catheters to open blocked fallopian tubes; a procedure used for some women with fertility problems.

Where to Find Help for Infertility and Adoption

These agencies can provide you with information about infertility and give referrals to specialists in your area:

American Society for Reproductive Medicine
(205) 978-5000
www.asrm.org

Planned Parenthood Federation of America
(800) 230-7526
www.plannedparenthood.org

RESOLVE
(703) 556-7172
www.resolve.org

These agencies can provide help to prospective adoptive parents:

The National Adoption Center
1-800-To-Adopt
www.adopt.org

National Council for Adoption
(703) 299-6633
www.adoptioncouncil.org

North American Council on Adoptable Children
(651) 644-3036
www.nacac.org

suggest that no more than two embryos be implanted in a woman under the age of 35.[28] Where do you stand on this issue?

Options for Infertile Couples

The process of coping with infertility problems can be an emotionally stressful experience for a couple. Fortunately, support groups have been established to assist couples with infertility problems. (Some of these groups are listed in the box "Where to Find Help for Infertility and Adoption.") There are a number of options to explore.

Adoption   For couples who have determined that biological childbirth is inadvisable or impossible, adoption offers a wonderful opportunity. Adopted children currently represent about 2.5 percent of all children in the United States.

Adoption is now a viable alternative for most adults. In the past, many states permitted only financially stable, heterosexual, young or midlife married couples to adopt children. Now, in many states, single persons can legally adopt children. Single gay and same-sex couples may also adopt in many areas of the country. (Visit the nonprofit organization www.familieslikeours.org website for more information.)

The most important factor in adoption seems to be the ability of the adopting person or couple to provide a stable, safe, and positive environment with sufficient space for the child. Adequate income is important, but being wealthy is not a requirement. (To find out more about adoption, visit www.childwelfare.gov, www.adopt.org, and www.davethomasfoundation.org.)

Foster Parenting   The number of children in foster care who are waiting to be reunited with their biological parents or awaiting adoption has risen steadily since the mid-1980s. Experts attribute the rise to family problems caused by parental drug abuse, unemployment, alcoholism, and other difficulties. Currently, about a half million children per year spend time in foster homes. Like adoption, foster parenting has presented a variety of ethical and legal issues, especially the debate over "the best interests of the child" versus parental rights.

Surrogate Parenting   *Surrogate parenting* is another option that has been explored, although the legal and ethical issues surrounding this method of conception have not been fully resolved. Surrogate parenting exists in a number of forms. Typically, an infertile couple will make a contract with a woman (the surrogate parent), who will then be artificially inseminated with semen from the expectant father. In some instances, the surrogate will receive an embryo from the donor parents. In some cases, women have served as surrogates for their close relatives. The surrogate will carry the fetus to term and return the newborn to the parents. Because of the concerns about true "ownership" of the baby, surrogate parenting may not be a particularly viable or legal option for many couples.

TALKING POINTS You have tried for a couple of years to get pregnant, and now you are ready to consider some of the newest options to increase the chances of conception. Your partner seems unwilling to spend much money for these high-tech procedures. You are ready to spend some of your retirement savings in this effort. How can you and your partner best come to an agreement on this issue?

Taking Charge of Your Health

- Use the Personal Assessment at the end of this chapter to help you determine which birth control method is best for you.

- Talk to your doctor about the health aspects of different types of birth control before making your decision.

- If the method of birth control you are currently using is unsatisfactory to you or your partner, explore other options.

- Reduce your risk of infertility by choosing a birth control method carefully, protecting yourself from infections of the reproductive organs, and maintaining good overall health.

- If you plan to have children, set a time frame that takes into account decreased fertility with advancing age.

SUMMARY

- Birth control refers to all the procedures that can prevent the birth of a child. Contraception refers to any procedure that prevents fertilization.
- Each birth control method has both a theoretical-effectiveness rate and a use-effectiveness rate. For some contraceptive approaches, these rates are similar (such as hormonal methods), and for others the rates are very different (such as condoms, diaphragms, and periodic abstinence).
- Many factors should be considered when deciding which contraceptive is best for you.
- Sterilization (vasectomy and tubal ligation) is generally considered an irreversible procedure.

- Abortion procedures vary according to the stage of the pregnancy.
- Several physiological factors can be either aids or obstacles to fertilization.
- Pregnant women should avoid agents that can harm the fetus.
- Childbirth takes place in three distinct stages.
- For couples with fertility problems, numerous strategies can be used to help conception take place.
- Adoption, foster parenting, and surrogate parenting are additional ways for adults to have children.

REVIEW QUESTIONS

1. Explain the difference between theoretical- and use-effectiveness rates. Which one is always higher?
2. Identify some of the factors that should be given careful consideration when selecting a contraceptive method. Explain each factor.
3. For each of the methods of birth control, explain how it works and its advantages and disadvantages.
4. How does the contraceptive patch differ from the contraceptive ring?
5. What is emergency contraception?
6. How are tubal ligation and vasectomy accomplished?

7. Identify and describe the different abortion procedures that are used during each trimester of pregnancy. What is a medication abortion?
8. What are some obstacles and aids to fertilization presented in this chapter? Can you think of others?
9. Identify and describe the events that occur during each of the three stages of childbirth. Approximately how long is each stage?
10. What can be done to reduce chances of infertility? Explain IVF-ET, GIFT, ZIFT, and ICSI procedures.

ANSWERS TO THE "WHAT DO YOU KNOW?" QUIZ

1. False   2. False   3. True   4. False   5. True   6. True   7. True

Visit the Online Learning Center (**www.mhhe.com/hahn11e**), where you will find tools to help you improve your grade including practice quizzes, key terms flashcards, audio chapter summaries for your MP3 player, and many other study aids.

SOURCE NOTES

1. Rosenbaum JE. Patient teenagers? A comparison of the sexual behaviors of virginity pledgers and matched nonpledgers. *Pediatrics* (online), 131(1), e110–e120, January 2009.

2. Hyde JS, DeLamater JD. *Understanding Human Sexuality* (11th ed.). New York: McGraw-Hill, 2011.

3. Crooks RL, Baur K. *Our Sexuality* (11th ed.). Belmont, CA: Wadsworth, Cengage Learning, 2011.

4. Hatcher RA, et al. *Contraceptive Technology* (19th ed.). New York: Ardent Media, 2007.

5. Planned Parenthood Federation of America. Birth control. www.plannedparenthood.org/health-topics/birth-control, accessed March 9, 2011.

6. Carroll JL. *Sexuality Now: Embracing Diversity* (3 rd ed.). Belmont, CA: Wadsworth, Cengage Learning, 2010.

7. DeNoon D. Best condoms still latex. WebMD Health, March 21, 2003. www.mywebmd.com.

8. Steiner MJ, et al. Contraceptive effectiveness of a polyurethane condom and a latex condom: a randomized controlled trial. *Obstetrics and Gynecology,* 101(3), 539–547, 2003.

9. Yarber WL, Sayad BW, Strong B. *Human Sexuality: Diversity in Contemporary America* (7th ed.). New York: McGraw-Hill, 2010.

10. Bayer Pharmaceuticals. What Mirena users may expect. www.mirenaus.com, accessed March 20, 2011.

11. WebMD. Comparing birth control pills. www.webmd.com, accessed March 17, 2011.

12. Schering-Plough Corporation. IMPLANON: how IMPLANON works. www.implanon.usa.com, accessed March 20, 2011.

13. Merck. NuvaRing: How does it work? www.nuvaring.com, accessed March 20, 2011.

14. Ortho-McNeil-Janssen Pharmaceuticals. What is ORTHO EVRA? www.orthoevra.com, accessed March 21, 2011.

15. Watson Pharma. What is *ellal*? www.ella-rx.com, accessed March 17, 2011.

16. Hologic. Benefits and risks of Adiana permanent contraception. www.adiana.com, accessed March 18, 2011.

17. Guttmacher Institute. In brief: facts on induced abortion in the United States, January 2011. www.guttmacher.org, accessed March 19, 2011.

18. National Cancer Institute, U.S. National Institutes of Health. *Fact Sheet: Abortion, Miscarriage, and Breast Cancer.* www.cancer.gov/cancertopics/factsheet/Risk/abortion-miscarriage, accessed March 31, 2011.

19. American Cancer Society. *Is Abortion Linked to Breast Cancer?* www.cancer.org/Cancer/Breast/Cancer/MoreInformation/is-abortion-linked-to-breast-cancer, accessed March 31, 2011.

20. Danco Laboratories, LLC. More facts about Mifeprex. www.earlyoptionpill.com, accessed March 21, 2011.

21. WebMD. Home pregnancy tests. www.webmd.com/baby/home-pregnancy-tests, accessed March 25, 2011.

22. Wardlaw GM, Smith AM. *Contemporary Nutrition* (8th ed.). New York: McGraw-Hill, 2011.

23. Martin, JA, et al. Births: final data for 2008. *National Vital Statistics Reports* 59(1). Hyattsville, MD: National Center for Health Statistics, December 2010.

24. RESOLVE: The National Infertility Association. *What are the risk factors?* www.resolve.org, accessed March 27, 2011.

25. WebMD. Ovulation calculator: 7 pregnancy tips. www.webmd.com/baby/healthtool-ovulation-calculator, accessed March 27, 2011.

26. WebMD. What drugs are used to treat infertility in women? www.webmd.com/infertility-and-reproduction/frequently-asked-questions-about-infertility, accessed March 27, 2011.

27. WebMD. Infertility and in vitro fertilization. www.webmd.com/infertility-and-reproduction/guide/in-vitro-fertilization, accessed March 27, 2011.

28. Landau E. Octuplets: eight times the ethical questions. www.cnn.com/2009/HEALTH/01/30/embryos.ethics/index, accessed January 31, 2009.

Personal Assessment

Which Birth Control Method Is Best for You?

To assess which birth control method would be best for you, answer the following questions, and check the interpretation section.

Do You: Yes   No

1. Need a contraceptive right away?   ____ ____

2. Want a contraceptive that can be used completely independent of sexual relations?   ____ ____

3. Need a contraceptive only once in a great while?   ____ ____

4. Want something with no harmful side effects?   ____ ____

5. Want to avoid going to the doctor?   ____ ____

6. Want something that will help protect against sexually transmitted diseases?   ____ ____

7. Have to be concerned about affordability?   ____ ____

8. Need to be virtually certain that pregnancy will not result?   ____ ____

9. Want to avoid pregnancy now but want to have a child sometime in the future?   ____ ____

10. Have any medical condition or lifestyle that may rule out some form of contraception?   ____ ____

Interpretation

If you have checked **Yes** to number:

1. Condoms, spermicides, and sponges may be easily purchased without prescription in any pharmacy.
2. Sterilization, oral contraceptives, hormone injections, rings, patches, implants, and periodic abstinence techniques do not require that anything be done just before sexual relations.
3. Diaphragms, condoms, sponges, and spermicides can be used by people who have coitus only once in a while. Periodic abstinence may also be appropriate but requires a high degree of skill and motivation.
4. IUD use should be carefully discussed with your physician, although IUDs are quite safe for most users. Sometimes the use of oral contraceptives

or hormone products results in some minor discomfort and, on rare occasions, may have harmful side effects.
5. Condoms, spermicides, sponges, and most kinds of emergency contraception do not require a prescription from a physician.
6. Condoms help protect against some sexually transmitted diseases. Nonoxynol-9 may increase STD transmission in some users. No method (except abstinence) can guarantee complete protection.
7. Be a wise consumer: Check prices, and ask pharmacists and physicians. The cost of sterilization is high, but there is no additional expense for a lifetime.
8. Sterilization provides near certainty. Hormone-based contraceptives, IUDs, and a diaphragm-condom-spermicide combination also give a high measure of reliable protection. Periodic abstinence, withdrawal, and douche methods should be avoided. Outercourse or abstinence may be a good alternative.
9. Although it is sometimes possible to reverse sterilization, it requires surgery and is more complex than simply stopping use of any of the other methods.
10. Smokers and people with a history of cardiovascular problems should probably not use oral contraceptives or other hormone approaches. Some people have allergic reactions to a specific spermicide or latex material. Some women cannot be fitted well with a diaphragm or cap. The woman and her health care provider will then need to select another suitable means of contraception.

TO CARRY THIS FURTHER . . .

There may be more than one method of birth control suitable for you. Always consider whether a method you select can also help you avoid an STD. Study the methods suggested above, and consult Table 13.1 to determine what techniques may be most appropriate. Consult with your physician, college health center, or local health clinic if you are uncertain or confused, or need additional information.

Source: Adapted from K. Haas and A. Haas, *Understanding Sexuality* (3rd ed.). St. Louis: Mosby, 1993. Used with permission by Adelaide Haas.

14

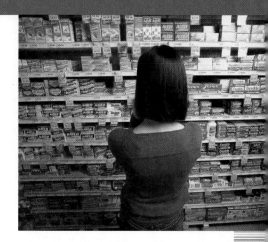

Becoming an Informed Health Care Consumer

What Do You Know About Health Care?

1. In terms of assessing the honesty of health-related advertising, testimonials represent the highest level of trustworthiness. True or False?

2. On the basis of current educational standards and state licensing examinations, a doctoral degree in allopathic medicine (MD) and a doctoral degree in osteopathic medicine (DO) are essentially interchangeable. True or False?

3. Nurse practitioners are primary care providers who are permitted to diagnose and treat patients, doing so under the supervision of physicians. True or False?

4. To be permitted to practice in the United States, practitioners in all fields of complementary and alternative medicine (CAM) must pass licensing examinations supervised by the U.S. Department of Health and Human Services. True or False?

5. The sale of a generic version of a nonbiologic or compounded prescription medication is permitted upon the expiration of the patent protection period of the brand-name medication. True or False?

6. You must have a prescription to purchase over-the-counter (OTC) medications in any state other than the state where you obtained your driver's license. True or False?

7. The safety and effectiveness of dietary supplements is established and carefully monitored by the Food and Drug Administration (FDA). True or False?

8. A federally orchestrated comprehensive health care plan was adopted, virtually intact, before the end of President Obama's first term in office. True or False?

Check your answers at the end of the chapter.

Before progressing further into this chapter, allow your authors to remind you of the role-fulfillment definition of health presented in Chapter 1 and their contention that the *health care system* that is familiar to Americans is, in fact, more accurately defined by the term *medical care system*. Your text will, however, most often use the familiar, but misnamed, *health care system*.

"Health" care providers often evaluate you by criteria from their areas of expertise. The nutritionist knows you by the food you eat. The physical fitness professional knows you by your body type and activity level. In the eyes of the expert in health consumerism, you are the product of the health information you believe, the health-influencing services you use, and the products you consume. When you make your decisions about health information, services, and products after careful study and consideration, your health will probably be improved. However, when your decisions lack insight, your health, as well as your pocketbook, may suffer.

That said, at this point an additional thought about health consumerism needs inclusion. The delivery of health care services (principally in the forms of medical care) could be undergoing changes in availability, method of delivery, and affordability that will make aspects of this chapter in need of changes that are not at this point determined. Your text can only sensitize you to the reality that the traditional American fee-for-services form of health care is no longer serving us as well as it should and that calls for change are growing increasingly louder. Certainly, the current administration in Washington is listening and plans for change have been formulated. At the time of this writing, the United States and South Africa are the only highly industrialized countries yet to adopt a more nationalized or regionalized form of medical care services. Check the Online Learning Center (www.mhhe.com/hahn11e) for the latest updates on government progress on reforming the health care system.

Health Information

The Informed Consumer

The Pew Charitable Trust's ongoing study of Internet use (Internet & American Life Project) provides current information on health-related Internet use.[1] The breadth of this activity is informative. Of the 95 million Americans who conducted health-related searches, 66 percent of the searchers sought information pertaining to specific conditions and problems, 51 percent to treatment and management of conditions, 51 percent to nutrition and diet, 42 percent to exercise and fitness, 40 percent to prescription medications and over-the-counter (OTC) products, and 30 percent to alternative treatments. Further, 31 percent sought information regarding health insurance, 18 percent investigated environmental health issues, and 11 percent pursued sexual health information. Among the 16 areas searched, only 8 percent sought information pertaining to drug and alcohol use, whereas 7 percent investigated information pertaining to smoking cessation, the area least visited.

A more recent study (2008) by the same project suggests that 75–80 percent of all Internet users do search the Web for health-related information.[2] An even more recent Pew Research Center study updated the 2004 findings only slightly, but added eight topical area questions.[3] Newly added were the areas of food safety and recalls (29 percent), medication safety and recalls (24 percent), pregnancy and childbirth (19 percent), memory loss (dementia) and Alzheimer's disease (17 percent), medical tests (16 percent), chronic pain management (14 percent), long-term care (12 percent), and end-of-life decisions (7 percent). When all the data are combined, over 80 percent of the American public seek health (medical)-related information via the Internet.

In light of the breadth of these interest areas and the complexity associated with each, it is very likely that most people also turn to a variety of sources for information. In the section that follows, you will be introduced to several sources of health-related information. Complete the Personal Assessment at the end of this chapter to rate your own skills as a consumer of health-related information, products, and services.

Sources of Information

Your sources of information on health topics are as diverse as the number of people you know, the number of publications you read, and the number of experts you see or hear. No single agency or profession regulates the quantity or quality of the health-related information you receive. Readers will quickly recognize that all are familiar sources and that some provide more accurate and honest information than others.

Family and Friends The accuracy of information you get from a friend or family member may be questionable. Too often the information your family and friends offer is based on "common knowledge" that is wrong. In addition, family members or friends may provide information they believe is in your best interest rather than facts that may have a more negative effect on you.

Advertisements and Commercials Many people spend much of every day watching television, listening to the radio, and reading newspapers or magazines. Because many advertisements are health oriented, these are significant sources of information. The primary purpose of advertising, however, is to sell products or services. One newer example of this intertwining of health information with marketing is the "infomercial," in which a compensated studio audience watches a skillfully produced program that trumpets the benefits of a particular product or service. In spite of the convincing nature of these info-mercials, however, the validity of their information is often questionable.

In contrast to advertisements and commercials, the mass media routinely offer public service messages, as mandated by the Federal Communication Commission (FCC), that give valuable health-related information. For example, the FCC, with the expertise of the Centers for Disease Control and Prevention, disseminated timely information to the American public, via an array of media, on various aspects of the novel-H1N1 (swine) flu during the 2009–2010 pandemic.

Labels and Directions Federal law requires that many consumer product labels, including all medications and many kinds of food (see Chapter 5), contain specific information. For example, when a pharmacist dispenses a prescription medication, he or she must provide a detailed information sheet describing the medication.

Many health care providers and agencies give consumers helpful information about their health problems or printed directions for preparing for screening procedures. Generally, information from these sources is accurate and current and is given with the health of the consumer foremost in mind.

Folklore Passed down from generation to generation, folklore about health is the primary source of health-related information for some people.

The accuracy of health-related information obtained from family members, neighbors, and coworkers is difficult to evaluate. As a general rule, however, one should exercise caution regarding its scientific soundness. A blanket dismissal is not warranted, however, because folk wisdom is occasionally supported by scientific evidence. In addition, the emotional support provided by the suppliers of this information could be the best medicine some people receive. In fact, for some ethnic groups, indigenous health care is central to overall health care. Even though many Americans would consider this form of care "folk medicine," it is highly valued and trusted by those who find it familiar.

Testimonials People want to share information that has benefited them. Others may base their decisions on such testimonials. However, the exaggerated testimonials that accompany the sales pitches of the medical "expert" or the "satisfied" customers appearing in advertisements and on commercials and infomercials should never be interpreted as valid endorsements. Particularly in regard to weight loss–related testimonials, note the disclaimer at the bottom of the screen or advertisement (in exceedingly small print) that states, "These results are not typical."

Although currently lacking a health-related name, beyond the current label *of social media*, Facebook, Twitter,

Communication Between Patients and Their Health Care Providers

In the complex world of modern health care, it is of critical importance that patients communicate important information to their health care providers and, in turn, that they understand as fully as possible the information they receive from the providers. Below are ten valuable suggestions from the joint commission on Accreditation of Healthcare Organizations and the U.S. government's Agency for Healthcare Research and Quality.

- Take part in every decision about your health care.

- If you are not prepared to ask questions on your own behalf, ask a family member or friend to fill this role for you.

- Tell your physician and pharmacist about every drug you are taking, including prescription drugs, OTC drugs, vitamins, supplements, and herbal products—bring them with you.

- Make certain that you get the results of every test and understand what they mean.

- If you do not hear about test results, never assume that everything is all right. Call your doctor's office and ask.

- Whenever possible, choose a hospital where many patients receive the same procedure that you are to receive. Ask your physician or the hospital for the actual numbers.

- Ask hospital personnel if they have washed their hands before they begin touching you.

- If you are having surgery, make sure that you, your physician, and your surgeon all agree on what will be done during the operation.

- Insist that your surgeon write his or her initials or words such as "yes" or "this side" on the part of the body to be operated on. Put "no" on the opposite body part.

- When you are discharged, ask your doctor to explain your treatment plan, including changes in medications, restrictions on activity, and additional therapies you will need.

In many situations involving medical care, carefully communicated comments and questions between providers and patients can be the basis of the successful resolution of a health problem, versus unnecessary delay, pain, discomfort, or even death.

Source: Ellis L. *How You Can Help Guard Against Errors,* June 28, 2002. Copyright 1996–2009. Reprinted with permission from Aetna InteliHealth (www.intelihealth.com).

and related technology-based services are playing an ever-growing role in the dissemination of information. In effect, these are the twenty-first century's transmission lines for testimonials and folklore. However, do not expect your primary care physician to accept your invitation to be "your friend" or to twitter you back while moving from one examination room to the next. Equally unlikely is that your physician will have a blog through which you can keep updated on your practitioner-patient status.

Mass Media Health programming on cable and satellite television stations, stories in lifestyle sections of newspapers, health care correspondents appearing on national network news shows, and the growing number of health-oriented magazines are sources of health information in the mass media.

In terms of the public's preferences for specific media sources of health information, a gradual evolution is occurring. As recently as 1999, television, followed by magazines and newspapers, were the three principal sources of health-related news for American adults. Now, these traditional sources of information are rapidly losing popularity to the Internet. Most likely, this trend will continue until a new information-sharing technology moves into the mainstream of American life.

Health-related information in the mass media is generally accurate, but it is sometimes presented so quickly or superficially that its usefulness is limited.

Practitioners The health care consumer also receives much information from individual medical practitioners and their professional associations. In fact, today's practitioners so clearly emphasize patient education that finding one who does not offer some information to a patient would be difficult. Education improves patient **compliance** with health care directives, which is important to the practitioner and the consumer (see the box "Communication Between Patients and Their Health Care Providers" on page 359 for more information).

Online Computer Services We have already discussed the rapidly growing utilization of the Internet as a primary source of health-related information. We have even, in a sense, concluded that you are or would be one of those users.

In spite of the fact that today's health care system depends on computer technology to diagnose and treat illness and injury, medical professionals are perhaps the professionals least likely to use the Internet to correspond with their clients. In a study of medical practitioners across a wide range of medical specialties, only 16 percent had ever used e-mail to correspond with patients, and less than 3 percent had done so with any frequency.[4]

In a 2011 perusal of the National Library of Medicine, using its public access portal (PubMed) and keywords *social media, Internet,* and *physician/patient communication,* fewer than 10 publications were identified. One article in particular suggested that physicians create a "sense of dual citizenship" when it comes to Internet-based use.[5] The authors recommend that a "professional" persona be used when providing medically related information and

when engaged in consultations with health care professionals, and a "private" (nonprofessional) persona when communicating with others—perhaps even when an "other" person could be a patient. In this latter persona, the physician could be perceived as being a nonphysician. Thus, this persona would protect confidentiality for all involved.

In a 2010 article in *USA Today,* primary care physician Kevin Pho suggests other reasons that physicians "ignore the Internet at their own peril."[6] Among these factors are the absence of professional standards for Internet use, issues of potential liability, loss of confidentiality, cost of IT support personnel, and the absence of a mechanism to bill patients for the physician's time.

Health Reference Publications A substantial portion of all households own or subscribe to a health reference publication, such as the *Encyclopedia of Complementary Health Practices,* the *Physicians' Desk Reference (PDR),* or a newsletter such as *The Harvard Medical School Health Letter* or *The Johns Hopkins Medical Letter: Health After 50.* Some consumers also use personal computer programs and DVDs featuring health-related information.

Reference Libraries Public and university libraries continue to be popular sources of health-related information. One can consult with reference librarians and check out audiovisual collections and printed materials. More and more of these holdings can be accessed through the home computer or through apps for tablet computers and smart phones.

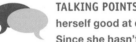 **TALKING POINTS** A family member considers herself good at diagnosing health problems. Since she hasn't been wrong in years, she no longer relies on physicians. What questions could you ask her to point out the dangers associated with her approach?

Consumer Advocacy Groups A variety of nonprofit consumer advocacy groups patrol the health care marketplace, such as those listed in Table 14.1. These groups produce and distribute information designed to help the consumer recognize questionable services and products. Large, well-organized groups, such as the National Consumers' League and Consumers Union, and smaller groups at the state and local levels champion the right of the consumer to receive valid and reliable information about health care products and services.

Voluntary Health Agencies Volunteerism and the traditional approach to health care and health promotion are virtually inseparable. Few countries besides the United States can boast so many national voluntary organizations, with state and local affiliates, dedicated to improving health through research, service, and public

Table 14.1 Consumer Protection Agencies and Organizations

These agencies and organizations can be found in a variety of forms. Many are located within the organizational makeup of various federal agencies, while others, taking the form of free-standing organizations, are sustained in part by the validity of products, services, and corporate "good citizenship" of companies engaged in retail sales. Yet a third arena of operation for consumer protective services is within the confines of a highly creditable professional organization, such as the American Medical Association. Several consumer protective agencies and organizations are listed below.

Federal Agencies

Office of Consumer Affairs, Food and Drug Administration
(301) 827-5006
www.fda.gov/oca/aboutoca.htm

Federal Trade Commission
(202) 326-2222
www.ftc.gov

Fraud Division, U.S. Postal Inspection Service
(202) 268-4299
www.usps.gov

Consumer Information Center
(719) 948-3334
www.pueblo.gsa.gov

U.S. Consumer Product Safety Commission Hotline
(800) 638-CPSC

Consumer Organizations

Consumers Union of the U.S., Inc.
(914) 378-2000
www.consumerreports.org

Professional Organizations

American Medical Association
(312) 464-5000
www.ama-assn.org

American Hospital Association
(312) 422-3000
www.aha.org

American Pharmaceutical Association
(202) 628-4410
www.aphanet.org

---

education. The American Cancer Society, the American Red Cross, and the American Heart Association are voluntary (not-for-profit) health agencies. Consumers can, in fact, expect to find a voluntary health agency for virtually every health problem. College students should also note that volunteerism on their part, perhaps with a health agency like the Red Cross or the AHA, is both a personally satisfying experience and an activity viewed favorably by potential employers.

Government Agencies Government agencies are also effective sources of information for the public. Through meetings and the release of information to the media, agencies such as the Food and Drug Administration, Department of Agriculture, Federal Trade Commission, U.S. Postal Service, and Environmental Protection Agency publicize health issues. Government agencies also control the quality of information sent out to the buying public, particularly through labeling, advertising, and mailings. The various divisions of the National Institutes of Health regularly release research findings and recommendations to clinical practices, which in turn reach the consumer through clinical practitioners.

State governments also distribute health-related information to the public. State agencies are primary sources of information, particularly in the areas of public health and environmental protection. (For an example of health care activism at work, see the box "Americans with Disabilities Act—New Places to Go.")

Qualified Health Educators Health educators work in a variety of settings and offer their services to diverse groups. Community health educators work with virtually all of the agencies mentioned in this section; patient educators function in primary care settings; and school health educators are found at all educational levels. Health educators are increasingly being employed in a wide range of wellness-based programs in community, hospital, corporate, and school settings.

Health Care Providers

The sources of health information just discussed can greatly help us make decisions as informed consumers. The choices we make about physicians, health services, and medical payment plans will reflect our commitment to remaining healthy and our trust in specific people who are trained in keeping us healthy. (See the box "Choosing a Physician" for advice on finding a physician who is right for you.)

Why We Consult Health Care Providers

Most of us seek care and advice from medical and health practitioners when we have a specific problem. A bad

> **Key Terms**
>
> **compliance** Willingness to follow the directions provided by another person.

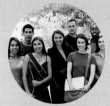
cold, a broken arm, or a newly discovered lump can motivate us to consult a health care professional. Yet *diagnosis* and *treatment* are only two reasons that we might require the services of health care providers.

We also might encounter health practitioners when we undergo *screening*. Screening most often involves a cursory (or noninvasive) collection of information that can quickly be compared to established standards often based on gender, age, race, or the presence of preexisting conditions. Your earliest experience with screening may have been in elementary school, where physicians, nurses, audiologists, and dentists sometimes examine children for normal growth and development patterns. As an adult, your screening is more likely to be done on an individual basis by a physician's staff as a routine portion of every office visit when they collect baseline information such as height, weight, and blood pressure measurements. You may also encounter community-based screening when you stop at your local shopping mall's health fair and have your blood pressure taken or cholesterol checked. Although screening should be considered much less precise than actual diagnosis, screening serves to identify people who should seek further medical examination.

Consultation is a fourth reason that knowledgeable consumers seek health care providers. A consultation is the use of two or more professionals to deliberate a person's specific health problem or condition. Consultations are especially helpful when **primary care health providers,** such as family practice physicians, gynecologists, pediatricians, internists, and general practice

dentists, require the opinion of specialists. Using additional practitioners as consultants can also help reassure patients who may have doubts about their own condition or about the abilities of their physician.

Prevention is a fifth reason we might seek a health care provider. With the current emphasis on trying to stop problems before they begin, using health care providers for prevention is becoming more common. People want information about how to avoid needless risks and promote their health, and they seek such advice from physicians, nurses, dentists, exercise physiologists, patient educators, and other health promotion specialists.

When prevention becomes a routine component of your personal health care, you will annually receive, in addition to the baseline measurements of height, weight, and blood pressure, more in-depth assessments such as a blood chemistry assessment, lipid profile, and cardiogram. Women will also likely receive a Pap test (of some version), breast examination, mammography, and pelvic examination, while men will likely receive a prostate-specific antigen (PSA) test, digital prostate examination, and testicular examination.

Physicians and Their Training

In every city and many smaller communities, the local telephone directory lists physicians in a variety of medical specialties. These health care providers hold the academic degree of doctor of medicine (MD) or doctor of osteopathy (DO).

We're moving to a new town at the beginning of the summer. What will my parents and I need to know about choosing a new doctor?

First, get some recommendations:

- Talk with people about their health care providers. Most likely they will identify some providers whom they would recommend or not recommend.
- Talk with people in the health care field. They will generally find ways to "suggest" practitioners without violating professional practice standards.
- Call local hospitals for recommendations. They will usually provide several names of physicians who they know are taking new patients.

Next, call the doctor's office and find out the following:

- Which hospitals does the doctor use?
- What are the office hours (when is the doctor available, and when can you speak to office staff)?
- Does the doctor or someone else in the office speak the language you are most comfortable speaking?
- How many other doctors "cover" for the doctor when he or she is not available? Who are they?
- How long does it usually take to get a routine appointment?
- How long might you need to wait in the office before seeing the doctor?
- What happens if you need to cancel an appointment? Will you have to pay for it anyway?
- Does the office send reminders about prevention tests—for example, Pap tests?

- What do you do if you need urgent care or have an emergency?
- Does the doctor (or a nurse or physician assistant) give advice over the phone for common medical problems?

The next step is to schedule a visit with your top choice. During that first visit, you will learn whether it is easy to talk with the doctor. You will also find out how well the doctor might meet your medical needs. After your initial visit, ask yourself: Did the doctor:

- Give me a chance to ask questions?
- Really listen to my questions?
- Answer in terms I understood?
- Show respect for me?
- Ask me questions?
- Make me feel comfortable?
- Address the health problem(s) I came with?
- Ask me my preferences about different kinds of treatments?
- Spend enough time with me?

If you answer yes to most of these questions, you have probably found a physician with whom you will feel comfortable. Trust your own reactions when deciding whether this doctor is the right one for you. But you also may want to give the relationship some time to develop. It takes more than one visit for you and your doctor to get to know each other.

Source: U.S. Department of Health and Human Services, Agency for Health-care Research and Quality, *Your Guide to Choosing Quality Health Care.* AHCPR Pub. No. 99-0012. Updated July 2001.

At one time, **allopathy** and **osteopathy** were clearly different health care professions in terms of their healing philosophies and modes of practice. Today, however, MDs and DOs receive similar educations and engage in very similar forms of practice. Both can function as primary care physicians or as board-certified specialists. Their differences are in the osteopathic physician's greater tendency to use manipulation in treating health problems. In addition, DOs often perceive themselves as being more holistically oriented than MDs are.

Medical and osteopathic physicians undergo a long training process. After they are accepted into professional schools, students generally spend four or more years in intensive training that includes advanced study in the preclinical medical sciences and clinical practice. When they complete this phase of training, the students are awarded the MD or DO degree and then take the state medical license examination.

Upon completion of their basic medical education, a *transitional year* residency program follows in which the physician moves through an array of clinical areas

in order to better define her or his area of specialized study. The period of specialized study that follows the transitional year, a more traditionally defined *residency*, will generally last an additional three to four years.

Key Terms

primary care health providers Health care providers who generally see patients on a routine basis, particularly for preventive health care.

allopathy (ah **lop** ah thee) A system of medical practice in which specific remedies (often pharmaceutical agents) are used to produce effects different from those produced by a disease or injury.

osteopathy (os tee **op** ah thee) A system of medical practice in which allopathic principles are combined with specific attention to postural mechanics of the body.

For many, but certainly not all, specialized physicians, an additional period of training, a *subspecialization,* will add more years of training. As of March 2010, a total of 147 areas of medical specialization were recognized in this country. For example, a newly graduated physician might next take a surgery-based transition-year program, followed by a specialization in cardiopulmonary surgery, eventually leading to a second full residency (subspecialization) in pediatric cardiopulmonary surgery. This sequence involves an additional decade or more of training beyond the completion of the premedical undergraduate degree.

In addition to state and specialty board certification, comprehensive national certification of physicians is a frequently discussed possibility. At this time, no nationally required and all-encompassing certification of physician competency is required.

During the past decade, this country has experienced a shortage of physicians, particularly those entering the field of primary care. In response to this shortage, the United States is relying heavily on foreign-trained physicians. According to the Association of American Medical Colleges, at today's rate of physician production, we will have 750,000 physicians in this country by 2025, while our needs would be for an additional 159,000 physicians. Although more applications are now being accepted, class sizes are expanding, and additional schools are being constructed, it is questionable whether the shortage problem will soon be resolved.

Complementary, Alternative, and Integrative Care Practitioners

In addition to medical and osteopathic physician care, several other forms of health care offer alternatives within the large health care market. Included within this group of complementary or alternative forms of practice are chiropractic, acupuncture, homeopathy, naturopathy, herbalism, reflexology, and ayurveda. Although the traditional medical community has long scoffed at these fields of practice as ineffective and unscientific, many people use these forms of health care and believe strongly that they are as effective as (or more effective than) allopathic and osteopathic medicine. As a result of this belief, today many physicians are better informed about complementary care methods and more comfortable discussing them with patients. Following are brief descriptions of some of the more popular of these complementary care fields and the practitioners who function within them.

Chiropractic Historically (and, to varying degrees, today) the underlying premise of **chiropractic** is that misalignment or subluxation of the spinal (vertebral) column is the primary cause of illness, and thus, its realignment is the appropriate treatment for illness.

Accordingly, chiropractic medical practice is primarily limited to vertebral adjustments, where manual manipulation of the spine is used to correct misalignments. With about 50,000 practitioners in the United States, chiropractic is the third-largest health profession, used by 15–20 million people. Some chiropractors use only spinal manipulation, whereas others use additional medical technologies, including dietary supplementation and various noninvasive technologies similar to those used by physical therapists and athletic trainers, including massage.

In spite of the fact that chiropractors undergo nearly the same number of years of initial medical school training (undergraduate plus four years to MD), and take courses closely aligned with those taken by physicians, current laws restrict the scope of chiropractic practice to noninvasive techniques initially consistent with the original theoretical basis of their discipline, "one cause—one cure of all illnesses and diseases." In 1998 the National Center for Complementary and Alternative Medicine (NCCAM) established a Comprehensive Center for Chiropractic Research (the eleventh alternative medical field to receive such a center) to establish scientific standards for the study of chiropractic effectiveness.[7] Should careful study of chiropractic demonstrate limited effectiveness, beyond the area of low-back pain, then chiropractic medicine is likely to remain a user-friendly, highly popular but highly limited approach to health care.

Acupuncture **Acupuncture** is, for Americans, the most familiar component of the 3,000-year-old Chinese medical system. This system is based on balancing the active and passive forces within the patient's body to strengthen the *qi* (chee), or life force. The system also involves herbs, food, diet, massage, and exercise.

Acupuncturists place hair-thin needles at certain points in the body to stimulate the patient's qi. These points are said to correspond to different organs and bodily functions and, when stimulated, help the body's own defenses fight illness.

Of all the Chinese therapies, acupuncture is the most widely accepted in the West. Researchers have produced persuasive evidence of acupuncture's effectiveness in treating low-back pain, adult postoperative pain, nausea and vomiting associated with chemotherapy, and pain following dental surgery. Acupuncture may also be effective in other areas such as addiction, headache, menstrual pain, fibromyalgia, osteoarthritis, and tennis elbow. However, because of the difficulty of conducting double-blind research that involves the insertion of needles, acupuncture research has been challenging to design; thus, its use may remain largely complementary. However, this limitation should be easily eliminated as pseudo-acupuncture needles, whose tips retract once the skin is initially punctured, have just become available, thus allowing double-blind studies to be conducted.

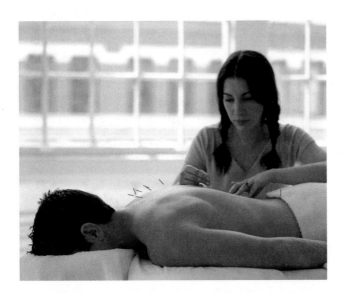

Acupuncture has received increasing acceptance within the Western medical community.

Manipulative Practices   Although chiropractic, osteopathic medicine, and physical therapy all fall under the heading of manipulative practices, this section addresses less widely used practices, including massage therapy, reflexology, rolfing, the Bowman technique, Trager bodywork, and a host of other practices that involve pressing on muscles, bones, joints, soft tissue, and underlying blood and lymphatic vessels.[8] So varied are the techniques, including location of pressure, depth of pressure, and interval between applications of pressure, that it is difficult to compare one with another. That said, all such techniques are based on the common agreement that the body is self-regulating and can heal itself, and that its parts are interdependent.

Although chiropractic, osteopathic, and physical therapy programs do sponsor research that appears in the medical literature (as identified by National Library of Medicine searches), the majority of the other techniques mentioned here have produced relatively little research, or research limited largely to patient observations and self-reporting. As a result, these practices remain "highly alternative" and are not covered by health insurance. On the positive side, relatively little risk is reported, particularly when practitioners are experienced.

Homeopathy   Widely accepted in Europe, **homeopathy** is the leading alternative therapy in France. Homeopathy uses infinitesimal doses of herbs, minerals, or even poisons to stimulate the body's curative powers. The theory on which homeopathy is based, the *law of similars,* contends that if large doses of a substance can cause a problem, tiny doses can trigger healing. A few small studies showed homeopathy to be at least somewhat effective in treating hay fever, diarrhea, and flu symptoms, but members of the scientific community call the studies flawed or preliminary and suggest that the placebo effect was occurring. It was further concluded that on the basis of these studies there was no strong evidence in favor of homeopathy over conventional treatment methods. The NCCAM recommended that larger, more carefully controlled studies be conducted.[9] Since the report on homeopathic medication was released by the NCCAM, studies continue to experience methodological difficulties, principally related to the small sample sizes used by researchers.

Naturopathy   The core of naturopathic medicine is what Hippocrates called *medicatrix naturae,* or the healing power of nature. Proponents of **naturopathy** believe that when the mind and the body are in balance and receiving proper care, with a healthy diet, adequate rest, and minimal stress, the body's own vital forces are sufficient to fight off disease. Getting rid of an ailment is only the first step toward correcting the underlying imbalance that allowed the ailment to take hold, naturists believe. Correcting the imbalance might be as simple as rectifying a shortage of a particular nutrient, or as complex as reducing overlong work hours, strengthening a weakened immune system, and identifying an inability to digest certain foods.

Herbalism   **Herbalism,** also known as herbology, phytotherapy, and herbal medicine, is without a doubt the most ancient form of medical treatment. As long ago as the Neandertal period (60,000 years ago), evidence indicates the use of plants for both food and medicine. Today herbalism is the principal form of medical treatment in developing areas of the world and is strongly supported in many developed areas as well. In the United States, botanicals provide the molecular models for many prescription medications and are principal players in the

> **Key Terms**
>
> **chiropractic** Manipulation of the vertebral column to relieve misalignments and cure illness.
>
> **acupuncture** Insertion of fine needles into the body to alter electroenergy fields and cure disease.
>
> **homeopathy** (hoe mee **op** ah thee) The use of minute doses of herbs, minerals, or other substances to stimulate healing.
>
> **naturopathy** (na chur **op** ah thee) A system of treatment that avoids drugs and surgery and emphasizes the use of natural agents, such as sunshine, to correct underlying imbalances.
>
> **herbalism** An ancient form of healing in which herbal preparations are used to treat illness and disease.

Researching and Evaluating CAM Practitioners

A campus flyer promotes acupuncture to relieve allergy symptoms. A close friend swears that the magnets built into her shoes relieve leg pain. A website for a local massage therapist advertises a specific type of massage to prevent migraines. What should you make of all these messages about complementary and alternative medicine (CAM)?

Information about CAM treatments and practitioners comes from many forms of media and can be difficult to evaluate. Compared to more traditional forms of medical care, there is often less scientific information available about CAM—and less regulation of CAM products and practitioners. It is important for you as a health care consumer to take an active role when you are considering CAM therapies. Don't rely on advertisements and testimonials as primary sources of information. The National Center for Complementary and Alternative Medicine (NCCAM) suggests the following strategies to assist you in your decision making about CAM.

Gathering Information

- If you are seeking a CAM practitioner, speak with your primary health care provider regarding the therapy you are interested in. Your doctor may know about the therapy and be able to advise you on its safety, use, and effectiveness, or possible interactions with any of your current medications.

- Make a list of CAM practitioners and gather information about each: Where did they receive their training? What licenses or certifications do they have? Contact a professional organization for the type of practitioner you are seeking; the National Library of Medicine's Directory of Information Resources (dirline.nlm.nih.gov) includes many relevant associations. Many states also have regulatory agencies or licensing boards for certain types of practitioners.

- Ask how much the treatment will cost. Check with your insurer to see if the therapy will be covered.

- Come to the first visit prepared to answer questions about your health history and all medicines, vitamins, and other supplements you take.

Having a Successful First Visit

Here are some questions you might want to ask during your first visit:

- What benefits can I expect from this therapy? What are the risks associated with this therapy? Do the benefits outweigh the risks for my disease or condition?

- What side effects can be expected? Will the therapy interfere with any of my daily activities?

- How long will treatment last? How often will my progress or treatment plan be assessed?

- Will I need to buy any equipment or supplies?

- How much will the therapy cost?

- Do you have scientific articles or references about using the treatment for my condition?

- Could the therapy interact with conventional treatments?

- Are there any conditions for which this treatment should not be used?

Making Decisions

Assess your first visit and decide if the practitioner is right for you:

- Was the practitioner easy to talk with? Were you comfortable asking questions, and did the practitioner answer your questions satisfactorily?

- Was the practitioner open to how both CAM therapy and conventional medicine might work together for your benefit?

- Do the treatment plan and its associated costs seem reasonable and acceptable to you?

Source: National Center for Complementary and Alternative Medicine, Selecting a CAM practitioner, NCCAM Publication No. D346, February 2007. http://nccam.nih.gov/health/practitioner/index.htm.

---

field of dietary supplementation. If prayer is excluded, herbal medicine is the most popular form of complementary and alternative medicine used in America.

Because plants contain active biochemical systems, they are known to produce a wide array of chemical compounds and bioactive metabolites. An experienced herbalist can prepare bioactive plant material for human use. However, as with any biologically active material, there is a risk of toxic reaction instead of therapeutic response.[10]

Herbal medications and supplements can be dispensed in a variety of forms, including teas, coffees, tinctures, fluid and solid extracts, poultices (plasters), ointments, oils, pills, capsules, and powders. Even though many prescription medications are botanically based, the FDA classifies herbal preparations as dietary supplements because their safety and effectiveness have not been subjected to rigorous testing. Consumers use these preparations knowing relatively little about their safety and effectiveness, processing, formulation, and packaging/labeling. These risks must be taken seriously, particularly by anyone who uses herbal supplements in large quantity or in combination with prescription medications. For readers interested in a quick tutorial regarding over 40 of the more commonly used herbs, the NCCAM offers *Herbs at a Glance,* accessible through the center's home page (http://nccam.nih.gov/).[11]

Ayurveda Even older than Chinese medicine, India's **ayurveda** takes a preventive approach to health care, through focusing on the interplay of body, mind, and spirit—and is, perhaps, the most holistic of the world's principal approaches to health care. In the Indian subcontinent, this is the medical care for the masses.

Important to ayurvedic medicine is the balanced nature of the constitution (or prakriti) appropriate to each individual. This constitution plays a critical role in how the individual expresses physiological processes, and thus maintains the internal and external balance needed for well-being. The prakriti, itself, is composed of three dosha (or qualities), each of which reflects combinations of the five basic elements of life—space, air, fire, water, and earth. Balance within each dosha, and among the three dosha, influences the balanced nature of the constitution or prakriti itself. The idea is that when balance exists, disease processes unique to each dosha will not develop. Dosha imbalances can result from lifestyle patterns, emotional factors such as stress, and environmental factors such as weather or the ambient germ pool.

Ayurvedic practitioners direct treatment toward *eliminating impurities* from the body through dietary changes, fasting, colonic cleansing of the gastrointestinal tract, and cleansing of the respiratory tract with nasal sprays and inhalations; *reducing symptoms* of imbalance through activities such as yoga, meditation, exercises, and relaxing in the sun, and through dietary changes; and *reducing worry and increasing harmony in life* by practicing peaceful thinking during exercising, yoga, and meditation. A fourth aspect of ayurvedic medical practice is the *elimination of existing physical and psychological discomfort* through massage directed at the 107 points where life's energy is stored within the body.

To date, no more than 1 percent of Americans have utilized the services of ayurvedic practitioners, and only a fraction of those using this form of health care have done so on a regular basis. Despite the limited awareness that most readers might initially have about ayurveda, this ancient but increasingly available form of complementary care could seem very attractive from a philosophical perspective and because of a virtual absence of invasive procedures. However, it is important to understand that ayurvedic medical preparations tend to include heavy metals, such as lead, mercury, and arsenic, which can lead to potentially serious levels of toxicity and reduce the effectiveness of medications important to allopathic medical practice.[12]

If you would like to consult a practitioner in one of the alternative disciplines but don't know where to start, see the box "Researching and Evaluating CAM Practitioners" for some tips.

National Center for Complementary and Alternative Medicine (NCCAM) At the urging of many people in both the medical and complementary health care fields, the National Institutes of Health requested federal funding to establish a scientific center for the study of alternative medical care. Today the NCCAM assembles information about alternative approaches to medical care and provides a framework for well-controlled research into the effectiveness of each approach.

It will be interesting to note whether all the branches of complementary medical care will want their theories of treatment and prevention tested under the rigorous criteria used by the National Center for Complementary and Alternative Medicine and to see how they respond if the results are not favorable.

Placebo Effects It seems safe to assume that most adults have some awareness of the positive effects of "sugar pills," as the term applies to the testing of new medications. In fact, in some cases, they hear that the "dummy" works as well as or, on occasion, better than the medication whose effectiveness is being evaluated. Upon learning the latter, some might question how medical doctors could know this and still actually be using such "medications" in their practices. Your textbook's response to this speculation is a simple reply—really? In fact, the concept of "true" and "perceived" placebos has been known for decades,[13] but is as yet less than totally understood from both a neurophysiological and a socioenvironmental perspective.

In the case of the first perspective, it is most likely that a basically inert material, in combination with emotional expectations that a physiologically active material may be involved, is capable of stimulating the cognitive basis of "effectiveness" through changes in the type or amount of neurotransmitters being produced in the central nervous system, or in terms of the level of "receptiveness" to these neurotransmitters within the cortical areas of the brain.[14] This is the "true" placebo effect in action.

The second perspective (socioenvironmental) is less easily described and less controllable in terms of clinical application since it requires the interplay of the patient's mindset, the nature of the physician-patient relationship, and multiple influences of the complex social environment in which the patient lives. To date, the controllability of these variables has not been easily assessed or established.[15]

In spite of the complexities associated with both aspects of the "total placebo effect," research continues and guidelines for its ethical application are being developed.

Key Terms

ayurveda (ai yur **vey** da) Traditional Indian medicine based on herbal remedies.

Restricted-Practice Health Care Providers

We receive much of our health care from medical physicians. However, most of us also use the services of various health care specialists who also have graduate-level training. Among these professionals are dentists, psychologists, podiatrists, and optometrists.

Nurse Professionals   Nurses constitute a large group of health professionals who practice in a variety of settings. Their responsibilities usually depend on their academic preparation. *Registered nurses* (RNs) are academically prepared at two levels: (1) the technical nurse and (2) the professional nurse. The technical nurse is educated in a two-year associate degree program. The professional nurse receives four years of education and earns a bachelor's degree. Both technical and professional nurses must successfully complete state licensing examinations before they can practice as RNs.

In light of the important role that nurse professionals play in today's health care system, it is worrisome that a significant shortage of nurses exists. On the basis of enrollment data for nursing programs in this country, and the number of nurses who have apparently left the workforce for various reasons, the current shortage of registered nurses is estimated to be 110,000. Projecting through 2012, it is estimated that 1.1 million new and replacement openings for nurses will exist in the United States,[16] a need that will most likely not be met. Unfortunately, for recent nursing school graduates and nurses wishing to return to the job market, the recession that began in 2009, and the slow recovery and high overall unemployment rate, has resulted in a significant reduction in the number of nurses finding positions. Today the hiring of nurses, particularly by hospitals and large group practices, has slowed to a standstill. Nursing homes, however, remain viable sites of employment. Whether the shortage so recently projected will return or not remains to be seen.

Many professional nurses continue their education and earn master's and doctoral degrees in nursing or other health-related fields. Some professional nurses specialize in a clinical area (such as pediatrics, gerontology, public health, or school health) and become certified as *advanced practice nurses* (APNs). Currently, four APN fields, including nurse midwives, nurse anesthetists, nurse practitioners, and nurse case managers, can be found in larger communities. Working in close association with physicians, APNs perform an array of diagnostic, treatment, and administrative activities once limited to physicians.

Allied Health Care Professionals   Our primary health care providers are supported by a large group of allied health care professionals, who are often responsible for highly technical services and procedures. These professionals include respiratory and inhalation therapists, radiographic technologists, nuclear medicine technologists, pathology technicians, general medical technologists, operating room technicians, emergency medical technicians, physical therapists, occupational therapists, cardiac rehabilitation therapists, dental technicians, physician assistants, and dental hygienists. Depending on the particular field, the training for these specialty support areas can take from one to five years of postsecondary school study. Programs include hospital-based training leading to a diploma through associate, bachelor's, and master's degrees. Most allied health care professionals must also pass state or national licensing examinations.

Self-Care/Home Care

The emergence of the **self-care movement** suggests that many people are becoming more responsible for maintaining their health. They are developing the expertise to prevent or manage many types of illness, injuries, and conditions. They are learning to assess their health status and treat, monitor, and rehabilitate themselves in a manner that was once thought possible only through a physician or some other health care specialist.

The benefits of this movement are that self-care can (1) reduce health care costs, (2) provide effective care for particular conditions, (3) free physicians and other health care specialists to spend time with other patients, and (4) increase interest in health-related activities.

Appropriate Self-Care   Self-care is an appropriate alternative to professional care in three areas. First, self-care may be appropriate for certain acute conditions that have familiar symptoms and are limited in their duration and seriousness. Common colds and flu, many home injuries, sore throats, and nonallergic insect bites are often easily managed with self-care. That said, there are some symptoms that might seem somewhat familiar that should not be responded to through self-care, but rather by seeing a physician promptly. These include a feeling of pressure or squeezing in the chest, a sudden severe headache, markedly blurred vision, difficulty talking or walking, dizziness and confusion, blood in urine or stool, unrelieved depression, and a cough with a yellow-green discharge.

A second area in which self-care might be appropriate is therapy. For example, many people administer injections for diabetes mellitus, multiple sclerosis, allergies,

---

> **Key Terms**
>
> **self-care movement**   The trend toward individuals taking increased responsibility for prevention or management of certain health conditions.

Good Health—What's It Worth, Now and Later?

The average life expectancy for women in the United States today is 80 years. For men, it's 76 years. That's a dramatic change from just a century ago. Thanks to tremendous advances in medical science and technology, many people are enjoying healthy, happy, and spiritually fulfilling lives well into their final years.

But this longevity comes with a price tag. It means that making healthful choices every day—including eating a balanced diet, getting exercise and adequate rest, and making opportunities for emotional and spiritual expression—takes on new importance. If you're going to live 10 "extra" years, what do you want to do with that time? Probably many of the things you're doing now, plus some different ones. Are you going to be able to meet the challenge—healthwise?

Taking charge of your health right now, when you're young and healthy, can be one of the most empowering things you do. By consciously choosing a healthy lifestyle—limiting your intake of alcohol,

avoiding drugs and cigarettes, and limiting your sex partners—you are building the foundation for good health in your later years.

If you should ever have a serious health problem, you'll be better equipped to handle it if you're used to taking care of yourself. You'll feel comfortable being involved in your treatment decisions and doing whatever you can to control the quality of your life. You'll see your health crisis as a challenge you need to deal with, instead of viewing yourself as a helpless victim.

Taking charge of your own health—by being an informed health care consumer, by choosing a healthy lifestyle, and by fostering a positive attitude—brings a sense of peace. It's knowing that you're doing everything you can to take care of yourself. It's enhancing the quality of your life today and preparing for an active and rewarding tomorrow.

---

and migraine headaches and continue physical therapy programs in their homes.

A third area in which self-care has appropriate application is health promotion. Weight loss programs, physical conditioning activities, smoking cessation, and stress reduction programs are particularly well suited to self-care (see the box "Good Health—What's It Worth, Now and Later?").

A potential fourth area in home care, self-diagnosis, is emerging, and not without some concern. Perhaps beginning with the thermometer and progressing to the home pregnancy test and the mail-in HIV diagnostic kit, today in-home genetic testing is available. These direct-to-consumer (DTC) genetic screening tests consist of a swab that is used to obtain a scraping of cells from the inner cheek and a mail-in envelope. Upon processing cells for their DNA, persons can obtain a genetic profile as it relates to specific disease predispositions. Principal concerns associated with the use of these tests are the shortcutting of primary care physicians (although some brands require physician consent) and the absence of genetic counselors to work with clients after they receive the results of their tests. Currently, in-home genetic screening tests cost $200–400 and are readily available over the Internet.

Over a thousand diseases can now be tested for using genetic screening. However, test results based on self-collected samples of genetic material are not necessarily reliable. For example, laboratories processing these materials do not consistently demonstrate analytical validity (getting the right technological outcome from the tissue sample submitted) and clinical validity (verifying that the DNA results are related to a medically recognized condition). Today there is little governmental supervision over this growing form of self-care.

Home Health Care As the U.S. population ages, it is becoming increasingly common for family members to provide home care to older relatives. As the number of frail older people increases, home care can significantly reduce the need for institutional care. Home care also can be delivered by home health care specialists. In fact, this form of care is proving so cost-effective that some insurance programs, including Medicare and Medicaid, cover portions of the cost of home health care for older adults.

Unfortunately, however, with the slow recovery from the recession of 2009, state-level participation in Medicaid is increasingly challenged and is fostering cost-saving strategies that have decreased funding for home health care services. These cost-saving actions have reduced the availability of professional expertise in the home setting and have increased the level of stress in caregivers, who are often older and/or have limited skill in patient care.

A decision to provide family-based home care, particularly for older adults, is often made for admirable and understandable reasons, including love for the relative who needs care and the high cost of professional home care and institutional care. For the millions of families who have made this decision, providing home health care can be highly rewarding. It also can be very demanding, however, because of the needs and limitations of the person who requires care and the compromises the caregivers must make.

Palliative Care Redefined

In the minds of most people, the term *palliative care* is associated with end-of-life care in which a terminally ill person, often in a hospice setting, is provided comfort measures, principally in the form of medications to minimize pain and other forms of discomfort. Today, however, *palliative care* is being defined in a manner more closely associated with broadly based forms of care and assistance that begins to be delivered soon after the diagnosis of an incurable condition and that continue through all stages of treatment. The goal of this redefined form of palliative care is to provide a wide array of services to maintain functionality, support ongoing medical care, yet enhance the quality of life and sustain the fullest sense of well-being under the circumstances.[17] The new palliative care, covered to various degrees by insurance and public assistance programs, does not replace the need for hospice care, but will hopefully delay its onset.

Health Care Facilities

Most of us have a general idea of what a hospital is. However, all hospitals are not alike. They usually fall into one of four categories—private, publicly funded, voluntary, or charitable. *Private hospitals* (or proprietary hospitals) function as profit-making institutions. They are not supported by tax monies and usually accept only clients who can pay all their expenses. Although there are some exceptions, these hospitals are generally smaller than tax-supported public hospitals. Commonly owned by a group of business investors, a large hospital corporation, or a group of physicians, these hospitals sometimes limit their services to a few specific types of illnesses.

Publicly funded hospitals are supported primarily by tax dollars. They can be operated by government agencies at the state level (such as state mental hospitals) or at the federal level (such as the Veterans Administration hospitals and various military service hospitals, such as Walter Reed Army Medical Center in Washington, DC, about which so much has been written in regard to conditions surrounding the care of wounded soldiers from the wars in Iraq and Afghanistan). Large county or city hospitals are frequently public hospitals. These hospitals routinely serve indigent segments of the population.

The most commonly recognized type of hospital is the *voluntary hospital.* Voluntary hospitals are maintained as nonprofit public institutions. Often supported by religious orders, fraternal groups, or charitable organizations, these hospitals usually offer a wider range of comprehensive services than do private hospitals or clinics. Voluntary hospitals are supported by patient fees (covered by health insurance), Medicare reimbursement, and Medicaid and public assistance reimbursement.

The fourth type of hospital, the *charity hospital,* is the least frequently found and may cease to exist in the face of today's medical care costs. Historically, these charitable institutions provided free care to those persons who had "fallen between the cracks" of the social safety net, as it existed at a particular point in time. Most often established and sustained by religious orders or county- or city-level

government, they provided the best care available for the relatively modest amount of funds to which they had access. In fact, during a good portion of the nineteenth and early twentieth centuries, they functioned as "teaching hospitals" for both public and private medical schools. Today, the remaining charity hospitals function more akin to nursing homes or free-standing emergency departments than the fuller-service hospitals they once were.

In the past decade, hospitals, particularly private and voluntary hospitals, have expanded their scope of services. Today hospitals often operate *wellness centers,* stress centers, cardiac rehabilitation centers, chemical dependence programs, health education centers, and satellite centers for well-baby care and care for the homeless. During the 1990s, two trends were observed in terms of hospital organization and ownership: (1) the acquisition of small hospitals (such as county hospitals and smaller community hospitals) by larger regional hospitals and (2) the reorganization of voluntary hospitals as for-profit hospitals. Both trends reflected the rapid movement of medical care in the direction of *managed care,* the term referring to the more profit-focused, cost-efficient, and third-party-controlled care reflective of the application of corporate strategies to the delivery of health care services.

The trend toward consolidation of the past decade, based on the cost-effectiveness of managed care, the increased income for newer, larger hospitals, and the costs of new technology, has its roots in hospitals' *desire to survive* as an institution. Today this trend to consolidate is more closely aligned with the financial difficulties surrounding the recent recession, the growing number of people who are uninsured or underinsured, the public demand for more affordable health care, and the growing focus on the "health care crisis" at all levels of government. Whether some of the innovative forms of health care delivery described later can be maintained during the current financial downturn remains to be seen, as these new delivery options face the same challenges faced by the more traditional hospitals.

Other health care facilities include clinics (both private and tax-supported), nursing homes (most of which are private enterprises), and rehabilitation centers. Rehabilitation centers are often supported by charitable organizations devoted to the care of chronically ill or handicapped people, orthopedically injured people, or burn victims. Increasingly, hospitals are decentralizing services into suburban areas.

In recent years, many private, 24-hour drop-in medical emergency and surgical centers have appeared. These clinics have their own professional staffs of physicians, nurses, and allied health professionals.

Regardless of the type of health care institutions in which you seek services, both you and the institutions have legally binding rights that structure your relationship. Table 14.2 details both your rights as a patient and their rights as licensed health care facilities.

Table 14.2 Patients' Institutional Rights

Regardless of the type of institution in which you are a patient, you have a variety of rights. These are intended to protect you from unnecessary harm and financial loss. The hospital, too, can expect your cooperation as a patient.

As a patient, you can expect all of the following from the institution:

- To be treated with respect and dignity
- To be afforded privacy and confidentiality consistent with federal and state laws, institutional policies, and the requirements of your insurance carrier
- To be provided services on request, as long as they are reasonable and consistent with appropriate care
- To be fully informed of the identity of the physicians and staff providing care
- To be kept fully updated about your condition, including its management and your prognosis for recovery
- To be informed of any experimental or other research/educational projects that may be utilized in your treatment and to be able to refuse such treatment
- To have the opportunity to specify advance directives (a living will, a life-prolonging statement, or the appointment of a health care representative) in order to facilitate health care decisions
- To receive an explanation of your bill for services regardless of the source of payment
- To present a complaint and receive a response about any aspect of your care or treatment and to have your complaint taken seriously
- To be involved in ethical considerations that arise during the course of your care

The institution can expect you, as a patient:

- To keep all appointments
- To provide all background information pertinent to your condition
- To treat hospital personnel with respect
- To ask questions and seek clarification about matters that affect you
- To follow the treatment prescribed by your physician
- To be considerate and respectful of other patients and to ensure that your visitors are considerate and respectful as well
- To satisfy your financial obligation to health care providers through the provision of insurance information and the credit where applicable

As a patient, you may at any time:

- Refuse treatment
- Seek a second opinion
- Discharge yourself from the institution

Beyond the "universal" patient/institutional rights listed above, a wide array of more specialized rights exists regarding care issues related to language-based needs, sensory perception deficiencies (including access to communication-based technologies), and availability of companionship for selected hospitalized patients. Information pertaining to these needs can be found in *Hospitals and Effective Communication,* Office for Civil Rights, U.S. Department of Health and Human Services, March 7, 2007, www.hhs.gov/ocr/hospitalcommunication.html.

Health (Medical) Care in America: For Better or For Worse

Paraphrasing a popular song from the film *The Sound of Music* ("How Do You Solve a Problem Like Marie?"), your authors simply replace Marie with "the American health (medical) care system?" Today that refrain is on the lips of people from the president to the average "Jane and Joe." The most recent (and apparently the last) World Health Organization (WHO) ranking of health care systems paints a disturbing picture of the American version.

Based on 2000 information gleaned from three sources (divisions of the WHO,[18] the World Bank,[19] and the CIA[20]), the U.S. system was ranked thirty-seventh when compared to its counterparts in 191 or 226 other countries, depending on the collection agencies named. Data from five quantifiable indices were the basis of the composite ranking reported by the WHO: (1) life expectancy at birth (31st), (2) health adjusted life expectancy or HALE (24th), (3) infant (birth–1 year)/ early childhood (1–5 years) life expectancy (33rd), (4) percentage of GDP spent on health care (value of goods and services produced by Americans) (1st) (16 percent), and (5) the annual expenditure on health care (1st) ($2.7 trillion).

Marie's problems were not ours, but ours have reached a critical, economy-crippling point that defies a single acceptable "fix" unless a true solution can be agreed on by the country's leadership and seen as acceptable and affordable by the majority of Americans. If an equitable solution could be found, it would, in the eyes of the Institute of Medicine of the National Academies of Science, be characterized by the following:

- Health [medical] care coverage would be universal.

- Health [medical] care coverage would be continuous.

- Health [medical] care coverage would be affordable to individuals and families.

- Health [medical] care coverage would be affordable for society.

- Health [medical] care coverage would enhance health and well-being by providing access to high-quality care that is effective, safe, patient-centered, and equitable.

The word "[medical]" has been added to each of the bulleted statements by your authors in support of the contention made in Chapter 1 that our health care system is far removed from the textbook's perception of health and is, in practice, a medical care system.

In our view, the current health care system cannot be sustained indefinitely. In 2009, President Obama introduced the Comprehensive Health Care Reform Act (H.R. 1495)[21] that, if sustained in or near its current configuration, would by 2018 significantly alter the health (medical) care model that is currently influencing virtually all aspects of American life. However, this legislation is so complex and multifaceted, as well as so bitterly opposed by large segments of the political spectrum, that we have assigned its initial configuration to the OLC for your consideration. Further, we urge you, as citizens and consumers of health care services, to follow the unpredictable unfolding of this legislation as it passes through the governance process so characteristic of politics in this country.

Health Insurance

Given the turmoil just described, it is possible that health insurance policies, currently written and sold to employers and individuals by insurance companies, may change in significant ways, particularly if the federal government becomes a principal payee for tomorrow's insurance policies. If, however, the structure of health insurance policies remains largely intact, then the description of health insurance that follows will be applicable.

Health insurance is a financial agreement between an insurance company and an individual or group for the payment of health care costs. After paying a premium to an insurance company, the policyholder is covered for specific benefits. Each policy is different in its coverage of illnesses and injuries. Merely having an insurance policy does not mean that all health care expenses will be covered. Most health insurance policies require various forms of payments by the policyholder, which includes cost-sharing of the premium with your employer, deductible amounts, fixed indemnity benefits, coinsurance, and exclusions.

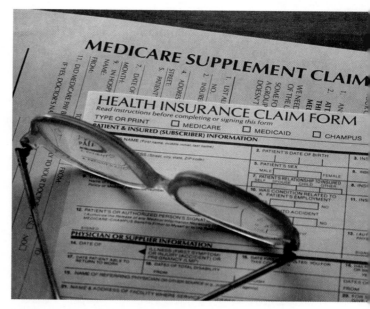

Health insurance helps consumers access quality health care, but millions of Americans have no insurance or have inadequate coverage.

A *deductible* amount is an established amount that the insuree must pay before the insurer reimburses for services. For example, a person or family may have to pay the first $1,000 of the year's medical expenses before insurance begins providing any coverage.

A policy with *fixed indemnity* benefits will pay only a specified amount for a particular procedure or service. If the policy pays only $1,000 for an appendectomy and the actual cost of the appendectomy was $1,500, then the policy owner will owe the health care provider $500. A policy with full-service benefits, which pays the entire cost of a particular procedure or service, may be worth the extra cost.

Policies that have *coinsurance* features require that the policyholder and the insurance company share the costs of certain covered services, usually on a percentage basis. One standard coinsurance plan requires that the policyholder pay 20 percent of the costs above a deductible amount, and the company pays the remaining 80 percent.

An *exclusion* is a service or expense that is not covered by the policy. Elective or cosmetic surgery procedures, unusual treatment protocols, prescription drugs, and certain kinds of consultations are common exclusions. Illnesses and injuries that already exist at the time of purchase (preexisting conditions) are often excluded. In today's turbulent health care climate, with looming governmental intervention, the insurance industry is "seeing the value" in curtailing the once-powerful preexisting-condition restrictions that characterized individual health insurance plans. In addition, injuries incurred during high-risk activities (ice hockey, hang gliding, mountain climbing, intramural sports) might not be covered by a policy.

Group Versus Individual Plans Health insurance can be obtained through individual policies or group plans. Group health insurance plans usually offer the widest range of coverage at the lowest price and are often purchased cooperatively by companies and their employees. In 2010, companies with health insurance benefits spent on average $13,770 for each employee's family health insurance plan, with the employer covering $9,723 of the $13,770 price, and the individual employee paying the remaining $3,997; a nonfamily policy (for a single employee) will cost the employer $4,181 and the employee $865, for total cost of $5,046.[22] In addition to family plans and individual (single-member) plans, an individual plus one plan is now available, allowing for more flexibility (and lower costs) when only a couple needs coverage. Fortunately, no employee is refused entry into a group insurance program. However, when employees leave the company, their previous group coverage can follow them for a prescribed period of time only, usually 18–24 months. Today, as many large American companies continue to lay off employees, the eventual loss of health insurance is becoming a serious personal and family issue. Fortunately, for persons who were employed by companies with 20 or more employees at the time of their job loss, the federal government allows them to carry their group health insurance for 18 months into the future. COBRA (Continuation of Health Coverage) costs, however, are paid entirely by the former employee, up to 102 percent of the plan's full cost.[23]

Individual policies (non-employer provided) can be purchased by one person (or a family) from an insurance company. These policies are often much more expensive than group plans and may provide much less coverage. Still, people who do not have access to a group plan should attempt to secure individual policies, because the financial burdens resulting from a severe accident or illness that is not covered by some form of health insurance can be devastating. Many colleges and universities offer annually renewable health insurance policies that students can purchase. Some questions to consider before purchasing a health insurance policy are these:

- Is the insurance company you're considering rated favorably by *Best's Insurance Reports* or your state insurance department?

- Have you compared health insurance policies from at least two other companies?

- Can you afford this insurance policy?

- Do you understand the factors that might raise the cost of this policy?

- Do you clearly understand which health conditions are covered and which are not?

- Do you clearly understand the deductible amounts of this policy?

- Do you clearly understand all information in this policy that refers to exclusions and preexisting conditions?

Although the health care insurance needs of most readers may already be met, such is not the case for a large minority of Americans. In fact, according to the U.S. Census Bureau, for an estimated 50.7 million Americans, the year 2010 was characterized by not being able to afford health care insurance at all, having health insurance for only a portion of the year, or having insurance so lacking in coverage that it was largely unusable (the underinsured). This depressing reality makes the United States almost completely unique among the world's most highly developed nations.

Modifications to Traditional Employer/Employee Insurance Plans In light of the uncertainty of today's health care environment, innovations in securing and paying for care are being seen. Three such innovations are (1) *open market* coverage, in which the employee places a need (such as knee replacement) online, providers submit cost data to the employer, and the employer/employee submits a cost-sharing plan to the employer's health insurance providers; (2) *private exchange* coverage, which involves a voucher issued by the employer indicating an amount that the employer will contribute to policies chosen by the employees; and (3) *concierge service,* which is not so much insurance as an opportunity for individuals to purchase "special attention" from health care providers. Generally, for an additional nonrefundable annual flat fee ($1,000), the payee obtains immediate access to her or his care provider, receives additional time when seeing the health provider, has annual health assessments and consultations beyond those normally provided, and gains access to other agreed-upon services not usually covered or less fully covered by health care insurance.

High-Deductible Health Plans with Health Savings Accounts Relatively new in the health care coverage arena are HDHP/HSA accounts in which pretax income is set aside into a "health saving account" (HSA) to be used exclusively for the payment of health care–related expenses, including enrollment in your employer's health insurance plan and expenses not covered by that plan. The HDHP component requires deductibles considerably higher than those normally required by health insurance plans—generally no lower than $1,000 for an individual plan and $2,000 for a family plan, but not to exceed $5,259 for an individual plan or $10,500 for a family plan. On the positive side, the money set aside on a monthly basis is not taxed, the cost of the insurance is less because of the high deductible, and the account can be transferred with changes in employment. These plans also emphasize coverage of preventive care, a feature not generally included in more traditional health insurance plans. The less attractive aspects of HDHP/HSA plans relate to the high deductibles and the unavailability of the pretaxed money for uses other than those intended.

Medicare

Since it was established in 1965, *Medicare* has been a key provider of health care coverage for the nation's older adults. Medicare is a federally funded health insurance program for persons 65 years of age and older, as well as for persons of any age who have particular disabilities or permanent kidney failure. Funding for Medicare comes primarily from federal payroll taxes (FICA) and is administered by the Health Care Financing Administration, within the U.S. Department of Health and Human Services.

In its current configuration, Medicare is divided into two portions. Part A (the hospital insurance portion) helps pay for care while in hospitals, as well as for care in skilled nursing facilities and hospice care, and for some home health care. Persons become eligible for Part A coverage on turning 65 years of age, on the basis of having paid Medicare taxes while working. Medicare Part A does require an annual deductible of $1,132 (historically deemed to be the equivalent of the first three days of hospital care).[24]

Part B is an optional portion of Medicare that can be chosen at the time of becoming eligible for Part A. Unlike Part A, there is a monthly charge for Part B coverage. Currently, that charge is $96.40 per month for individuals making $85,000 or less or a couple making $170,000 or less,[24] but is subject to annual adjustment. Persons earning above these amounts paid $115.40 per month in 2011. Part B helps pay for doctors' services, outpatient hospital care, and some home medical services not covered under Part A, including physical and occupational therapy, medical devices, and some home health care. Routine dental and vision care are not covered. Like Part A, Medicare Part B also has a deductible, currently $162.[24]

Because of the universal nature of Medicare Part A and the affordable monthly charge for Part B, group health insurance plans to which many retirees belong require that Medicare be the "first payer" for services, thus allowing the group plan to be responsible for only that portion of health-related charges not covered by Medicare.

The Medicare Prescription Drug Improvement and Modernization Act of 2003 (now referred to as Part D) provides new prescription coverage options for Medicare recipients. As of 2011, it provides prescription coverage through third-party providers for a premium of $32.34 per month. As of 2011, after meeting an annual deductible of $310, Medicare covers 75 percent of the costs of prescription drugs, up to $2,840 per year; there is then a gap (the "donut hole") in coverage until out-of-pocket expenses reach $4,550 in a single year, at which point

Medicare kicks in again and covers 95 percent of further costs for the remainder of the year.[24] In 2011, individuals who were in the donut hole received a single $250 payment to assist in purchasing their needed medications. The Medicare prescription drug program is expected to cost the Medicare system $724 billion during the first decade of its existence.

After its initial implementation in 2006, Medicare Part D remains confusing for many older persons, for a number of reasons. But at this point, many eligible persons have accepted Part D, and first-year costs were slightly lower than initially anticipated. Further refinements in Medicare-based drug coverage will likely occur with time.

Medigap and Advantage Medicare Plans Because Medicare Parts A and B have deductibles and copays, along with areas that are not covered, most Medicare recipients select additional insurance coverage to assist them in covering the out-of-pocket expenses associated with Medicare Parts A and B. These programs, featuring multiple levels of coverage and approved for sale by private sector insurance companies, are often referred to as *Medigap* policies. The cost of individual policies vary widely, depending on the limitations found in less expensive policies and on the more comprehensive coverage of therefore more expensive versions.

A second form of supplemental coverage for Medicare recipients is the *Advantage* programs. These programs also come in a variety of forms and at differing costs, but have in common aspects of both drug coverage (Medicare Part D) and Medigap or supplemental coverage related to Part A and Part B deductibles and uncovered services.

Medicaid

Unlike Medicare, a program that is almost exclusively for persons 65 and older, as well as persons on disability and those with specific conditions such as end-stage renal failure[24] and ALS (Lou Gehrig's disease),[24] *Medicaid* is a program designed to assist in meeting the health care needs of qualified persons regardless of age. Also unlike Medicare, which is a federal program entirely funded through Medicare tax withholdings (Part A) and user-paid elected enrollment fees (Part B), Medicaid is a federal- and state-funded program administered by each of the individual states.

Qualification for receiving Medicaid assistance can be perplexing. Federal Medicaid law sets mandatory eligibility standards, while optional eligibility standards allow each state to tailor many aspects of the program to fit its unique needs. Central to the majority of the federally mandated eligibility standards is the current federal poverty level (FPL), as well as the standards related to the Aid to Families with Dependent Children (AFDC) program and the Temporary Assistance to Needy Families (TANF) program. Optional eligibility standards allow states to define some aspects of eligibility for pregnant women, disabled children, certain working disabled persons, and those designated as medically needy.

Federally mandated Medicaid services are wide ranging and include hospital services, physician services, laboratory/x-ray procedures, immunizations, family planning services, home health care services, transportation for medical care services, and nursing home services. This final service is of critical importance to older adults in that it pays for the majority of nursing home care required by this age group. Optional services, which are under state control, include prescription drugs, rehabilitation and physical therapy services, prosthetic devices, vision services, hearing services, and dental services, to include a few.

Health Maintenance Organizations

Health maintenance organizations (HMOs) are health care delivery plans under which health care providers agree to meet the covered medical needs of subscribers for a prepaid amount of money. For a fixed monthly fee, enrollees are given comprehensive health care with an emphasis on preventive health care. Enrollees receive their care from physicians, specialists, allied health professionals, and educators who are hired (group model) or contractually retained (network model) by the HMO.

Managed care, and HMOs in particular, was a reaction to the sharply climbing costs of health care that began in the 1980s. Businesses, which paid a large portion of health care costs through employee benefit plans, complained that no one in the health care loop had an incentive to control costs. Employers pointed out that consumers paid only a deductible and a small copayment, giving them little cause to question prices; doctors faced little financial oversight; and insurance companies merely rubber-stamped the bills.

When HMOs presented an alternative, employers began offering their workers incentives to select HMOs over traditional fee-for-service coverage and thus attempted to rein in the runaway costs of health care. HMOs now cover nearly 66.8 million Americans. In 2009, when viewed on a state-by-state basis, the leading HMO enrollment states were California with 15.6 million members, New York with 5.9 million, Florida with 3.6 million, and Pennsylvania with 3.2 million.[25]

HMOs are usually the least expensive but most restrictive type of managed care. The premiums are 8–10 percent lower than those for traditional plans, they charge no deductibles or coinsurance payments, and copayments are $15–20 per visit. However, you are limited to using the doctors and hospitals in the HMO's network, and you must get approval for treatments and referrals.

In theory, HMOs were to be the ideal blend of medical care and health promotion. Today, however, many observers are concerned that too many HMOs are being too tightly controlled by a profit motive in which physicians are being paid large bonuses to *not* refer patients to specialists or are prevented by "gag rules" from discussing certain treatment options with patients because of their costs to the HMOs.

In spite of the problems just mentioned, HMOs remain, in theory, more cost-efficient than the traditional fee-for-service health care model. Cost containment is achieved, in part, because most of the medical services within a group model HMO are centralized, and there is little duplication of facilities, equipment, or support staff.

Other new approaches to reducing health costs are *independent practice associations* (IPAs) and *preferred provider organizations* (PPOs). An IPA is a modified form of an HMO that uses a group of doctors who offer prepaid services out of their own offices and not in a central HMO facility. IPAs are viewed as "HMOs without walls." A PPO is a group of private practitioners who sell their services at reduced rates to insurance companies. When a policyholder chooses a physician who is in that company's PPO network, the insurance company pays the entire physician's fee, less the deductible and copay amounts. When a policyholder selects a non-PPO physician, the insurance company pays a smaller portion of that physician's fee. Today, more than 80 percent of Americans with health benefits are enrolled in a managed care plan (HMO, IPA, or PPO).

Extended or Long-Term Care Insurance

With the aging of the population and the greater likelihood that nursing home care will be required (a medium cost of $77,747 per year in 2011 for a semiprivate room), insurers have developed extended care policies.[26] When purchased at an early age (by mid-50s), these policies are much more affordable than if purchased when a spouse or family member will soon require institutional care. However, not all older adults will need extensive nursing home care, so an extended or long-term care policy could be an unnecessary expenditure.

Health-Related Products

As you might imagine, prescription and over-the-counter (OTC) drugs constitute an important part of any discussion of health-related products.

Prescription Drugs

Caution: Federal law prohibits dispensing without prescription. This FDA warning appears on the labels of approximately three-fourths of all medications. Prescription drugs must be ordered for patients by a licensed practitioner. Because these compounds are legally controlled and may require special skills in their administration, the public's access to them is limited.

Although the *Physicians' Desk Reference* lists more than 2,500 compounds that can be prescribed by a physician, only 260 drugs made up the bulk of the nearly 3,679 million new prescriptions and refills dispensed by online, supermarket, mass-market, corporate, and independent pharmacies in 2009.[27] Total retail prescription sales of $217 billion for 2009 represent a 1.3 percent increase over 2007 sales.[27] Pharmaceutical sales growth in this range is far below the reliable 6–9 percent annual increases enjoyed for many consecutive years and suggests a downturn for the coming years. This reversal of fortunes for the pharmaceutical industry reflects a number of factors, including a decreasing number of new drugs coming into the market, a significant number of brand-name drugs moving out of patent protection and into generic sales, and the negative influences of the financial climate on the ability of many people to have prescriptions filled or refilled. It is projected that by the year 2015, approximately $446 billion will be spent on prescription medications.

Research and Development of New Drugs

As consumers of prescription drugs, you may be curious about the process by which drugs gain FDA approval. The rigor of this process may be the reason that only about 21 new drugs were approved in 2008, the lowest number in several years, although 2009 saw 25 approved, and 2010 had 21 new approvals. This reduction from the former average of closer to 30 new drugs per year is believed to reflect the newer FDA stance (Quality First) that arose following the removal of medications after longer-term use found them to be less safe than initially believed.

The nation's pharmaceutical companies constantly explore the molecular structure of various chemical compounds in an attempt to discover important new compounds with desired types and levels of biological activity. Once these new compounds are identified, companies begin extensive in-house research with computer simulations and animal testing to determine whether clinical trials with humans are warranted. Of the 125,000 or more compounds under study each year, only a few thousand receive such extensive preclinical evaluation. Even fewer of these are then taken to the FDA to begin the evaluation process necessary to gain approval for further research with humans. When the FDA approves a drug for clinical trials, a pharmaceutical company can obtain a patent, which prevents the drug from being manufactured by other companies for the next 17 years.

If the seven years of work needed to bring a new drug into the marketplace go well, a pharmaceutical company enjoys the remaining 10 years of legally protected retail sales. Today new "fast-track" approval procedures at the FDA are progressively reducing the development period, particularly for desperately needed breakthrough drugs like those used to treat AIDS. Concern was expressed in 2000 that this "rush to approval" forced the FDA to utilize the services of independent evaluators, many of whom had ties to the pharmaceutical industry that could have influenced their assessments of a drug's readiness for marketing. Even today, conflict-of-interest issues based on financial ties between review panels and the pharmaceutical industry exist, and are a possible factor in the growing backlog of approvals required in the development and marketing of new medications and biologics.

Figure 14-1 maps the long, arduous, and expensive process whereby a scant few of the tens of thousands of compounds, often derived from botanical sources, are, after nearly seven years of testing and review, approved for market as the newest prescription medications. During these carefully monitored stages, pharmaceutical companies take biologically active molecules through computer modeling, synthesizing, testing in vitro, testing in animals, and human trials, and eventually some are approved for marketing. Note that in this example, of the 5,000 compounds initially introduced into the process, only 1 successfully completes the approval process to become a marketable prescription medication. For more information on the drug approvals process, visit the website for the FDA Center for Drug Evaluation and Research (www.fda.gov/cder/handbook).

As a point of interest, it should be noted that in spite of the near-universal acceptance of American pharmaceuticals, over 80 percent of the pharmacologically active substances in compounded American prescription medications are produced overseas, principally in China, India, and Germany.

For decades the process of testing and reviewing new prescription medications involved human testing only on adult males (medical students, prisoners, and patients). In the latter decades of the twentieth century, concerns were raised about the absence of women, and then children and older adults, in the testing process, and most recently testing using pregnant women. Today, when deemed appropriate for the best use of a new medication, these groups are included in the human testing protocol. Now when a new medication comes onto the market, it is no longer necessary to extrapolate from adult male dosages in order to determine safe and effective use with women, children, or older adults.

Despite the importance of modern drugs and biologics in today's practice of medicine, the American public is far from pleased with the pharmaceutical manufacturing industry. According to a joint survey by the Harvard School of Public Health, the Kaiser Family Foundation, and *USA Today*, 79 percent of those surveyed believed that the costs of prescriptions were unreasonable, 79 percent

	Preclinical Testing		Clinical Trials				FDA		Phase IV
			Phase I	Phase II	Phase III				
Years	3.5		1	2	3		2.5	12 Total	
Test Population	Laboratory and animal studies	File IND at FDA	20 to 80 healthy volunteers	100 to 300 patient volunteers	1,000 to 3,000 patient volunteers	File NDA at FDA			Additional post-marketing testing required by FDA
Purpose	Assess safety and biological activity		Determine safety and dosage	Evaluate effectiveness, look for side effects	Verify effectiveness, monitor adverse reactions from long-term use		Review process/approval		
Success Rate	5,000 compounds evaluated		5 enter trials				1 approved		

Figure 14-1 New Drug Development and Approval   Only about 5 of 5,000 investigated compounds make it to human testing (clinical trials), and only about 1 in 5 of drugs tested in people is eventually approved. The FDA is involved in two stages of drug development: A company files an Investigational New Drug Application (IND) to request approval to test a new drug in humans. If clinical trials indicate that a drug is safe and effective, a drug developer will then file a New Drug Application (NDA) seeking FDA approval to make the drug available for physicians to prescribe to patients. Additional testing and surveillance may be required after drug approval in order to evaluate long-term effects.

Source: Used with permission by Pharmaceutical Research and Manufacturers of America.

thought that unacceptably high costs were principally the fault of the drug companies, 74 percent felt that these companies were making excessive profits, and 51 percent and 60 percent felt that too much was being spent on marketing to doctors and on public advertisements.[28] The final two issues, under the strong urging of Congress, will be sharply curtailed over the coming years, thus ending for doctors the free pens and note pads, paid trips to professional meetings held on tropical islands, free computer bags emblazoned with drug company logos, and industry-underwritten grand rounds where medical students see respected clinicians using the drugs of a particular company.

Biologics and Biosimilar Medications

In the last 20 years, new forms of treatment modalities have emerged employing modifications of living materials, principally in the form of genetically modified immune system proteins. These noncompounded prescription medications, or *biologics,* represent the "cutting edge" in the treatment of a growing number of conditions, including cancer, rheumatoid arthritis, multiple sclerosis, and irritable bowel diseases, such as Crohn's. Although highly effective, these medications are extremely expensive in comparison to traditional prescription medications. Further, due to the unique nature of the development and manufacturing of these modalities, the FDA was encouraged to set aside laws limiting patent protection times

applicable to compounded medications. In the absence of future generics, biologics were destined to forever be "top-dollar" modalities. In recent years, however, competitors, in the form of *biosimilar modalities* (aka *follow-on biologics*), have emerged from within the domestic and international pharmaceutical industry to challenge legally protective exclusivity of the original biologics, thus promising more competitive pricing.

Generic Versus Brand-Name Drugs

When a new drug comes into the marketplace, it carries three names: its **chemical name,** its **generic name,** and its **brand name.** While the 17-year patent is in effect, no other drug with the same chemical formulation can be sold. When the patent expires, other companies can manufacture a drug of equivalent chemical composition and market it under the brand-name drug's original

Key Terms

chemical name Name used to describe the molecular structure of a drug.

generic name Common or nonproprietary name of a drug.

brand name Specific patented name assigned to a drug by its manufacturer.

generic name. Because extensive research and development are unnecessary at this point, producing generic drugs is far less costly than is developing the original brand-name drug. Nearly all states allow pharmacists to substitute generic drugs for brand-name drugs, as long as the prescribing physician approves. For those interested in viewing all of the currently approved generics, the FDA updates daily its Generic Drug Approvals list.[29]

Today there is a sizable backlog of applications, being held by the FDA, for the marketing of new generics. To facilitate the approval process, the generic manufacturers have proposed that the FDA establish a generic user fee in their industry to raise additional FDA funds. This money could be used to form more review panels and to employ more FDA overseas inspectors for better quality control of the active ingredients used in the manufacturing of virtually all American prescription medications.

 TALKING POINTS Your mother insists on using the brand-name drug that she has used for years to control her arthritis pain, even though her doctor has prescribed a generic version that has recently become available. What might you say to help her consider the less expensive option?

Over-the-Counter Drugs

When people are asked when they last took some form of medication, for many the answer might be "I took aspirin (or a cold pill, or a laxative) this morning." In making this decision, people engaged in self-diagnosis, determined a course for their own treatment, self-administered their treatment, and freed a physician to serve people whose illnesses were more serious than theirs. None of this would have been possible without readily available, inexpensive, and effective OTC drugs.

Although 2,500 prescription drugs are available in this country, there are easily as many as 100,000 OTC products, now classified as belonging to one or more of 80 categories—such as acne medications, laxatives, skin-bleaching agents, cold and cough suppressants, diaper rash ointments, and wart removal compounds. Incorporated into these thousands of products are 1 or more of the 800 FDA-approved (as safe and effective) active ingredients. Like prescription drugs, nonprescription drugs are regulated by the FDA. However, for OTC drugs, the marketplace is a more powerful determinant of success.

The regulation of OTC drugs is based on a provision in a 1972 amendment to the 1938 Food, Drug, and Cosmetic Act. As a result of that action, OTC drugs were placed in three categories (I, II, and III) based on the safety and effectiveness of their active ingredient(s). Today, only category I OTC drugs that are safe, effective, and truthfully labeled are to be sold without a

prescription. The FDA's drug classification process also allows some OTC drugs to be made stronger and some prescription drugs to become nonprescription drugs by reducing their strength through reformulation.

Like the label shown in Figure 14-2, current labels for OTC products reflect FDA requirements. The labels must clearly state the type and quantity of active ingredients, alcohol content, side effects, instructions for appropriate use, warning against inappropriate use, and risks of using the product with other drugs (polydrug use). Unsubstantiated claims must be carefully avoided in advertisements of these products. In addition, under new labeling laws, the use of "black boxes" will be required when it is known that OTC medications hold risks, particularly when used in combination with other medications. An example of this occurred in 2008 when OTC cough remedies were found to be ineffective and in fact dangerous when used by young children. In response to the concerns of the pediatric community, the OTC manufacturers agreed to "black box" the use of these popular products for children 4 years of age and younger, while in 2011, new dosing standards were added (black boxed) regarding the appropriate use of liquid cold medications, particularly for children 2 years of age or younger. When used on a routine basis, OTC medications should be carefully discussed with a physician or a pharmacist.

Dietary Supplements

Currently, more than 50 percent of American adults are using an array of vitamins, minerals, herbal products, hormones, amino acids, and glandular extracts in their quest for improved health. People turn to dietary supplements rather than the dietary recommendations discussed in Chapter 5 for many reasons, including concern over their own morbidity and mortality, dissatisfaction with today's impersonal health care system, distrust in the safety of the food supply, and increasing inability to control other aspects of their lives. As a result, we are now spending an estimated $27 billion annually on dietary supplements—many of which appear unnecessary and some of which may be unsafe and ineffective. Recall that dietary supplement makers are not required to submit evidence of safety or effectiveness to the Food and Drug Administration, as is the case with prescription medications and, to a lesser degree, OTC products.

In spite of the lack of available data on safety and effectiveness, the traditional medical community is showing increasing interest in the potential benefits of dietary supplements. A growing number of teaching hospitals are establishing departments of complementary medicine, and medical students are learning about the documented role (to the extent that it is known) that these supplements can play in promoting health.

Drug Facts

Active Ingredient (in each tablet)   **Purpose**
Chlorpheniramine maleate 2 mg   Antihistamine

Uses temporarily relieves these symptoms due to hay fever or other upper respiratory allergies:
■ sneezing ■ runny nose ■ itchy, watery eyes ■ itchy throat

Warnings
Ask a doctor before use if you have
■ glaucoma ■ a breathing problem such as emphysema or chronic bronchitis
■ trouble urinating due to an enlarged prostate gland

Ask a doctor or pharmacist before use if you are taking tranquilizers or sedatives

When using this product
■ you may get drowsy   ■ avoid alcoholic drinks
■ alcohol, sedatives, and tranquilizers may increase drowsiness
■ be careful when driving a motor vehicle or operating machinery
■ excitability may occur, especially in children

If pregnant or breast-feeding, ask a health professional before use.
Keep out of reach of children. In case of overdose, get medical help or contact a Poison Control Center right away.

Directions

adults and children 12 years and over	take 2 tablets every 4 to 6 hours; not more than 12 tablets in 24 hours
children 6 years to under 12 years	take 1 tablet every 4 to 6 hours; not more than 6 tablets in 24 hours
children under 6 years	ask a doctor

Other information
■ store at 20-25°C (68-77°F)   ■ protect from excessive moisture

Inactive ingredients D&C yellow no. 10, lactose, magnesium stearate, microcrystalline cellulose, pregelatinized starch

Figure 14-2 Over-the-Counter Drug Label   The FDA requires over-the-counter drugs to carry standardized labels, such as the one above.

However, the extent to which the National Center for Complementary and Alternative Medicine (within the National Institutes of Health) will undertake carefully controlled studies of dietary supplements remains uncertain.

In light of the NCCAM's inability to carefully research the multitude of products currently defined as dietary supplements, and the FDA's inability to meaningfully regulate their safety and effectiveness, the dietary supplement industry remains largely self-regulated. Only its advertising falls under federal regulation.

In the 1994 Dietary Supplement Health and Education Act, the regulation of advertising of dietary supplements was assigned to the Federal Trade Commission (FTC). However, the FTC has a broad arena of responsibility, and critics doubt that the FTC assertively scrutinizes information supplied by dietary supplement manufacturers in the promotion of their products. However, the FTC has issued some guidelines regarding questionable claims in this advertising and urges concerned consumers to contact the FTC. Following are examples of advertising claims that would be the basis of such reporting:[30]

- A claim that the product is an effective cure-all for a wide variety of diseases or can function as a diagnostic tool for identifying a health problem
- A claim that the product can treat or cure a specific disease or condition
- Phrasing such as "scientific breakthrough," "miraculous cure," or "ancient remedy"
- Technologically unfamiliar words such as *thermogenesis, hypothalamic appetite center,* or *metabolic substrates*
- Undocumented personal testimonials from patients or practitioners claiming spectacular results
- A claim that availability is limited or that a "holding deposit" is needed
- A promise of a no-risk guarantee

For readers seeking accurate information on dietary supplements, your textbook recommends *IBIDS*, the database on dietary supplements, from the Office of Dietary Supplements of the National Institutes of Health (NIH), which can be found at http://grande.nal.usda.gov/ibids/index.php.[31]

Health Care Consumer Fraud

A person who earns money by marketing inaccurate health information, unreliable health care, or ineffective health products is called a fraud, a **quack,** or a charlatan. **Consumer fraud** flourished with the old-fashioned medicine shows of the late 1800s. Unfortunately, consumer fraud still flourishes. You need look no further than large city newspapers to see questionable advertisements for disease cures and weight loss products. Quacks have found in health and illness the perfect avenues to indulge in **quackery**—to make maximum gain with minimum effort. Fraud can even occur after death (see the box "Modern 'Grave Robbing'").

Key Terms

quack A person who earns money by purposely marketing inaccurate health information, unreliable health care, or ineffective health products.

consumer fraud Marketing of unreliable and ineffective services, products, or information under the guise of curing disease or improving health; quackery.

quackery The practice of disseminating or supplying inaccurate health information, unreliable health care, or ineffective health products for the purposes of defrauding another person.

Modern "Grave Robbing"

Perhaps one of the most distressing examples of health-related consumer fraud reached headline status in 2006 when it was discovered that a body-parts procurement business was working in conjunction with a mortuary (or individual mortuary employees) to harvest marketable human body parts for sale to medical schools for medical research or to hospitals for transplantation into living recipients. Modern "grave robbing" is, of course, illegal. All organ donations must be authorized by the donor or by the immediate family of the deceased. In addition to stealing and selling body parts, the mortuary deceived the survivors of the deceased into believing that the body had been handled properly in preparation for viewing before burial or cremation. This scandal reached public attention when investigators released x-rays showing that the mortuary had inserted PVC pipes and other "filler" to normalize the appearance of the body in areas where parts had been illegally removed.

In light of the high demand for, and limited supply of, human body parts for use in modern medical education, medical research, and medical practice, a cadaver is worth thousands of dollars, as virtually every type of tissue, individual body part, anatomical region (pelvis, intact leg, head, and so on), and, of course, the intact body, can be used. This said, how can a family be assured that no illegal harvesting has occurred? The answer, beyond only using the services of a "trusted" mortuary in the local community, is to request viewing of the prepared body before dressing and placement in the casket or in the retort prior to cremation—something many a grieving family member would be uncomfortable doing.

When people are in poor health, they may be afraid of becoming disabled or dying. So powerful are their desires to live and avoid suffering that people are vulnerable to promises of health improvement or a cure. Even though many people have great faith in their physicians, they also want access to experimental treatments or products touted as being superior to currently available therapies. When tempted by the promise of help, people sometimes abandon traditional medical care. Of course, quacks recognize this vulnerability and present a variety of "reasons" to seek their help. Gullibility, blind faith, impatience, superstition, ignorance, or hostility toward professional expertise eventually carry the day. In spite of the best efforts of agencies at all levels, no branch of government can protect consumers from their own errors of judgment that so easily play into the hands of quacks and charlatans.

Regardless of the motivation that leads people into consumer fraud, the outcome is frequently the same. First, the consumers lose money. The services or products are grossly overpriced, and consumers have little recourse to help them recover their money. Second, the consumers often feel disappointed, guilty, and angered by their own carelessness as consumers. Far too frequently, consumer fraud may lead to unnecessary suffering.

Taking Charge of Your Health

- Keep yourself well informed about current health issues and new developments in health care.
- Analyze the credibility of the health information you receive before putting it into practice.
- Select your health care providers by using a balanced set of criteria (see pages 363 and 366).
- Explore alternative forms of health care, and consider using them as a complement to traditional health care.
- In selecting a health insurance policy, compare various plans on the basis of several key factors, not simply cost (see page 373).
- Assemble a complete personal/family health history as soon as possible.

Be sure to include information from older family members.
- Comply with all directions regarding the appropriate use of prescription and OTC medications.

SUMMARY

- Physicians can be either doctors of medicine (MDs) or doctors of osteopathy (DOs). They receive similar training and engage in similar forms of practice.
- Although alternative health care providers, including chiropractors, naturopaths, herbalists, and acupuncturists, meet the health care needs of many people, systematic study of these forms of health care is only now under way.
- Nursing at all levels is a critical health care profession. Advanced practice nurses represent the highest level of training within nursing.
- Self-care is often a viable approach to preventing illness and reducing the use of health care providers.
- Our growing inability to afford medical care services has reached crisis proportions in the United States.

- Health insurance is critical to our ability to afford modern health care services.
- Medicare and Medicaid are governmental plans for paying for health care services.
- The development of prescription medication is a long and expensive process for pharmaceutical manufacturers. The cost of prescription medication is the most rapidly increasing aspect of health care affordability.
- OTC products have a role to play in the treatment of illness, but their safe use is based on following label directions.
- Critical health consumerism, including avoiding health quackery, requires careful selection of health-related information, products, and services.

REVIEW QUESTIONS

1. Identify and describe some sources of health-related information presented in this chapter. What factors should you consider when using these sources?
2. Describe the similarities between allopathic and osteopathic physicians. What is an alternative health care practitioner? Give examples of the types of alternative practitioners.
3. What are the theories underlying acupuncture and ayurveda?
4. In what ways is the trend toward self-care evident? What are some reasons for the popularity of this movement?
5. How do private, publicly owned, voluntary (proprietary), and charity hospitals differ?
6. What is health insurance? Explain the following terms relating to health insurance: *deductible amount, fixed*

indemnity benefits, full-service benefits, coinsurance, exclusion, and *preexisting condition.*

7. What is a health maintenance organization? How do HMO plans reduce the costs of health care? What are IPAs and PPOs?
8. What role does Medicare and Medicaid play in meeting the health care needs of the American public? Which portion of Medicare is universal? What elective option does Medicare offer?
9. What is a biologic medication, and how would it differ from traditional prescription medications?
10. What are the three criteria that must be met by an OTC drug?
11. What is health quackery? What can a consumer do to avoid consumer fraud?

ANSWERS TO THE "WHAT DO YOU KNOW?" QUIZ

1. False   2. True   3. True   4. False   5. True   6. False   7. False   8. False

Visit the Online Learning Center (**www.mhhe.com/hahn11e**), where you will find tools to help you improve your grade including practice quizzes, key terms flashcards, audio chapter summaries for your MP3 player, and many other study aids.

SOURCE NOTES

1. *Health Information Online.* Pew Internet & American Life Project, May 17, 2005. www.pewinternet.org/PPF/r/156/report_display.asp.
2. *The Engaged E-Patient Population.* Pew Internet & American Life Project, August 26, 2008. www.ihealthbeat/org/.
3. Health topics: 80% of Internet users look for health information online. Pew Internet & American Life Project, February 1, 2011. www.pewinternet.org/Reports/2011/HealthTopics.aspx.
4. Physicians' use of email with patients: factors influencing electronic communication and adherence to best practices. *Journal of Medical Internet Research,* 8(1), e2, 2006. www.jmir.org/2006/1/e2.
5. Mostgaghimi A, Crotty BH. Professionalism in the digital age. *Annals of Internal Medicine,* 154(8), 560–562, 2011.
6. Pho K. Doctors ignore Internet at their own peril. *USA Today,* A11, January 27, 2010.

7. National Center for Complementary and Alternative Medicine (NCCAM), National Institutes of Health, Health and Human Services, March 24, 2011. www.info@nccam.nih.gov.
8. *BackGround: Manipulative and Body-Based Practices: An Overview.* National Center for Complementary and Alternative Medicine, National Institutes of Health, U.S. Department of Health and Human Services, January 23, 2007. www.nccam.nih.gov/health/backgrounds/manipulative.htm.
9. National Center for Complementary and Alternative Medicine (NCCAM). Homeopathy: an introduction, August 2010 (update). www.nccam.nih.gov/health/homeopathy/.
10. Lee JS. Medicinal plants: a powerful health aid? *Science Creative Quarterly,* (2), 1–7, 2007. www.scq.ubs.ca/?p=49.

11. *Herbs at a Glance.* National Center for Complementary and Alternative Medicine (NCCAM), National Institutes of Health, Health and Human Services, April 9, 2009.

12. Saper RB, Phillips RS, Sehgal A, et al. Lead, mercury, and arsenic in U.S. and Indian-manufactured Ayurvedic medication sold via the Internet. *Journal of the American Medical Association,* 300(8), 915–923, 2008.

13. Ernst E, Resch KL. Concept of true and perceived placebo effect. *British Medical Journal,* 311(7004), 551–553, 1995.

14. Ernst E. Placebo: new insights into an old enigma. *Drug Discoveries Today,* 12(9–10), 413–418, 2007.

15. Manchikanti L, Giordano J, Fellows, et al. Placebo and nocebo in interventional pain management: a friend or a foe—or simply foes? *Pain Physician,* 14(2), 157–175, 2011.

16. Department for Professional Employees. Nurse: vital signs. AFL-CIO, 2004. www.dpeaflcio.org/policy/factsheets/fs_2004nurses.htm.

17. National Institute of Nursing Research, National Institutes of Health (NIH). *Palliative Care: The Relief You Need When You're Experiencing the Symptoms of Serious Illness,* June 2009, NIH Publication No. 08-6415.

18. Press release WHO/44. *World Health Organization Assesses the World's Health Systems,* June 21, 2000. www.photius.com/rankings/who_health_ranks.html.

19. Draft document—2010.

20. Central Intelligence Agency. *The World Factbook* (updated weekly). www.cia.gov/library/publications/the-world-factbook/index.html.

21. 111th Congress, 1st session. H.R. 1495: Comprehensive Health Care Reform Act of 2009. www.thomas.loc.gov/cgi/query/z?c111:H.R.1495.IH.

22. Henry J. Kaiser Family Foundation, Health Research and Education Trust Survey of employer health benefits 2010, Slide 2 and Exhibit 5, September 2, 2010. www.ehbs.kff.org/.

23. *Continuation of Health Coverage—COBRA.* U.S. Department of Labor, Centers for Medicare & Medicaid Services, 2009 CMS Publication No. 10050-53. 2008.

24. *Medicare & You 2011.* Centers for Medicare and Medicaid Services. CMS publication No. 10050-53, 2010.

25. Henry J. Kaiser Family Foundation. *Total HMO Enrollment— Kaiser State Health Facts,* July 2009. www.statehealthfacts.org/comparemaptabloe.jsp?cat=7ind=348.

26. Genworth. *Executive Summary Genworth 2011 Cost of Care Survey.* www.genworth.com/content/products/long_term_care/long_term_care/cost_care.html.

27. Henry J. Kaiser Family Foundation, Health Costs and Budgets. *United States: Prescription Drugs, 2010.* May 15, 2011. www.statehealthfacts.org/profileind.jsp?66&rgn=l&cat=5.

28. *USA Today*/Kaiser Family Foundation/Harvard School of Public Health. *The Public on Prescription Drugs and Pharmaceutical Companies* (conducted January 3–23), March 4, 2008. www.kff.org/-kaiserpolls/pomr030408pkg.cfm.

29. *Approved Drug Products with Therapeutic Equivalence Evaluations: Orange Book.* Center for Drug Evaluation and Research. Food and Drug Administration, U.S. Department of Health and Human Services, 2011. www.accessdata.fda.gov/scripts/cder/ob/default.cfm. Accessed May 16, 2011 (Updated daily by the FDA).

30. "Miracle" health claims: Add a dose of skepticism. Federal Trade Commission, September 2001. www.ftc.gov/bcp/conline/pubs/health/frdheal.htm.

31. International Bibliographic Information on Dietary Supplements (IBIDS) Database. Office of Dietary Supplements, National Institutes of Health, 2009. www.ods.od.nih/gov/Health_Information/IBIDS.aspx.

Personal Assessment

Are You a Skilled Health Care Consumer?

Circle the selection that best describes your practice. Then total your points for an interpretation of your health consumer skills.

1 = Never
2 = Occasionally
3 = Most of the time
4 = All of the time

1. I read all warranties and then file them for safekeeping.
   1   2   3   4

2. I read labels for information pertaining to the nutritional quality of food.
   1   2   3   4

3. I practice comparative shopping and use unit pricing, when available.
   1   2   3   4

4. I read health-related advertisements in a critical and careful manner.
   1   2   3   4

5. I challenge all claims pertaining to secret cures or revolutionary new health devices.
   1   2   3   4

6. I engage in appropriate medical self-care screening procedures.
   1   2   3   4

7. I maintain a patient-provider relationship with a variety of health care providers.
   1   2   3   4

8. I inquire about the fees charged before using a health care provider's services.
   1   2   3   4

9. I maintain adequate health insurance coverage.
   1   2   3   4

10. I consult reputable medical self-care information before seeing a physician.
    1   2   3   4

11. I ask pertinent questions of health care providers when I am uncertain about the information I have received.
    1   2   3   4

12. I seek second opinions when the diagnosis of a condition or the recommended treatment seems questionable.
    1   2   3   4

13. I follow directions pertaining to the use of prescription drugs, including continuing their use for the entire period prescribed.
    1   2   3   4

14. I buy generic drugs when they are available.
    1   2   3   4

15. I follow directions pertaining to the use of OTC drugs.
    1   2   3   4

16. I maintain a well-supplied medicine cabinet.
    1   2   3   4

TOTAL POINTS _____

Interpretation

16 to 24 points—A very poorly skilled health consumer
25 to 40 points—An inadequately skilled health consumer
41 to 56 points—An adequately skilled health consumer
57 to 64 points—A highly skilled health consumer

TO CARRY THIS FURTHER . . .

Could you ever have been the victim of consumer fraud? What will you need to do to be a skilled consumer?

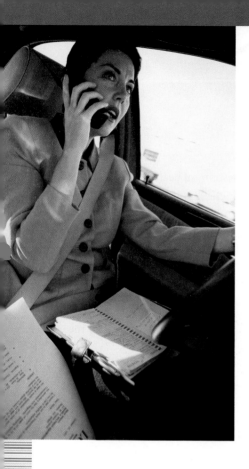

15

Preventing Injuries

What Do You Know About Preventing Injuries?

1. More injuries occur at home than in any other location. True or False?

2. Motor vehicle injuries take more lives than any other type of injury. True or False?

3. Male and female drivers with BACs of 0.08 or greater die in motor vehicle crashes at about the same rate. True or False?

4. The death rate for motorcycle riders is about 30 times higher than that for car riders. True or False?

5. Falls are the leading cause of fatal injuries in the home. True or False?

6. The violent crime rate in the United States is higher now than ever before. True or False?

7. Less than half of all violent crimes are reported to police. True or False?

Check your answers at the end of the chapter.

If you are a traditional-age college or university student (18–24 years of age), your chances of dying at this time are relatively low. But if you were to die, you would be more likely to die as a result of an injury than any other cause. Injuries are the leading cause of death for those from 1-44 years old and kill more people in the 15–24 age group than *all* other causes of death combined.[1] Injuries are the fifth-leading cause of death in this country, and if homicides are included, injuries rank third. Injuries are also the number-one reason people visit hospital emergency departments. In 2009 in the United States, there were 36.8 million injuries and poisonings for which individuals sought or received medical care.[2] Clearly, injuries are an important personal health concern, one that causes significant pain and suffering not only to the victims but also to the victims' families and friends.

Injuries are part of living in an imperfect world, and we cannot expect to eliminate all injuries that occur in our lives. But we can take steps as individuals and as a society to reduce the number and seriousness of injuries. In this chapter, we explain how and why injuries occur and offer thoughts on injury prevention and control. As you read the chapter, keep in mind that many federal, state, and local agencies are also working to minimize the toll injuries take on individuals, families, and society. Among these agencies are the National Center for Injury Prevention and Control, the National Center for Occupational Safety and Health, the National Highway Safety Administration, the Federal Trade Commission, the Department of Justice, the Department of Homeland Security, the U.S. Coast

Guard, numerous law enforcement agencies, and many voluntary, nongovernmental agencies.

We begin this chapter with a discussion of unintentional injuries, injuries that occur with no one intending that harm be done, and we describe ways you can lower your risk of injury. We then discuss intentional injuries, injuries that result from interpersonal violence, and we suggest ways to protect yourself from these injuries. Our goal is to help you, the student, protect your health by reducing your risk of becoming an injury victim. Complete the Personal Assessment at the end of this chapter to see whether you are adequately protecting yourself from injuries.

Unintentional Injuries

The vast majority of injuries that occur each year are **unintentional injuries,** injuries that occur without anyone intending harm. More than half of all these injuries occur in or around the home.[2] Nearly twice as many injuries occur in the home as occur outside, and falls are the leading cause of medically consulted injuries in the home. The next most common locations for injuries are recreation areas, and streets and highways.[2] Even though we spend a lot of time at schools and places of work, these venues are relatively safe.

Unintentional injuries and poisonings account for about two-thirds of all injury deaths annually in the United States. Of the 117,176 unintentional injury deaths reported in 2009, 32 percent were caused by unintentional poisonings, 31 percent by motor vehicle crashes, and 21 percent by falls. Other causes included exposure to smoke and flames, drowning, and the discharge of firearms.[1] The annual cost of such injuries to society is estimated at $702 billion, including $355 billion in lost wages, $145 billion in medical expenses, $122 billion in insurance administrative costs, and $42 billion in motor vehicle damage and other costs.[3]

Motor Vehicle Injuries

Motor vehicle crashes are the leading cause of injury deaths for the 16- to 24-year age group (the age group that includes most college and university students), and the second-leading cause of injury deaths overall. In 2009, approximately 36,284 people were killed in motor vehicle crashes in the United States.[1] In addition, an estimated 1.5 million people were injured, many of them seriously.[4] The rates of involvement in crashes with a fatality in 2009 were highest in the 16- to 20-year and 21- to 24-year age groups; the fatal injury rate for males is twice as high as that for females at every age (see Figure 15-1).[4] Nights and weekends are more dangerous driving times than daylight or weekday hours. Midnight to 3 a.m. on Saturdays and Sundays is the most dangerous time to be on the road.[4]

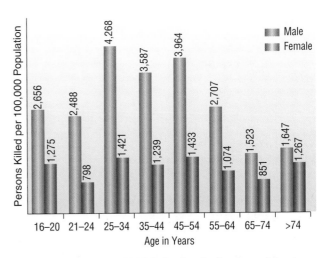

Figure 15-1 Fatal Motor Vehicle Crashes by Gender and Age
Males are more likely than females to be involved in fatal motor vehicle crashes; rates are highest among young drivers. What could be done to reduce the number of driving fatalities in young men?
Source: National Highway Traffic Safety Administration, *Traffic Safety Facts 2009.* Washington, DC: U.S. Department of Transportation.

Alcohol is frequently a contributing factor to the number and seriousness of unintentional injuries. This is especially true for motor vehicle crashes. Alcohol involvement increases the likelihood that a crash will occur and that it will result in a fatality. Twenty-seven percent of drivers and motorcycle riders involved in fatal crashes had blood alcohol concentrations (BACs) of 0.01 gram per deciliter or higher; 22 percent had BACs of 0.08 or higher. Among 21- to 24-year-olds, this figure climbs to 35 percent (see Figure 15-2). The percentage of male drivers with a BAC of 0.08 or higher (25 percent) who died in crashes was nearly twice as high as that of female drivers (14 percent).[4]

Alcohol impairment can increase the severity of injuries in motor vehicle crashes in another way. Alcohol-impaired drivers are less likely to use their seat belts and, if transporting a child, are less likely to have him or her properly restrained. Only 32 percent of children who died while riding with drinking drivers were properly restrained at the time of the crash.[5] Clearly, enforcement of child safety seat and safety belt laws is needed. The good news is that by 2008, self-reported seat belt use in the United States had increased to 85 percent overall and to 88 percent in states with primary enforcement laws (laws that

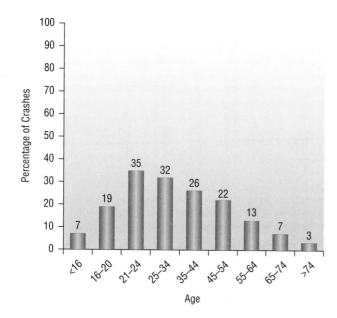

Figure 15-2 Alcohol and Fatal Motor Vehicle Crashes
Percentage of drivers and motorcycle riders with blood alcohol concentration of 0.08 or higher involved in fatal crashes.

Source: National Highway Traffic Safety Administration, *Traffic Safety Facts 2009.* Washington, DC: U.S. Department of Transportation.

allow police officers to stop drivers and issue tickets solely because the drivers are unbelted).[6] Since seat belt use reduces the likelihood of serious injury in a crash by about 50 percent, it makes good sense to buckle up.

Alcohol, while a major contributor to motor vehicle crashes, is not the only way driving performance can be impaired. In recent years, increasing attention has been paid to driver distraction as a roadway hazard. Drivers become distracted when their behaviors take their attention from the roadway (see the box "Cell Phone Safety and Distracted Driving").

Many college and university students commute to and from campus, or otherwise spend a lot of time driving or riding in cars and trucks. Make sure that you are not a "distracted driver," and if you are the passenger, help your driver be a safe driver. In addition to following commonsense driving rules, here are some safety tips:

- Make sure that everyone in your vehicle wears a seat belt *all the time.*

- If children are being transported, make sure that each child is restrained in the *appropriate type* of child safety seat *all the time.*

- If you are driving or riding on a motorcycle, *wear a helmet.*

- Do *not* answer a cell phone if you are driving. If you must make a call, pull off the highway into a safe place and then make the call.

- Do *not* use any other electronic devices while driving.

- Avoid adjusting the radio or CD player while driving.

- Do *not* drive if you are tired or sleepy. If you become sleepy while driving, let someone else drive or get off the road until you feel rested and alert.

Remember, the first goal of any trip is to arrive safely at your destination. Poor decisions about driving affect not only you and your riders but also your families and friends and, of course, others on the road. Wise decisions will save lives and prevent physical and emotional injuries for everyone.

Motorcycle Injuries   Some emergency room physicians call motorcycles "murder-cycles" because of their experiences with motorcycle crash victims. The statistics support this grim view. With the death rate for motorcycles at 37 per million vehicle miles of travel, compared to a death rate for cars of 1.3, motorcycles are 29 times more deadly.[4] Therefore, our first recommendation is to not operate or ride on the back of a motorcycle. If you do choose to ride a motorcycle, you can reduce your risk of injury or death by following these suggestions:

- If you are a new rider, know your bike and get proper training before you ride, especially before you carry a passenger.

- *Always* wear a helmet.

- Wear boots, gloves, and heavy clothing to protect your skin.

- *Never* ride after drinking alcohol or taking any medication that can reduce your alertness or driving performance.

- *Always* ride defensively. Assume that other drivers do *not* see you and will *not* give you the right-of-way.

Motor vehicle crashes, including motorcycle crashes, that involve injuries usually adversely affect people other than the drivers and passengers directly involved. Among the loved ones whose lives may be permanently altered by a motor vehicle–related injury or death are husbands, wives, parents, children, siblings, and close friends. The value of preventing motor vehicle–related injuries and deaths is self-evident.

Preventing Injuries at Home

More injuries of all types occur at home than anywhere else. Approximately 1 person in 10 is injured each year at home. It is not that our homes (residence halls, apartments, houses) are particularly dangerous; it is simply that we spend more time at home than anywhere else. Injuries that occur where we live include poisonings, falls, burns, and suffocations.

Cell Phone Safety and Distracted Driving

Cell phones and other personal electronic devices are becoming ubiquitous; there are some 310 million in use in the United States and 5 billion in use worldwide. But using a cell phone while driving a motor vehicle is clearly dangerous. A variety of studies and reports indicate a four- to ninefold increase in the potential for motor vehicle crashes associated with the driver's use of a cell phone. Since the first statewide ban on the use of handheld cell phones while driving was passed in New York in 2001, 30 other states have passed laws regulating cell phone use while operating a motor vehicle. States continue to collect data on crashes and cell phone usage as a basis for developing appropriate legislation. Highlights of the current cell phone restrictions include the following[*]:

- No state bans all cell phone use by all drivers.

- Twenty-eight states and the District of Columbia ban all cell phone use by novice drivers.

- Eighteen states ban cell phone use by school bus drivers when passengers are present.

- Thirty states, Guam, and the District of Columbia ban text messaging by all drivers.

- Eight additional states prohibit text messaging by novice drivers.

- Six states have "preemptive laws" that prohibit local jurisdictions from enacting such restrictions through local ordinances.

Some states consider cell phone use to be a part of a greater problem—distracted driving, which has become a recognized roadway hazard for everyone. Distracted driving is any nondriving activity in which a driver engages that might divert her or his attention from the primary task of driving. In a recent survey, more than 1 in 3 interviewees responded that they felt less safe on the highways today than before; 3 in 10 indicated that distracted driving was the single most important reason they felt this way.[†,‡] In the past decade, the number of personal electronic devices in use—cell phones (including iphones), personal digital assistants (PDAs), BlackBerries, laptops, electronic notebooks, Kindles, Nooks, and global positioning devices—has mushroomed. There are also more in-car entertainment devices, such as DVD players and gaming devices. Distracted driving also occurs when those who are driving eat or drink, search for something in a purse or elsewhere in the car, tune the radio, tend to children, apply makeup, or read a map. In 2010, 34 states collected data on crashes in which distracted driving was a factor; collecting such data may soon become a federal requirement.[§]

Texting and e-mailing while driving are simply the most recent driver distractions. Twenty-one percent of drivers surveyed admitted to having read or sent a text message or e-mail within the past 30 days according to a recent survey. For drivers under 35 years of age, the percentage jumped to 40 percent, and for drivers ages 16–19, it was 51 percent.[†] Forty-one states have initiated some type of campaign aimed at reducing these percentages through education and/or legislation.[**]

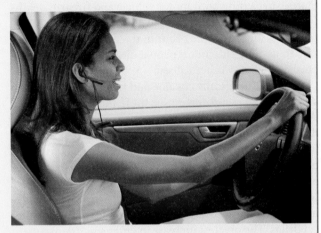

Anything that distracts a driver—talking on a phone, reading a map or notes, eating and drinking, or adjusting vehicle controls—can decrease concentration and slow reaction time. Driver distraction is a key contributing factor in many crashes.

Here are some basic guidelines for cell phone and other personal electronic device use in the car if you are driving:

- Before you start your car or truck, make any calls you might need to make during your trip. Then turn your cell phone off (just as you would if you were attending a lecture or performance). After you have arrived at your destination and turned off your motor, turn your cell phone back on.

- Never make or answer a call while driving.

- Never send or receive a text or e-mail message while driving.

- If you must make or return a call or text message, leave the highway and park your vehicle before you do so.

- If you use a global positioning system, ask a passenger to help you; otherwise, pull off the road to use it.

If you are a passenger, make sure your driver is not distracted by you or an electronic device. Be prepared to ask your driver whether he or she plans to turn their cell phone off or have you answer it for them. Encourage your driver to focus on the task of driving. It could save your life.

*Governors Highway Safety Association, Cell phone and texting laws, March 2011. www.ghsa.org.
†AAA Foundation for Traffic Safety, 2009 traffic safety culture index. Washington, DC: Author. www.AAAFoundation.org.
‡Centers for Disease Control and Prevention, Distracted driving, 2010. http://www.cdc.gov/MotorVehicleSafety/distracted_driving/index.html.
§Vermette E, Curbing distracted driving: 2010 survey of state safety programs. Washington, DC: Governors Highway Safety Association. http://www.ghsa.org/html/publications/survey/index.html.
**National Highway Traffic Safety Administration, Policy statement and compiled FAQs on distracted driving, 2010. http://www.nhtsa.gov/Driving+Safety/Distracted+Driving/Policy+Statement+and+Compiled+FAQs+on+Distracted+Driving.

Poisonings   By 2009, poisonings had become the leading cause of unintentional injury deaths in the United States, surpassing both motor vehicle and firearm deaths (see Figure 15-3).[1] Since the vast majority of unintentional poisoning deaths occur in the home, it is no longer safe to assume that more people die from motor vehicle crashes than any other cause.

Drugs, specifically cocaine and narcotics, are responsible for the largest portion of these poisoning deaths.[7,8] Between 1999 and 2006, the number of drug overdose deaths doubled. During the period 2004–2008, the estimated number of emergency department visits for non-medical use of opioid analgesics (narcotics) increased 111 percent (from 144,600 to 305,900 visits). In 2008, there were just as many emergency department visits involving legal drugs used nonmedically as there were for illegal drugs. The greatest increase in emergency department visits from poisonings was attributable to three drugs: oxycodone (OxyContin), hydrocodone (Vicodin), and methadone.[9]

Prevention of poisoning by prescription drugs requires an understanding of the potency of these agents, particularly the opioid analgesics such as oxycodone. These and similar drugs depress respiration to the point where there is insufficient oxygen in the body to sustain a heartbeat.

To reduce your risk of a drug overdose, adhere to the following precautions:

- Always read all information provided with your prescription.
- Always precisely follow the directions for taking prescription medications.
- Never exceed the prescribed dosage.
- Never try to obtain prescriptions for the same illness from different physicians.
- Never mix prescription drugs.
- Never drink alcohol while taking prescription drugs.
- Never take someone else's drugs or give your drugs to someone else.
- Always keep prescription medications in their original container.
- Keep the poison control center telephone number handy.

Other Unintentional Residential Injuries   Falls are the second-leading cause of injury deaths and the leading cause of nonfatal injuries in the home. Falls primarily affect the very young and very old, who may be more seriously injured and who may be slower to recover

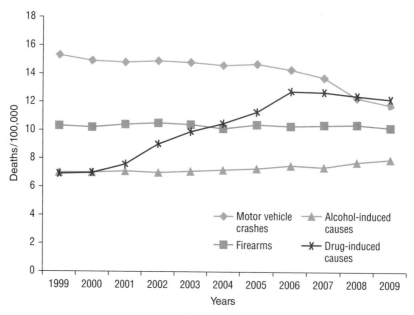

Figure 15-3 Death Rates for Four Types of Injuries, 1999–2009—United States

Sources: Xu J, Kochanek KD, Murphy SL, Betzaida T-V, Deaths: final data for 2007. *National Vital Statistics Reports,* 48(19), 1–136. National Center for Health Statistics, Centers for Disease Control and Prevention, U.S Department of Health and Human Services, May 20, 2010; U.S. Department of Transportation, National Highway Traffic Safety Administration, *Traffic Safety Facts 2009 (Early Edition): A Compilation of Motor Vehicle Crash Data from the Fatality Analysis Reporting System and the General Estimates System.* Washington, DC: Author, 2008. http://www.nrd.nhtsa.dot.gov/Pubs/811402EE.pdf. Accessed March 2, 2011; Miniño AM, Xu JQ, Kochanek KD, Deaths: preliminary data for 2008. *National Vital Statistics Reports,* 59(2). Hyattsville, MD: National Center for Health Statistics, 2010. http://www.cdc.gov/nchs/data/nvsr/nvsr59/nvsr59_02.pdf. Accessed March 24, 2011; Kochanek KD, Xu JQ, Murphy SL, Miniño AM, Kung HC, Deaths: preliminary data for 2009. *National Vital Statistics Reports,* 59(4). Hyattsville, MD: Author, 2011. http://www.cdc.gov/nchs/data/nvsr/nvsr59/nvsr59_04.pdf. Accessed March 24, 2011.

from nonfatal falls. Making sure that flooring is in good repair and that stairways are well lighted and equipped with handrails can reduce the risk of falls.

Exposure to heat, smoke, and flames is another leading cause of residential deaths; installation of smoke detectors and fire extinguishers can reduce the risk of injuries resulting from a fire. Suffocation affects mostly young children, who can suffocate on a toy or other object left within their reach. Another dangerous object found in many homes is a firearm. While only 2–3 percent of all firearm deaths are classified as unintentional, these deaths are, nonetheless, tragic and unnecessary.

Because we spend more time at home than at any other single location, safety in the home is an important component of our personal health. The National Home Safety Council provides a top-10 list of tips for preventing unintended injuries in the home.[10] As you review this list, note that many, but not all, of the items are aimed at protecting the very young and very old. The list, while not all-inclusive, suggests the leading causes of unintentional injuries in the home and provides a starting point for your efforts to ensure a safe home environment. How many of these suggestions would make sense in your home? How many would make sense in your parents' or grandparents' homes?

Prevent Falls

1. Install grab bars in the tub and shower. Use nonslip mats.
2. Have bright lights over stairs and steps and on landings. Keep stairs clear of clutter.

Prevent Poisonings

3. Keep cleaners, medication, and beauty products in a place where children can't reach them. Use child safety locks.
4. For Poison Help call 1-800-222-1222. Call if you need help or want information about poisons. Call 911 if someone needs to go to the hospital right away.

Prevent Fires and Burns

5. Have working smoke alarms and hold fire drills. If you build a new home, install fire sprinklers.
6. Stay by the stove when cooking, especially when you are frying food.
7. Keep your hot water at 120°F to prevent burns. Use back burners and turn pot handles toward the back of your stove. Use a travel mug when you drink something hot.

Prevent Choking and Suffocation

8. Be aware that things that can fit through a toilet paper tube can cause a young child to choke. Keep coins, latex balloons, and hard, round foods, such as peanuts and hard candy, where children cannot see or touch them.

9. Place babies to sleep on their backs, alone in their crib. Don't put pillows, blankets, comforters, or toys in cribs. These things can sometimes keep a baby from breathing.
10. When your children are in or near water, watch them very carefully. Stay close enough to reach out and touch them. This includes bathtubs, toilets, pools, and spas—even buckets of water.

Firearms, present in many American homes, are another potential source of injury. As noted previously, while only 2–3 percent of all firearm deaths are classified as unintentional, this represents hundreds of tragic and avoidable deaths, many of which occur in the home. Guns represent a unique health concern because a relatively high proportion of gunshot injuries are fatal. Below we list some commonly accepted safety rules associated with keeping a firearm in the home:

- Keep the gun and any ammunition out of sight of children.
- Keep the gun locked up and unloaded.
- Keep the ammunition locked up and in a separate location from the gun.
- Store the keys for the gun and the ammunition in a different area from where you store household keys, and out of reach of children.
- Lock up gun-cleaning supplies, which are often poisonous.
- Teach children to follow these rules from the National Rifle Association (NRA). If they come into contact with a gun, they should:
  - Stop.
  - Don't touch.
  - Leave the area.
  - Tell an adult.

Another source of injuries around the home is dogs. Even though most dog owners will say that their pet "wouldn't bite anyone," more than 4.7 million people are bitten each year, and 800,000 dog bite victims seek medical attention for their bites; half of these are children.[11] To reduce the likelihood of a dog bite, consider several things before getting a dog: (1) Check with an expert about the most suitable dog for your household; (2) do not acquire a dog that has a history of aggression, especially if children will be present; (3) spend time with the dog before buying or adopting it; (4) never leave an infant or toddler alone with a dog; (5) make sure the dog is properly socialized or trained; and (6) immediately seek professional help if the dog develops aggressive or undesirable behaviors. Children should be taught basic safety around dogs: (1) Do not approach an unfamiliar dog; (2) do not scream and run from a dog; (3) when approached by an unfamiliar dog, remain motionless;

(4) do not pet a dog without allowing it to see and sniff you first; (5) report stray dogs to an adult; and (6) report a dog bite to an adult.[11]

Preventing Recreational Injuries

The thrills we get from risk taking are an essential part of our recreational endeavors. It is indicative of the amount of leisure time we have that recreational areas are the third-leading location for unintentional injuries. Injuries can occur during organized sporting events and practices and also during individual pursuits, such as hiking or biking. Bicycle riding, which accounted for 500,000 emergency department visits in 2008, was the leading cause of recreational injuries that year. Basketball accounted for the second-highest number of visits to emergency departments.[3]

Preventing Bicycle Injuries   Communities and individuals vary greatly in their acceptance and tolerance of bicycles and bicycle riders. Bicycle riders should know their community and always choose the safest routes to ride. We offer the following suggestions to reduce the number and seriousness of injuries from bicycling:

- Wear a helmet; it could save your life.
- Obey traffic signals just as if you were in any other vehicle. Do not run through stop signs and red lights.
- Wear brightly colored clothing when riding during the day.
- Use a bright head light and a red tail light, and wear reflective clothing when riding at night.
- Refrain from carrying passengers; if you must carry a child, make sure the child is strapped into an approved seat and is wearing an approved helmet.
- Pay attention to weather conditions that could degrade the road surface.
- Make sure your bicycle is in good working order, especially the brakes.
- Equip your bike with a bell or other audible warning device if you are riding where pedestrians are present.

Preventing Boating Injuries   Boating is an enjoyable recreational endeavor for those living close to rivers, lakes, reservoirs, or the ocean. But each year hundreds of people drown. Many of these deaths occur because the victim was not wearing a personal flotation device (PFD). Of the 543 boaters who drowned in 2009, most could have been saved if they had been wearing a PFD, according to the U.S. Coast Guard. Two-thirds of the victims in fatal boating accidents drowned and 84 percent that year were not wearing life jackets.[12] Alcohol is also a risk factor; intoxication is a factor in more than half of all boating accidents.

The major cause of boating injuries and fatalities is "operator error," including (1) inattention (not looking in the direction the craft is traveling), (2) carelessness (boating in bad weather or water conditions), (3) speeding, and (4) boating while intoxicated with alcohol or other drugs. Drinking and boating, like drinking and driving, are a dangerous combination. Alcohol is a factor in more than half of all boating mishaps and, in 2009, was the direct or indirect cause of 30 percent of the boating mishaps in which a fatality occurred.[12] Below are some suggestions for preventing boating injuries:

Operators

- Know your craft; know how it responds under all weather conditions.
- Be alert for sudden changes in the weather.
- Before your passengers board your craft, make sure all safety gear is on board, in working order, and easily accessible.
- Never consume alcohol immediately before or while you operate your craft.
- Monitor the alcohol consumption and behavior of your passengers.

Passengers

- Wear a life jacket; it could save your life.
- Obey all safety rules.
- Realize that alcohol consumption reduces your chances of survival should you end up in the water.

Intentional Injuries

Intentional injuries are injuries purposely inflicted either by the victim or by another person. Each year in the United States, intentional acts of violence, including suicides, result in more than 50,000 deaths and another 2 million nonfatal injuries.[13] Included in these 50,000 fatal intentional injuries are more than 30,000 suicides, the leading cause of intentional injury deaths, and approximately 20,000 fatalities resulting from *interpersonal violence*. (See Chapter 2 for more information about suicide and suicide prevention.) In this chapter, we discuss only those intentional injuries that result from interpersonal violence.

Interpersonal Violence

Interpersonal violence occurs in our homes and communities, including our schools, places of work, and college campuses. Interpersonal violence can be perpetrated by family members, friends, colleagues, acquaintances, strangers, or gang members. Motivations for these acts include material gain, power, anger, jealousy, and religious, racial, or ethnic hatred.

In 2009, an estimated 4.3 million violent crimes were committed against U.S. residents 12 years of age and older. This is equivalent to 17 violent crime victims for every 1,000 people living in the United States. While this figure may seem high, it remains less than half the 1994 rate.[14] An estimated 1.8 million persons were treated for nonfatal physical-assault-related injuries in emergency departments in 2006.[15] Although the physical assault rate is higher for males, the rate of assault-related emergency department visits is higher for females. The highest rates of intentional injury for both genders were for the 20- to 24-year-old age group.[14]

Homicide   The spectrum of interpersonal violence includes homicide, robbery, rape and sexual assault, and simple and aggravated assault (assaults with a weapon). **Homicide,** or murder, is the intentional taking of one person's life by another person. Sadly, the United States leads the industrialized world in homicide rates. The homicide rate for 2009 was 5.8 per 100,000.[1] Homicide ranked as the fifteenth-leading cause of death in the United States in 2009, accounting for 17,859 deaths. Among 15- to 24-year-olds, 4,820 of whom were murdered, homicide was the second-leading cause of death in 2009.[1] Seventy-nine percent of all homicide victims are males.

The U.S. homicide rate is higher than that of any European country, but it has significantly declined since 1991, when it was 9.8 per 100,000 population.[16] Nonetheless, there are reasons to be concerned. Easy access to firearms in this country facilitates their use in violent acts. The latest injury data reveal that 50 percent of suicides and 69 percent of homicides in the United States are committed with firearms.[1,13] At highest risk for homicide and suicide involving firearms are adolescent boys and young men, ages 15–24.

While high school and college campuses are generally considered to be relatively safe social environments, the presence of guns on these campuses suggests otherwise. According to a recent survey, 6 percent of high school males had carried a weapon to school at least once in the previous month.[17] In a random sample of 10,000 college students, 4.3 percent reported that they had a working firearm at college, and 1.6 percent said that they had been threatened by a gun while at college.[18] In the past, the standard practice of college and university administrations was to ban guns on campus. A recent study revealed that virtually all campuses have such a policy in place.[19] However, this practice has been successfully challenged in Utah where, in 2006, the state supreme court ruled that the University of Utah could not bar guns from campus.[20] The next state that may allow students and professors to carry guns on campus

appears to be Texas. If the Texas legislature passes the bill allowing concealed handguns on college and university campuses, 500,000 students in 38 public universities will be involved.[21] This is a serious concern when one considers that one-fourth of campus police officers have not been trained to deal with an "active shooter" on campus and that most faculty members have not been trained to handle "troubled" students.[19] Is the answer to gun violence on campus more guns? The "vast majority (86 percent) of campus police chiefs surveyed believed that allowing students to carry concealed firearms on campus would not prevent some or all campus killings."[19]

College students are under considerable stress from financial concerns, relationship problems, and academic issues. Recall from Chapter 2 that suicide is the second-leading cause of death among college students. Each year about 10 percent of college students seriously think about suicide.[22] Since 50 percent of suicides involve the use of firearms, do we really want to allow troubled students, who may need counseling, easy access to handguns? Finally, as you learned in Chapter 7, nearly 50 percent of college students binge drink. A recent report revealed that 83 percent of college arrests involve alcohol.[23] Allowing college students to possess/carry guns on campus virtually guarantees that campus violence will become more deadly.

Other Types of Interpersonal Violence   Homicide is just one type of interpersonal violence. There are also robberies, rapes, sexual assaults, and aggravated and simple assaults. Since 1993 the rate of violent victimization has fallen from 50 to 17 violent victimizations per 1,000 persons in 2009.[14] Victims of violent crimes tend to be male, Black, and under 25 years of age. In 2009, males experienced higher rates of robbery and aggravated assault (assault with a weapon) than females; females were more likely than males to be victims of rape or sexual assault. Blacks were more likely to be victims of a violent crime than people of other races, but people of two or more races had the highest victimization rates among races. Females were also more likely to be victimized by someone they knew. The greatest disparity in violent crime committed against males and females was intimate partner violence. Less than half of all violent crimes are reported to police.[14]

> **Key Terms**
>
> **intentional injuries**   Injuries that are purposely inflicted, either by the victim or by another person.
>
> **homicide**   The intentional taking of one person's life by another person.

Stalking

In recent years, the crime of stalking has received considerable attention. **Stalking** has been defined as "a course of conduct directed at a specific person involving repeated visual or physical proximity; nonconsensual communication; verbal, written, or implied threats; or a combination thereof that would cause fear in a reasonable person, with 'repeated' meaning on two or more occasions."[24] Many stalkers are excessively possessive or jealous and pursue people with whom they formerly had a relationship. Other stalkers pursue people with whom they have had only an imaginary relationship. A third type is the vengeful stalker; this person needs to "get even" for real or imagined slight.

Stalkers often go to great lengths to locate their intended victims and frequently know their daily whereabouts. Although not all stalkers plan to batter or kill the person they are pursuing, their presence and potential for violence can create an extremely frightening environment for the intended victim and family. Some stalkers serve time in prison for their offense, waiting years to "get back at" their victims.

In one 12-month period, 3.4 million persons age 18 and over were victims of stalking. Females are three times more likely to be a victim of stalking.[25,26,27] Among these victims are many college students.[28] About 13 percent of college women are stalked in a given year.[28] If you think you are being stalked, report it to the police (or call your local crisis intervention hot line) immediately. Stalking is a crime in all 50 states.

Stalking can be carried out through electronic means as well as in person, by **cyberstalking**—the use of technology (phone, fax, GPS, Internet, computer spyware, or electronic monitoring with digital cameras or listening devices) to stalk victims.[26] Fortunately, since 1990, virtually all states have enacted or tightened their laws relating to stalking and have imposed stiff penalties for those convicted of stalking. If you think you are being stalked, report it immediately (see the box "Cyberstalking").

 TALKING POINTS You suspect that someone is stalking you, but your friends think you're being dramatic. How would you get objective advice on what to do?

Key Terms

stalking A crime involving repeated visual or physical proximity, nonconsensual communication, or threats that would cause fear in a reasonable person.

cyberstalking The unsolicited contacting, pursuing, or harassing of others, usually through the Internet or e-mail.

Table 15.1 Rape: Myth Versus Fact

Myth	Fact
Only women are raped.	Nearly 16 percent of reported rape victims (19,820) in 2009 were males.
Most rapists are strangers.	Twenty-six percent of male victims and 79 percent of female victims describe the offender as a nonstranger (intimate, other relative, or friend/acquaintance).
Most rapes occur in streets, alleys, and deserted places.	Ninety percent of rapes occur in living quarters—60 percent in the victim's residence.
Rapists are easily identified by their demeanor or psychological profile.	Most experts indicate that rapists do not differ significantly from nonrapists.
Rape is an overreported crime.	Only one-half of rapes are reported.
Rape happens only to people in low socioeconomic classes.	Rape occurs in all socioeconomic classes. Each person, male or female, young or old, is a potential victim.
There is a standard way to avoid rape.	Each rape situation is different. No single method to avoid rape can work in every potential rape situation. Because of this we encourage personal health classes to invite speakers from a local rape prevention services bureau to discuss approaches to rape prevention.

Rape and Other Sexual Assault   Ideally, sexual intimacy is a mutual, enjoyable form of communication between two people. Far too often, however, relationships are approached in an aggressive, hostile manner. Victims of *rape* and *sexual assault* include young and old, male and female. They can be the mentally retarded, prisoners, hospital patients, or college students. We all are potential victims, and self-protection is critical.

Rape involves both completed and attempted forced sexual intercourse, using both psychological coercion and physical force. This includes "vaginal, anal or oral penetration by the offender(s)," including penetration by a foreign object. This definition covers attempted rapes and rapes by same-sex or opposite-sex perpetrators.[24,25,26] Victims of rape fall into no single category; anyone can become a rape victim. The crime of rape is shrouded in myths, some of which are presented in Table 15.1.

Rape is an all-too-common occurrence on college campuses.[28,29] High levels of alcohol consumption and other drug use foster a campus environment in which violence can result. Among this violence are frequent instances of unplanned and unwanted sex, including attempted and completed rapes. Many of these assaults occur at house parties and are sometimes called *date rape* or *acquaintance rape.*

According to one estimate, 50–70 percent of all sexual assaults on college campuses involve alcohol.[30] In a 2005 study of 5,446 college women from two large, four-year schools, nearly 20 percent reported completed or attempted sexual assault since entering college. A report by the Bureau of Justice Statistics puts the figure at about 3 percent per year. A majority of the assaults occurred after women voluntarily consumed alcohol. A much smaller group of women experienced a sexual assault after having been given a drug without their knowledge or consent.[31] Among the drugs used to incapacitate the rape victim are Rohypnol (roofies), ketamine hydrochloride (Special K), and gamma-hydroxybutyrate (GHB) (see Chapter 7). The effects of these drugs, which can be easily incorporated into drinks without the intended victim's knowledge, are disinhibition, confusion, relaxation of voluntary muscles, and eventual unconsciousness.[32] The amnesic effect of the drugs reduces the ability of victims to supply information needed to apprehend the perpetrator. Although these "date rape" drugs garner publicity from time to time, alcohol remains the number-one date rape drug.

Psychologists believe that, aside from the physical harm of date rape, a greater amount of emotional damage may occur. Such damage stems from the concept of broken trust. Date rape victims feel particularly violated because the perpetrator was not a stranger; it was someone they initially trusted, at least to some degree. Once that trust is broken, developing new relationships with other people becomes much more difficult for the date rape victim.

Nearly all victims of date rape seem to suffer from *posttraumatic stress disorder.* They may have anxiety, sleeplessness, eating disorders, and nightmares. Guilt concerning their own behavior, loss of self-esteem, and judgment of other people can be overwhelming, and the individual may require professional counseling. Because of the seriousness of these consequences, all students should be aware of the existence of date rape.

Wise students "party" responsibly. To lower your risk of all types of injuries, either refrain from alcohol consumption or drink only moderately (one or two drinks).

Doing "shots" or binge drinking will reduce your judgment and increase your risk of injury. For more suggestions on how to lower your risk of becoming a victim of rape and sexual assault, see the box above.

Counseling services are provided to college and university students, usually at no cost. If you have been a victim of sexual violence, do not hesitate to take advantage of these services. A trained counselor can provide guidance and support to you as you resolve your feelings about the incident and then try to refocus on pursuing your personal and academic goals.

Sexual Harassment *Sexual harassment* consists of unwanted attention of a sexual nature that creates embarrassment or stress. Examples of sexual harassment include unwanted physical contact, excessive pressure for dates, sexually explicit humor, sexual innuendos or remarks, offers of job advancement based on sexual favors, and sexual assault. Unlike more overt forms of sexual victimization, sexual harassment may be applied in a subtle manner and can, in some cases, go unnoticed by coworkers and fellow students. Still, sexual harassment produces stress that cannot be resolved until the harasser is identified and forced to stop. Both men and women can be victims of sexual harassment.

Sexual harassment can occur in many settings, including employment and academic settings. On the college campus, harassment may be primarily in terms of the offer of sex for grades. If this occurs to you, think carefully about the situation and document the specific times, events, and places where the harassment took place. Consult your college's policy concerning harassment. Next, you could report these events to the appropriate administrative officer (perhaps the affirmative action officer, dean of academic affairs, or dean of students). You may also want to discuss the situation with a staff member of the university counseling center.

If harassment occurs in the work environment, the victim should document the occurrences and report them to the appropriate management or personnel official. Reporting procedures will vary from setting to setting. Sexual harassment is a form of illegal sex discrimination and violates Title VII of the Civil Rights Act of 1964.

In 1986 the U.S. Supreme Court ruled that the creation of a "hostile environment" in a work setting was sufficient evidence to support the claim of sexual harassment. This action served as an impetus for thousands of women to step forward with sexual harassment allegations. Additionally, some men are filing sexual harassment lawsuits against female supervisors.

Not surprisingly, this rising number of complaints has served as a wake-up call for employers. From university settings, to factory production lines, to corporate board rooms, employers are scrambling to make certain that employees are fully aware of actions that could lead to a sexual harassment lawsuit. Sexual harassment workshops and educational seminars on harassment are now common and serve to educate both men and women about this complex problem.

Bias and Hate Crimes

One sad aspect of any society is how some segments of the majority treat certain people in the minority. Nowhere is this more obvious than in **bias and hate crimes.** These crimes, which account for just 3 percent of all violent

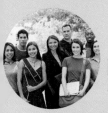

Learning from Our Diversity

Violence Against People with Disabilities

No one is totally free from the risk of senseless violence—children, adults, or college students. No single group, however, is a more tragic target of violence than people with disabilities. Despite the protective efforts of laws such as the Fair Housing Amendments Act, the Americans with Disabilities Act, and the Rehabilitation Act, people with disabilities remain an easily victimized segment of the population.

Because of the high level of vulnerability that disabled persons face, national advocacy groups, such as All Walks of Life, are working to assist the disabled, their caregivers, and the general population in reducing the risk of violence to this group. However, much can also be accomplished on an individual basis. If you are an able-bodied college student, you can probably implement the following suggestions on your campus:

- Encourage your peers who have disabilities to remain vigilant by staying tuned in to their environment. Remind them that simply because they appear to have a disability does not guarantee that they will be protected from harm.
- Support your friends with disabilities in overcoming the challenges imposed by their limitations, particularly when they are in unfamiliar environments or experiencing unusual situations.
- Suggest that your peers with disabilities carry or wear a personal alarm device. Such devices, also frequently carried by able-bodied

students, can be purchased in bookstores or sporting goods stores.
- Remind your friends who have disabilities to inform others about their schedule plans—for example, when they will be away from school and when they are likely to return.
- Encourage people with disabilities to seek the assistance of an escort (security personnel) when leaving a campus building or a shopping mall to enter a large parking area.
- Be an advocate for your friends with disabilities. For example, if residence hall room doors do not have peepholes at wheelchair height, find out if the doors can be modified.

One additional approach remains controversial: That is the teaching of self-defense techniques to people with disabilities. Groups that advocate instruction to the disabled in the martial arts, such as judo, remind us that "doing nothing will produce nothing." Others contend that a limited ability to use a martial art leads to a false sense of confidence that encourages a disregard for other forms of protection. They further argue that if persons with disabilities try to counter aggression with ineffectively delivered martial arts techniques, they may anger their attacker and actually increase the aggression against themselves.

---

crimes, are defined as crimes that occur "when offenders choose a victim because of some characteristic—for example, race, ethnicity, or religion—and provide evidence that the hate prompted them to commit the crime."[33] More than half (55 percent) of these crimes were motivated by race, another 31 percent were motivated by the victims' association with persons with certain characteristics such as multiracial marriage, 29 percent by ethnicity, 18 percent by sexual orientation, 13 percent by religion, and 11 percent by disability (see the box "Violence Against People with Disabilities"). The targeted individual or group may be attacked verbally or physically, have their property damaged, may be threatened with violence, or may be forced to move from a neighborhood or community.

Typically, the offenders in bias or hate crimes are fringe elements of the larger society who believe that the mere presence of someone with a racial, ethnic, sexual orientation, religious difference, or disability is inherently bad for the community, state, or country. Examples in the United States include skinheads, the Ku Klux Klan, and other white supremacist groups. (The case of Matthew Shepard—see the box "Violence Based on Sexual Orientation" on page 396—drew worldwide attention to hate crimes.) Increasingly, state and federal laws have been enacted to make bias and hate crimes serious offenses.

Family Violence

Unfortunately, some victims of interpersonal violence are family members. **Family violence** is the use of physical force by one family member against another, with the intent to hurt, injure, or cause harm. The spectrum of family violence includes intimate partner violence, maltreatment of children, sibling violence, and violence directed at elder family members. One in every six homicides is the result of family violence.

Intimate Partner Violence **Intimate partner violence (IPV)** is interpersonal violence perpetrated by current or former dates, spouses, or cohabiting partners

---

> **Key Terms**
>
> **bias and hate crimes** Criminal acts directed at a person or group solely because of a specific characteristic, such as race, religion, sexual orientation, ethnic background, or disability.
>
> **family violence** The use of physical force by one family member against another, with the intent to hurt, injure, or harm.
>
> **intimate partner violence (IPV)** Interpersonal violence perpetrated by a current or former spouse, date, or cohabiting partner.

Violence Based on Sexual Orientation

Recent news reports indicate that violence based on sexual orientation continues to occur in the United States. Nowhere is this more clear than in the case of Matthew Shepard, an openly gay University of Wyoming freshman who was murdered in October 1998. Shepard was lured from a Laramie, Wyoming, bar by two young adult men posing as homosexuals. These men beat Shepard severely, stole $20 from him, and tied him to a fence post, where he was left to die. The men were later convicted of kidnapping and murder.

In July 1999, Barry Winchell, an Army private at Fort Campbell, Kentucky, was bludgeoned to death with a bat wielded by fellow private Calvin Glover. Glover, who said he was intoxicated when he committed the crime, was later convicted of premeditated murder in a military court and sentenced to life in prison, with the possibility of

parole. Another soldier, charged as an accessory to the crime, apparently had spread rumors among members of the Army unit that Winchell was gay. This accomplice also tried to clean up the scene of the crime. He was sentenced to 12 years in prison.

Both of these deaths served as a reminder that the federal government has not yet passed the Hate Crimes Prevention Act. This proposed legislation would add acts of hatred motivated by sexual orientation, gender, and disability to the list of hate crimes already covered by federal law. Among these crimes already covered are

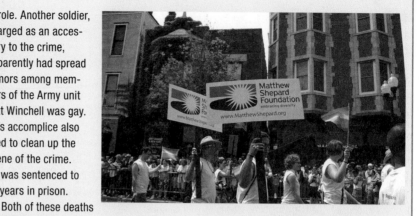

ones motivated by prejudice based on race, religion, color, or national origin.

It will be interesting to see whether this proposed federal legislation will be enacted soon. The public outcry following the deaths of Matthew Shepard and Barry Winchell indicates that much support exists for some version of a Hate Crimes Prevention Act.

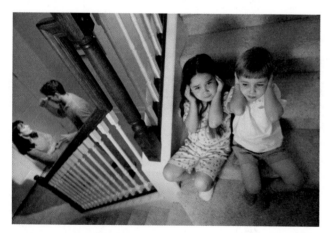

Witnessing violence in the home makes children feel unsafe, afraid, and/or guilty.

("cohabiting" meaning living together at least some of the time as a couple).[24] IPV can include physical and sexual abuse; simple, aggravated, and sexual assault; rape; stalking; and robbery. Acts of physical abuse range from a slap on the face, a punch, or a kick, to murder.

Females are five and one-half times more likely than males to be a victim of intimate partner violence. More than a half-million women were victims of intimate partner violence in 2008. Nonfatal intimate partner violence against both sexes has declined by more than 50 percent since 1993. Simple assault (assault without a weapon) is

the leading type of intimate partner violence.[25] Not all instances of intimate partner violence are reported. In 2008, 72 percent of intimate partner violence against males and 49 percent of intimate partner violence against females was reported to police.[25] Intimate partner violence is underreported because (1) the victim may believe her or his own behavior perpetrated the violent act, (2) domestic violence is seen as a personal, private matter, and/or (3) the victim fears reprisal for reporting the violence. Not reporting intimate partner violence increases the risk that the violence will become more severe.

In 2007, 2,340 homicide victims were killed by an intimate partner; intimate partners committed 14 percent of all homicides that year. Females made up 70 percent of victims killed by an intimate partner. Although rates of intimate partner homicide for both males and females have fallen since 1993, they have not fallen as fast as the overall U.S. homicide rate during the same period.[25]

Instances of children witnessing intimate partner violence are not uncommon. One study found that in 36 percent of the cases that came to court, children were present. In 60 percent of the cases where they were present, the children directly witnessed the violence.[25] Witnessing violence makes children feel unsafe, afraid, and/or guilty. They may adopt unhealthy or aggressive behaviors, have trouble in school, or have difficulty getting along with others. The National Center for Children Exposed to Violence (NCCEV) has as its mission "to increase the capacity of individuals and communities to reduce the incidence and impact of violence on children and families; to train and support the professionals who provide intervention and treatment to children and families affected by violence; and, to increase professional and public awareness of the effects of violence on children, families, communities and society."[34]

Psychological abuse is another form of spouse abuse. Psychological abuse includes verbally threatening or berating an intimate partner, starting rumors or telling lies about an intimate partner, turning the victim's children against the victim, and/or neglecting the victim emotionally. Psychological abuse often accompanies intimate partner violence, but it is harmful even in the absence of physical violence. It can lead to disability, causing missed days of work, and health problems, including chronic pain, migraines and other headaches, stammering, stomach ulcers, spastic colon, indigestion, diarrhea, and/or constipation.[35]

However, help is available for victims of intimate abuse. Most communities have family support or domestic violence hot lines that abused people can call for help. Many have shelters where abused women and their children can seek safety while their cases are being handled by the police or court officials. If you are being abused or know of someone who is being injured by domestic violence, don't hesitate to use the services of these local hot lines or shelters. Also, check the resources listed in the Health Reference Guide at the back of this text.

 TALKING POINTS A close friend confides that her boyfriend sometimes "gets rough" with her. She's afraid to talk to him about it because she thinks that will make things worse. What immediate steps would you tell her to take?

Maltreatment of Children Like intimate partner violence, **child maltreatment** tends to be a silent crime. It is estimated that nearly three-quarters of a million children are survivors of child abuse and neglect each year.[36] Some children are survivors of repeated crimes, and since many survivors do not report these crimes, the actual incidence of child abuse is difficult to determine.

Child maltreatment includes child abuse and child neglect. Children are abused in various ways. Physical abuse reflects physical injury, such as bruises, burns, abrasions, cuts, and fractures of the bones and skull. Sexual abuse includes acts that lead to sexual gratification of the abuser. Examples include fondling, touching, and various acts involved in rape, sodomy, and incest. Psychological abuse is another form of child abuse. Certainly, children are scarred by family members and others who routinely damage their psychological development. However, this form of abuse is especially difficult to identify and measure.

Child neglect is failure to provide a child with adequate clothing, food, shelter, and medical attention. The incidence of child neglect is approximately three times that of physical abuse and about seven times the incidence of child sexual abuse. Furthermore, child maltreatment deaths are more often associated with neglect than with any other type of abuse.[36] Educational neglect, such as failure to see that a child attends school regularly, is one of the most common types of child neglect. Each form of abuse can have devastating consequences for the child—both short term and long term. Abused children are more likely to suffer from poor educational performance, increased health problems, and low levels of overall achievement. Recent research points out that abused and neglected children are significantly more likely than nonabused children to become involved in adult crime and violent criminal behavior.

The key to reducing the frequency and severity of child maltreatment is timely detection, reporting, and intervention. Teachers, social workers and police, and public health personnel are required to report suspected cases of child maltreatment, and nearly half of all cases are reported by these professionals. Relatives, friends, and other adults must not hesitate to report suspected cases to their local police or Child Protective Services. As long as the report is filed in good conscience (without malice), there will be no negative ramifications for the person filing it. When an individual has abused a child once, he or she is likely to do it again. So prompt intervention may save the life of a child.

Many community agencies, such as YMCAs, churches, and recreation centers, offer parenting courses. Adults who were abused as children may tend to become abusive parents themselves. By participating in a parenting class, these adults can learn alternative approaches to child rearing. Even new parents who were not raised in abusive situations can learn much about parenting by enrolling in one of these courses. These courses teach parents and other caregivers how to resolve conflicts, improve communication, cope with anger, and use nonviolent methods to discipline their children. While not a substitute for such a course, the box "Twelve Alternatives to Lashing Out at Your Child" provides a few helpful guidelines for parents.

Maltreatment of Elders Among the 40 million adults 65 years of age and older, between 1 and 2 million have been injured, exploited, or otherwise mistreated.[37,38]

Key Terms
child maltreatment The act or failure to act by a parent or caregiver that results in abuse or neglect of a child which places the child in imminent risk of serious harm.

Particularly vulnerable are women and those of advanced age. More than 65 percent of elder abuse victims were female, and nearly half of the victims were 80 years of age or older. The most common relationships of the perpetrators to the victims were adult-child (32.6 percent) and other family member (21.5 percent).[39]

Many elderly people are hit, kicked, attacked with knives, denied food and medical care, and have their Social Security checks and automobiles stolen. This problem reflects a combination of factors, particularly the stress of caring for failing older people by middle-aged children who are also faced with the demands of dependent children and careers. In many cases, the middle-aged children were themselves abused, or there may be a chemical dependence problem. The alternative, institutionalization, is so expensive that it is often not an option for either the abused or the abusers.

Although protective services are available in most communities through welfare departments, elder abuse is frequently unseen and unreported. In many cases, the elderly people themselves are afraid to report their children's behavior because of the fear of embarrassment that they were not good parents to their children. Regardless of the cause, however, elder abuse must be reported to the appropriate protective service so that intervention can occur.

Violence in Our Communities

When family members go to school, attend college, or participate in other community activities, we do not expect them to be injured by the intentional acts of another.

School Violence Usually, students are safe at school, but occasional, highly publicized fatal school shootings, like the ones at Columbine High School and Red Lake Indian Reservation, cause parents to ask how safe their children are at school. The National Center for Educational Statistics collects data to determine the frequency, seriousness, and incidence of violence in elementary and high schools. During the 2008–2009 school year, 85 percent of public schools reported one or more violent incidents, serious violent incidents, thefts of items valued at $10 or greater, or other crimes occurring at their school. This amounted to 2 million crimes, a rate of 43 crimes per 1,000 enrolled students. Additionally, 25 percent of public schools reported that bullying was a daily or weekly problem. In 2009, 31 percent of 9th- to 12th-grade students reported they had been in a fight anywhere, and 14 percent said they had been in a fight on school property during the previous 12 months. Also, 17 percent reported that they had carried a weapon in the past 30 days, and 6 percent reported they had carried a weapon in the past 30 days on school property.[17,40] The fact that 1 in 20 high school children carried a weapon to school within the past 30 days is frightening.

Weapon carrying is related to another form of interpersonal violence at school—bullying. Bullying includes making fun of another person; spreading rumors about a person; threatening to harm another person; pushing, shoving, tripping, or spitting on another person; pressuring someone to do something they don't want to do; excluding another person; or destroying their property. In 2007, 32 percent of 12- to 18-year-olds reported that they were bullied at school during the school year.

Another type of bullying has become all too common—cyberbullying, the electronic harassment or bullying among minors, usually within a school context. This behavior can be very troubling to children, who are just learning to form friendship groups among their peers, and to whom acceptance or rejection can mean everything. Victims of cyberbullying can experience psychological and physical damage to their health, including changes in sleeping and eating patterns, anxiety and fear for safety, hypervigilance, and feelings of helplessness. Instances of cyberbullying must be reported immediately,

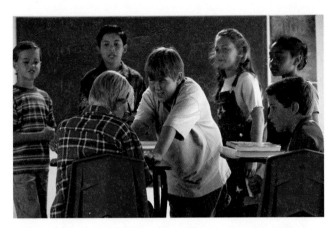

Bullying includes making fun of another person, spreading rumors about that person, and threatening to harm another person. Thirty-two percent of 12- to 18-year-olds reported that they were bullied at school.

just like any other form of child maltreatment. If you are a parent, make sure your child knows about cyberbullying, knows never to reply, and knows to tell you immediately if anyone sends him or her a nasty or hate message, or threatens him or her on a cell phone or computer. Teach your child to "stop, block, and tell"—that is, stop what he or she is doing, block the person who sent the message, and tell a trusted adult. If a child feels unsafe and unable to confide his or her problems to a parent, he or she might decide to respond to bullying or cyberbullying by carrying a weapon to school or joining a gang.

In spite of the statistics cited above, the odds of a student suffering a school-associated violent death are less than one in a million. From July 1, 2008, through June 30, 2009, only 15 homicides and 7 suicides of school-aged youth occurred at school. This translates into 1 homicide or suicide of a school-aged youth at school per 3.6 million students enrolled during the 2008–2009 school year.[40] So, while violence at schools has captured the headlines, schools are really a relatively safe place for children to be.

Violence at College   In spite of media headlines about shootings on campuses, colleges and universities are a relatively safe place to be. College students (ages 18–24) experience less violence than do nonstudents in the same age group.

Simple assault (assault without a weapon) accounts for 63 percent of the violent victimizations, whereas rape/sexual assault accounts for 6 percent. Males are about twice as likely to be victims of violence as females were. About 93 percent of the crimes occur off campus, 72 percent occur at night, and 41 percent of victims perceive that the offenders were using alcohol or drugs at the time of the offense.[29]

One factor that increases the risk of interpersonal violence on American college campuses is the consumption

of alcohol and other drugs. More than 40 percent of victims of violent crimes in college settings perceived their offenders to be using drugs or alcohol. The percentage was even higher for aggravated and simple assault.[29] It should be noted that this is higher than the level of drug use perceived by victims in all settings.[41] To reduce your risk of becoming a victim of interpersonal violence, consider reducing your alcohol intake and pay attention to the alcohol consumption of those around you, and stay away from places where people are drinking heavily.

Campus Safety and Violence Prevention   Although many of the topics in this chapter are unsettling, students and faculty must continue to lead normal lives in the campus environment despite potential threats to our health. The first step in being able to function adequately is knowing about these potential threats. You have read about these threats in this chapter; now you must think about how this information applies to your campus situation.

The campus environment is not immune to many of the social ills that plague our society. At one time the university campus was thought to be a haven from the real world. Now there is plenty of evidence to indicate that significant intentional and unintentional injuries can happen to anyone at any time on the college campus.

For this reason, you must make it a habit to think constructively about protecting your safety. In addition to the personal safety tips presented earlier in this chapter, remember to use the safety assistance resources available on your campus. One of these might be your use of university-approved escort services, especially in the evenings as you move from one campus location to another. Another resource is the campus security department (campus police). Typically, campus police have a 24-hour emergency phone number. If you think you need help, don't hesitate to call this number. Campus security departments frequently offer short seminars on safety topics to student organizations or residence hall groups. Your counseling center on campus might also offer programs on rape prevention and personal protection.

If you are motivated to make your campus environment safer, you might wish to contact Security on Campus, an organization that focuses on campus security (www.securityoncampus.org). We encourage you to become active in making your campus a safer place to live.

Youth and Gang Violence   Youth gangs have been around for decades, especially in cities. A *gang* is a self-formed association of peers bound together by mutual interests, with identifiable leadership and well-defined lines of authority. Members of the gang act together to achieve a purpose—to control a specific geographic territory or enterprise, for example—and their acts usually include illegal activities and may involve criminal violence. In the 1950s and 1960s, gangs used fists, chains, tire irons, and occasionally cheap hand-guns to defend their territory or enterprise. Beginning in the 1980s, warfare between gangs over the lucrative drug trade increasingly involved the use of semi-automatic weapons. The violence became much more deadly, and the national homicide rate rose accordingly. During the latter 1990s, the prevalence of gangs and gang violence declined. It rose again slightly during 2002–2005, but has remained steady since then. In 2008, an estimated 774,000 gang members and 27,900 gangs were active in the United States. About one-third of jurisdictions surveyed reported gang activity. The largest increases in gang activity in 2007–2008 occurred in urban areas with populations greater than 250,000.[42]

Attempting to control gang and youth violence is problematic for communities. For every gang-related homicide, there are about 100 nonfatal gang-related intentional injuries, so gang violence becomes an expensive health care proposition. Furthermore, gang and youth violence takes an enormous financial and human toll on law enforcement, judicial, and corrections departments. Reducing gang and youth violence is a daunting task for the nation.

Factors That Contribute to Intentional Injuries

A major contributing factor to interpersonal violence leading to intentional injuries is the presence of alcohol or other psychoactive drugs. (You may wish to refer again to Chapters 7 and 8.) It is estimated that nearly 2 million state and local arrests are made for drug abuse each year.[43] In 2007, 3.9 percent of the 14,831 homicides committed were drug related.[44] About 26 percent of victims of violent crimes perceived that the perpetrator was influenced by alcohol or drugs at the time of the crime. This figure rises to 41 percent for violent crimes committed on college campuses.[29]

A psychological manifestation of alcohol intoxication is the lowering of inhibitions, and for some individuals, this loss of behavior control results in acts of interpersonal violence. A drunk or drugged person is more likely than a sober person to become either a perpetrator or a victim of violence.

Another factor that contributes to the deadliness of interpersonal violence is the availability of firearms. It is estimated that 40–50 percent of American homes have guns. In 2009, firearms were the second-leading cause of death (after automobiles) in the 15–24 age group, accounting for nearly 14 percent of all deaths in that group.[1] Colleges are not immune to gun violence; 4.3 percent of college students have a working firearm at school. As mentioned earlier in this chapter, at least one university administration's rules prohibiting firearms have been found unconstitutional. Leaders on other campuses are anxiously wondering if their states will strike down prohibitions against firearms on their campuses.

You can take steps to prevent or reduce your risk of a violent injury where you live by taking a few precautions:

- If possible, avoid living in a first-floor apartment.
- Change locks when moving into a new apartment or home.
- Use initials for first names on mailboxes and in phone books.
- Install a peephole and deadbolt locks on outside doors.
- Make sure you can lock all windows.
- Require repair and delivery people to show valid identification.
- Get to know your neighbors, and agree to be vigilant and share information about neighborhood safety issues.
- Do not provide personal information over the phone or on the computer.
- Be cautious around garages, parking lots, and laundry rooms (especially at night), and make sure these areas are well lighted and clear of hiding places.
- Keep important telephone numbers near your phone or listed in your cell phone directory so you can call them quickly.
- If there is a person whom you wish to have contacted in case you are injured, enter that person's number in your cell phone directory under the heading of ICE ("in case of emergency").

Identity Theft

Identity theft has been on the rise since the early 1990s. In 2008, 11.7 million households (5 percent of all persons age 16 or older in the United States) discovered that they had become victims of identity theft during the previous two-year period. The financial loss from identity theft totaled more than $17 billion.[45] The most common type of identity theft was unauthorized use of an existing credit card; the next most prevalent type of theft involved another existing account, such as a bank account. More than a million victims discovered identity theft involving misuse of personal information. This might involve opening a new account, fraudulently obtaining medical care or government benefits, or providing fake identification to law enforcement during a crime or traffic stop. Persons living in households with incomes of $75,000 or higher were at higher risk for identity theft, as were persons ages 16–24. Households headed by persons 65 and older and rural households were at lower risk.[44] Thieves use falsely obtained names, addresses, and Social Security numbers to open credit card accounts and bank accounts, purchase cell phone services, and secure loans to buy automobiles and other big-ticket items. They might even avoid paying taxes by working under false Social Security numbers, or use your identity for other purposes—if they are arrested, for example. Identity thefts can drain a person's bank account and ruin her credit rating before she knows she's become a victim. Often the crime is not discovered until a person wants to make a major purchase—such as a house or a car—which requires a credit check.

Here are some of the common ways ID theft occurs. Identity thieves (1) rummage through trash looking for bills and other papers bearing your personal information ("dumpster diving"), (2) steal credit or debit card numbers using a special storage device when processing your card ("skimming"), (3) pretend to be a financial institution or other business and try to get you to reveal personal information ("phishing"), (4) divert your mail by submitting a change of address form for you, or (5) simply steal your wallet, purse, or mail, such as preapproved credit offers, new checks, or other papers. Another way is "pretexting," a process of getting your personal information under false pretenses. They might also steal your information from your employer by bribing a dishonest employee who has access to it.

There are several steps that you can take to avoid becoming a victim of identity theft. The most important step involves ordering copies of your credit reports each year to make sure that there are no fraudulent accounts in your name.

The Federal Trade Commission provides useful information on its website (www.ftc.gov/idtheft) and recommends the following strategies for protecting yourself from identity theft [46]:

Deter Thieves by Safeguarding Your Information:

- Shred financial documents with personal information before you throw them out.

- Protect your Social Security number by not giving it out unless absolutely necessary. Don't carry it in your wallet or write it on your checks; if a business requests it, ask to use another identifier.

- Don't give out personal information unless you know whom you are dealing with.

- Never click on links sent in unsolicited e-mails. Use up-to-date firewalls and antispyware and antivirus software to protect your home computer. Refer back to the material on spamming and phishing in Chapter 3 for additional information about e-mail safety.

- Don't use an obvious password like your birth date, your mother's maiden name, or the last four digits of your Social Security number.

Detect Suspicious Activity:

- Be aware if bills do not arrive as expected, you receive unexpected credit cards or account statements, you are denied credit for no apparent reason, or you receive calls or letters about purchases you did not make.

- Inspect your credit report. The law requires the major consumer reporting companies (Equifax,

Experian, and TransUnion) to give you a free copy of your credit report annually.

- Inspect your financial accounts and billing statements regularly for charges you did not make.

Defend Against Identity Theft as Soon as You Suspect It:

- Place a "fraud alert" on your credit reports; this tells creditors to follow certain procedures before they open new accounts in your name or make changes to your existing accounts.

- Close any accounts that have been tampered with or established fraudulently. Call the security or fraud departments of each relevant company and follow up in writing. Keep copies of documents and records of your conversations about the theft.

- File a police report and report the theft to the Federal Trade Commission at http://ftc.gov/idtheft.

Terrorism

Although definitions vary, the United Nations defines **terrorism** as any act "intended to cause death or serious bodily harm to civilians or noncombatants with the purpose of intimidating a populace or compelling a government or an international organization to do or abstain from doing any act."[47] Over the past 30 years the world has witnessed dozens of acts of terrorism in countries such as Germany, Spain, Indonesia, Sudan, Kenya, England, Northern Ireland, Japan, and Russia. The United States has not been immune from terrorist acts, including the World Trade Center bombing in 1993, the Oklahoma City bombing in 1995, the Olympic Park bombing in Atlanta in 1996, and the attacks on the World Trade Center and Pentagon in 2001.

By their very nature, terrorist acts are difficult to prevent. However, it is less likely that your health will be affected by a terrorist act than by your everyday health behavior. As an educated person, you should become knowledgeable about world events and support federal, state, and local security efforts. If you travel abroad, keep in mind that American-style restaurants and nightclubs might be more attractive targets for anti-American terrorist acts than locally owned or natively owned establishments.

Key Terms

identity theft A crime involving the fraudulent use of a person's name, Social Security number, credit line, or other personal, financial, or identifying information.

terrorism Any actions intended to harm or kill civilians in order to intimidate a populace or force a government to take some action.

Taking Charge of Your Health

- Use the Personal Assessment at the end of this chapter to determine how well you protect yourself from injuries.
- Find out about the security services available on your campus, and take advantage of them. Post the 24-hour-help phone number in your room and carry it with you.

- Minimize your risk for identity theft by taking the steps outlined on pages 400–401.
- Review the motor vehicle safety tips on page 386. If you need to make changes to your car or your driving, begin working on them at once.
- Check your residence for the safety strategies listed on pages 388–389. Make

the necessary changes to correct any deficiencies.
- Check the recommendations for recreational safety on page 389 and put them into practice. Be assertive about using these measures when you are participating in activities with others.

SUMMARY

- Injuries are the leading cause of death for those from 1 to 44 years old and kill more people in the 15–24 age group than all other causes of death combined.
- Injuries are the number-one reason people visit hospital emergency departments.
- Deaths from unintentional injuries—injuries that occur with no one intending harm be done—account for two-thirds of all injury deaths.
- More unintentional injuries and injury deaths occur in the home than anywhere else.
- Distracted driving, including cell phone use while driving, is a serious roadway hazard for everyone.
- Unintentional poisonings have surpassed motor vehicle crashes as the leading cause of injury deaths.
- Falls remain the leading cause of nonfatal injuries.
- Bicycles are the leading cause of emergency department visits due to recreational injuries.
- You can take steps to reduce your risk of unintentional injuries in the home and on the road.
- Intentional injuries are those that result from self-directed or interpersonal violence.
- The spectrum of interpersonal violence includes homicide, robbery, rape and other sexual assault, and simple and aggravated assault.

- The victimization rate from interpersonal violence has declined significantly in the United States over the past 20 years.
- Date rape, acquaintance rape, alcohol- and drug-facilitated rape, and sexual assault are serious interpersonal violence concerns on college campuses.
- Stalking, including cyberstalking, is a crime in all 50 states.
- Bias and hate crimes are crimes directed at persons or groups solely because of a specific characteristic, such as race, religion, sexual orientation, ethnic background, or disability.
- Family violence includes intimate partner violence, maltreatment of children, and maltreatment of elders.
- Alcohol consumption, other drug use, and the availability of firearms are important factors that contribute to the prevalence and deadliness of interpersonal violence in America.
- To reduce the risk of identity theft, shred all documents with personal information before discarding them, refrain from sharing personal information, carefully inspect your bills and accounts, and report suspicious incidents immediately.

REVIEW QUESTIONS

1. Explain the difference between intentional and unintentional injuries. Give three examples of each category of injury.
2. Where do most nonfatal unintentional injuries occur? Where do most fatal unintentional injuries occur?
3. What is the leading cause of unintentional injury deaths? What is the second-leading cause?
4. What is distracted driving? List the ways drivers become distracted.
5. List 10 ways to make your home safer.
6. List nine ways you can avoid a drug overdose at home.
7. List some rules for gun safety in the home.
8. Bicycles are the leading cause of recreational injuries. What is the number-one preventive measure to take to

avoid an injury while riding a bicycle? List at least four other guidelines for safe biking.
9. List the precautions to take to minimize your risk of injury while boating.
10. What is meant by the term *interpersonal violence*? What types of acts are considered interpersonal violence?
11. What is stalking? How common is it? What should you do if you become a victim of stalking?
12. Date rape, acquaintance rape, and drug/alcohol-facilitated rape are an acknowledged problem on college campuses. What are some ways to lower your risk of becoming a victim?
13. Define *sexual harassment*. Identify some acts that could be considered sexual harassment.

14. What are bias and hate crimes? Who are the perpetrators? Who are the victims?
15. What is included in the category of family violence? How widespread is the problem? Who are the perpetrators and who are the victims?
16. Overall, the violent crime rate has declined in our communities over the past 20 years. Provide at least three explanations for this.
17. List all the ways you can think of to protect yourself from identity theft.
18. Define *terrorism*.

ANSWERS TO THE "WHAT DO YOU KNOW?" QUIZ

1. True   2. False   3. False   4. True   5. False   6. False   7. True

Visit the Online Learning Center (**www.mhhe.com/hahn11e**), where you will find tools to help you improve your grade including practice quizzes, key terms flashcards, audio chapter summaries for your MP3 player, and many other study aids.

SOURCE NOTES

1. Kochanek KD, Xu J, Murphy SL, Miniño AM, Kung H-C. Deaths: preliminary data for 2009. *National Vital Statistics Reports,* 59(4), 1–68. National Center for Health Statistics, Centers for Disease Control and Prevention, U.S. Department of Health and Human Services, March 16, 2011. http://www.cdc.gov/nchs/data/nvsr/nvsr59/nvsr59_04.pdf. Accessed March 24, 2011.
2. Adams PF, Martinez ME, Vickerie JL. Summary health statistics for the U.S. population: National Health Interview Survey, 2009. *Vital and Health Statistics,* 10(248). Hyattsville, MD: National Center for Health Statistics, Centers for Disease Control and Prevention, U.S. Department of Health and Human Services. DHHS Publication No. (PHS) 2011-1576, December 2010.
3. National Safety Council. *Injury Facts 2008 Edition.* Itasca, IL: Author, 2008.
4. U.S. Department of Transportation, National Highway Traffic Safety Administration. *Traffic Safety Facts 2009 (Early Edition): A Compilation of Motor Vehicle Crash Data from the Fatality Analysis Reporting System and the General Estimates System.* Washington, DC: Author, 2008. http://www.nrd.nhtsa.dot.gov/Pubs/811402EE.pdf. Accessed March 2, 2011.
5. Centers for Disease Control and Prevention. Child passenger deaths involving drinking drivers—United States, 1997–2002. *Morbidity and Mortality Weekly Report,* 53(4), 77–79, 2004.
6. Centers for Disease Control and Prevention. Vital signs: nonfatal, motor vehicle-occupant injuries (2009) and seat belt use (2008) among adults—United States. *Morbidity and Mortality Weekly Report,* 59(51 and 52), 1681–86, 2011.
7. Centers for Disease Control and Prevention, Center for Injury Prevention and Control. Unintentional drug poisoning in the United States. http://www.cdc.gov/HomeandRecreationalSafety/pdf/poison-issue-brief.pdf. Accessed March 26, 2011.
8. Warner M, Chen LH, Makuc DM. Increase in fatal poisonings involving opioid analgesics in the United States, 1999–2006. *NCHS Data Brief,* 22, September 2009. Centers for Disease Control and Prevention, National Center for Health Statistics. http://www.cdc.gov/nchs/products/databriefs.htm. Accessed March 3, 2011.
9. Centers for Disease Control and Prevention. Emergency department visits involving nonmedical use of selected prescription drugs—United States, 2004–2008. *Morbidity and Mortality Weekly Report,* 59(23), 705–709, 2010.
10. Home Safety Council. *Top 10 List.* http://www.homesafetycouncil.org/safetyguide/sg_topten_w001.asp. Accessed March 4, 2011.
11. Centers for Disease Control and Prevention. Dog bite: fact sheet. http://www.cdc.gov/HomeandRecreationalSafety/Dog-Bites/biteprevention.html. Accessed March 25, 2011.
12. U.S. Department of Homeland Security, U.S. Coast Guard, Office of Auxiliary and Boating Safety. *Recreational Boating Statistics 2009.*

COMDTPUB P16754.23. http://www.uscgboating.org/statistics/accident_statistics.aspx. Accessed March 3, 2011.
13. Centers for Disease Control and Prevention, National Center for Injury Prevention and Control, WISQARS (Web-based Injury Surveillance Query and Reporting System). http://www.cdc.gov/injury/wisqars/index.html. Accessed March 5, 2011.
14. Truman JL, Rand MR. National crime victimization survey: criminal victimization, 2009. U.S. Department of Justice, Office of Justice Programs. *Bureau of Justice Statistics: Bulletin,* NCJ 231327, October 2010.
15. Niska RW, Bhuiya F, Xu J. National hospital ambulatory medical care survey: 2007 emergency department summary. *National Health Statistics Reports,* 7. Hyattsville, MD: National Center for Health Statistics, 2010.
16. Fox JA. *Homicide Trends in the U.S.* Department of Justice, Office of Justice Programs, Bureau of Justice Statistics, 2006. http://bjs.ojp.usdoj.gov/content/pub/pdf/htius.pdf. Accessed March 5,2011.
17. Centers for Disease Control and Prevention. Youth risk behavior surveillance—United States, 2009. *Morbidity and Mortality Weekly Report,* 59(SS-5), 1–146, 2010. http://www.cdc.gov/mmwr/pdf/ss/ss5905.pdf. Accessed March 7, 2011.
18. Miller MD, Hemenway D, Wechsler H. Guns and gun threats at college. *Journal of American College Health,* 51(2), 57–65, 2002.
19. Thompson A, Price JH, Mrdjenovich AJ, Khubchandani J. Reducing firearm-related violence on college campuses—police chiefs' perceptions and practices. *Journal of American College Health,* 58(3), 247–254, 2009.
20. Jaschik S. Gun rights vs. college rights. *Inside Higher Education,* 2006. http://www.insidehighered.com/news/2006/09/11/guns. Accessed June 10, 2010.
21. USA Today: Texas to allow guns on campus. *The Star Press,* A10, February 21, 2011.
22. Schwartz V, Kay J, Appelbaum P. Keep guns off college campuses. *The Huffington Post* (posted May 12, 2010). http://www.huffingtonpost.com/victor-schwartz/keep-guns-off-college-cam_b_573634.html. Accessed June 10, 2010.
23. The National Center on Addiction and Substance Abuse at Columbia University. *Wasting the Best and the Brightest: Substance Abuse at America's Colleges and Universities.* New York: Author, 2007.
24. Tjaden P, Thoennes N. *Extent, Nature, and Consequences of Intimate Partner Violence: Findings from the National Violence Against Women Survey.* NCJ 181867. Washington, DC: National Institute of Justice, 2000.
25. Catalano SE, Smith E, Snider H, Rand M. *Female Victims of Violence.* U.S. Department of Justice, Bureau of Justice Statistics, Selected Findings. NCJ 228356, 2009. http://bjs.ojp.usdoj.gov/. Accessed March 17, 2011.

26. Baum K, Catalano S, Rand M, Rose K. Stalking victimization in the United States. U.S. Department of Justice, Office of Justice Programs, Bureau of Justice Statistics Special Report, *National Crime Victimization Survey*. NCJ 224527, January 2009. http://bjs.ojp.usdoj.gov/content/pub/pdf/svus.pdf. Accessed March 17, 2011.

27. U.S. Department of Justice, Office of Justice Programs, National Institute of Justice, Research, Development, and Evaluation Agency. Stalking. http://www.ojp.usdoj.gov/nij/topics/crime/stalking/welcome.htm. Accessed March 17, 2011.

28. Fisher BS, Cullen FT, Turner MG. *The Sexual Victimization of College Women*. U.S. Department of Justice, Bureau of Justice Statistics. NCJ 182369, 2001.

29. Baum K, Klaus P. Violent victimization of college students, 1995–2002. U.S. Department of Justice, Office of Justice Programs, Bureau of Justice Statistics *Special Report: National Crime Victimization Survey*. NCJ 206836, January 2005. www.ojp.usdoj.gov/bjs/pub/pdf/vvcs02.pdf. Accessed January 9, 2009.

30. American College Health Association. *Shifting the Paradigm: Primary prevention of sexual violence*. Baltimore: Author, 2008.

31. Krebs CP, Lindquist CH, Warner TD, Fisher BS, Martin SL. College women's experiences with physically forced, alcohol- or other drug-enabled, and drug-facilitated sexual assault before and since entering college. *Journal of American College Health*, 57(6), 639–647, 2009.

32. Schwartz RH, Milteer R, LeBeau MA. Drug-facilitated sexual assault ("date rape"). *South Medical Journal*, 93(6), 558–561, 2000.

33. Harlow CW. Hate crimes reported by victims and police. Bureau of Justice, *Special Report: National Criminal Victimization Survey and Uniform Crime Reporting*. U.S. Department of Justice, Office of Justice Programs. NCJ 209911, 2005.

34. National Center for Children Exposed to Violence, Yale University Child Study Center. http:/www.nccev.org/. Accessed March 10, 2011.

35. Coker AL, Smith PH, Bethea L, King MR, McKeown RE. Physical health consequences of physical and psychological intimate partner violence. *Archives of Family Medicine*, 9(5), 451–457, 2000.

36. United States Department of Health and Human Services, Administration for Children and Families, Administration on Children, Youth and Families, Children's Bureau. *Child Maltreatment 2009*. http://www.acf.hhs.gov/programs/cb/pubs/cm09/cm09.pdf. Accessed March 9, 2011.

37. U.S. Census Bureau. *An Older and More Diverse Nation by Midcentury*. http://www.census.gov/newsroom/releases/archives/population/cb08-123.html. Accessed March 9, 2011.

38. National Research Council. *Elder Mistreatment: Abuse, Neglect and Exploitation in an Aging America*. Washington, DC: National Academies Press, 2003.

39. National Committee for the Prevention of Elder Abuse and the National Adult Protective Services Administration. *The 2004 Survey of State Adult Protective Services: Abuse of Adults 60 Years of Age and Older*, 2006. http://www.ncea.aoa.gov/NCFAroot/Main_Site/pdf/2-14-06%20FINAL%2060+REPORT.pdf. Accessed March 9, 2011.

40. United States Department of Education, National Center for Education Statistics. *Indicators of School Crime and Safety: 2010*. NCES 2011-002, 2007. http://nces.ed.gov/pubs2011/2011002.pdf. Accessed March 9, 2011.

41. U.S. Department of Justice, Bureau of Justice Statistics. *Criminal Victimization in the United States, 2006, Statistical Tables*. Table 32. Percent distribution of victimizations by perceived drug or alcohol use by offender. NCJ 223436, 2008. http://bjs.ojp.usdoj.gov/content/pub/pdf/cvus06.pdf. Accessed: October 18, 2011.

42. Egley Jr. A, Howell JC, Moore JP. Highlights of the 2008 National Youth Gang Survey. *OJJDP Fact Sheet*. U.S. Department of Justice, Office of Justice Programs, Office of Juvenile Justice and Delinquency Prevention, March 2010. http://www.ncjrs.gov/pdffiles1/ojjdp/229249.pdf. Accessed March 15, 2011.

43. U.S. Department of Justice, Office of Justice Programs. Substance abuse and crime. http://www.ojp.usdoj.gov/programs/substance.htm. Accessed March 15, 2011.

44. Dorsey TL, Middleton P. *Drugs and Crime Facts*. U.S. Department of Justice, Office of Justice Program, Bureau of Justice Statistics. NCJ 165148. http:bjs.ojp.usdoj.gov/content/pub/pdf/dcf.pdf. Accessed March 15, 2011.

45. Langton L, Planty M. Victims of identity theft, 2008. U.S. Department of Justice, Bureau of Justice Statistics, Special Report. *National Crime Victimization Survey Supplement*. NCJ 231680, December 2010. http://bjs.ojp.usdoj.gov/content/pub/pdf/vit08.pdf. Accessed March 15, 2011.

46. Federal Trade Commission. Deter·Detect·Defend: Avoid ID theft: fighting back against identity theft. www.ftc.gov/idtheft. Accessed January 15, 2009.

47. Annan, K. [In the second part of the report titled] Larger freedom. A commentary issued by the United Nations at the Security Council Meeting, March 17, 2005. www.un.org/unifeed/script.asp?scriptId=73. Accessed February 17, 2007.

Personal Assessment

How Well Do You Protect Yourself from Injuries?

This quiz will help you measure how well you protect yourself from unintentional and intentional injuries. For each item, circle the number that reflects the frequency with which you take the following injury prevention actions. Then total your individual scores and check the interpretation at the end.

3 = Regularly
2 = Sometimes
1 = Rarely

1. I wear my seat belt.   3   2   1
2. I refrain from talking on a cell phone while I am driving.   3   2   1
3. I refrain from sending or receiving e-mail or text messages while I am driving.   3   2   1
4. I refrain from driving a motor vehicle after I have been drinking alcohol.   3   2   1
5. I refrain from riding in a car or truck, or on a motorcycle with a driver who has been drinking alcohol.   3   2   1
6. I drive my car or truck, or ride my motorcycle safely and defensively.   3   2   1
7. My motor vehicle is in good mechanical condition.   3   2   1
8. I lock my car doors.   3   2   1
9. I keep an emergency first-aid kit in my car, and I have a plan of action if my car should break down.   3   2   1
10. I have deadbolt locks on the doors of my home and safety locks on the windows.   3   2   1
11. I keep all drugs in my home in their original containers and out of reach of children.   3   2   1
12. I change the batteries in my home smoke detector once a year.   3   2   1
13. I have installed a carbon monoxide detector in my home.   3   2   1
14. There is adequate lighting in areas around my home and garage.   3   2   1
15. I have the electrical, heating, and cooling systems in my home inspected annually for safety and efficiency.   3   2   1
16. I keep emergency numbers near my land-based phone and on my cell phone.   3   2   1
17. I refrain from keeping a loaded gun in my home.   3   2   1
18. I carefully monitor weather conditions and know how to respond to weather emergencies.   3   2   1
19. I use appropriate safety equipment, such as a life jacket or flotation device, while boating.   3   2   1
20. I can swim well enough to save myself in most situations.   3   2   1
21. I wear a helmet when I bike.   3   2   1
22. I carefully monitor my alcohol intake, especially at parties.   3   2   1
23. I don't accept drinks from people I don't know well, and I keep an eye on my drinks at parties.   3   2   1
24. When I attend parties or go to clubs, I go with trusted friends.   3   2   1
25. I avoid locations where interpersonal violence is likely to occur.   3   2   1
26. I am aware of my surroundings and do not get lost.   3   2   1
27. When I walk across campus at night, I walk with others.   3   2   1
28. I use a crosscut shredder to shred documents with my personal information before discarding them.   3   2   1
29. I refrain from sharing my personal information (address, phone number, Social Security number, my daily schedule) with people I do not know well.   3   2   1
30. I check my receipts and bank account balances regularly to make sure my accounts are secure.   3   2   1

TOTAL POINTS _____

Personal Assessment—*continued*

Interpretation

81 to 90 points—You appear to carefully protect your personal safety.

74 to 80 points—You adequately protect many aspects of your personal safety.

67 to 73 points—You should consider improving some of your safety-related behaviors.

Below 67 points—You must consider improving some of your safety-related behaviors.

TO CARRY THIS FURTHER . . .

Although no one can be completely safe from personal injury or possible random violence, there are ways to minimize the risks to your safety. Refer to the text and this assessment to provide you with useful suggestions to enhance your personal safety. Which safety tips will you use today?

16

The Environment and Your Health

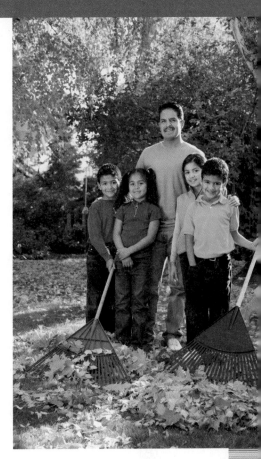

What Do You Know About Environmental Health?

1. The vast majority of your exposure to potentially harmful pollutants occurs in the home and workplace. True or False?

2. Electromagnetic radiation from electrical power lines, microwave ovens, and cell phones has been shown to cause cancer. True or False?

3. If you live in an old house, you and your family are at greater risk for lead poisoning, which can reduce intelligence and increase behavior problems in young children. True or False?

4. The government has tested all chemicals used in household and personal hygiene products to ensure that they do not cause adverse health effects in people. True or False?

5. If you suffer from asthma or other lung diseases, it would be good for your health to move to Los Angeles. True or False?

6. Tap water from a municipal water supplier can contain measurable amounts of potentially harmful pollutants. True or False?

7. Warming of Earth's climate associated with increasing carbon dioxide in the atmosphere from burning fossil fuels can have a negative impact on your health. True or False?

Check your answers at the end of the chapter.

Many college-age students are aware of how human activities damage the health of the environment, but how many know of the risks that their environment poses to their own health? You likely have heard that global warming associated with burning of fossil fuels to power our modern society is causing polar ice caps to melt, endangering the polar bear. You may be aware that overhunting and habitat destruction associated with logging, farming, urban development, and pollution destroys or degrades natural habitats and puts many species at risk of extinction. But do you know what potentially harmful substances or organisms are in the air you breathe, the water you drink, and the food you eat? Do you know which products you purchase and bring into your home can increase your risk of developing cancer

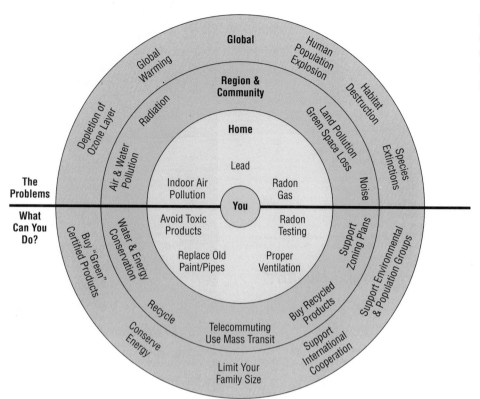

Figure 16-1 Environmental Problems and Solutions This model shows spatial scales of environmental health risks and appropriate personal responses to environmental problems.

or having a child with birth defects? Are you aware of the materials and appliances in your home that emit noxious or dangerous fumes? Do you know how to maintain your home to minimize your exposure to disease- or allergy-producing organisms? Have you ever felt sad, angry, or hopeless when you read or heard about the loss of a species or a beautiful natural habitat but didn't know what you could do about it? The main focus of this chapter is to make you aware of those components of your environment that may adversely affect your personal health and to provide you with suggestions for how you can manage these environmental factors.

Your **environment** includes a range of conditions that can influence your health, such as the availability of resources (oxygen, water, food), and environmental characteristics, such as temperature, humidity, toxins, allergens, pathogens, noise, and radiation. Conditions in your environment operate across a wide range of spatial scales, from the air immediately surrounding your body to the global earth, air, and ocean system. Your physical health is influenced primarily by your *personal environment,* which comprises conditions in the home, neighborhood, and workplace, including indoor air, drinking water, toxic building materials, and noise. This personal environment is influenced by conditions in the larger *community* and *regional environment,* including such conditions as air pollution and water pollution. These local and regional conditions are influenced by conditions of the *global environment,* such as climate and solar radiation.

The goal of this chapter is to help you identify aspects of your environment that can significantly affect your health and to suggest ways that you can exert personal control over these environmental influences. Different environmental conditions and personal responses will be important at the various spatial scales (home/workplace, community/region, and global). Figure 16-1 displays some environmental problems at various spatial scales and a range of personal responses that might be appropriate at each level.

The Personal Environment: Home, Neighborhood, Workplace

On average you spend about 90 percent of your time in your home, workplace, local stores, and entertainment venues.[1] The indoor air you breathe, the water you drink

---

Key Terms

environment The physical conditions (temperature, humidity, light, presence of substances) and other living organisms that exist around your body.

indoor air quality Characteristics of air within homes, workplaces, and public buildings, including the presence and amount of oxygen, water vapor, and a wide range of substances that can have adverse effects on your health.

---

from the tap, the food you eat, and the radiation and noise in your immediate surroundings are environmental factors that have the most direct impact on your health. Some indoor environmental problems cause immediate health effects, such as headaches, dizziness, nausea, or allergic reactions. Other environmental problems act in subtle, cumulative ways, causing major health problems such as cancer or neurological damage that may not become apparent until permanent harm is done.

Of all the different environmental influences on your health, you have the greatest control over factors in your personal environment. You are responsible for maintaining appliances so that they do not produce excessive air pollution. You control the ventilation in your home, allowing you to vent pollutants outside. You select the foods you eat. You choose which products you purchase and can avoid products that contain toxic chemicals. You can eliminate tobacco smoke from your home and workspace. You can identify sources of health risk in the workplace and notify those responsible for environmental safety.

In this section, you will learn to identify important environmental health risks in your personal environment, learn the effects of these environmental factors on your health, and see what you can do to minimize associated risks of health problems. Table 16.1 identifies notable pollutants in the personal environment, and Table 16.2 outlines how to minimize your exposure to these pollutants.

Indoor Air Quality

Indoor air quality can be influenced by a wide range of factors, including ventilation, humidity, gases given off by building construction materials, furniture and flooring materials, and combustion by-products from stoves and furnaces. When there is a problem with one or more of these factors, people in the affected building can experience a wide range of symptoms, from headaches and itchy eyes to unconsciousness and death. This section covers some of the most important health risks associated with indoor air quality.

Table 16.1 Pollutants in the Personal Environment

Pollutant	Sources	Health Effects
Carbon monoxide	Poorly functioning furnaces, space heaters, water heaters, gas stoves; gasoline/diesel engine exhaust	*At 70–150 ppm:* headache, dizziness, mental confusion, nausea *Above 150 ppm:* death
Volatile organic compounds (VOCs)	Oil paints and paint stripper, cleaning solvents, wood preservatives, aerosol sprays, cleaners, disinfectants, stored fuels, automotive fluids	*Immediate effects:* irritation to eyes, nose, throat, nausea *Long-term effects:* damage to liver, kidney, central nervous system; some VOCs are carcinogenic
Formaldehyde	Home insulation foam, carpet adhesives, plywood, paneling, particleboard, fiberboard, furniture made from these	Irritation to eyes, nose, throat, lungs; long-term exposure may cause lung cancer
Asbestos	Building materials such as floor tiles, noise-dampening tiles, fireproofing	Inhaled asbestos fibers can cause lung damage, emphysema, lung cancer
Lead	Pre-1980 house paint, plumbing solder, dust from nearby highways	Damages nervous system, kidneys, blood; in children, causes lower IQ, delayed physical and mental development
Biological pollutants (including *E. coli*)	Disease-causing viruses and bacteria in air or water, dust mites, plant pollen, mold, pet dander, rodent and cockroach feces	Colds and flu; allergic reactions that include itchy eyes, runny nose, sneezing, headache, skin rashes; may induce asthma; waterborne organisms may cause nausea, diarrhea, fever
Radon	Naturally occurring radioactive substances in soil around the home	Major cause of lung cancer
Nitrate	Agricultural fertilizer contamination of groundwater wells	Interferes with oxygen transport by blood; damages reproductive system; may cause several cancers
Vinyl chloride	Pre-1977 PVC pipe in plumbing	Causes cancer
Pesticides	Contamination of water supplies, food	Damages nervous system; interferes with reproductive development; carcinogenic
Phthalates and bisphenol A	Soft plastics in food containers, shampoos and soaps, cosmetics, paints, adhesives, wallpaper, carpet	Interferes with reproductive development; causes cancer, birth defects

Table 16.2 Managing Pollutants in the Personal Environment

Pollutant	How to Minimize Exposure
Carbon monoxide	Properly maintain appliances that burn natural gas. Ensure proper use and ventilation of fuel-burning space heaters, cooking grills, fireplaces. Avoid breathing exhaust fumes from autos or powerboats. Install a carbon monoxide detector in your home.
Volatile organic compounds (VOCs)	Minimize use of products that emit these substances (e.g., use latex paint instead of oil paint) or use only in well-ventilated area. Never mix household chemicals (might react to produce VOCs). Do not store VOC-emitting products in your home; dispose of excess product properly.
Formaldehyde	Use only "low-emission" formaldehyde-containing products (carpet, paneling, adhesives). Have adequate ventilation of personal environment spaces.
Asbestos	Never disturb intact asbestos-containing materials. Hire qualified contractors to remove asbestos from your home; *never* do this yourself. If your home was built before 1978, have interior paint tested for lead (ask local health department for guidance). Do not disturb intact lead-containing paint; hire qualified contractor to remove deteriorated lead-containing paint. Keep children and pregnant women away from areas with deteriorated lead-containing paint. Beware of cheap metal toy jewelry for children as this often contains lead.
Biological pollutants	Use exhaust fans or dehumidifiers to maintain relative humidity of your home at 30–50 percent to minimize growth of mold. Remove all water-damaged carpet and drywall to prevent mold. Regularly clean/vacuum home and eliminate cockroaches and rodents to minimize exposure to allergens. Have tap water tested for *E. coli* and install chlorination or filtration system if present.
Radon	Test home for presence of radon. If test is positive, install radon reduction system in home.
Nitrate	If your water source is a well and you live in an agricultural area, have your water tested. If nitrate is present, drink bottled water or install reverse osmosis water system in your home.
Vinyl chloride	If your house was built before 1977 and has PVC pipes for the water supply, replace these pipes.
Pesticides	Test your well water or get water quality report from water company, drink bottled water or install reverse osmosis system if pesticides found in tap water. Eat organically produced food.
Phthalates and BPA	Reduce use of personal hygiene products and cosmetics that list the words "phthalate" in the ingredients. Avoid food and drink containers made of soft plastic; use water bottles made of glass, metal, or plastic labeled as BPA-free. Eliminate all exposure to these if you are pregnant. Do not give soft plastic toys or plastic bottles to your small children unless these items are labeled as phthalate- and BPA-free.

Carbon Monoxide **Carbon monoxide** is a highly toxic gas that is colorless, odorless, and tasteless, and so is not detectable by the unaided senses. Health effects of carbon monoxide begin with mild discomfort, including headache or light-headedness at first and flulike symptoms (nausea and lethargy) with continued exposure to low levels. Persons who suffer from heart disease may feel chest pain. These symptoms rapidly disappear after you leave the location where you are exposed to the gas. Exposure to high levels of this gas can be lethal, causing first unconsciousness and then death:[1,2] According to the U.S. Consumer Product Safety Commission, about 170 people per year die from household exposure to carbon monoxide, many from using portable generators, fireplaces, or charcoal grills indoors.

Volatile Organic Compounds **Volatile organic compounds (VOCs)** are gases emitted to indoor air from a wide range of household products. These gases often have a "chemical" smell (for example, gasoline or paint stripper). *Formaldehyde* is a specific VOC that is emitted by many building products (plywood, particleboard, fiberboard, urea foam insulation, building/carpet adhesives).[2] This indoor air pollutant was the main reason victims of Hurricane Katrina had to be relocated out of travel trailer housing provided by FEMA. In hundreds of these travel trailers, indoor air concentrations of formaldehyde were 4–50 times greater than normal levels in homes and well above levels known to cause adverse health effects.[3] People living in these trailers complained of a range of symptoms, including irritated eyes, headaches, and dizziness.

The health effects of volatile organic compounds vary depending on which specific substance is involved, ranging from irritation to the eyes and respiratory system, to organ damage, to cancer.

You can control your exposure to toxic volatile organic compounds through your choices of which products you bring into your home and by using VOC-emitting products only in well-ventilated areas.

Tobacco Smoke Secondhand tobacco smoke is an indoor air pollutant widely recognized as a major health risk, especially for children. For example, this pollutant can increase the risk for acute asthma attacks that require hospital emergency care. Some evidence indicates that regular exposure to tobacco smoke increases the risk of developing asthma in the first place.[4] Exposure to tobacco smoke in the home is also associated with increased risk of sudden infant death syndrome (SIDS); childhood bronchitis, pneumonia, and ear infections; cardiovascular disease; and cancer. The health effects of indoor tobacco smoke are covered in more detail in Chapter 9.

Asbestos **Asbestos** is a building material that was widely used for its insulation, fire retardant, and noise-dampening properties. When the serious health risks associated with exposure to asbestos fibers became known, governmental agencies banned several asbestos products, and manufacturers voluntarily limited other uses of asbestos. Today, asbestos is most commonly found in older buildings, including homes, schools, and factories. Health effects of asbestos exposure most commonly occur only after many years of exposure, usually in the workplace.[5] Currently, your greatest risk of exposure to asbestos occurs when insulation, floor tiles, and other asbestos-containing substances deteriorate or are damaged during building renovation. These activities release the asbestos fibers to the air, from which they are inhaled into the lungs. However, intact and undisturbed, asbestos-containing products are relatively safe.[5]

Lead Lead is a toxic metal that was widely used in house paint, as a gasoline additive, and in plumbing solder for metal pipes. As the health consequences of lead toxicity became known, most of these uses of lead were banned. However, lead is a stable substance that remains in the environment today.[6] Lead exposure most commonly occurs in

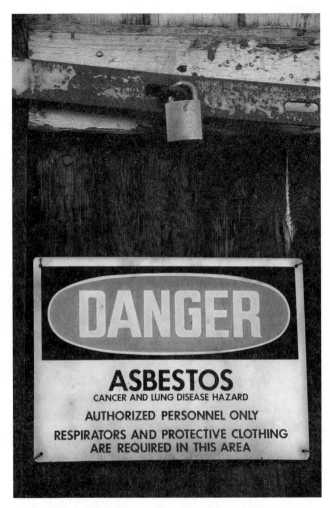

If released from damaged building materials, asbestos can injure the lungs and cause cancer. Asbestos-containing materials should be removed by professionals using proper safety gear and precautions.

homes built before 1978 that contain lead-based wall paint. In late 1991, more than 10 years after lead-based paint was banned, the U.S. Department of Health and Human Services called lead "the number one environmental threat to the health of children in the United States."[7] Exposure to lead from old paint occurs when the paint breaks down into paint flakes and dust, which are then inhaled or swallowed. This risk is especially high for young children, who often put their hands in their mouth.

Lead has serious health effects when ingested or inhaled, especially for children. Blood lead levels as low as 10 micrograms per deciliter in children can delay development, lower IQ, reduce attention span, and increase behavioral problems. Lead is not readily excreted by the body and will tend to accumulate over time. There are drugs that help the body to excrete lead, but they have adverse side effects and are used only to treat acute lead toxicity.[7] See Table 16.2 for ways to avoid exposure to lead in the home.

Key Terms

carbon monoxide A gaseous by-product of the incomplete combustion of natural gas, kerosene, heating oil, wood, coal, gasoline, and tobacco; a compound that can "inactivate" red blood cells.

volatile organic compounds (VOCs) A wide variety of chemicals that contain carbon and readily evaporate into the air.

asbestos A class of minerals that have a fibrous crystal structure; a known carcinogen when inhaled.

Is a "Too-Clean" Environment Bad for Your Health?

Improved sanitation, treatment of drinking water supplies, and use of antibiotics and antiseptics have dramatically reduced the incidence of infectious disease and intestinal parasites in the economically developed countries of North America and western Europe. However, a large body of scientific research indicates that these improvements have come at the cost of dramatic (200–400 percent) increases in the incidence of allergic and autoimmune diseases such as asthma, type 1 diabetes, multiple sclerosis, rheumatoid arthritis, eczema, food and pet allergies, hay fever, and inflammatory bowel diseases such as Crohn's disease and ulcerative colitis.[*] Autoimmune diseases are caused by the body's immune system attacking and damaging its own tissues. Allergies are also due to an immune system malfunction that results in overresponse to otherwise innocuous foreign substances in the environment, such as certain foods, pet dander, insect dander, or pollen. A number of researchers have proposed that insufficient exposure to pathogens and innocuous parasites and microbes during early childhood results in abnormal development of the immune system, which is the underlying cause for many allergies and autoimmune diseases.[*,†] This is generally referred to as the "hygiene hypothesis."

Evidence in support of the hygiene hypothesis comes in many forms. The recent increase in the incidence of allergies and autoimmune diseases in developed countries did not occur in underdeveloped countries that still have a high incidence of infectious and parasitic diseases. Within developed countries, low-income people, who often live in less sanitary conditions, have a lower incidence of allergies and autoimmune diseases. Children who had siblings prior to age 5 years or who went to daycare centers had a lower incidence of allergies and asthma, presumably due to experiencing a greater number of infections. Likewise, people who spent time as young children on a farm with livestock have a lower incidence of allergies and autoimmune diseases than people who were raised in cities, presumably due to exposure to various microbes from the livestock. Blood tests indicate that people who were exposed early to infectious diseases have markers associated with better regulation of the immune system.[†] Mice strains genetically predisposed to develop autoimmune diseases were more likely to develop these diseases if raised in a germ-free environment than if raised in a normal environment.[‡] Inflammation associated with immune system malfunction has also been linked to development of several types of cancer.[‡,§] Preliminary experiments have documented that individuals who suffer from ulcerative colitis or asthma exhibited reduced symptoms after they were given innocuous intestinal worms or "probiotic" microbes.[**,††] These components of the natural intestinal flora have coevolved with humans for thousands of years and produce chemicals that suppress the overactive immune system of these patients that causes their diseases.

Many people in the United States appear to believe that keeping a sterile home is good for their family's health; witness the popularity of bactericidal soaps and cleaning products.

The large body of scientific research that supports the hygiene hypothesis indicates that this overemphasis on cleanliness may actually be bad for your health and, even more important, bad for the health of your children. Most of the positive influence of microbes normally found in the environment occurs during early childhood when the immune system is actively developing. The human immune system is a wonder of nature, amazingly adaptive and able to protect us from most of the pathogens and parasites in our environment. However, the "hygiene hypothesis" research indicates that if the immune system is not given the opportunity to interact with its natural adversaries, it has a tendency to attack its own body. So keep a clean house, but pass on the bactericidal products and use antibiotics only if necessary.

[*]Bach JF, The effect of infections on susceptibility to autoimmune and allergic diseases, *New England Journal of Medicine,* 347, 911–920, 2002.
[†]Seppa N, Worming your way to better health, *Science News,* 179(3), 26–29, 2011.
[‡]Tlaskalova-Hogenova H, and others, The role of gut microbiota (commensal bacteria) and the mucosal barrier in the pathogenesis of inflammatory and auto-immune diseases and cancer: contribution of germ-free and gnotobiotic animal models of human diseases, *Cellular & Molecular Immunology,* 8, 110–120, 2011.
[§]Rook G, Dalgleish A, Infection, immunoregulation and cancer, *Immunological Reviews,* 240, 141–159, 2011.
[**]Summers RW, Elliott DE, Urban JF, Thompson RA, Weinstock JV, Trichuris suis therapy for active ulcerative colitis: a randomized controlled trial. *Gastroenterology,* 128(4), 825–832, 2005.
[††]Gutkowski P, and others, Effect of orally administered probiotic strains Lactobacillus and Bifidobacterium in children with atopic asthma, *Central European Journal of Immunology,* 35(4), 233–238, 2010.

Biological Pollutants There are many sources of **biological air pollutants** within your personal environment. Disease-causing viruses and bacteria (common cold, flu, measles) are put into the air when infected people or animals sneeze or cough. Contaminated central air handling systems can be breeding grounds for mold, mildew, and bacteria and can then distribute these contaminants throughout the home. Some people have allergic reactions to spores from mold that grows on moist surfaces inside buildings. Some research indicates that exposure to indoor mold can more than double your risk of developing adult-onset asthma.[4] Pollen from plants around the home or workplace can cause allergic reactions (hay fever) in many people. Household pets, rats, mice, and cockroaches are sources of saliva, urine, feces, and skin dander that can also stimulate strong allergic reactions.[8] The best way for you to minimize biological pollutants is to keep a clean, dry home free of mold and sources of allergens. However, there is a growing body of research indicating that people who grow up in a "too clean" environment are more likely to develop allergies or autoimmune diseases (see the box "Is a 'Too-Clean' Environment Bad for Your Health?").

Radon **Radon** is a naturally occurring gas that forms as a result of the decay of radioactive minerals in soils that are found in all 50 states. It seeps from the soil into buildings through the foundation, and this is how most people are exposed. Radon is colorless, odorless, and tasteless, and can be detected only by using a radon detector. It is estimated that indoor radon levels sufficient to increase risk of lung cancer occur in 7 percent of homes in the United States, and radon is the second leading cause of lung cancer.[9,10] You can view state-by-state maps of radon risk zones at the U.S. Environmental Protection Agency's radon website (for example, to view a map for Indiana, go to www. epa.gov/radon/zonemap/indiana). The key to minimizing the health risk of radon is to have your home tested. Inexpensive "do-it-yourself" test kits are available in hardware stores. You can also purchase test kits from the National Safety Council's Radon Hotline (800-767-7236). If unsafe levels of radon are detected in your home, you should install a radon venting system below and around the house foundation. If you plan to build a new home in a region where high radon levels are common, you should tell your contractor to install radon-resistant features during construction, reducing costs by as much as 400 percent.[9]

Toxic Substances in the Workplace

Exposure to dangerous indoor air pollutants often occurs in the workplace, especially in mining and manufacturing facilities. Workers in manufacturing plants are often exposed to asbestos, toxic metals, VOCs, strong acids, and a variety of carcinogens. Sometimes the adverse health effects of these substances were not known until after workers were exposed. In some cases, the adverse health effects were known, but this information was not made available to workers.

One example of such a workplace is the Bannister Federal Complex in Kansas City, Missouri, also known as the Benndix, Allied Signal, or Honeywell Plant for the companies that managed it at various times under government contract. This plant produced many components used in nuclear weapons and aerospace programs from 1949 until it was closed in 2009. The U.S. Department of Labor lists 785 toxic substances that were used at the plant during this time, and $65 million was spent prior to 2009 to clean up residual hazardous materials. A local newspaper article documented the life-altering effects on past employees resulting from their work-related exposure to these toxic substances, including severe allergies, debilitating respiratory diseases, arthritis, cancers in both workers and their children, and premature deaths.[11] One woman was exposed to a toxic metal as a 16-year-old working a summer job at the plant; she was pregnant at the time. Her son died of cancer at age 27, and she now suffers from a respiratory disease that substantially degrades her quality of life and will ultimately kill her. A lawyer considered organizing ex-workers in a class action lawsuit but knew that the litigation would take more years than his clients were likely to survive. Many workers interviewed described puzzling instructions from managers to wear a face mask or cover their skin, with no additional explanation, suggesting that

knowledge of potentially dangerous substances was not always shared with low-level workers. A lesson one might take from this story is that if something doesn't seem right in a workplace environment, it might be best to look for another job; no amount of money can make up for the loss of health and well-being.

Nonionizing Radiation

Common sources of **nonionizing radiation** in the personal environment are sunlight, electrical devices, electric power transmission lines, and cell phones. This part of the electromagnetic spectrum includes ultraviolet and infrared radiation (in sunlight) and radio frequency radiation (from electronic devices). Most documented health effects of nonionizing radiation are associated with heating tissues or sunburn.

Some have proposed that certain forms of nonionizing radiation may have more serious health effects. A few small studies have documented DNA damage in brain cells of rats exposed to high levels of radiofrequency radiation (RFR) similar to that emitted by early mobile phones. However, other animal studies did not find similar effects. A large-scale study of 420,000 people in Denmark who have been using cell phones for more than 10 years found that they were no more likely to have cancer in the brain, ear, salivary glands, or eye (tissues close to where the cell phone is placed when in use) than people who did not use cell phones.[12] However, a smaller study in Sweden found that people with malignant brain tumors were more likely to have been heavy users of cell phones (analog or digital) or cordless home phones over long periods than were randomly chosen people without cancer.[13] Cell phones are a relatively new technology, and the authors of the Swedish study note that cancers caused by RFR may take many years to develop. Hence, there has not yet been sufficient time to study effects of long-term exposure to RFR.[14] As people use cell phones more, beginning at an ever-younger age, some suggest that it may be prudent to reduce exposure to RFR from these devices.[13] This can be easily done by using a headset attachment to the cell phone to move the cell phone transmitter away from the brain. Advances in cell phone technology are also reducing the amount of RFR emitted by newer cell phones.

Key Terms

biological air pollutants Living organisms or substances produced by living organisms that cause disease or allergic reactions, including bacteria, molds, mildew, viruses, dust mites, plant pollen, and animal dander, urine, or feces.

radon A naturally occurring radioactive gas that is emitted during the decay of uranium in soil, rock, and water.

nonionizing radiation Forms of electromagnetic radiation that cannot break chemical bonds but may excite electrons or heat biological materials.

Another common source of nonionizing radiation in the human environment is electricity flowing through wires and electronic devices, and electricity transmission lines. A few studies have suggested that exposure to non-ionizing radiation around electric devices such as microwave ovens, televisions, tanning lamps, and electric blankets, and electricity transmission lines may slightly increase risk for some cancers.[15,16] However, attempts to replicate and confirm these small studies have failed, and the vast majority of studies have failed to find any increased risk of adverse health effects associated with household electronics or living near power lines.[14,17]

Drinking Water

The safety of drinking water in your home is affected by environmental factors both in the home or neighborhood and in the larger community. The water supply for rural homes is often a well that draws from groundwater and can be much affected by environmental conditions around the home and neighborhood. In urban areas, municipal water supply systems treat the water to make it safe to drink. The community/regional environment plays the dominant role in determining the safety of water from municipal suppliers. However, municipal water can be contaminated by the personal environment as it passes through pipes in the home. Environmental health issues relating to drinking water as influenced by conditions in your home and neighborhood will be covered here. Issues related to municipal water supply are discussed later in this chapter.

Approximately 23 million people in the United States obtain their drinking water from groundwater (that is, from private wells), streams, or cisterns that collect rain water.[18] These households are responsible for ensuring the safety of their own drinking water. Private drinking water supplies that rely on surface waters, or shallow wells, are at risk of contamination from home septic systems, leaking underground fuel storage tanks, improperly disposed household chemicals (cleaners, automotive fluids), and fertilizers and pesticides applied to surrounding farm fields. *Nitrate* from agricultural fertilizer that leaches into shallow groundwater supplies poses a widespread health risk in rural areas. The U.S. Geological Survey estimates that 10–20 percent of groundwater sources of drinking water may have levels of nitrate contamination that pose risks to human health.[19] Rural wells contaminated by nitrate may also have high levels of other agricultural chemicals. See the section "Endocrine Disrupters" for information on the health effects of pesticides and herbicides.

Leaching of substances from pipes in the plumbing of older homes is another potential source of contamination to drinking water in the home.[20] Metallic pipes can release toxic metals such as lead and copper into the water. Polyvinyl chloride (PVC) pipes manufactured before 1977 may release toxic vinyl chloride into

the water. Vinyl chloride is a known human carcinogen. Leaching of toxic substances from pipes into tap water is greatest in pipes with less than a 2-inch diameter when water temperature is high and the water is stagnant in the pipes for more than 24 hours.[20] To reduce your exposure to these contaminants from household plumbing, let the tap run for a couple of minutes before taking water to drink, especially first thing in the morning or if you have been away from home for a long time. In some cases, it may be advisable to replace the old plumbing, but this can be very expensive.

Sources of Drinking Water   Private water supplies should be tested annually for nitrate and fecal coliform bacteria. If you suspect there may be a problem with radon or pesticide contamination, you may need to test your water even more frequently.[18] Testing will require that you send samples to a laboratory. You can get a listing of local certified laboratories from your local or state public health department. Some local health departments test private water for free. A private laboratory will charge $10–20 to perform a nitrate and bacteria test. Testing for pesticides or organic chemicals may cost from several hundred to several thousand dollars.

If your drinking water contains contaminants that exceed safety standards, you should immediately contact your public health department for assistance. High bacteria concentrations can be easily controlled by disinfecting a well. Water filters may also remove some contaminants. However, other problems may require a new source of water, such as a deeper well. You may need to rely on bottled water until a new water source can be obtained.[18] You can obtain technical assistance with residential drinking water supply problems from the organization Farm*A*Syst/Home*A*Syst (see the websites www.uwex.edu/farmasyst or www.uwex.edu/homeasyst).

Endocrine Disrupters

Endocrine-disrupting chemicals include a number of infamously dangerous pollutants (dioxin, PCBs, DDT) and various pesticides, herbicides, antiseptics, and chemicals used in the manufacture of plastics (phthalates, bisphenol A or BPA) and Teflon (perfluorooctanoic acid or PFOA). These chemicals enter the home and work environment as contaminants of air, food, and water in household plastics, nonstick cookware, and a range of personal products, such as cosmetics, hair spray, perfumes, soap, and shampoo. Many of these substances are not readily eliminated from the body and tend to accumulate; large proportions of people in the United States have measurable amounts of these substances in their bodies.[21]

Agricultural pesticides and herbicides that act as endocrine disrupters include some of the most widely used chemicals in our food production system (for example, the herbicide Atrazine). Your exposure to these chemicals can occur via pesticide residues on fruit and vegetables or contamination of well water (in locations with large areas of farmland). These chemicals have been linked to testicular and breast cancer, reduced sperm production in men, and nervous disorders in children.[22]

Phthalates are a class of endocrine disrupters that have become a recent source of concern after analyses of urine from a random sample of people in the United States indicated that virtually the entire population has measurable quantities of one or more of these chemicals in their bodies.[21] This is likely because of the almost ubiquitous use of phthalates in soft plastics used for food packaging, toys, and many personal hygiene products. Phthalates are released from plastics to air, water, and food and are readily absorbed across the skin and via the lungs and digestive tract. Phthalates disrupt the action of the sex hormones estrogen and testosterone, affecting both reproductive development of fetuses and children and reproductive function of adults.[23] Disruption of hormonal balance at critical stages in the development of a fetus or child can have long-lasting effects.[24] Some have suggested that increases in the occurrence of breast and testicular cancer, and decreases in human sperm quality, in recent decades may be linked to exposure to endocrine-disrupting chemicals such as phthalates.[25] As these health risks associated with phthalates have become better documented, major retail stores (such as WalMart, Toys R Us, and Target) have required their suppliers to reduce or eliminate these chemicals from the plastics used for children's toys.

Bisphenol A (BPA) is a component of polycarbonate plastic containers used for food and drink and epoxy resins used to line food and drink cans. This substance can leach from the container wall into the food or drink within, which is then consumed. A recent report documented that 93 percent of the U.S. population has measurable amounts of BPA in their body fluids, with the highest levels measured in children and women.[26] The health effects of BPA are currently a source of controversy. The U.S. Food and Drug Administration (FDA) released a report in April 2008 stating that current evidence indicates BPA is safe at current levels of exposure.[27] However, a paper later published in a prestigious medical journal indicated that current BPA exposure may increase risk of developing type 2 diabetes and heart and liver disease.[28]

BPA is an estrogenlike chemical that may also interfere with the male sex hormone testosterone, and it has been linked to adverse effects on male sex organs and fertility. However, it is difficult to isolate the suspected effects of BPA from other factors, and claims of these adverse health effects are controversial. To address the uncertainties associated with inconsistent results from studies of BPA's health effects, the National Institute for Environmental Health Sciences launched a multimillion-dollar research initiative for 2010–2011.[29] In the meantime, the FDA issued interim guidelines in January 2010 to limit the use of BPA in baby bottles and containers for foodstuffs intended for infants. Pregnant women might also avoid canned foods, which usually have BPA in the liners.

It can be difficult for you to avoid exposure to endocrine-disrupting chemicals when the health effects of many chemicals widely used in consumer products are not yet well known. Both phthalates and BPA have been widely used for decades. Initial studies indicated that these substances were not toxic to humans, and so they were deemed safe. Widespread use in various products has resulted in most of the U.S. population having some amounts of these substances in their bodies. Later research has shown that these chemicals may have subtle adverse health effects that develop only after long-term exposure. There are many such chemicals in the various modern consumer products that you bring into your personal environment. These chemicals provide a wide range of benefits. But with the benefits, you may also incur risks. The best way to protect yourself is to be aware of health-related news and to act when new information identifies risks that you can reduce or eliminate from your life.

Noise

Noise can be defined as any undesirable sound. What constitutes "undesirable sound" will vary from one person to the next, but it often involves loud sounds that occur at irregular intervals and cannot be controlled by the listener.[30] In the personal environment, noise may include overly loud music, barking dogs, motorcycles and cars with broken mufflers, loud machinery, appliances and power tools, airplanes flying overhead, and train whistles.

Health Effects of Noise   The health effects of environmental noise depend on the intensity, frequency, and nature of the noise. Excessively loud noise can cause physical damage to sensory tissues in your ears, resulting in partial or total hearing loss that can be temporary or permanent. This physical damage will depend on both the intensity (as measured in decibels) and the duration of exposure to the loud noise. A common source of loud sound that causes hearing loss in many young people is long-term exposure to amplified music. A study of college students in New York City indicated that over 50 percent listen to their MP3 players at a combination of

---

Key Terms

endocrine-disrupting chemicals A large class of substances that can interact with the system of glands, hormones, and tissues that regulate many physiological processes in humans, including growth, development from fetus to adult, regulation of metabolic rate and blood sugar, function of the reproductive system, and development of the brain and nervous systems.

volume and duration sufficient to cause permanent degradation of hearing.[31] Many incorrectly believe that their MP3 player has a volume limiter to prevent hearing damage and set the volume to its maximum.

Even noise at lower levels can cause adverse health effects. The American Speech-Language-Hearing Association reports that low-level noise can elevate blood pressure, reduce sleep, cause fatigue, and disturb digestion. These physical effects of low-level noise can diminish emotional, intellectual, social, and occupational health. Effects reported by the World Health Organization include increased frustration and anxiety, impaired ability to concentrate, reduced productivity and ability to learn, and increased absenteeism and accidents. These effects of noise can increase your feelings of stress and cause you to exhibit anger and aggression that are out of proportion to the immediate source of your irritation.[30] This antisocial behavior may have negative consequences in your personal relationships and occupational health (see the box "Reducing Health Risks of Noise Pollution").

 TALKING POINTS How can you encourage your children to develop sound habits regarding their environment and their personal health? What changes can you make in your own habits to serve as a better example for them?

The Community and Regional Environment

The community and regional environment is composed of the outdoor air you breathe, local rivers and lakes that provide water and recreation opportunities, surrounding lands (urban, industrial, suburban, rural, agricultural, natural communities), and all the people and other

species that live in these areas. A wide range of human activities can degrade this community environment in ways that affect personal health. Air, water, and land pollution include many substances that have significant negative effects on physical health. Loss of natural areas and other recreational and aesthetic "green space" to roads, cities, and industrial development can adversely affect your perceived quality of life, with negative effects on emotional and spiritual health. Degraded environmental conditions in many communities discourage new economic development and may limit occupational health.

While you can exert some influence on the environmental conditions in your community, the influence of any one individual is usually small. Your control over how the community environment affects your personal health is often limited to controlling your exposure to known health risks, such as contaminated water and land or outdoor air pollution. You can also choose to reduce your own contributions to community/regional air, water, and land pollution through conservation of energy and water and the recycling of solid waste.

Because one person cannot have a significant impact on community environmental problems, many people join organizations that work to improve the environment and quality of life in their community. By working with others of like mind in the political process and in environmental organizations, you become "part of the solution" to major environmental problems that can affect your health and that of your family. For many people, getting involved in solving local environmental problems can provide significant benefits to emotional and spiritual health.

In this section, you will learn about aspects of the community and regional environment that can affect your health, and things you can do to exert some level of personal control over these environmental influences.

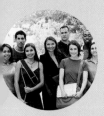

Learning from Our Diversity

Race, Economic Status, and Exposure to Pollution

While it is impossible to prevent all pollution, it is important to know if the risk of adverse health effects due to exposure is fairly distributed across the population. The "environmental justice" movement studies whether people of color and people who are economically or politically disadvantaged are disproportionately exposed to environmental hazards and more likely to suffer associated injury or disease than the general population. This movement gained prominence after a report found that new hazardous waste dumps were being disproportionately located in communities with high proportions of racial minorities and low-income families.[*] In the years since, researchers have studied this issue in various regions of the United States. Many, but not all, studies have found evidence that environmental hazards are more likely to be found near areas with a high percentage of minority and low-income population.

Two hypotheses have been proposed for this association between race, class, and pollution: (1) *industrial siting decisions:* pollution producers prefer to locate their facilities in areas that have cheap real estate and/or where the community is less able to resist (poor and uneducated); and (2) *move-in decisions:* hazardous pollution sources reduce the value of surrounding housing and land, attracting low-income renters and homeowners who tend to be disproportionately racial and ethnic minorities.[†] While there is evidence for both phenomena, siting decisions appear to be the primary factor.

Issues of environmental justice are not restricted to industrial pollution and hazardous waste dumps. In recent years, the siting of large confined-animal feeding operations (CAFOs) has stirred much controversy in rural areas of the United States. These mainly corporate-affiliated facilities generate millions of gallons of animal waste that is stored in sewage lagoons. Sewage lagoons can emit large amounts of hydrogen sulfide (rotten egg smell) and ammonia into the atmosphere. These very unpleasant-smelling air pollutants result in adverse physical health effects, diminished quality of life, and reduced land value in the area around the CAFO.[‡] Studies in the southeastern United States have provided evidence that new hog CAFOs were being preferentially sited in areas with high proportions of African American and low-income families.[§]

Studies of the impact of increased exposure to air pollutants in low-income and minority-dominated communities have documented increased risk of cancer and respiratory distress and decreased academic performance of students in schools located in these communities.[**] This latter effect acts to strengthen the cycle of poverty, as lowered academic performance by children in poor neighborhoods contributes to reduced future opportunities for economic advancement.

These and other studies have motivated a social and political environmental justice movement that helps disadvantaged communities resist attempts to locate new pollutant sources near their neighborhoods. Governmental recognition of the environmental justice issue has resulted in new laws and regulations for land-use planning and permits that require builders of new pollutant sources to specifically address issues of disproportionate pollution exposure of minority and low-income populations. If we all benefit from the products made by industries that produce pollutants, fairness requires that we also share equally the health costs of associated pollutants. If we all share equally the costs and benefits of industry, perhaps there will be greater motivation to develop less-polluting technologies.

---

[*]United Church of Christ, *A National Report on the Racial and Socio-Economic Characteristics of Communities with Hazardous Waste Sites,* UCC Committee for Racial Justice, New York, 1987.
[†]Pastor M, et al., Which came first? toxic facilities, minority move-in, and environmental justice, *Journal of Urban Affairs,* 23(1), 1–21, 2001.
[‡]Donham K, et al., Community health and socioeconomic issues surrounding concentrated animal feeding operations, *Environmental Health Perspectives,* 115, 317–320, 2006.
[§]Wing S, et al., Environmental justice in North Carolina's hog industry, *Environmental Health Perspectives,* 108, 225–231, 2000.
[**]Pastor M, et al., Reading, writing, and toxics: children's health, academic performance, and environmental justice in Los Angeles, *Environment and Planning C: Government and Policy,* 22, 271–290, 2004.

Air Pollution

Air pollution includes substances that naturally occur in the air (pollen, microbes, dust, sea salt, volcanic ash) and substances produced by human activities (engine exhaust, ozone, various volatile organic compounds, acid rain). In this section on community and regional environmental influences on health, we focus on those components of air pollution that are produced within a specific region and that have substantial health effects within that community or region.

Sources of Air Pollutants The primary sources of human-caused air pollutants are various kinds of internal combustion engines associated with electric power plants, industry, and transportation (trucks, automobiles, farm/ construction equipment). Oil refineries and chemical production factories also contribute to air pollution in some communities. Electric power stations, industrial facilities, and chemical factories are classified as *point sources* that produce large amounts of pollution from a single location (see the box "Race, Economic Status, and Exposure to Pollution"). Automobiles, trucks, heavy construction/

> **Key Terms**
>
> **air pollution** Substances in the atmosphere that can have adverse effects on human health, crop productivity, and natural communities.

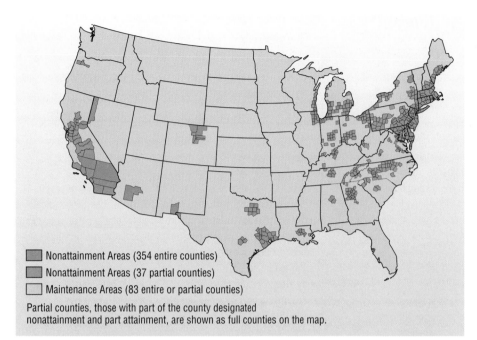

Figure 16-2 Exposure to Unhealthy Air
This map shows counties classified by the EPA as in "nonattainment" of ozone standards in the year 2007, meaning levels of ozone exceeded the limit set by the EPA.
Source: U.S. Environmental Protection Agency.

Nonattainment Areas (354 entire counties)

Nonattainment Areas (37 partial counties)

Maintenance Areas (83 entire or partial counties)

Partial counties, those with part of the county designated nonattainment and part attainment, are shown as full counties on the map.

farm equipment, gas stations, lawn mowers, and charcoal grills are *nonpoint sources* of air pollutants. Individually, nonpoint sources produce relatively small amounts of pollution but, when added together, account for a large proportion of community air pollution.

Health Effects of Air Pollutants   Air pollutants that are directly produced by internal combustion engines include *carbon monoxide, nitrogen dioxide, sulfur dioxide, polycyclic aromatic hydrocarbons,* and *particulate matter.* Carbon monoxide is a toxic gas that impairs respiration, as described under indoor air quality in the earlier section. Nitrogen and sulfur oxides interact with water vapor in the air to form small particulates (diameter <2.5 micrograms) that are inhaled into the deepest parts of the lungs. These substances can damage lung tissues, reduce lung capacity, and cause coughing and chronic bronchitis, and they may worsen such ailments as hypersensitivity to allergens, asthma, emphysema, and heart disease. The EPA estimates that over 70 million people in the United States live in counties where levels of small-particulate air pollutants exceed human health standards for at least some part of the year.[32] It has been estimated that small-particulate air pollution causes as many as 50,000–100,000 premature deaths in the United States per year.[33]

Polycyclic aromatic hydrocarbons (PAHs)   have been shown to be carcinogenic to both test animals and humans. Several studies indicate that PAHs can cross the placenta and have adverse health effects on a developing human fetus.[34,35] Increased maternal exposure to PAHs was associated with lower birth weight, smaller head

circumference, and reduced birth length of newborn children.[34] Another study documented a significant association between maternal exposure to PAHs and PAH-linked DNA damage in newborns that is associated with increased risk of cancer.[35]

Tropospheric ozone is produced when hydrocarbons, nitrogen oxides, and other small-particulate matter chemically interact in the presence of sunlight. The result is a brownish haze over affected cities, often called *smog.* Ozone levels are particularly high in locations with warm, sunny climates (southern California) and where natural vegetation produces volatile organic compounds that contribute to the photochemical process that produces ozone (eastern United States). The EPA estimates that over 110 million people in the United States live in counties where ozone levels exceed human health standards for at least part of the year.[32] Most of these people live in southern California and near the East Coast between Virginia and southern Maine (see Figure 16-2).

Inhalation of ozone can cause lung damage that reduces lung capacity. This is a particular health risk to individuals who suffer from asthma, emphysema, or heart disease. On days when ozone concentrations are highest, local hospital emergency room visits associated with respiratory distress increase from 10 to 20 percent.[33] There is also some evidence that childhood exposure to ozone can actually cause children to become asthmatic.[36]

Air toxics are a diverse collection of hazardous air pollutants produced by electric power plants, industrial sources, and internal combustion engines that constitute an environmental health risk to people. Some of these substances are carcinogenic, some can cause birth defects, and others cause damage to lungs, nervous system, liver, and other organ systems. The most recent inventory of air toxics by the EPA, based on air quality data collected through 2002, assessed 181 different pollutants.[37] Emissions of air toxics have decreased by 40 percent since passage of the 1990 Clean Air Act, but it is estimated that 1 in every 28,000 people in the U.S. population could develop cancer as a result of exposure to air toxics, if they are exposed to 2002 pollution levels over their entire lifetime. However, people living in air toxics "hotspots" near local industrial point sources have a substantially higher risk of developing cancer; approximately 25 percent of the national increased cancer risk associated with air toxics is accounted for by these local hotspots. Air toxics from mobile sources (transportation), mainly benzene, account for 30 percent of the overall increased cancer risk associated with air toxics. This report also indicated that air toxics increase risk for noncancer health problems. Adverse respiratory effects were mainly due to a single pollutant, acrolein, which is used in the manufacture of some plastics and also as an herbicide for aquatic weeds. Adverse neurological effects associated with air toxics were mainly due to manganese, cyanide, and mercury compounds. Elevated risk of cancer and respiratory disease due to air toxics was indicated mainly for large urban areas, West Coast states, Florida, and the Washington, DC–Boston urban corridor. Areas with elevated risk for neurological diseases associated with air toxics were highly localized to a few specific sites, affecting fewer than 350,000 people. Of course, this is cold comfort for the people who live in those places.

Taking Action on Air Pollution Unfortunately, the degree to which you can control your own exposure to regional air pollution and the associated health risks is limited. In larger urban areas where air pollution levels are high, weather reports often include information about air pollution. If you live in a large city, you should pay attention to air pollution information, often conveyed in color-coded alerts. A "yellow" air pollution alert means that people who suffer from respiratory or cardiac diseases, or hypersensitivity to allergens, should stay indoors. An "orange" alert indicates that everyone should limit their outdoor activities to the minimum possible. If you want to avoid exposure to harmful air pollutants altogether, the EPA website includes maps of air pollution levels for counties within the contiguous United States; with this information, you can choose to live where the air and water are least polluted.

You can also help to lower regional air pollution levels by reducing your own contributions to this problem. Here are some suggestions:

- Carpool, use mass transit, or telecommute (work at home via a computer network) to reduce air pollution from automobile exhaust.

- Fill your gas tank, mow your lawn, and use your grill during cooler evening hours to reduce your contribution to tropospheric ozone.

- Conserve electricity to reduce emissions from electric power plants.

In areas of the United States where air pollution is especially problematic, local laws may require that you do some of these things on days when conditions result in a "pollution emergency."

Water Pollution

We humans have had a very "schizophrenic" relationship with our rivers and lakes. Water is an essential resource for all living things on our planet, including humans and the plants and animals we use for food. We also value our rivers and lakes for the recreational benefits they provide. Yet for decades we used these water bodies as convenient dumps for our sewage and industrial wastes.

The problem of water pollution came to national attention on a day in 1968 when children playing with matches set on fire chemical pollutants that covered the Cuyahoga River in Ohio. The subsequent public outcry resulted in major national legislation, including the Clean Water Act of 1972 and the Safe Drinking Water Act of 1974. Since then, substantial progress has been made in reducing water pollution and ensuring safe drinking water supplies. However, the job of cleaning up rivers and lakes in the United States is not complete, and worldwide almost 900 million people do not have access to clean drinking water. Over 3.5 million people per year die from waterborne diseases.

Sources of Water Pollution Water pollutants in surface waters come from obvious point sources (sewer overflows, confined livestock feedlot operations [sometimes called "factory farms"]) and from nonpoint sources such as water runoff from urban streets and agricultural areas that carry various chemicals and animal waste into

---

Key Terms

polycyclic aromatic hydrocarbons (PAHs) Air pollutants from fossil fuel combustion.

tropospheric ozone Ozone comprises three oxygen atoms that are bound into a single molecule; tropospheric ozone refers to this substance as it occurs in the lower layer of the atmosphere, close to the ground.

air toxics A class of 181 toxic air pollutants identified by the U.S. Environmental Protection Agency as known or suspected causes of cancer or other serious health effects.

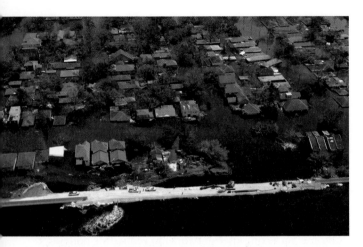

Agricultural runoff and the flow of untreated sewage into rivers during urban flooding are key sources of biological water pollutants.

local rivers. In some areas, water drainage from mines carries toxic metals into nearby streams. Some of the most troublesome water pollutants in the United States today are described here.

Biological water pollutants from untreated sewage and drainage from leaking home septic systems include various species of disease-causing viruses, bacteria, and protozoa found in rivers and lakes. The largest sources of biological water pollutants in U.S. surface waters today are overflows from urban combined septic and storm sewers during heavy rainfall events and animal wastes that are carried by runoff of rainfall from agricultural areas. Although much has already been done to eliminate biological contamination from municipal sewer systems, billions of dollars are still required to dig up old combined sewer systems and replace them with separate systems for sewage and storm water runoff. As large animal factory farms have become more common in rural America, government agencies have established regulations for the proper handling of the huge amounts of animal sewage they generate. Even so, violations of regulations and occasional accidents result in contamination of local surface waters with animal waste.

A wide variety of **toxic pollutants** can be found in surface and groundwater sources of drinking water. These substances include naturally occurring toxic elements (such as arsenic and mercury) produced by breakdown of minerals in certain kinds of rock. Various industrial and agricultural activities produce a wide range of toxic chemicals that find their way into U.S. surface waters, including metals, solvents, plastics, and PCBs (polychlorinated biphenyls). Some toxic substances, including arsenic and mercury, have both natural and human-caused sources. While the dumping of toxic substances into surface waters is now illegal, some of these toxins are very stable and can be found in large

quantities in the sediments of rivers and lakes that were polluted before 1972. Cleaning up these toxic sediments can be very costly. A recent decision to dredge and dispose of PCB-contaminated sediments in the Hudson River near Albany, New York, will cost hundreds of millions of dollars.

Agricultural pesticides can be significant toxic water pollutants in parts of the United States where large areas of land are used for crop production. These chemicals include insecticides, fungicides, and herbicides to kill organisms that consume or compete with crop plants. Rainfall can carry these chemicals from croplands into local streams and rivers.

Health Effects of Water Pollution Organisms present in biological pollution cause diseases that are at best uncomfortable (diarrhea) and at worst potentially lethal (dysentery, hepatitis, typhoid fever, cholera). In the late 1800s, diseases associated with drinking water contaminated by biological pollution were the third-leading cause of death in the United States.[38] When surface water polluted with these organisms is used for crop irrigation of fruit and vegetables, these foods can become contaminated and cause disease or death (as seen in recent foodborne *E. coli* outbreaks).

Health effects of agricultural chemicals and other toxic substances depend on the specific chemical.[38] Taken as a group, these substances have been linked to adverse effects on the blood, liver, spleen, kidney, adrenal gland, thyroid gland, reproductive system (fertility), and cardiovascular system. Some are known or suspected human *carcinogens* (substances that cause cancer), *mutagens* (substances that cause cell mutations), or *teratogens* (substances that cause birth defects). Obvious health effects that occur immediately after exposure to high concentrations of these substances include nausea, fatigue, headache, skin and eye irritation, and tremors. The risks for these immediate adverse health effects are

---

Key Terms

biological water pollutants Disease-causing organisms that are found in water.

toxic pollutants Substances known to cause or suspected of causing cancer or other serious health problems.

fecal coliform bacteria A category of bacteria that live within the intestines of warm-blooded animals; the presence of these bacteria is used as an indicator that water has been contaminated by feces.

ionizing radiation Electromagnetic radiation that is capable of breaking chemical bonds, such as x-rays and gamma rays.

greatest for workers who come in direct contact with the concentrated chemicals. More insidious are health effects such as cancer and birth defects that develop slowly, imperceptibly, after long-term exposure to low concentrations of these chemicals in the environment.

Taking Action on Water Pollution At present, your personal risk of exposure to biological water pollution in the United States is relatively small. Public health departments monitor local surface waters for the presence of **fecal coliform bacteria** in every U.S. county. While they may or may not cause illness or disease, the presence of fecal coliform organisms is an indicator that water has been contaminated by sewage. All municipal drinking water systems, and many private households, in the United States treat their water to kill pathogenic organisms. By the end of the twentieth century, deaths due to water pathogens in the drinking water supply were very rare in the United States.[38] It is also important to wash fresh vegetables before eating them, just in case they have been contaminated by polluted irrigation water.

The best way for you to minimize physical health risks posed by waterborne biological or toxic contaminants is to be well informed. Read the annual water quality report from your municipal water supplier that lists the amounts of biological contaminants, agricultural pesticides, and toxic substances detected in its water. You can access this report at www.epa.gov/safewater/dwinfo. Look at the maximum value for each contaminant to determine if your water system occasionally fails to adequately remove any regulated contaminants. If your water supplier fails to meet health standards, consider installing a reverse osmosis water filter under the kitchen sink to remove most contaminants from drinking water at a cost of pennies per gallon. Many people who are concerned about possible contaminants in municipal water supplies (tap water) instead drink bottled water. However, almost 50 percent of bottled water is actually just packaged tap water. A 2009 Government Accountability Office report to Congress (www.gao.gov/new.items/d09861t) found that tap water was more stringently regulated by the EPA than bottled water was regulated by the FDA. Not only is tap water actually safer than most bottled water, but it is free and does not pollute the environment with billions of disposable plastic bottles.

You can also be exposed to toxic water pollutants by eating contaminated fish. Some toxic substances, such as mercury and PCBs, accumulate to high levels in the bodies of shellfish and fish that live in contaminated water. This problem can occur even in remote, apparently pristine areas if there are natural sources of toxic substances such as mercury. People who regularly consume fish from contaminated waters may be at high risk of adverse health effects (see Chapter 5 for information on seafood safety).

You can also be exposed to waterborne pollutants as a result of recreational activities, such as swimming, boating, and backpacking. You can limit your personal risk of exposure to health risks from contaminated water by being aware of "Don't swim" warnings for your local rivers and lakes, usually issued by the public health department. If you are backpacking in an apparently pristine wilderness area, never assume that crystal-clear water in the mountain stream is safe to drink. Backpackers should always filter, boil, or chemically treat drinking water to kill pathogens that may be present even in such remote water sources.

Ionizing Radiation

Sources and Effects of Radiation *Radiation* is a general term that refers to various forms of energy, including radio waves, infrared waves, heat, visible light, ultraviolet waves, x-rays, and gamma rays. Each of the various kinds of radiation has different effects on human health. The most dangerous form of radiation is **ionizing radiation,** which can damage DNA and body tissues and even cause death. Ionizing radiation is produced by nuclear reactions, and sources include medical x-rays and CAT scans, naturally occurring radioactive substances such as uranium and radon, various radioactive materials used by industry, nuclear power plant accidents, and nuclear bomb explosions.

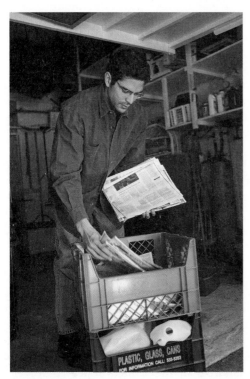

Recycling can reduce land pollution and consumption of natural resources.

The health effects of exposure to ionizing radiation depend on many factors, including the type, duration, and dose of radiation, and your individual sensitivity. The most common sources of exposure to ionizing radiation are medical imaging (x-ray and CAT scan) and radon (discussed in the "Indoor Air Quality" section). These sources rarely result in immediate adverse health effects, but have been shown to increase the risk of developing cancer.

In recent history, the most common cause of ionizing radiation that resulted in significant disease and death has been nuclear bomb explosions and accidents at nuclear power plants. A comprehensive, long-term study of people who survived the nuclear bomb blasts at Hiroshima and Nagasaki, Japan, indicated a 45 percent increase in the incidence of leukemia and an 11 percent increase in solid cancers. Studies of populations in the United States immediately downwind of atmospheric nuclear bomb test sites documented an increased incidence of thyroid cancer. In 1979, there was a partial core meltdown of a nuclear reactor at the Three Mile Island power plant near Harrisburg, Pennsylvania. While radioactive gases were released to the environment, subsequent studies have failed to detect any adverse health effects in the surrounding human population.

In 1986, the largest nuclear accident in history occurred at the Chernobyl nuclear power station near Kiev, Ukraine. During this accident, a full reactor core meltdown and major explosions released massive quantities of highly radioactive material into the environment. Contamination to the local environment was so great that entire cities were abandoned, permanently displacing over 350,000 people, many of these areas remain closed to this day. Winds carried these radioactive materials afar, contaminating large areas of eastern Europe and Scandinavia. Assessments of the health effects of the Chernobyl nuclear accident have produced widely varying estimates and have been highly controversial. A study by the United Nations Committee on the Effects of Atomic Radiation documented 57 immediate deaths due to radiation poisoning among emergency personnel who worked to bring the disaster under control and estimated an additional 4,000–6,000 thyroid cancer cases, mainly among individuals who were children at the time of the event and drank milk contaminated with radioactive iodine. However, studies by other groups have estimated that the disaster caused hundreds of thousands of cancers and an unknown, but presumably large, number of premature deaths, as well as increased incidence of birth defects. Perhaps the most difficult aspect of contamination by radioactive substances is that their effects on individuals are potentially catastrophic, but distinguishing these effects from background levels in populations is difficult. This leaves people worrying about a health risk that may or may not exist.

The 2011 accident at the Fukushima power plant in Japan, damaged by a strong earthquake and tsunami, has been compared to the Chernobyl disaster. While containment structures limited release of radioactive materials from the reactor cores (unlike Chernobyl), loss of cooling water from nuclear waste storage pools resulted in fires and the release of radioactive iodine, cesium, and plutonium to the local environment. Both iodine and cesium are readily absorbed by the body and incorporated into tissues. Radioactive iodine damages the thyroid gland while cesium tends to be deposited in bones; both can cause cancers of these tissues. But whereas radioactive iodine rapidly decays to harmless forms, cesium requires years to decay and plutonium requires thousands of years. Unlike at Chernobyl, large-scale releases of radioactive materials from the Fukushima accident have been mainly limited to the local environment, with little or none reaching other countries. The health consequences of this Japanese nuclear accident will likely not be known for many years, and as with Chernobyl, assessments of these health effects will likely be highly controversial.[39]

Land Pollution

We do not physically consume land or soil the way we do air and water, but pollution of land can still result in serious adverse health effects. Disposal of toxic wastes often involves burying them in the ground. When done with proper safeguards, this disposal method can be safe. If done improperly, toxic pollutants leach into groundwater or are carried by runoff into surface waters, resulting in significant human health risks.

Sources and Components of Solid Waste   Most land pollution today is associated with the disposal of **solid waste.** *Municipal solid waste* consists of everyday items such as product packaging, grass clippings, furniture, clothing, bottles, food scraps, newspapers, appliances, paint, and batteries. Other solid waste produced by business and industry includes waste tires; concrete, asphalt, bricks, lumber, and shingles from demolished buildings; and *sewage sludge* (solids remaining after wastewater treatment). In 2009, the U.S. population produced 243 million tons of solid waste, or about 4.3 pounds of waste per person per day (or 1,570 pounds per person per year).[40] The top four components of this solid waste were paper (33 percent), yard trimmings (13 percent), food scraps (13 percent), and plastic (12 percent).

Disposal of Solid Waste   Municipal sanitation departments and private disposal companies are very efficient at removing these wastes from our homes and businesses and putting them someplace where we don't see them. Much of this waste (54 percent) is deposited in sanitary landfills where it is buried.[40] There are currently 3,091 active landfills in the United States, and over 10,000 municipal landfills that have reached their capacity and been closed.[40]

Many older landfills are major sources of toxic substances that contaminate groundwater and emit methane, which is a very potent greenhouse gas. By law, new landfills must have impermeable plastic liners, waterproof caps, and leachate collection systems to limit groundwater contamination, and must capture and/or burn the methane gas. However, some have questioned the long-term reliability of barriers that protect groundwater. Another disposal method for solid waste is burning it in incinerators; 12 percent of solid waste in the United States is burned, often in a system that uses the heat to generate electricity.[40] However, concerns have been raised about incinerators because they can release toxic substances to the air, and the ash left after burning contains concentrated toxic chemicals in forms that could readily leach into the groundwater. This ash must be handled as hazardous waste, and proper disposal is expensive.

Taking Action on Land Pollution Most of the potential health effects of land pollution have already been discussed in this chapter in the sections on air and water pollution; people are usually exposed to toxic substances from solid waste via air or water. You can limit your exposure to this source of pollution by being aware of the locations of landfills and other waste disposal sites in your community, past and present. You should pay particular attention to this if your home water source is a private well that draws from groundwater that might be contaminated.

You can reduce your personal contribution to the solid waste problem of your community by following the three R's:

- *Reduce* waste by consuming less, accepting less packing on the products you buy, and composting yard waste or using a lawn mower with a mulching blade to eliminate grass clippings and leaves.

- *Reuse* bottles, zipper-closure storage bags, cloth shopping bags, and cloth diapers.

- *Recycle* newspapers, magazines, aluminum and steel cans, glass bottles, and many plastic containers instead of disposing of them in the trash. As of 2009, 34 percent of solid waste in the United States was recycled, double the rate in 1985.[40] Recycling reduces the volume of waste going to landfills and also reduces the demand for natural resources like wood, water, metal ore, and energy. In a market-based economy, such as that in the United States, recycling efforts are sustainable only if consumers are willing to buy products that use recycled materials. When you buy products made with recycled paper, plastic, and wood, you support recycling.

Electronic equipment (computers, cell phones, televisions) pose special waste and recycling challenges as these products contain a number of highly toxic substances (for example, lead, mercury, arsenic, and PCBs, just to name a few). A number of these substances readily leach into groundwater, and many states have banned the disposal of electronic waste in landfills. You should never dispose of these products in your regular household solid waste. The EPA provides information about recycling programs for electronics, including local, manufacturer, and retailer programs (see www.epa.gov/osw/conserve/materials/ecycling/donate).

Loss of Green Space

Loss of **green space** represents another kind of land pollution that can affect your quality of life and health. In many parts of the United States, green space is being converted to housing developments, shopping malls, industrial sites, and highways. Wildlife species disappear from your community and surroundings as their habitats are destroyed.

While development of green space for human uses may provide job opportunities, the "urban sprawl" nature of development can adversely impact your physical, emotional, and spiritual health. Recent studies have shown that urban development that increases commute times to work or school is associated with decreased physical activity and increased prevalence of obesity and high blood pressure.[41] Development of green space and urban sprawl can also adversely affect your emotional health and quality of life when you no longer see wild animals in your backyard or you feel that your community is becoming ugly.

Some communities have created land-use (zoning) plans that regulate development to protect recreational and aesthetic values in their communities. These zoning plans try to balance the rights of private property owners with the welfare of the entire community. You can help protect environmental quality in your community by supporting land-use planning and zoning laws.

 TALKING POINTS How can you approach your political representatives about environmental policy? What are some effective ways of keeping health-related environmental issues on the national agenda?

> ### Key Terms
>
> **solid waste** Pollutants that are in solid form, including nonhazardous household trash, industrial wastes, mining wastes, and sewage sludge from wastewater treatment plants.
>
> **green space** Areas of land that are dominated by domesticated or natural vegetation, including rural farmland, city lawns and parks, and nature preserves.

The Global Environment

The global environment is made up of the atmosphere, oceans, continental land masses, and all the living organisms that exist on Earth. Interactions among these components of the global environment influence the characteristics of solar radiation at the ground level, climate (temperature, precipitation, seasonal variation), production of food plants and animals, availability of freshwater, energy requirements for heating and cooling of human habitations, the geographic distribution of diseases, the composition of natural communities (deserts, tundra, rain forests), and the survival and extinction of species.

Some of the characteristics of the global environment have obvious and direct effects on human physical health, such as the presence of disease-causing organisms or solar UV radiation that can increase the risk of skin cancer. Other effects of the global environment on personal health are less well documented, such as the adverse effects on emotional or spiritual health associated with the extinction of species or destruction of natural communities. Many scientists warn that the global environment is being degraded by the combined forces of ever more powerful technology being used by a rapidly increasing human population. In this section, we briefly describe major concerns regarding the global environment and how these might affect personal health.

Human Population Explosion

Many scientists warn that the human population is increasing at a rate that cannot be sustained by the resources of the Earth (see Figure 16-3). There are currently close to 7 billion people in the global human population, and this is projected to increase to over 10 billion in the next 50 years.

Every year the world's population grows by about 77 million people, with 97 percent born in the poorest countries.[42]

Effects of Population Growth The effects of the human population explosion on personal health depend on who you are and where you live. Many of the poorer nations of Asia, Africa, and South America will not be able to feed their people; starvation and associated diseases will be major health problems for these populations. Growing populations in dry regions are exceeding their freshwater supply, and hundreds of millions of people must drink from contaminated water sources. Every year, 5 million children die from waterborne diarrhea diseases associated with unsanitary drinking water.[42] By 2025, 2.5 billion people may live in regions where available freshwater is insufficient to meet their needs.

In many extremely poor countries, hungry people will destroy most or all of the remaining natural communities (tropical rain forests, African savanna) in vain efforts to grow food on lands that are not suited for agriculture. Overcultivation of farmlands has already degraded the fertility of a land area equivalent to that of the United States and Canada combined.[42] Hungry people on oceanic islands destroy their coral reefs by using dynamite or cyanide to catch fish. In Africa hungry people hunt wild game for food, putting more species at risk of extinction.

Competition among nations for limited supplies of food, water, and oil is often a root cause of political tensions, terrorism, and war. Recent political upheaval in the Middle East has been linked to increased food prices and high unemployment caused by too many young people and too few jobs. The genocide that killed hundreds of thousands in Rwanda in 1994–1995 has been traced to inequitable distribution of land and associated hunger in some parts of that country.[43]

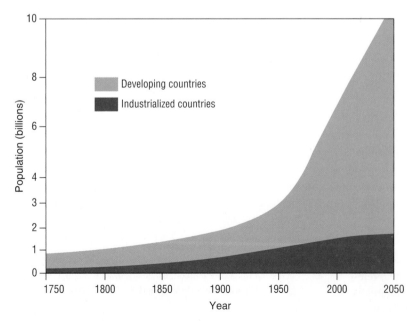

Figure 16-3 World Population Development

Source: World population development. In UNEP/GRID-Arendal Maps and Graphics Library. Retrieved July 17, 2011 from http://maps.grida.no/go/graphic/world_population_development.

Reducing Human Population Growth Solutions to reduce human population growth are simple in theory, but often complex in implementation. Basic ecological theory states that population growth is reduced if (1) women have fewer children and (2) they delay the birth of their first child. Another, somewhat counterintuitive, pattern is that improved health care leading to reduced infant mortality also slows population growth. When women are confident their children will survive, they often choose to have fewer children.[42]

Simply providing education and employment opportunities to females can result in substantial, long-lasting reductions in population growth. Educated women marry and begin families later than their uneducated sisters.[42] Educated women have greater opportunity to be employed outside the home, which is also associated with women choosing to have fewer children. Educated working women have higher social status and greater influence in determining how many children they will have. Of course, universal access to birth control information and affordable contraception is also needed to allow women to have only as many children as they desire. These commonsense policies are sometimes resisted by social and political powers that adhere to traditional values and gender roles. Nonetheless, the result of these policies is that many women freely choose to have fewer children; coercive approaches such as China's "one-child" policy are not necessary to reduce population growth. In fact, during the decade just prior to China's imposing this policy (1970–1979), the birth rate decreased from 34 per 1,000 population to 22 per 1,000, and the population growth rate decreased by more than half, from 2.76 percent per year to 1.33 percent. During the first decade of the one-child policy, there was no trend of decreasing birth rate or reduced population growth rate. However, during the period of economic development in China after 1990, the birth rate had dropped to 12 per 1,000 population, and the population growth rate had dropped to 0.5 percent per year as of 2008 (based on United Nations data from www.gapminder.org). It is unclear if this recent decrease in the birth and population growth rates in China can be attributed to the coercive one-child policy or to the widely observed phenomenon that people tend to freely choose smaller family size when economic conditions and opportunities improve. For more information on issues related to population growth, visit the websites listed in the box "Organizations Related to Environmental and Population Control Concerns" on page 428.

Global Climate Change

Greenhouse Gases Many human activities add **greenhouse gases** to the atmosphere that trap heat and increase the temperatures on Earth. This is called the "greenhouse effect" or "global warming." Human-caused sources of greenhouse gases include carbon dioxide from both industrial and agricultural activities, conversion of natural communities (grasslands, forests, wetlands) to human uses, methane emissions from leaking natural gas pipelines, large herds of cattle, flooded rice fields, tropospheric ozone (described earlier in this chapter), chlorofluorocarbons from air-conditioner fluids, and nitrous oxide from agricultural fertilizer use. The average concentration of carbon dioxide in the atmosphere has increased 36 percent since the 1700s, mostly due to the burning of fossil fuels, and concentrations of the other greenhouse gases have also increased during this period.[44]

There is growing evidence that increases in atmospheric greenhouse gases are associated with changes in global climate. Chemical analyses of gas bubbles in glacial ice core samples from the polar ice caps indicate that atmospheric carbon dioxide and methane concentrations have been closely related to changes in global temperature through several cycles of ice ages and warm periods during the past 420,000 years; when carbon dioxide and methane concentrations increased, so did atmospheric temperature.[44] The current increase in greenhouse gases is also associated with increasing global temperature. According to the websites of the National Oceanic and Atmospheric Administration (NOAA) and the World Meteorological Association, 9 of the 10 warmest years in the instrumental record have occurred during the period 2001–2010. The rate of increase in temperature has been accelerating since the mid-1970s.

Most scientists around the world believe that the changes in global climate described earlier are the first evidence of global climate change related to human activities. However, a vocal minority of scientists still question the relative contributions of humans versus natural processes, and whether this warming trend is a short-term phenomenon or the beginning of a long-term trend (see the box "Hype Versus Useful Information").

Effects of Climate Change Because climate is such a fundamental characteristic of the environment, global warming is expected to have diverse and widespread effects, including melting of the polar ice caps, which will raise sea levels and flood coastal areas (including major coastal cities), and increased frequency and severity of hurricanes and other destructive weather events. Effects of climate change on human health include increased heat stress, loss of life in storms and floods, expansion of the ranges of disease-carrying insects (such as mosquitoes)

Key Terms

greenhouse gases A category of gases in the atmosphere that allow solar radiation to pass through the atmosphere to the Earth but then trap the heat that is radiated from the Earth back toward space; greenhouse gases include water vapor, carbon dioxide, methane, nitrous oxide, and tropospheric ozone.

Hype Versus Useful Information

"The media" is one of the most powerful forces in American society. In the past 20 years, the media has experienced two very divergent trends: consolidation of "mainstream media" (newspapers, magazines, radio, television) by a small number of corporations and fragmentation of media as more people create and view media via the Internet. Mainstream media controlled by for-profit corporations often filters news for its entertainment value. What is deemed sufficiently entertaining is hyped and repeated; uninteresting information is simply ignored. The explosion of Internet-based media has produced legions of bloggers and websites that present opinion and special-interest perspectives with little or no objectivity or error-checking. It is left to the consumer of Internet media to determine the credibility of the various sources of information.

The "entertainment filter" of mainstream media may not interact well with issues of environmental health. Many environmental problems are complex and affect human health in subtle ways over long periods. For example, the U.S. population is being exposed to hundreds, if not thousands, of chemicals that have not been tested for human toxicity. They are found in our air, water, and food supply. They are found in our bodily fluids and hair. Some cause cancer and birth defects in laboratory animals. The EPA estimates that air pollution contributes to thousands of deaths from respiratory and cardiovascular disease each year. In the last 20–30 years, cancer rates in the U.S. population have increased substantially, while fertility of men as measured by sperm counts has been declining by 1–3 percent per year. When was the last time you heard about these issues on the evening news or read about them in a newspaper? By way of comparison, many people know that the polar bear is endangered by global warming and melting of the polar ice cap.

When the mainstream media does cover an environmental health story, it is often presented as a debate to make it more interesting. All too often, these debates give the misperception that an environmental health issue is unresolved, leading to inaction. For example, 97 percent of climate scientists agree that the climate is warming and human activities are part of the cause.* Only a small, but vocal, minority dispute this, and many receive funding from the fossil fuel industry.[†] News programs that present one representative from each side of this issue claim to be "fair and balanced," but actually give a mistaken impression that the state of science regarding global warming is not sufficiently settled to justify action.

On the positive side, it has never been easier to obtain information about environmental health issues on the Internet. However, when you Google an environmental health issue, you will need to exercise judgment about what you believe. Advocacy groups and industrial groups all have their own web presence where they promote their perspectives. See the "Building Media Literacy Skills" box in Chapter 1 for suggestions about how to be a discerning user of information on the Web. These skills will help you identify important issues and questions and give you a better basis on which to make informed decisions for yourself.

*Doran P, Zimmerman M, Survey: scientists agree human-induced warming is real. *Eos, Transactions, American Geophysical Union,* 20(3), 2009.
[†]Union of Concerned Scientists, Smoke, mirrors, and hot air: how Exxon-Mobile uses Big Tobacco's tactics to manufacture uncertainty on climate science, 2007. http://www.ucsusa.org/assets/documents/global_warming/exxon_report.pdf.

from subtropical regions into temperate regions (such as the United States), increased abundance of waterborne pathogens, decreased air and water quality, and decreased food availability associated with severe weather and water shortages. In 2003, a highly unusual heat wave in western Europe killed 35,000 people. While it is unknown if this event was linked to global warming, it proved the potential for severe climate events to have major impacts, even in economically developed countries. In less developed countries, millions of people have died from drought-related famine and severe storms (hurricanes and typhoons).

Taking Action on Climate Change Your ability as an individual to take personal responsibility for addressing the global warming problem is limited, but all good things must start with individuals willing to do the right thing. Ways you can reduce your personal contribution to global warming include the following:

- Go to the Nature Conservancy's "carbon footprint" calculator to get a rough estimate of your personal contribution to greenhouse gas emissions and recommendations for ways to reduce your impact (www.nature.org/greenliving/carboncalculator).

- Conserve electricity at home by purchasing the most efficient appliances and heating/cooling systems and lighting. Compact fluorescent lighting consumes only 10 percent of the electricity compared with incandescent or halogen lighting.

- Insulate and weatherproof your home, and set your thermostat to lower temperatures in winter and higher temperatures in summer to reduce energy use for heating and cooling.

- Drive the most fuel-efficient vehicle that meets your needs, use mass transit if available, or telecommute to work if possible.

- Reduce, reuse, and recycle to reduce demand for and production of consumer products.

- Use alternative energy sources (solar, wind, geothermal) as they become available at prices you can afford.

- Support governmental action to encourage development of alternative energy sources and discourage emission of greenhouse gases. This is most effectively done through organized actions of groups dedicated to these causes and through active participation in the political process.

Stratospheric Ozone Depletion

The *stratospheric ozone layer* is a concentration of ozone molecules located about 10–25 miles above the Earth's surface. This "ozone layer" contains about 90 percent of the planet's ozone. Stratospheric ozone is a naturally occurring gas formed by the interaction of atmospheric oxygen and components of solar radiation. Unlike tropospheric (low-elevation) ozone, which has many adverse health and ecological effects, the stratospheric ozone layer has the beneficial health effect of protecting living organisms on the Earth's surface from harmful solar ultraviolet (UV) radiation.

Causes of Ozone Depletion   Chemical reactions between stratospheric ozone and certain human-made air pollutants can significantly reduce the ozone layer, causing increased UV radiation at the Earth's surface. The chemicals that cause ozone depletion include chlorofluorocarbons (CFCs, used as coolants in many air-conditioning and refrigeration systems, in insulating foams, and as solvents), halons (used in fire suppression systems), and methyl bromide (used in pesticides). When these substances are released to the atmosphere and rise to the stratosphere, they release either chlorine or bromine molecules. One chlorine molecule can destroy 100,000 ozone molecules, and these substances can remain in the atmosphere for years.[45]

The vast majority of depletion of the ozone layer occurs in the atmosphere above the north and south poles;

the colder temperatures and ice crystals in the atmosphere over the poles increase the breakdown of ozone. In 2006 the Antarctic "ozone hole" reached a record size of 10.6 million square miles. Thankfully, the Arctic ozone hole, which is much closer to major human population centers in Europe and North America, was not nearly so large. The decrease in the stratospheric ozone layer has been associated with as much as a 50 percent increase in UV radiation at the ground level in Antarctica.[45] The ozone layer above the United States has decreased by only 5–10 percent.

Effects of Ozone Layer Depletion and Increased UV Radiation   For people, overexposure to UV rays can lead to skin cancer, cataracts (clouding of the lens of the eye), and weakened immune systems. Increased UV can also lead to reduced crop yield and reduced plant production in natural communities. The latter can result in less food for all the other species in the communities and disruption of the ocean's food chain.

Taking Action on Ozone Depletion   In response to the well-documented links between certain air pollutants and depletion of the ozone layer, a complete ban on the production of halons and CFCs went into effect in the mid-1990s. As the amounts of ozone-depleting chemicals in the atmosphere decrease, the ozone layer is projected to recover to natural levels by the year 2050.[45] However, there remain thousands of tons of CFCs in older refrigeration and air-conditioning systems, including those in older automobiles. You can contribute to reducing ozone-depleting chemicals in the atmosphere by always having your refrigerator and air-conditioning systems serviced by licensed technicians who have the equipment to capture and properly dispose of old CFC chemicals.

To reduce your risk of skin cancer and other UV-related health problems that can be exacerbated by ozone layer depletion, you should limit your exposure to direct sunlight, and when you are outside you should wear sunscreen on exposed skin. You should also wear sunglasses that are rated as eliminating over 95 percent of UV radiation.

 TALKING POINTS Your sister is a sun worshipper who loves the look of a deep, dark tan. How might you persuade her to protect her skin from the rays of the sun?

Loss of Natural Habitats and Species Extinctions

Causes of Habitat Destruction and Species Extinctions   On every continent, an exploding human population armed with powerful technology is altering or completely taking over the habitats of other species. Over 20 percent of the total land surface of Earth has been converted entirely for human uses, and as much as 40–50 percent has been degraded by human activities.[46]

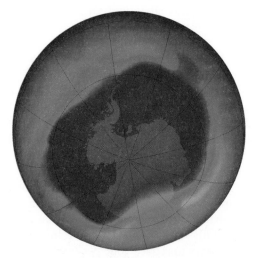

The "ozone hole" over Antarctica in 2006 was the largest to date. The depleted ozone layer in the atmosphere is expected to recover, but the process is slow and will likely take until about 2050.

Organizations Related to Environmental and Population Control Concerns

Population Issues
United Nations Population Fund
www.unfpa.org

International Planned Parenthood
Federation
www.ippf.org

The Population Institute
www.populationinstitute.org

Environmental Political Advocacy Groups
Sierra Club
www.sierraclub.org

Wilderness Society
www.wilderness.org

National Wildlife Federation
www.nwf.org

Natural Resources Defense Council
www.nrdc.org

Environmental Defense
www.environmentaldefense.org

The League of Conservation Voters
www.lcv.org

**Conservation of Natural Communities and
Endangered Species**
The Nature Conservancy
www.nature.org

World Wildlife Fund
www.panda.org

Source of Environmental Information
World Watch Institute
www.worldwatch.org

U.S. Environmental Protection Agency
www.epa.gov

Humans currently use 50 percent of the Earth's freshwater runoff, and dams for electric power generation have impacted 94 percent of rivers in the world.[47]

Human impact on the biosphere is not limited to the land. Humans consume 25–35 percent of the energy flow in coastal ocean waters.[46] As of 2003, 29 percent of all ocean fish populations exploited for human consumption had collapsed due to overharvesting. If current trends continue, all populations of ocean fish currently used for human food production will collapse by the year 2050.[48] Worldwide, 30 percent of all coral reefs have been destroyed by human activities. Coastal water pollution causes fish kills and massive "dead zones" where nothing else can live.[47]

The cumulative effects of all these human-caused changes to the Earth's land and oceans have increased the species extinction rate by 100–1,000 times over rates estimated for the period before human domination. The primary causes of these extinctions are habitat loss due to human activities and overharvesting of species by humans.[47]

Personal Health Effects of Habitat Destruction and Species Extinctions The effects of degradation and loss of the natural systems and species of the Earth are highly variable from person to person. For some, these losses undermine the systems that provide sustenance or employment, or degrade systems that function to make Earth a livable planet, contributing to problems such as climate change, freshwater shortages, loss of farmland, and increased frequency of destructive storms and floods.

Some have proposed that human psychological health depends on some degree of exposure to intact natural systems. In his book *Biophilia,* E. O. Wilson proposed that human evolution on the savannas of Africa predisposes us to be most happy when we are surrounded by natural beauty (the scattered trees and grass of many urban parks are reminiscent of the African savanna). The famous

conservationist John Muir wrote of the psychological benefits of spending time in his beloved Sierra Nevada mountains: "Climb the mountains and get their good tidings. Nature's peace will flow into you as sunshine flows into trees. The winds will blow their own freshness into you, and the storms their energy, while cares drop off like autumn leaves." While many people will never venture into remote wild places the way that Muir did, they still benefit from the knowledge that such places exist and enjoy pictures and stories of unspoiled nature. In the opening passage of the Wilderness Act of 1964, which created a system of intact wilderness areas in the United States, the historian and environmentalist Wallace Stegner wrote, "We simply need that wild country available to us, even if we never do more than drive to its edge and look in. For it can be a means of reassuring ourselves of our sanity as creatures, as part of the geography of hope." For many, widespread destruction of the natural beauty and wonders of the Earth could have profoundly adverse emotional, spiritual, and psychological effects, causing anger, depression, and despair.[49]

Taking Action on Habitat Destruction and Species Extinction How can you exert any degree of personal control over such a great and complex threat to your physical, emotional, and spiritual health? Start with the little things. Conserve energy, limit your consumption of resources to what you need, and join with others to support organizations that are working to solve these big problems (see the box "Organizations Working to Address Environmental and Population Concerns"). If you want to make a bigger personal commitment to solving global environmental problems, you could limit your own family size to at most two children. For a list of many more ways to reduce your personal impact on the Earth, go to the website www.earthshare.org/greentips.

Another way you can reduce the negative environmental effects of your personal consumption of natural resources is to "buy green" when you can. Environmental organizations have begun certification programs so that the consumer can identify which products are produced by "Earth-friendly" means (for more information, see www.newdream.org/buy). Examples of such products include sustainably harvested lumber, shade-grown coffee, and organic food and cotton. These products are often more expensive, because they are produced by methods that lack the efficiency of environmentally destructive production systems. When you "buy green," you support Earth-friendly producers and reduce economic pressure to destroy natural communities.

The combined actions of 7 billion people making personal choices will determine the future of the Earth's environment and thus the future of humankind. The solutions to the great environmental problems looming in the future begin with you, today. Your positive actions and faith in fellow humans to do the right thing will not only benefit the future but also enhance your emotional well-being in the present.

Taking Charge of Your Health

All environmental problems and their associated health risks begin with personal choices regarding resource consumption, waste disposal, and election of leaders who set policies and regulations. When you make your choices, consider the environmental consequences and act in ways that promote a healthy environment for all people and other living things on Earth.

- Be aware of environmental hazards in the air, water, and materials in your personal environment, and work to minimize or eliminate these hazards.
- Reduce your own consumption of natural resources, and dispose of wastes responsibly.
- Be aware of government policies regarding natural resource exploitation, pollution, and habitat destruction.
- Vote for leaders who are more concerned with the quality of the environment of all people and other species than they are for economic special interests.

- When that small voice inside you says, "Forget it, there is nothing I can do," don't listen! That voice is leading you toward a life of cynicism and despair. For your own psychological, emotional, and spiritual well-being, have faith that the actions of individuals can accumulate to bring about world change.*

*Ellison K, A question of faith, *Frontiers in Ecology and the Environment*, 1(1), 56, 2003.

SUMMARY

- Environmental influences on personal health operate over a wide range of spatial scales, from the personal spaces of your home and workplace, to the common spaces of your community and region, to the global environment that supports all life on Earth.
- You can exert the greatest degree of control over your exposure to pollutants within the personal environment of your home and workplace. You can identify environmental health risks in your personal environment and then eliminate or reduce these risks by changing your buying habits and eliminating pollutant sources.
- Air pollution in major urban areas can cause serious adverse health effects, especially for people who suffer from respiratory or cardiac disease.
- Much progress has been made in reducing community water pollution, but water and fish in many rivers and lakes still contain chemicals and pathogens that can adversely affect your health.
- Loss of green space in your community and regional environment, associated with urban sprawl and unregulated land development, can diminish your perceived quality of life and reduce opportunities for exercise, which is important for maintaining good physical health.

- While you have limited personal control over the environment of your community and region, you can still work to enhance your environment by joining others of like mind in groups that advocate for environmental protection through the democratic political process.
- At the current rate of human population growth, most scientists of the world warn of increased starvation and disease, decreased standards of living, and increased conflict over diminished supplies of natural resources.
- Pollutants produced by humans are responsible for changes in the atmosphere that are altering climate patterns and allowing harmful solar radiation to reach the surface of the Earth.
- Changes in the global environment have the potential to increase risks to human health and to significantly harm many other species and natural communities.
- While individuals can do little to address global environmental problems, the solutions all start with individual choices about family size, resource consumption, and political candidates. The best path to a livable future for humankind is to do your part and have faith that others will do theirs.

REVIEW QUESTIONS

1. Identify the sources and the potential health effects of the following common indoor air pollutants: carbon monoxide, volatile organic compounds, and biological pollutants such as mold, mildew, pollen, and pet dander. Describe actions you could take to minimize health risks from these pollutants.
2. What health risks are associated with lead and asbestos? What actions can you take to minimize these risks?
3. Describe actions you should take to safeguard drinking from a well on your own property.
4. Tropospheric ozone and small-particulate matter are community and regional air pollutants that have been linked to serious health risks. For each of these substances, describe the main human source(s), the effect(s) on human physical health, and the actions you could take to minimize your own risk of adverse health effects from these air pollutants.
5. What are "air toxics," and where are you most likely to be exposed to these substances? What can you do to minimize your personal health risk from air toxics?
6. What are some pollutants that might be in drinking water from a tap in your home? What are the main sources of these pollutants? What can you do to minimize the risk to your personal health from water pollutants?
7. What is "green space," and why is it important to your personal health? What personal actions could you take to protect green space in your community or region?
8. What policies should U.S. foreign aid agencies implement in poor, underdeveloped countries to help them reduce their population growth rate? Explain how these policies would work toward this goal.
9. Global warming and stratospheric ozone depletion are large-scale changes in the global environment with uncertain, but potentially significant, health consequences. For each of these global changes, describe the cause(s) of environmental change, the potential health effects, and what might be done to minimize these effects.
10. Loss of natural habitats and species extinctions are major ecological problems, but do these phenomena represent any risk to *your* personal health? Your answer should reflect your own perceptions and should provide some explanation for your assessment.
11. A well-known environmentalist slogan is "Think globally, but act locally." Based on what you've learned in this chapter, describe how you think this slogan applies to your personal actions in response to environmental health risks.

ANSWERS TO THE "WHAT DO YOU KNOW?" QUIZ

1. True   2. False   3. True   4. False   5. False   6. True   7. True

Visit the Online Learning Center (**www.mhhe.com/hahn11e**), where you will find tools to help you improve your grade including practice quizzes, key terms flashcards, audio chapter summaries for your MP3 player, and many other study aids.

SOURCE NOTES

1. U.S. Environmental Protection Agency. *Healthy Buildings, Healthy People: A Vision for the 21st Century,* 2003. http://www.epa.gov/iaq/hbhp/index.html.
2. U.S. Environmental Protection Agency. *The Inside Story: A Guide to Indoor Air Quality,* 1995. http://www.epa.gov/iaq/pubs/insidest.html.
3. U.S. Centers for Disease Control. *Final Report on Formaldehyde Levels in FEMA-Supplied Travel Trailers, Park Models and Mobile Homes,* 2008. http://www.cdc.gov/nceh/ehhe/trailerstudy.
4. Thorn J, et al. Adult-onset asthma linked to mold and tobacco smoke exposure. *Allergy,* 56, 287–292, 2001.
5. U.S. Environmental Protection Agency. *Sources of Indoors Air Pollution: Asbestos,* 2003. http://www.epa.gov/iaq/asbestos.html.
6. U.S. Environmental Protection Agency. *Sources of Indoor Air Pollution: Lead (Pb),* 2003. www.epa.gov/iaq/lead.html.
7. U.S. Department of Health and Human Services, Public Health Service, Agency for Toxic Substances and Disease Registry. *Case Studies in Environmental Medicine: Lead Toxicity,* 1995. www.atsdr.cdc.gov/HEC/CSEM/lead.
8. U.S. Environmental Protection Agency. *Sources of Indoors Air Pollution: Biological Pollutants,* 2003. http://www.epa.gov/iaq/-biologic.html.
9. National Safety Council. *Radon,* 2002. http://www.nsc.org/ehc/radon.htm.
10. National Academy of Science. *The Health Effects of Exposure to Radon (BEIR VI),* 1999. National Academy Press. http://books.nap.edu/books/0309056454.html/.
11. Pflaum N. As Honeywell closes its 60-year-old site, workers are dealing with the fatal aftereffects, 2009. http://www.pitch.com/content/printVersion/1214364/.
12. Schüz J, et al. Cellular telephone use and cancer: update of a nationwide Danish cohort. *Journal of the National Cancer Institute,* 98(23), 1707–13, 2006.
13. Hardell L, et al. Pooled analysis of two case-control studies on use of cellular and cordless telephones and the risk for malignant brain tumors diagnosed in 1997–2003. *International Archives of Occupational and Environmental Health,* 79(8), 630–639, 2006.
14. Ahlbom A, et al. Epidemiology of health effects of radiofrequency exposure. *Environmental Health Perspectives,* 112(17), 2004.
15. UK Childhood Cancer Study Investigators. Childhood cancer and residential proximity to power lines. *British Journal of Cancer,* 83, 1573–80, 2000.
16. Greenland S, et al. A pooled analysis of magnetic fields, wirecodes, and childhood leukemia. *Epidemiology,* 11, 624–634, 2000.
17. U.S. Food and Drug Administration, Center for Devices and Radiological Health, 2008. http://www.fda.gov/cdrh/wireless/research.html.
18. U.S. Environmental Protection Agency. Water on tap: what you need to know, 2003. http://www.epa.gov/safewater/.
19. U.S. Environmental Protection Agency. *Factsheet on: Nitrate/Nitrite,* 2002. http://www.epa.gov/safewater/dwh/t-ioc/nitrates.html.

20. U.S. Environmental Protection Agency. *Permeation and Leaching,* 2002. http://www.epa.gov/ogwdw/disinfection/tcr/pdfs/whitepaper_tcr_permeation-leaching.pdf.

21. U.S. Centers for Disease Control and Prevention. *Third National Report on Human Exposure to Environmental Chemicals,* 2005. http://www.cdc.gov/exposurereport/report.htm.

22. Gray LE, Ostby J. Effects of pesticides and toxic substances on behavioral and morphological reproductive development: endocrine versus no-endocrine mechanisms. *Toxicology and Industrial Health,* 14, 159–184, 1998.

23. U.S. Environmental Protection Agency. *Endocrine Disrupting Chemicals Risk Management Research.* http://www.epa.gov/ord/NRMRL/EDC.

24. Adibi J, et al. Pre-natal exposures to phthalates among women in New York City and Krakow, Poland. *Environmental Health Perspectives,* 111(14), 1719–22, 2003.

25. Landrigan P, Garg A, Droller D. Assessing the effects of endocrine disruptors in the National Children's Study. *Environmental Health Perspectives,* 111(13), 1678–82, 2003.

26. U.S. Centers for Disease Control and Prevention. *National Report on Human Exposure to Environmental Chemicals: Spotlight on Bisphenol A,* 2008. http://www.cdc.gov/exposurereport/pdf/factsheet_bisphenol.pdf.

27. U.S. Food and Drug Administration. *Bisphenol A,* 2009. http://www.fda.gov/oc/opacom/hottopics/bpa.html.

28. Lang IA, et al. Association of urinary bisphenol A concentration with medical disorders and laboratory anomalies in adults. *Journal of the American Medical Association,* 300(11), 1303–10, 2008.

29. Borrell B. The big test for bisphenol A. *Nature* 464(22), 1122–24, 2010.

30. Bell P. Noise, pollution, and psychopathology. In Ghadirian A, Lehmann H (Eds.), *Environment and Psychopathology.* New York: Springer, 1993.

31. Levey S, Levey T, Fligor B. Noise exposure estimates of urban MP3 player users. *Journal of Speech, Language, and Hearing Research,* 54, 263–277, 2011.

32. U.S. Environmental Protection Agency. *Report on the Environment,* 2008. http://www.epa.gov/indicators.

33. Dockery D, Pope C III. Acute respiratory effects of particulate air pollution. *Annual Review of Public Health,* 15, 107–132, 1994.

34. Perera F, et al. Effects of transplacental exposure to environmental pollutants on birth outcomes in a multiethnic population. *Environmental Health Perspectives,* 111(2), 201–205, 2003.

35. Perera F, et al. DNA damage from polycyclic aromatic hydrocarbons measured by benzo[a] pyrene-DNA adducts in mothers and newborns from northern Manhattan, the World Trade Center area, Poland, and China. *Cancer, Epidemiology Biomarkers & Prevention,* 14, 709–714, 2005.

36. National Institute of Environmental Health Sciences. *Asthma,* 2008. http://www.niehs.nih.gov/health/topics/conditions/asthma/index.cfm.

37. U.S. Environmental Protection Agency. *The National Air Toxics Assessment,* 2008. http://www.epa.gov/ttn/atw/nata2002/index.html.

38. U.S. Environmental Protection Agency. *Drinking Water and Your Health, What You Need to Know, List of Drinking Water Contaminants & MCL's,* 2003. http://www.epa.gov/safewater/mcl.html#1.

39. Kaiser J. Radiation risks outlined by bombs, weapons work, and accidents. *Science,* 331, 1504–5, 2011.

40. U.S. Environmental Protection Agency. *Non-Hazardous Waste—Municipal Solid Waste,* 2008. http://www.epa.gov/osw/basic-solid.htm.

41. Ewing R, et al. Relationship between urban sprawl and physical activity, obesity and morbidity. *American Journal of Health Promotion,* 18(1), 47–57, 2003.

42. The Population Institute. http://www.populationinstitute.org/.

43. Gasana, J. Remember Rwanda? *World Watch,* 15(5), 24–33, 2002.

44. Intergovernmental Panel on Climate Change. *IPCC Fourth Assessment Report: Working Group 1 Report, The Physical Science Basis,* 2007. http://www.ipcc.ch/ipccreports/ar4-wg1.htm.

45. U.S. Environmental Protection Agency. *The Science of Ozone Depletion,* 2003. http://www.epa.gov/docs/ozone/science/index.html.

46. Vitousek P, et al. Human domination of Earth's ecosystems. *Science,* 277, 494–499, 1997.

47. World Resources Institute. 2003. http://www.wri.org.

48. Worm B, et al. Impacts of biodiversity loss on ocean ecosystem services. *Science,* 314, 787–790, 2006.

49. Gardner GT, Stern PC. *Environmental Problems and Human Behavior.* Needham Heights, MA: Allyn & Bacon, 1996.

Personal Assessment

Are You an Environmentalist?

When asked, many people will say that they are an "environmentalist," including political leaders who are widely criticized for decisions perceived by others to be environmentally destructive. So what is an "environmentalist"? One definition of environmentalism is that it is an ideology that values and reveres Nature, and works to protect and preserve natural systems both for ethical reasons and because humankind depends on these systems for life. However, beyond this general statement, environmentalists encompass a wide diversity of beliefs and practices. For some, their environmental beliefs are a form of religion, others function mainly in the political process, and some operate like terrorist groups who use violence to fight human economic development on behalf of Earth.* The wide diversity of beliefs and practices encompassed under "environmentalism" creates a situation whereby almost anyone could claim to be an environmentalist. Perhaps more useful criteria for determining if you are an environmentalist would be (1) your awareness of how various human activities create environmental health hazards or degrade natural systems, (2) your willingness to consider your own role in creating environmental problems, and (3) your willingness to act in ways that reduce your personal risk from environmental hazards and your contribution to the causes of these hazards. These three criteria define a hierarchy of commitment to environmental protection. First, you have to know a problem exists. Then you have to recognize your own part in creating that problem. The last, and most difficult, step is that you must be willing to reduce or eliminate your contribution to environmental problems. Your answers to the following questions will help you think about where you really stand on protecting the environment for yourself, your community, and all the rest of life on Earth.

Awareness of Environmental Problems

1. If your drinking water is from a well, do you know about potential sources of contamination (waste disposal sites, agricultural areas) in your watershed?
2. Do you know if your community wastewater treatment system occasionally dumps raw sewage into the local rivers?
3. Have you ever made a note of air pollution alerts in a local newspaper or on local TV news?
4. Are you aware of health advisories regarding contaminants in fish (for example, mercury or PCBs)?

5. When you listen to loud music, do you think about the nuisance noise you create for your neighbors?
6. Do you know if your community (city, county, state) has a land-use management (zoning) plan?
7. When you see new economic developments (malls, housing developments), do you wonder if wildlife habitats were destroyed?
8. Do you know the human causes of global warming and the potential consequences of climate change?
9. Do you know the causes and potential health effects of stratospheric ozone depletion?
10. Do you know the link between the wood you buy at a store like Menard's, Lowe's, or Home Depot and species extinctions?

Willingness to Consider Your Personal Environmental Impact

11. When you think about having a family of your own, do you worry about contributing to a rapidly growing human population?
12. When you think about purchasing a vehicle, do you consider fuel efficiency more important than "image" sold by advertisers?
13. When you consider purchasing any product, do you consider the resources used, and pollution created, to produce that product?
14. When you purchase an electric appliance or a gas-powered device, do you consider energy efficiency?
15. When you use or dispose of household, yard, and automotive chemicals and fluids, do you consider that you may be contributing to local water pollution?
16. When you hear about global warming, do you recognize that your own use of electricity and gas-powered vehicles contributes to this problem?
17. Did you know that if you vent your home or automotive air-conditioning system coolant while performing do-it-yourself maintenance, you are contributing to the depletion of the stratospheric ozone layer?
18. When you purchase lumber, do you wonder if the wood you are buying was harvested using environmentally sound practices?
19. Do you consider how your vote in public elections can affect government policies that impact the environment?

Willingness to Alter Your Lifestyle to Protect Yourself and the Environment

20. Would you limit the number of your own children to one or two so as to reduce your contribution to the problem of global human population explosion?
21. When you purchase a vehicle, is energy efficiency your main concern?
22. Would you use mass transit to travel from home to work, to reduce your contribution to local air pollution?
23. When you buy a home, would you try to minimize the distance from work and schools to reduce gas consumption and minimize air pollution?
24. When you buy a home, would you look for a smaller, energy-efficient home?
25. When you buy lighting, do you buy energy-efficient lightbulbs (compact fluorescent and LED)?
26. When furnishing your home, would you seek out water-efficient toilets, faucets, and showerheads that conserve freshwater and reduce demands on wastewater treatment systems?
27. Do you set the thermostat in your home to cooler temperatures in winter and warmer temperatures in summer to conserve energy?
28. Would you be willing to pay more for organically grown foods that were produced without the use of pesticides and fertilizers that pollute the surrounding environment?
29. Would you buy locally grown foods to support local farmers (and their green spaces) and reduce energy spent on long-distance transport?
30. When purchasing wood products, would you buy more expensive wood that is certified to have been harvested using environmentally sound practices?
31. Would you limit your personal consumption of material goods to mainly those things you need, so as to reduce exploitation of natural resources?

32. When you dispose of household chemicals, automotive fluids, and spent batteries, do you make the extra effort to dispose of them properly?
33. Do you make the effort to recycle paper, glass, plastic, and metals?
34. When you make purchases, do you look for products made from recycled materials?
35. Do you limit the noise that you produce (loud music, loud car or motorcycle engines, barking dogs) to reduce noise pollution in your neighborhood?
36. Do you contribute financial support to environmental groups that promote conservation and protection of natural resources through the legal and political systems?
37. When you consider candidates for public office, do you vote for the candidates who have strong records or position statements for environmental protection?

Interpretation

If the majority of your answers to questions 1–10 are yes, you are likely "environmentally aware." That is, you pay attention to news stories about environmental issues or have taken an environmental science course.

If most of your answers to questions 11–19 are yes, you are "environmentally conscious." That is, you are not only aware of the problems but also beginning to think about how these problems are related to your own lifestyle.

If the majority of your answers to questions 20–37 are yes, you are likely "environmentally active." That is, you are personally involved in efforts to address environmental problems through your own lifestyle choices and through the political process.

*Wikipedia (The Free Encyclopedia). www.wikipedia.org/wiki/environmentalism.

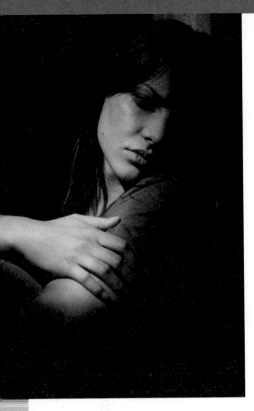

Accepting Dying and Death

What Do You Know About Dying and Death?

1. Signing a donor card or the organ-donor option on your driver's license ensures that your organs will be donated when you die. *True or False?*

2. Death is defined as a state when one's heartbeat can no longer be detected and breathing has ceased. *True or False?*

3. There are only two states in the United States where physician-assisted suicide is legal. *True or False?*

4. It is advisable to bring children to funerals to help them better understand and accept death. *True or False?*

5. Hospice care is provided primarily in the patient's home. *True or False?*

6. The average cost for a funeral service is around $7,500. *True or False?*

7. People are choosing cremation for disposal of their bodies less frequently than in the past. *True or False?*

Check your answers at the end of the chapter.

The Experience of Dying

The primary goal of this chapter is to help people realize that the reality of death can motivate us to live a more enjoyable, healthy, productive, and contributive life. Each day in our lives becomes even more meaningful when we have fully accepted the reality that someday we are going to die. We can then live each day to its fullest.

Our personal awareness of death can provide us with a framework from which to appreciate and conduct our lives. It helps us to prioritize our activities so that we can accomplish our goals (in our academic work, our relationships with others, and our recreation) before we die. Quite simply, death can help us to appreciate living.

Dying in Today's Society

Since shortly after the turn of the twentieth century, the manner in which people experience death in this society has changed significantly. Formerly, most people died in their own homes, surrounded by family and friends. Young children frequently lived in the same home with their aging grandparents and saw them grow older and eventually die. Death was seen as a natural extension of life. Children grew up with a keen sense of what death meant, both to the dying person and to the grieving survivors.

Times have indeed changed. Today approximately 80 percent of people die in hospitals, nursing homes, and assisted living care facilities, not in their own homes. The extended family is seldom at the bedside of the dying person.[1] Frequently, frantic efforts are made to keep a dying person from death. Although medical technology has improved our lives, some people believe that it has reduced our ability to die with dignity. Some are convinced that our way of dying has become more artificial and less natural than it used to be. The trend toward hospice care may be a positive response to this high-tech manner of dying.

As the Baby Boomers age over the next 30 years, the number of people age 85 and older will more than double to 9 million. This means that the topic of death and dying will become increasingly common and relevant for us all as we cope with the loss of our parents, grandparents, friends, and other family members.

Definitions of Death

Before many of the scientific advancements of the past 30 years, *death* was relatively easy to define. People were considered dead when a heartbeat could no longer be detected and when breathing ceased. Now, with the technological advancements in medicine, especially emergency medicine, some patients who give every indication of being dead can be resuscitated. Critically ill people, even those in comas, can now be kept alive for years with many of their bodily functions maintained by medical devices, including feeding tubes and respirators.

Thus, death can be a very difficult concept to define.[2] Numerous professional associations and ad hoc interdisciplinary committees have struggled with this problem and have developed criteria by which to establish death. The Uniform Determination of Death Act of 1981 is adhered to by most states in defining death. It states, "An individual who has sustained either (1) irreversible cessation of circulatory and respiratory functions, or (2) irreversible cessation of all functions of the entire brain, including the brain stem, is dead."[3]

Clinical determinants of death refer to measures of bodily functions. Often judged by a physician, who can then sign a legal document called a *medical death certificate,* these clinical criteria include the following:

- Lack of heartbeat and breathing.
- Lack of central nervous system function, including all reflex activity and environmental responsiveness. Often this can be confirmed by an *electroencephalograph* reading. If there is no brain wave activity after an initial measurement and a second measurement after 24 hours, the person is said to have undergone *brain death.*
- The presence of *rigor mortis,* indicating that body tissues and organs are no longer functioning at the cellular level. This is sometimes referred to as *cellular death.*

The *legal determinants* used by government officials are established by state law. A person is not legally dead until a death certificate has been signed by a physician, *coroner,* or health department officer. However, some argue that death should be defined as occurring when there is an irreparable lack of consciousness or loss of the structures that support thinking, even if the brain stem is still functioning. This would allow faster harvesting of donor organs, such as hearts, for transplant patients.

Psychological Stages of Dying

A process of self-adjustment has been observed in people who have a terminal illness. The stages in this process have helped form the basis for the modern movement of death education. An awareness of these stages may help you understand how people adjust to other important losses in their lives.

Perhaps the most widely recognized name in the area of death education is Dr. Elisabeth Kübler-Ross. As a psychiatrist working closely with terminally ill patients at the University of Chicago's Billings Hospital, Kübler-Ross was able to observe the emotional reactions of dying people. In her classic book *On Death and Dying,* Kübler-Ross summarized the psychological stages that dying people often experience.[4]

- *Denial.* This is the stage of disbelief. Patients refuse to believe that they actually will die. Denial can serve as a temporary defense mechanism and can allow patients the time to accept their prognosis on their own terms.
- *Anger.* A common emotional reaction after denial is anger. Patients can feel as if they have been cheated. By expressing anger, patients are able to vent some of their fears, jealousies, anxieties, and frustrations. Patients often direct their anger at relatives, physicians and nurses, religious figures, and healthy people.
- *Bargaining.* Terminally ill people follow the anger stage with a stage characterized by bargaining. In an effort to avoid their inevitable death, they attempt to strike bargains—often with God or a church leader.

Some people undergo religious conversions. The goal is to buy time by promising to repent for past sins, to restructure and rededicate their lives, or to make a large financial contribution to a religious cause.

- *Depression.* When patients realize that, at best, bargaining can only postpone their fate, they may begin an unpredictable period of depression. In a sense, terminally ill people are grieving for their own anticipated death. They may become quite withdrawn and refuse to visit with close relatives and friends. Prolonged periods of silence or crying are normal components of this stage and should not be discouraged.

- *Acceptance.* During the acceptance stage, patients fully realize that they are going to die. Acceptance ensures a relative sense of peace for most dying people. Anger, resentment, and depression are usually gone. Kübler-Ross describes this stage as one without much feeling. Patients feel neither happy nor sad. Many are calm and introspective and prefer to be left either alone or with a few close relatives or friends.

One or two additional points should be made about the psychological stages of dying. Just as each person's life is totally unique, so is each person's death. Unfolding deaths vary as much as do unfolding lives. Some people move through Kübler-Ross's stages of dying very predictably, but others do not. It is not uncommon for some dying people to avoid one or more of these stages entirely or to revisit a stage more than once.

The second important point to be made about Kübler-Ross's stages of dying is that the family members or friends of dying people often pass through similar stages as they observe their loved ones dying. When informed that a close friend or relative is dying, many people also experience varying degrees of denial, anger, bargaining, depression, and acceptance. Because of this, as caring people, we need to recognize that the emotional needs of the living must be fulfilled in ways that do not differ appreciably from those of the dying.[5]

Near-Death Experiences

As Bob lay on the gymnasium floor in apparent cardiac arrest, he watched from above as the team trainer and coaches performed CPR. After observing his own attempted resuscitation, he began walking in the direction of his uncle's voice. The last time he had heard his uncle's voice was a few days before his death four years earlier. Suddenly, his uncle instructed Bob to stop and turn back because Bob was not yet ready to join him. Over 24 hours later, Bob regained consciousness in the cardiac intensive care unit of The Ohio State University Hospital.

A great deal of research has been conducted on *near-death experiences,* which is when someone almost dies or is pronounced clinically dead but then revives. People reporting these experiences don't register a pulse or breathe for up to 60 minutes and then are resuscitated. It is estimated that 5 percent of American adults, or 8 million people, have had a near-death experience. Inexplicably, these individuals do not suffer any brain damage. The classic work of Raymond Moody, who examined reports of people who had near-death experiences, suggests that we may have less to fear about dying than we have generally thought.[6]

In a comprehensive study of more than 100 people who had near-death experiences, Kenneth Ring reported that these people shared a core experience.[6] This experience was composed of some or all of the following stages:

1. Hearing the pronouncement of death
2. Having an out-of-body experience in which the dying person floats above his or her body and is able to witness the activities that are occurring
3. Moving into a dark tunnel
4. Encountering loved ones who have died
5. Seeing a shaft of intense light that generally leads upward or lies in the distance
6. Experiencing a sense of well-being and peace
7. Reviewing one's life
8. Reaching a boundary or border
9. Returning to the body, sometimes reluctantly
10. Feeling a sense of warmth when returning to the body

The events that occurred when the person "died" have been verified by physicians, nurses, family, and friends, such as what happened after the person died, how the family was told and reacted, and what was done to the body after the person was pronounced dead.

Experts are not in agreement as to whether near-death experiences are truly associated with death or more closely associated with the depersonalization that is experienced by some people during particularly frightening situations. In a scientific sense, near-death experiences are impossible to prove. However, there has also been research suggesting that oxygen deprivation may cause these near-death experiences. Science can neither verify nor deny the existence of out-of-body experiences.[1]

Near-death experiences are life-changing events for most people. Some report that they feel grateful and privileged to have had this experience and want to tell anyone who will listen, while others have more negative reactions, such as depression and disappointment that they returned to their bodies. Often people change jobs and have a different outlook on their lives after going through a near-death experience.

Interacting with Dying People

Facing the impending death of a friend, relative, or loved one is a difficult experience. If you have yet to go through this

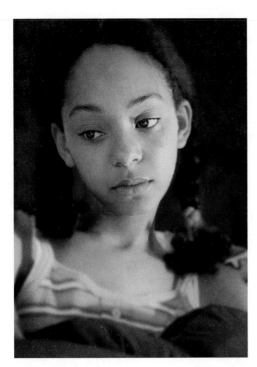

Talking honestly, answering questions, and providing support can help a child cope with loss.

situation, be assured that, as you grow older, your opportunities will increase. This is part of the reality of living.

It is important that counselors, physicians, nurses, and ministers who spend time with terminally ill people display honesty, respect, and compassion when interacting with them. Just the thought of talking with a dying person may make you feel uncomfortable. Sometimes, to make ourselves feel less anxious or depressed, we may tend to deny that the person we are with is dying. Our words and nonverbal behavior indicate that we prefer not to face the truth. Our words become stilted as we gloss over the facts and merely attempt to cheer up both our dying friend and ourselves. This behavior is rarely beneficial or supportive—for either party.

Often people say they don't know how to behave or what to say when with a person who is dying. It is helpful to be as genuine and emotionally supportive as possible. Sometimes people try to avoid talking about death or the severity of the person's illness, but this is not being honest or genuine. It can be comforting for terminally ill patients to be able to talk openly about what is happening to them, to be able to express any thoughts or feelings and talk about funeral arrangements. It can be stressful to pretend that the situation is not as serious as it is, and the dying person may be trying to put on a "brave face" for everyone else and take care of others and make them feel comfortable. Talking about daily events, reading the newspaper or a book, holding hands, giving a back massage, and providing music to listen to are other helpful ways of interacting with dying people.

Talking with Children About Death

Because most children are curious about everything, it is not surprising that they are also fascinated with death. From very young ages, children are exposed to death through mass media (cartoons, pictures in newspapers and magazines, news reports), adult conversations ("Aunt Emily died today," "Uncle George is very ill"), and their discoveries (a dead bird, a crushed bug, the death of a pet). The manner in which children learn about death will have an important effect on their ability to recognize and accept their own mortality and to cope with the deaths of others.

Psychologists encourage parents and older friends to avoid shielding children from or misleading children about the reality of death. Young children need to realize that death is not temporary and is not like sleeping. Parents should make certain they understand children's questions about death before they give an answer. Most children want simple, direct answers to their questions, not long, detailed dissertations, which often confuse the issues. For example, when a 4-year-old asks her father, "Why is Tommy's dog dead?" an appropriate answer might be "Because he got very, very sick and his heart stopped beating." Getting involved in a lengthy discussion about "doggy heaven" or the causes of specific canine diseases may not be necessary or appropriate.

Parents should answer questions when they arise and always respond with openness and honesty. In this way, young children can learn that death is a real part of life and that sad feelings are a normal part of accepting the death of a loved one.[7]

End-of-Life Options and Decisions

Many decisions related to dying and death can be anticipated and discussed with family members. Areas to consider include the type of care you'd like at the end of your life and whether you plan to donate organs.

Palliative Care

Palliative care involves receiving treatment from physicians, nurses, counselors, and other health care providers, at any stage in the patient's illness and for as long as the patient wishes. The illness doesn't have to be a terminal one. Usually, the care is provided in a hospital, nursing home, or long-term care facility. Research shows that palliative care patients live longer and have a higher quality of life than those who do not receive these services.[8]

Hospice Care

The thought of dying in a hospital ward, with institutional furniture, medical equipment, and strict visiting hours, is not the way most people envision spending the last days of their life. Perhaps this thought alone has helped encourage the concept of **hospice care.** Hospice care provides an alternative approach to dying for terminally ill patients and their families. Over a third of patients who died in 2008 were in hospice care at the time, and a little over three months was the average duration of such services. In order to qualify to receive hospice care, the patient must have been given a terminal diagnosis or a life expectancy of 6 to 12 months. The goal of hospice care is to maximize the quality of life for dying people and their family members. Popularized in England during the 1960s, the hospice helps people die comfortably and with dignity by using one or more of the following strategies:

- *Pain control.* Patients are not treated for their terminal disease; they are provided with appropriate drugs to keep them free from pain, alert, and in control of their faculties. Drug dependence is of little concern, and patients can receive pain medication when they feel they need it.

- *Family involvement.* Family members and friends are trained and encouraged to interact with the patient and with each other. Family members often care for the dying person at home. If the hospice arrangement includes a hospice ward in a hospital or a separate building (also called a *hospice*), the family members have no restrictions on visitation.

- *Multidisciplinary approach.* The hospice concept promotes a team approach.[3] Specially trained physicians, nurses, social workers, counselors, and volunteers work with the patient and family to fulfill important needs. The needs of the family receive nearly the same priority as those of the patient.

- *Patient decisions.* Contrary to most hospital approaches, hospice programs encourage patients to make their own decisions. The patient decides when to eat, sleep, go for a walk, and just be alone. By maintaining a personal schedule, the patient is more apt to feel in control of his or her life, even as that life is slipping away.

Another way in which the hospice differs from the hospital approach concerns the care given to the survivors. The family receive bereavement services for up to a year after the patient's death. Helping families with their grief is an important role for the hospice team.[1]

There are 4,850 hospices in the United States.[9] People seem to be convinced that the hospice system does work. Part of this approval may be linked to the cost factor. The cost of caring for a dying person in a hospice is usually less than the cost of full (inpatient) services provided by a hospital. Although insurance companies are delighted to see the lower cost for hospice care, many are still uncertain as to how to define hospice care. Thus, not all insurance companies are fully reimbursing patients for their hospice care. Before discussing the possibility of hospice care for members of your family, you should consider the extent of hospice coverage in your health insurance policy.

Euthanasia

There are two types of euthanasia: **indirect (passive) euthanasia** and **direct (active) euthanasia.**

Indirect Euthanasia Indirect euthanasia, or passive euthanasia, is when people are allowed to die without being subjected to life-sustaining efforts such as being placed on life support. Examples of indirect euthanasia include physicians' orders of "do not resuscitate" (DNR) and "comfort measures only" (CMO).

Indirect euthanasia is increasingly occurring in a number of hospitals, nursing homes, and medical centers. Physicians who withhold heroic lifesaving techniques or drug therapy treatments or who disconnect life support systems from terminally ill patients are practicing indirect euthanasia. Although some people still consider this form of euthanasia a type of murder, indirect euthanasia seems to be gaining legal and public acceptance for people with certain terminal illnesses—near-death cancer patients, brain-dead accident victims, and hopelessly ill newborn babies.

Direct Euthanasia Direct euthanasia, or active euthanasia, is when people are intentionally put to death. It usually involves the administration of large amounts of depressant drugs, which eventually causes all central nervous system functioning to stop. Although direct euthanasia is commonly practiced on house pets and laboratory animals, it is illegal for humans in the United States, Canada, and other developed countries. However, in 1992, the Netherlands became the first developed country to enact legislation that permits euthanasia under strict guidelines. Belgium, Germany, and Switzerland have enacted similar laws.

 TALKING POINTS You're having a class discussion on euthanasia. How would you argue different viewpoints—including euthanasia as murder and euthanasia as an act of mercy?

> ### Key Terms
>
> **hospice care** (**hos** pis) An approach to caring for terminally ill patients that maximizes the quality of life and allows death with dignity.
>
> **indirect (passive) euthanasia** Allowing people to die without the use of life-sustaining procedures.
>
> **direct (active) euthanasia** Intentionally causing death.

Figure 17-1 Sample Living Will Living wills and other advance directives must conform to specific state laws. To obtain a copy of the living will for your state, visit the website for the National Hospice and Palliative Care Organization (www.caringinfo.org).

Source: Copyright © 2007 National Hospice and Palliative Care Organization. All rights reserved. Reproduction and distribution by an organization or organized group without the written permission of the National Hospice and Palliative Care Organization is expressly forbidden.

Physician-Assisted Suicide

In recent years, physician-assisted suicide has been the focus of some important news stories. In July 1997, the U.S. Supreme Court unanimously ruled that dying people have no fundamental constitutional right to physician-assisted suicide. In effect, this ruling left the decision to individual states to permit or prohibit physician-assisted suicide.

By April 1999, more than 30 states had enacted laws prohibiting assisted suicide, and many other states had essentially prohibited it through common law.[10] Three states allow physician-assisted suicide. Oregon passed a law in 1994 that legalized assisted suicide, referred to as the Death with Dignity Act. In November 2008, Washington followed suit by passing the Washington Initiative 1000, allowing physician-assisted suicides. This allows doctors to prescribe fatal doses of barbiturates and other drugs to adults of sound mind who have less than six months to live. It requires the patient to be at least 18 years

of age and of sound mind, make two oral and one written request for the medication with 15 days between the first request and the final one, consult with two physicians, and notify pharmacists and state health authorities before proceeding with physician-assisted suicide. A fatal drug is prescribed, and the patient may ingest it orally at his or her discretion, with or without the doctor present. It remains illegal for physicians to administer lethal injections. There were 59 deaths recorded from physician-assisted suicides in Oregon in 2009.[11] In 2009, Montana became the third state to allow physician-assisted suicide.[10]

Even though physician-assisted suicide is legal in Oregon, Washington, and Montana, many physicians are unwilling to prescribe the lethal medication. Being confined to their bed or home, living a long way from a large urban area, experiencing difficulty finding a willing physician, dying before completing the requirements of the law, and encountering opposition from family and friends are some of the reasons greater numbers of terminally ill patients are not obtaining medication to end their lives.

Interestingly, most physicians will not inform patients if they are terminally ill. A recent study showed that only one-third of doctors reported that they routinely tell their patients that they are dying. This lack of information can make it difficult for the dying person, family, and friends to make decisions and prepare for this event.

 TALKING POINTS Would you want to know that you were dying if your doctor knew you were terminally ill? How would this information change the way you spent the rest of your life and the decisions you would make?

Advance Health Care Directives

Because some physicians and families find it difficult to support indirect euthanasia, many people are starting to use legal documents called *advance health care directives.*[12] One of these health care directives is the **living will.** A living will is a legal document in which the patient has outlined specific directives as to whether he or she will allow the use of life support, feeding tubes, and other medical devices or treatment by health care providers and caregivers. A living will is invoked only when the patient is incapacitated to the extent that he or she is unable to give consent or refusal for treatment. A living will can be very specific or very general. An example of a statement sometimes found in a living will is "If I suffer an incurable, irreversible illness, disease, or condition and my attending physician determines that my condition is terminal, I direct that life-sustaining measures that would serve only to prolong my dying be withheld or discontinued."[13] (see Figure 17-1). Living will statutes exist in all 50 states and the District of Columbia.[13] The living will requires that physicians or family members carry out a person's wishes to die naturally, without receiving life-sustaining treatments. An estimated 41 percent of U.S. adults have signed living wills.[12]

President Obama was the first U.S. president to publicly announce that he has a living will, and he has encouraged others to have one as well. One problem that has surfaced with living wills is the lack of knowledge by physicians, family, and friends about the existence of a patient's living will, and so it is not followed. Other complications with living wills are that they sometimes don't address medical issues and questions that arise or are in conflict with standard medical practices. This is the reason that a second type of advance health care directive came into being—the **durable power of attorney for health care,** also called the medical power of attorney or health care proxy appointment. This legal document authorizes another person to make specific health care decisions about treatment and care when the patient is incapacitated and cannot communicate her or his medical wishes. This document helps inform hospitals and physicians about which person will help make the critical medical decisions. It is recommended that people complete both a living will and a durable power of attorney for health care document.

A third type of advance directive is called the *Five Wishes directive,* but it is not valid in eight states. It was introduced in 1997 by the Robert Wood Johnson Foundation and is distributed by the Aging with Dignity organization. It is designed to take the place of a living will or durable power of attorney. The patient describes his or her wishes (see the box "The Five Wishes"), which some criticize as not as compelling as directives. The American Medical Association has stated that it doesn't meet their standards for addressing pain management. Another criticism of this directive is that it allows the appointed health care representative to decline this role and doesn't allow a spouse who is separated to make these decisions even if he or she is listed as one of the people authorized to do so, which has some legal implications.

Organ Donation

For some, the decision to donate body tissue and organs is rewarding and comforting. Organ donors understand that their small sacrifice can help give life or improve the quality of life for another person. In this sense, their death can mean life for others (see the box "Organ Donation" on page 442).

Organ/Tissue Donor Card

I wish to donate my organs and tissues. I wish to give:

☐ any needed organs and tissues ☐ only the following organs and tissues: _____

Donor
Signature _____ Date _____
Witness _____
Witness _____

You can request a free national donor card like the one shown here at www.organdonor.gov. You can also contact the United Network for Organ Sharing (UNOS) at 1-888-894-6361 or www.unos.org.

Key Terms

living will A legal document that requires physicians or family members to carry out a person's wishes to die naturally, without receiving sustaining treatments.

durable power of attorney for health care A legal document that designates who will make health care decisions for people unable to do so.

Many states permit people to state on their driver's license that they wish to donate their organs. There is a new, more convenient way to register for organ donation through a nonprofit organization called Donate Life America at www.donatelife.net. Most states have agreed to have this online registration option. However, family consent (by next of kin) is also required at the time of death for organ or tissue donation to proceed. Recently, hospitals have been required by federal law to inform the family of a deceased person about organ donation at the time of death. Thus, those who wish to donate organs at the time of death should discuss these wishes with their family as soon as possible so that family members will support the donation after the individual has died. The need for donor organs is much greater than our current supply. There is also an increase in the types of transplants that can be performed. For example, the first face transplant in the United States was performed in 2008, the fourth such transplant performed worldwide since 2005. Some believe that instead of signing up to be an organ donor, the default should be that everyone is automatically an organ donor unless they explicitly opted out. This would increase the number of organ donors significantly. New York, Pennsylvania, and Delaware are considering passing this measure. Interestingly, a study in New York showed that while 67 percent of people supported organ donation, only 13 percent had signed up to do so.[14]

Grief and Coping

The emotional feelings that people experience after the death of a friend or relative are collectively called *grief.* *Mourning* is the process of experiencing these emotional feelings in a culturally defined manner. (See the box "The Grieving Process" for more information.)

Grief and the Resolution of Grief

The expression of grief is seen as a valuable process that gradually permits people to accept the loss of the deceased. Expressing grief, then, is a sign of good health.

Although people experience grief in remarkably different ways, most people have some of the following sensations and emotions:

- *Physical discomfort.* Shortly after the death of a loved one, grieving people display a rather similar pattern of physical discomfort. This discomfort is characterized by "sensations of somatic distress occurring in waves lasting from 20 minutes to an hour at a time, a feeling of tightness in the throat, choking with shortness of breath, need for sighing, and an empty feeling in the abdomen, lack of muscular power, and an intense subjective distress described as a tension or mental pain. The person soon learns that these waves of discomfort can be precipitated by visits, by mentioning the deceased, and by receiving sympathy."[5]

- *Sense of numbness.* Grieving people may feel as if they are numb or in a state of shock. They may deny the death of their loved one.

- *Feelings of detachment from others.* Grieving people see other people as being distant from them, perhaps because the others cannot feel the loss. A person in grief can feel very lonely. This is a common response.

Building Media Literacy Skills

Organ Donation: Fact or Fiction?

From people not really being dead when their organs are harvested, to medical personnel not doing all that they can to save people's lives in order to obtain more organ donors, there are many myths surrounding organ donation. Perhaps this is one of the biggest reasons the need for donated organs surpasses the number of available organs. Here are some common myths and facts about organ donation.

Myth To be an organ donor, I just have to sign an organ donor card or indicate my preference on my driver's license.

Reality By signing a donor card, you indicate your wish to be a donor. However, at the time of death, your next-of-kin will still be asked to sign a consent form for donation. If you wish to be an organ donor, it is important to tell your family about this decision so that your wishes will be honored at the time of death. It is estimated that about 35 percent of potential donors never become donors because family members refuse to give consent.

Myth Donating organs will cost my family money.

Reality Your family pays for your medical care and funeral costs, but not for organ donation. Costs related to donation are paid by the recipient, usually through insurance, Medicare, or Medicaid.

Myth Being an organ donor can help only one other person.

Reality Each organ and tissue donor saves or improves the lives of as many as 50 people.

Myth I won't be able to have an open-casket funeral.

Reality Donation does not interfere with having an open-casket service. Surgical techniques are used to retrieve organs and tissues, and all incisions are closed.

Myth I have to be 18 years old or older to donate.

Reality All individuals can indicate their intent to donate, although persons younger than 18 years of age must have a parent's or guardian's consent. Newborns as well as senior citizens have been organ donors.

Myth I have to have had no previous medical conditions in order to be an organ donor.

Reality False. Transplant professionals will evaluate the condition of your organs at the time of your death and determine if your organs are suitable for donation. You should consider yourself a potential organ and tissue donor; indicate your intent to donate on your driver's license, donor card, or state donor registry; and discuss your decision with family members.

Myth If I sign a donor card, it will affect the quality of medical care I receive at the hospital.

Reality No! The medical team trying to save your life is separate from the transplant team. Every effort is made to save your life before donation is considered.

Myth It would be against my religion's beliefs.

Reality Virtually all religious denominations approve of organ and tissue donation as representing the highest humanitarian ideals and the ultimate charitable act.

Myth The need for organs is the same across all ethnicities.

Reality Minorities overall have a particularly high need for organ transplants because some diseases of the kidneys, heart, lungs, pancreas, and liver are found more frequently in racial and ethnic minority populations than in the general population. For example, African Americans, Asians and Pacific Islanders, and Hispanics are three times more likely than Whites to suffer from end-stage renal (kidney) disease, often as the result of high blood pressure and other conditions that can damage the kidneys. In addition, similar blood type is essential in matching donors to recipients. Because certain blood types are more common in ethnic minority populations, increasing the number of minority donors can increase the frequency of minority transplants.

It is hoped that knowing the facts will ease people's minds about the process and enable them to make well-informed choices about organ donation and perhaps save another person's life.

Sources: Adapted from U.S. Department of Health and Human Services, Health Resources and Services Administration, Find answers: organ donation and transplantation, http://answers.hrsa.gov/, November 3, 2009; Congressional Kidney Caucus, 25 facts about organ donation and transplantation, http://www.house.gov/mcdermott/kidneycaucus/25facts.html, February 2002.

- *Preoccupation with the image of the deceased.* The grieving person may not be able to complete daily tasks without constantly thinking about the deceased.

- *Guilt.* The survivor may be overwhelmed with guilt. Thoughts may center on how the deceased was neglected or ignored. Sensitive survivors feel guilt merely because they are still alive. Indeed, guilt is a common emotion.

- *Hostility.* Survivors may express feelings of loss and remorse through hostility, which they direct at other family members, physicians, lawyers, and others.

- *Disruption in daily schedule.* Grieving people often find it difficult to complete daily routines. They can suffer from an anxious type of depression. Seemingly easy tasks take a great deal of effort. Initiation of new activities and relationships can be difficult. Social interaction skills can temporarily be lost.

- *Delayed grief.* In some people, the typical pattern of grief can be delayed for weeks, months, and even years.

The grief process continues until the bereaved person can establish new relationships, feel comfortable with others, and look back on the life of the deceased person with positive feelings (see the box "Helping the Bereaved" on page 445). Although the duration of the grief resolution process will vary with the emotional attachments one has to a deceased person, the grieving process usually lasts for 18 months. Professional help should be sought when grieving is characterized by unresolved guilt, extreme hostility,

The Grieving Process

The grieving process consists of four phases, each of which is variable in length and unique in form to the individual. These phases are composed of the following:

1. *Internalization of the deceased person's image.* By forming an idealized mental picture of the dead person, the grieving person is freed from dealing too quickly with the reality of the death.
2. *Intellectualization of the death.* Mental processing of the death and the events leading up to its occurrence move the

grieving person to a clear understanding that death has occurred.

3. *Emotional reconciliation.* During this third and often delayed phase, the grieving person allows conflicting feelings and thoughts to be expressed and eventually reconciled with the reality of the death.
4. *Behavioral reconciliation.* Finally, the grieving person is able to comfortably return to a life in which the death has been fully reconciled. Old routines are reestablished and new patterns of living

are adopted where necessary. The grieving person has largely recovered.

A mistake that might be made by the friends of a grieving person is encouraging a return to normal behavior too quickly. When friends urge the grieving person to return to work right away, make new friends, or become involved in time-consuming projects, they may be preventing necessary grieving from occurring. It is not easy or desirable to forget about the fact that a spouse, friend, or child has recently died.

physical illness, significant depression, and a lack of other meaningful relationships. Trained counselors, physicians, and hospice workers can all play significant roles in helping people through the stages of grief.

Coping with Death from Specific Causes

Coping with Death from a Terminal Illness Watching a family member or friend slowly die can bring mixed emotions, from being glad to have that person with you as long as possible to wishing that the person would not have to suffer. It can be painful to see the person you know gradually slip away. In addition, he or she may become someone who seems more like a stranger to you and may not even recognize you or acknowledge your presence. Some people say that they are thankful for the time they have with this person and for the opportunity to say good-bye. However, others may feel a false sense of hopefulness that the person is beating the illness only to feel shocked and devastated when the illness begins to progress at a faster rate. The research does suggest that we cope better with loss when we are expecting it, when we have time to prepare and take whatever action we feel necessary in response to it. In this way, a protracted illness can facilitate the ability to cope that people who experience loss through accidental death, natural disaster, suicide, or murder do not have.

Coping with Death from Accident, Natural Disaster, Terrorism, or War Deaths that occur from natural disasters or accidental deaths bring some unique challenges. Accidental death is the number-one cause of death for 15- to 34-year-olds, and so college students may encounter this more often than terminal illnesses. Though any type of trauma or crisis is more difficult to deal with when it is unexpected, accidental death seems particularly devastating in that you are unprepared for and shocked by the news. Often people have more trouble

accepting this type of death because it is so unexpected that it seems unreal.

Deaths from natural disasters are typically uncommon and unlikely and so are even more difficult to comprehend and accept. We tend to cope better with events we can understand and explain. Yet this may be impossible to do with accidental deaths such as from a car accident or from incidents without a clear cause of death. Part of finding an explanation can also involve blaming someone: "I should have known he was too tired to drive." People can feel more vulnerable and fearful after accidents and disasters and become more hesitant in their day-to-day living. Things that you may not have questioned begin to seem potentially dangerous, such as going swimming after a friend has drowned or driving after a car accident.

Death associated with terrorism was something that Americans generally did not have to face, as other countries have, until 9/11. Since that time, Americans have felt less safe on their own soil and abroad. People have changed their lifestyles in terms of taking trips, having a survival kit at home, stockpiling food and water, and encountering stringent security. Organizations, hospitals, and government agencies are developing responses to bioterrorism and other types of terrorist attacks.

Those who say good-bye to a soldier going off to combat may dread that the soldier will die in the war. Even though we know this is a possibility, such a death is very difficult to accept, especially when the soldier is young, as so many are. Those who have lost a loved one to war may have mixed emotions—pride at the person's courage, heroics, and sacrifice, and anger at the enemy or the government. When a soldier is missing in action, loved ones lack closure and may remain hopeful that he or she will be found alive and well. When people die in a war thousands of miles away, their deaths can seem unreal because of the distance and the different worlds people and their loved ones have been living in.

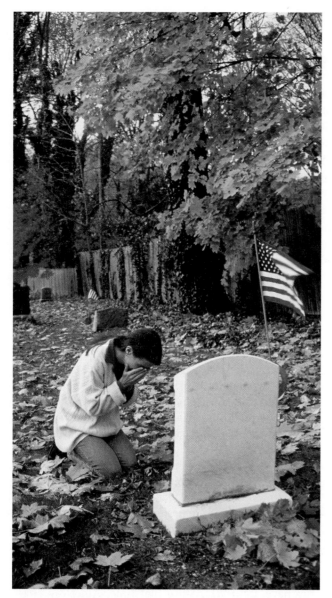

The cause and manner of death can affect the experience of grief. The death of a young soldier in war can be difficult to accept and can lead to a mix of emotions—pride, anger, and profound loss.

Coping with Death by Suicide People react similarly to suicides as they do to accidental death, because both means of death are sudden and unexpected. Making sense of these types of death is difficult, and coping with a completed suicide brings the added burden of trying to understand the reasons and motivations behind the death. If you hold religious beliefs that tell you committing suicide is a sin, this can lead to additional misunderstanding and anger. As with death by murder, this type of death is a crime, and so there are legal as well as religious and moral implications in accepting a person's decision to take his or her own life.

Family members frequently say they feel ashamed and embarrassed by the suicide because of these connotations. They worry that others will see them and their family as crazy. These concerns usually mean that coping with death by suicide can be a longer process than coping with other types of death. It is helpful for people to understand the events that led up to and contributed to a person's choosing to take his or her life.

Chapter 2 discussed the warning signs and factors that contribute to suicide. Often people blame themselves for not seeing the warning signs or not acting on those they did see. There can also be a sense of feeling unimportant or unloved by this person because you tell yourself, "If she really cared about me, she would have fought to stay with me and not left me." Survivors of suicide often feel abandoned and rejected. If your relationship with this person was distant, if you hadn't talked to him or her for a while, or if you had recently had an argument, you may feel guilty and blame yourself, saying, "If only I had been nicer or called her more often, this might not have happened."

Coping with Death by Murder Shock, anger, guilt, confusion, and vulnerability are some of the emotions people commonly experience when they cope with a murder. You don't expect murder to happen—certainly not to someone you know. It can be difficult to comprehend the taking of someone's life, which makes it even more difficult to accept such a loss. You may blame yourself for not protecting the victim in some way or not doing something to prevent it from happening. If the suspect hasn't been identified or apprehended, you may feel angry at the police for not doing more or feel scared that you live in a world that seems suddenly very unsafe and frightening. If the murderer has been apprehended, it can take years before the trial is over, making it hard to have a sense of closure.

Coping with the Death of a Child

Adults face not only the death of their parents and friends but perhaps also the death of a child. Whether because of sudden infant death syndrome (SIDS), chronic illness, accident, or suicide, children die and adults are forced to grieve the loss of someone who was "too young to die."

Coping with the death of a child is particularly difficult because it seems so unnatural and wrong for a child to precede his or her parents in death. The death of a child can be the most devastating loss parents can experience, and many say that they feel a part of them died with their child. Experts agree that grieving adults, particularly the parents, should express their grief fully and proceed cautiously on their return to normal routines. Many pitfalls can be avoided. Adults who are grieving for dead children should do the following:

- *Avoid trying to cope by using alcohol or drugs.*
- *Make no important life changes.* Moving to a different home, relocating, or changing jobs usually doesn't help parents deal any better with the grief they are experiencing.

I know someone whose brother just died. I want to help without getting in the way at this difficult time. What's the best approach?

Leming and Dickinson point out that the peak time of grief begins in the week after a loved one's funeral. Realizing that there is no one guaranteed formula for helping the bereaved, you can help by doing some or all of the following:

- Make few demands on the bereaved; allow him or her to grieve.
- Help with the household tasks.
- Recognize that the bereaved person may vent anguish and anger and that some of it may be directed at you.
- Recognize that the bereaved person has painful and difficult tasks to complete; mourning cannot be rushed or avoided.

- Do not be afraid to talk about the deceased person; this lets the bereaved know that you care for the deceased.
- Express your own genuine feelings of sadness, but avoid pity. Speak from the heart.
- Reassure bereaved people that the intensity of their emotions is very natural.
- Advise the bereaved to get additional help if you suspect continuing severe emotional or physical distress.
- Keep in regular contact with the bereaved; let him or her know you continue to care.

Source: Based on information in Leming MR, Dickinson GE, *Understanding Dying, Death, and Bereavement* (5th ed.). Fort Worth: Harcourt College Publishers. Copyright © Thomson Learning, Inc., 2002.

- *Share feelings with others.* Grieving adults should share their feelings particularly with other adults who have experienced a similar loss. Group support is available in many communities.
- *Avoid trying to erase the death.* Giving away clothing and possessions that belonged to the child cannot erase the memories the adult has of the child.
- *Take the time and space to grieve.* On the anniversary of the child's death or on the child's birthday, grievers should give themselves special time just for grieving.
- *Don't attempt to replace the child.* Do not quickly have another child or use the deceased child's name for another child.

For most adults, grieving over the death of a child will require an extended period. Eventually, however, life can return to normal.

Coping with the Death of a Parent, Spouse, or Sibling

In some ways, coping with the death of a parent, spouse, or sibling is similar to coping with the death of a child. In each case, survivors must live with the significant loss of a family member. Each death produces some degree of emotional trauma for each survivor, followed by a period of grief. Gradually, the force of the grieving process lessens as the survivors put the death into a perspective that they can live with. Despite the similarities, there are some differences involving the death of a parent, spouse, or sibling.

Death of a Parent The death of a parent can be especially difficult because parents have formed a foundation in most people's lives. In a sense, parents have always

"been there." There is a sense of a loss of security that a parent provided for his or her children. A "safety net" for the children disappears. Perhaps for the first time, adult children genuinely see themselves as getting older. When a parent dies, the children realize they have become the new matriarchs and patriarchs, the leaders of their families.

When a parent dies, adult children are reminded of their own mortality.[3] It is not unusual for this realization to push adult children into serious reflection about their own lives. They may, for the first time, evaluate their lives to determine whether the dreams they had as young adults have materialized. This evaluation can be a positive experience for midlife adults, if it encourages them to refocus on the real priorities in their lives.

Death of a Spouse There is great variability in the way a person adapts to the death of a spouse depending on the length of the marriage (or relationship), the age of the person at death, the children from that marriage, financial resources, the vitality of the relationship, the manner in which the spouse died, and the health status of the widow or widower.

Some couples become so interconnected that the death of one leaves the survivor feeling utterly alone and not whole. A spouse's death might also create a single-parent family, thereby making day-to-day activities quite challenging for the survivor. Some couples may need to assume roles and responsibilities that are unfamiliar and difficult for them, such as handling finances and doing home repairs.

The death of a spouse can also result in the loss of a primary source of one's social interactions.[3] It is important for the remaining spouse to maintain a network of family and friends for social support and interaction (see the box "Aftercare"). This social support will be crucial in determining how well the survivor adjusts to his or her new situation. Fortunately, there are support groups for recently widowed persons. These can be found in local communities through churches or social support agencies. Support groups also exist on the Internet for those who wish to seek an online form of support.

Death of a Sibling The death of a brother or a sister can be very difficult for the surviving sibling(s). It is common for children to feel great guilt for outliving their sibling. They may wonder why the death happened to the sibling rather than them. They may start to question their own mortality and feel more vulnerable to death themselves. Survivors may feel overwhelmed with guilt and believe that they, in some strange way, caused the death. For example, the surviving child who frequently had wished "that his brother was dead" (a common sibling rivalry wish) may believe that his wish caused the car accident that killed his brother.

The manner in which parents communicate and respond to the situation can help the surviving child come to terms with the sibling death. Parents need to keep the lines of communication open, listen to the child's concerns, avoid becoming overly protective of the child, and avoid attempting to re-create in the living child certain qualities of the deceased child.[3] Children must be allowed to express their feelings. Talking with mental health experts in the field of grief and bereavement can be especially helpful to children. Individual counseling sessions and group sessions are available in most communities.

Rituals of Death

Our society has established a number of rituals associated with death that help the survivors accept the reality of death, ease the pain associated with the grief process, and provide a safe disposal of the body. Our rituals give us the chance to formalize our good-byes to a person and to receive emotional support and strength from family members and friends (see the box "Cultural Differences in Death Rituals"). In recent years, more of our rituals seem to be celebrating the life of the deceased. In doing this, our rituals also reaffirm the value of our own lives.

Most of our funeral rituals take place in funeral homes, churches, and cemeteries. *Funeral homes* (or *mortuaries*) are business establishments that provide a variety of services to the families and friends of the deceased. The services are carried out by funeral directors, who are licensed by the state in which they operate. Most funeral directors are responsible for preparing the bodies for viewing, filing death certificates, preparing obituary notices, establishing calling hours, assisting in the preparation and details of the funeral, selecting casket, transporting mourners to and from the cemetery, and counseling the family. Although licensing procedures vary from state to state, most new funeral directors must complete one year of college, one year of mortuary school, and one year of internship with a funeral home before taking a state licensing examination.

Full Funeral Services

An ethical funeral director will attempt to follow the wishes of the deceased's family and provide only the services requested by the family. Most families want traditional **full funeral services.** Three significant components of the full funeral services are as follows.

> **Key Terms**
>
> **full funeral services** All the professional services provided by funeral directors.

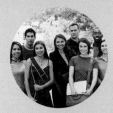

Learning from Our Diversity

Cultural Differences in Death Rituals

Death rituals vary considerably among ethnic and religious groups. Even within the broad categories of ethnic, racial, or religious distinction, differences exist in how groups of people dispose of their deceased. For example, funeral rituals may differ between Orthodox Jews and Conservative Jews. Furthermore, groups of people living in the United States may not be able to follow the traditional funeral rituals of their home countries because they lack the necessary resources and community support. However, some general cultural differences in funeral rituals can be seen in the following examples.

Funeral rituals by the Amish are carried out in the deceased person's home. The church community takes care of the arrangements for visitors, relieving the grieving family of these tasks. In some Amish communities, a wakelike "sitting up" takes place in which family members are supported by friends throughout the night. The funeral itself is simple, with burial in an unadorned wooden coffin, often made by the local Amish carpenter. Children are encouraged to see death as a transition to a better life. Although the Amish clearly feel the pain of their loss, they often may not express this grief openly.

Muslim death rituals are based on their belief that death is the result of God's will. Death is foreordained. For Muslims (and for members of many other religious groups), life in this world is seen as a preparation for eternal life. At death, the deceased's bed is turned to face the Holy City of Mecca, and verses of hope and acceptance are read from the Qur'an. The dead body is washed three times by a Muslim of the same sex as the deceased and then is wrapped in white material and buried as soon as possible, usually in a brick- or cement-lined grave facing Mecca. Prayers are offered for the dead at the cemetery, at the mosque, or at the home. Unless the deceased is a husband or close relative, women usually do not attend the burial. Cremation is not practiced among Muslims.

In Judaism, death is seen as part of the life cycle. Traditional Jews believe in an afterlife in which a person's soul continues to flourish. In this afterlife, people are judged by their actions in life. People who have lived righteous lives are likely to be rewarded in the next world. Judaism does not have a form of last rites; any Jew may ask for God's forgiveness.

At traditional Jewish funerals, the body is rarely embalmed, unless there are unusual circumstances causing burial to be delayed. Burial routinely takes place within a short time after death. Cosmetic restoration is used minimally, if at all. The body is wrapped in a shroud and placed in an unadorned wooden casket. Traditionally, flowers are not displayed at the funeral or at the cemetery. The funeral service is directed at honoring the deceased while praising God and encouraging people to reaffirm their faith. Traditionally, a seven-day period of immediate mourning (*shiva*) takes place after the burial. After this period there are established mourning periods. For example, mourning for a relative typically lasts 30 days; for a parent, one year.

Source: Labar S, Youngblunt J, Brooton D, Cross-cultural beliefs, ceremonies, and rituals surrounding death of a loved one. *Pediatric Nursing*, 32(1), 44–50, 2006.

Embalming Embalming is the process of using formaldehyde-based fluids to replace the blood components. Embalming helps preserve the body and return it to a natural look. Embalming permits friends and family members to view the body without being subjected to the odors associated with tissue decomposition. Embalming is often an optional procedure, except when death results from specific communicable diseases or when body *disposition* (disposal) is delayed.

Calling Hours Sometimes called a *wake,* this is an established time when friends and family members can gather in a room to share their emotions and common experiences about the deceased. Generally in the same room, the body will be in a casket, with the lid open or closed. Open caskets help some people to confirm that death truly did occur. Some families prefer not to have any calling hours, sometimes called *visiting hours.*

Funeral Service Funeral services vary according to religious preference and the emotional needs of the survivors. Although some services are held in a church, most funeral services today take place in a funeral home, where a special room might serve as a chapel. Some services are held at the graveside.

Memorial Service

Families may also choose to have a *memorial service* weeks or months after the funeral. Completing the Personal Assessment at the end of this chapter will help you think about what kind of funeral arrangements you would prefer for yourself.

Disposition of the Body

Ground Burial Bodies are disposed of in one of four ways. *Ground burial* is the most common method. About 63 percent of all bodies are placed in ground burial. The casket is almost always placed in a metal or concrete vault before being buried. The vault serves to further protect the body (a need only of the survivors) and to prevent collapse of ground because of the decaying of caskets. Use of a vault is required by most cemeteries.

Entombment A second type of disposition is *entombment.* Entombment refers to nonground burial, most often in structures called **mausoleums.** A mausoleum has a series of shelves where caskets can be sealed in vaultlike areas called *niches.* Entombment can also occur

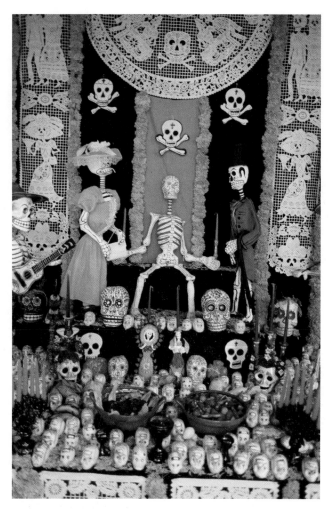

There are cultural differences in the rituals associated with death. Day of the Dead, which originated in Mexico, is a celebration of the dead and the continuation of life, characterized by both sadness and joy. Graves may be decorated with orange marigolds, the deceased's favorite foods, sugared skulls, and figurines of skeletons.

in the basements of buildings, especially in old, large churches. The bodies of famous church leaders are sometimes entombed in vaultlike spaces called **crypts.**

Cremation *Cremation* is a third type of body disposition. In the United States, 37 percent of all bodies are cremated.[15] This practice is increasing. Generally, both the body and casket (or cardboard cremation box) are incinerated so that only the bone ash from the body remains. The body of an average adult produces about 5–7 pounds of bone ash. These ashes can then be placed in containers called *urns,* and then buried, entombed, or scattered, if permitted by state law. Urns can be shaped into almost anything, such as a motorcycle gas tank, a fiddle, a heart, or a car. One company makes teddy bears with a pouch that holds the ashes. Ashes can also be compressed into diamonds for jewelry or put into a pendant, ring, or earring.

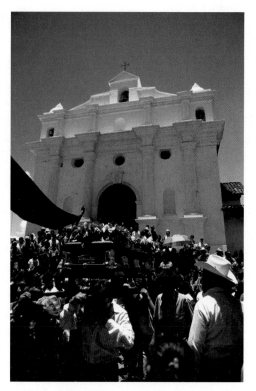

Guatemalan funerals, such as this one, have their own cultural rituals.

Ashes have also been put into key chains or crushed into balls and placed in the ocean. The average cost of cremation ($600–1,000) is much less than that of ground burial. Some families choose to cremate after having full funeral services.[16]

Anatomical Donation A fourth method of body disposition is *anatomical donation.* Separate organs (such as corneal tissue, kidneys, or the heart) can be donated to a medical school, research facility, or organ donor network.

Some people choose to donate their entire body to medical science. Often this is done through prior arrangements with medical schools. Bodies still require embalming. After they are studied, the remains are often cremated and returned to the family, if requested.

Costs

The full funeral services, also referred to as death care services, offered by a funeral home cost upward of $7,500,

---

Key Terms

mausoleum (moz oh **lee** um) An above-ground structure, which frequently resembles a small stone house, into which caskets can be placed for disposition.

crypts Burial locations generally underneath churches.

with other expenses added to this price. Casket prices vary significantly, with the average cost between $1,500 and $2,500. Costs can vary tremendously depending on the type of casket, funeral services, and other arrangements. Some people are opting to have plastic surgery as part of the funeral preparations, which would certainly increase the death care service costs. When all the expenses associated with a typical funeral are added up, the average cost is $7,500.[17]

Regardless of the rituals you select for the handling of your body (or the body of someone in your care), people are encouraged to prearrange their plans. Before you die, you can ease your survivors' burden by putting your wishes in writing. *Funeral prearrangements* relieve the survivors of many of the details that must be handled at the time of your death. You can gather much of the information for your obituary notice and your wishes for the disposition of your body. Prearrangements can be made with a funeral director, family member, or attorney. Many individuals also prepay the costs of their funeral. By making arrangements in advance of need, you can have peace of mind. Currently, about 30–40 percent of funerals are preplanned or prepaid or both.[17] However, there may be some risk involved with prepaying funeral arrangements, such as if the funeral home goes out of business, sells the business to another owner who doesn't honor these arrangements, or items are not available or included at the time of the funeral service.

Personal Preparation for Death

This chapter is designed to help you to develop a new framework about death and form your own personal perspective on death and dying. Remember that the ultimate goal of death education is a positive one—to help you best live and enjoy your life. Becoming aware of the reality of your own mortality is a step in the right direction. Reading about the process of dying, grief resolution, and the rituals surrounding death can also help you accept that someday you too will die.

There are some additional ways in which you can prepare for the reality of your own death. Preparing a will, purchasing a life insurance policy, making funeral prearrangements, preparing a living will, and considering an anatomical or organ donation are measures that help you prepare for your own death. At the appropriate time, you might also wish to talk with family and friends about your own death. You may discover that an upbeat, positive discussion about death can help relieve some of your apprehensions and those of others around you.

Another suggestion to help you emotionally prepare for your death is to prepare your *obituary notice* or **eulogy.** Include all the things you would like to have said about you and your life. Now compare your obituary notice and eulogy with the current direction your life seems to be taking. Are you doing the kinds of activities for which you want to be known? If so, great! If not, perhaps you will want to consider why your current direction does not reflect how you would like to be remembered. Should you make some changes to restructure your life's agenda in a more personally meaningful fashion?

Another suggestion to help make you aware of your own eventual death is to write your own **epitaph.** Before doing this, you might want to visit a cemetery. Reading the epitaphs of others may help you develop yours.

Further awareness of your own death might come from attempting to answer these questions: (1) If I had only one day to live, how would I spend it? (2) What one accomplishment would I like to achieve before I die? (3) Once I am dead, what two or three things will people miss most about me? By answering these questions and accomplishing a few of the tasks suggested in this section, you will have a good start on accepting your own death and understanding the value of life itself.

Taking Charge of Your Health

- Start considering how you might plan for your funeral by completing the Personal Assessment at the end of this chapter.
- Consider completing a living will and designating a health care agent or proxy. Discuss your wishes with your family and friends.

- Consider completing an organ donor card, purchase life insurance, and/or prepare a will.
- If you don't already know, ask your family about their end-of-life wishes.
- Write your own eulogy, epitaph, or obituary.

- If you have experienced a loss, think about where you would place yourself in the psychological stages of grief. If appropriate, explore with a trusted friend, family member, spiritual leader, or counselor how you can move closer to a sense of acceptance of this loss.

SUMMARY

- Death is determined primarily by clinical and legal factors.
- Euthanasia can be undertaken with either direct or indirect measures.
- The most current advance health care directives are the living will and the durable power of attorney for health care. Both documents permit critically ill people (especially those who cannot communicate) to die with dignity.
- Denial, anger, bargaining, depression, and acceptance are the five classic psychological stages that dying people commonly experience, according to Kübler-Ross.
- Hospice care provides an alternative approach to dying for terminally ill people and their families.
- The expression of grief is a common experience that can be expected when a friend or relative dies. The grief process can vary in intensity and duration.

- Death in our society is associated with a number of rituals to help survivors cope with the loss of a loved one and to ensure proper disposal of the body.
- In the past, most people died at home, whereas now the majority of people die in hospitals, nursing homes, and assisted-living facilities.
- The shortage of organ donations is the biggest problem facing people who need a transplant to save their lives.
- Hospice care is an alternative end-of-life health care option for terminally ill patients and their families.
- We dispose of bodies in four ways: ground burial, entombment, cremation, and anatomical donation.

REVIEW QUESTIONS

1. How does the experience of dying today differ from that in the early 1900s?
2. Identify and explain the clinical and legal determinants of death, and indicate who establishes each of them.
3. Explain the difference between direct and indirect euthanasia.
4. How does a living will differ from a durable power of attorney as a health care document? Why are these advance health care directives becoming increasingly popular?
5. Identify the five psychological stages that dying people tend to experience. Explain each stage.
6. Identify and explain the four strategies that form the basis of hospice care. What are the advantages of hospice care for the patient and the family?
7. Explain what is meant by the term *grief*. Identify and explain the sensations and emotions most people have when they experience grief. When does the grieving process end?
8. What purposes do the rituals of death serve? What are the significant components of the full funeral service?
9. What are the four ways in which bodies are disposed?
10. What activities can we undertake to become better aware of our own mortality?

ANSWERS TO THE "WHAT DO YOU KNOW?" QUIZ

1. False   2. False   3. False   4. True   5. True   6. True   7. False

Visit the Online Learning Center (**www.mhhe.com/hahn11e**), where you will find tools to help you improve your grade including practice quizzes, key terms flashcards, audio chapter summaries for your MP3 player, and many other study aids.

SOURCE NOTES

1. Leming MR, Dickinson GE. *Understanding Dying, Death, and Bereavement* (7th ed.). New York: Harcourt, 2011.
2. Kastenbaum RJ. *Death, Society, and Human Experience* (10th ed.). Boston: Allyn & Bacon, 2008.
3. DeSpelder L, Strickland A. *The Last Dance: Encountering Death and Dying* (8th ed.). New York: McGraw-Hill, 2008.
4. Kübler-Ross E. *On Death and Dying* (reprint ed.). New York: Collier Books, 1997.
5. Kübler-Ross E. *To Live Until We Say Goodbye* (reprint ed.). Upper Saddle River, NJ: Prentice-Hall, 1997.
6. Atwater P. *The Big Book of Near Death Experiences: The Ultimate Guide to What Happens When We Die.* Charlottesville, VA: Hampton Roads, 2007.
7. Staudacher C. *Beyond Grief.* Oakland, CA: New Harbinger Publications, 2000.
8. Palliative care focuses on life. *USA Today,* February 23, 2011.
9. National Hospice and Palliative Care Organization. NHPCO *Facts and Figures.* www.nhpco.org, 2009.
10. Montana 3rd state to allow doctor-assisted suicide. *USA Today,* January 2, 2010.
11. Oregon Department of Human Services. Annual Report 2010, Oregon's Death with Dignity Act.
12. Choice in Dying (now: Partnership in Caring). *Choice in Dying: An historical perspective.* CID 1035 30th Street, NW, Washington, DC, 2007.
13. Jones C. With living wills gaining in popularity, push grows for more extensive directive. *Crain's Cleveland Business,* August 20, 2007.
14. Organ donation: an opt-out policy? *USA Today,* June 30, 2010.
15. Cremation Association of North America. *2008 statistics and projections to the year 2025: 2009 Preliminary Data,* August 2010.
16. Cremation Association of North America. *2008 statistics and projections to the year 2025: 2009 Preliminary Data,* August 2010.
17. Plan funeral now to make sure you have the final word. *USA Today,* July 28, 2006.

Personal Assessment

Planning Your Funeral

In line with this chapter's positive theme of the value of personal death awareness, here is a funeral service assessment that we frequently give to our health classes. This inventory can help you assess your thoughts about the funeral arrangements you would prefer for yourself.

After answering each of the following questions, you might wish to discuss your responses with a friend or close relative.

1. Have you ever considered how you would like your body to be handled after your death?
   _____ Yes   _____ No

2. Have you already made funeral arrangements for yourself?
   _____ Yes   _____ No

3. Have you considered a specific funeral home or mortuary to handle your arrangements?
   _____ Yes   _____ No

4. If you were to die today, which of the following would you prefer?
   _____ Embalming   _____ Ground burial
   _____ Cremation   _____ Entombment
   _____ Donation to medical science

5. If you prefer to be cremated, what do you want done with your ashes?
   _____ Buried   _____ Entombed
   _____ Scattered
   _____ Other; please specify _____

6. If your funeral plans involve a casket, which of the following ones do you prefer?
   _____ Plywood (cloth covered)
   _____ Hardwood (oak, cherry, mahogany, maple, etc.)
   _____ Steel (sealer or nonsealer type)
   _____ Stainless steel
   _____ Copper or bronze
   _____ Other; please specify _____

7. How important is a funeral service for you?
   _____ Very important
   _____ Somewhat important
   _____ Somewhat unimportant
   _____ Very unimportant
   _____ No opinion

8. What kind of funeral service do you want for yourself?
   _____ No service at all
   _____ Visitation (calling hours) the day before the funeral service; funeral held at church or funeral home
   _____ Graveside service only (no visitation)
   _____ Memorial service (after body disposition)
   _____ Other; please specify _____

9. How many people do you want to attend your funeral service or memorial service?
   _____ I do not want a funeral or memorial service
   _____ 1–10 people
   _____ 11–25 people
   _____ 26–50 people
   _____ Over 50 people
   _____ I do not care how many people attend

10. What format would you prefer at your funeral service or memorial service? Select any of the following that you like:

	Yes	No
Religious music	_____	_____
Nonreligious music	_____	_____
Clergy present	_____	_____
Flower arrangements	_____	_____
Family member eulogy	_____	_____
Eulogy by friend(s)	_____	_____
Open casket	_____	_____
Religious format	_____	_____
Other; please specify _____		

11. Using today's prices, how much do you expect to pay for your total funeral arrangements, including cemetery expenses (if applicable)?
   _____ Less than $4,500
   _____ Between $4,501 and $6,000
   _____ Between $6,001 and $7,500
   _____ Between $7,501 and $9,000
   _____ Between $9,001 and $13,000
   _____ Above $13,000

TO CARRY THIS FURTHER . . .

Which items had you not thought about before? Were you surprised at the arrangements you selected? Will you share your responses with anyone else? If so, whom?

A

abortion Induced premature termination of a pregnancy.

absorption The passage of nutrients or alcohol through the walls of the stomach or the intestinal tract into the bloodstream.

abuse Any use of a drug in a way that is detrimental to health.

acquired immunity (AI) A form of immunity resulting from exposure to foreign protein (most often wild, weakened, or killed pathogenic organisms).

acupuncture Insertion of fine needles into the body to alter electroenergy fields and cure disease.

acute alcohol intoxication A potentially fatal elevation of the BAC, often resulting from heavy, rapid consumption of alcohol.

acute rhinitis The common cold; the sudden onset of nasal inflammation.

adaptive thermogenesis The physiological response of the body to adjust its metabolic rate to the presence of food.

additive effect The combined (but not exaggerated) effect produced by the concurrent use of two or more drugs.

adipose tissue Tissue made up of fibrous strands around which specialized cells designed to store liquefied fat are arranged.

aerobic energy production The body's means of energy production when the respiratory and circulatory systems are able to process and transport a sufficient amount of oxygen to muscle cells.

agent The causal pathogen of a particular disease.

air pollution Substances in the atmosphere that can have adverse effects on human health, crop productivity, and natural communities.

air toxics A class of 181 toxic air pollutants identified by the U.S. Environmental Protection Agency as known or suspected causes of cancer or other serious health effects.

alarm stage The first stage of the stress response, involving physiological, involuntary changes that are controlled by the hormonal and nervous systems; the fight or flight response is activated in this stage.

alcohol abuse Patterns of alcohol use that create problems for the drinker's school and job performance, other responsibilities, and interpersonal relationships. Also called *problem drinking*.

alcohol dependence Tolerance, withdrawal, and a pattern of compulsive use of alcohol. A primary, chronic disease with genetic, psychosocial, and environmental factors influencing its development. Also called *alcoholism*.

allopathy (ah **lop** ah thee) A system of medical practice in which specific remedies (often pharmaceutical agents) are used to produce effects different from those produced by a disease or injury.

alveoli (al **vee** oh lie) Thin, saclike terminal ends of the airways; the sites at which gases are exchanged between the blood and lungs.

Alzheimer's disease Gradual development of memory loss, confusion, and loss of reasoning; eventually leads to total intellectual incapacitation, brain degeneration, and death.

amenorrhea The absence of menstruation.

amino acids The building blocks of protein; can be manufactured by the body or obtained from dietary sources.

amotivational syndrome Behavioral pattern characterized by lack of interest in productive activities.

anabolic steroids Drugs that function like testosterone to produce increases in muscle mass, strength, endurance, and aggressiveness.

anaerobic energy production The body's means of energy production when the necessary amount of oxygen is not available.

anal intercourse A sexual act in which the erect penis is inserted into the rectum of a partner.

angina pectoris (an **jie** nuh **peck** tor is) Chest pain that results from impaired blood supply to the heart muscle.

anorexia nervosa An eating disorder in which the individual weighs less than 85 percent of the expected weight for his or her age, gender, and height; has an intense fear of gaining weight; and, in females, ceases to menstruate for at least three consecutive months. People with anorexia perceive themselves as overweight, even though they are underweight.

anovulatory (an **oh** vyu luh tory) Not ovulating.

antagonistic effect Effect produced when one drug reduces or offsets the effects of a second drug.

antibodies Chemical compounds produced by the body's immune system to destroy antigens and their toxins.

antioxidants Substances that may prevent cancer by interacting with and stabilizing unstable molecules known as free radicals.

artificially acquired immunity (AAI) A type of acquired immunity resulting from the body's response to pathogens introduced into the body through immunizations.

asbestos A class of minerals that have a fibrous crystal structure; a known carcinogen when inhaled.

asphyxiation Death resulting from lack of oxygen to the brain.

atherosclerosis Buildup of plaque on the inner walls of arteries.

attention deficit hyperactivity disorder (ADHD) Above-normal rate of physical movement; often accompanied by an inability to concentrate on a specified task; also called *hyperactivity*.

autoimmune An immune response against the tissues of a person's own body.

axon The portion of a neuron that conducts electrical impulses to the dendrites of adjacent neurons; neurons typically have one axon.

ayurveda (ai yur **vey** da) Traditional Indian medicine based on herbal remedies.

B

ballistic stretching A "bouncing" form of stretching in which a muscle group is lengthened repetitively to produce multiple quick, forceful stretches.

basal metabolic rate (BMR) The amount of energy, expressed in calories, that the body requires to maintain basic functions.

basic needs Deficiency needs that are viewed as essential and fundamental, including physiological, safety and security, belonging and love, and esteem needs.

benign Noncancerous; localized nonmalignant tumors contained within a fibrous membrane.

beta blockers Drugs that reduce the workload of the heart, which decreases occurrence of angina pectoris and helps control blood pressure.

beta endorphins Mood-enhancing, pain-reducing, opiatelike chemicals produced within the smoker's body in response to the presence of nicotine.

bias and hate crimes Criminal acts directed at a person or group solely because of a specific characteristic, such as race, religion, sexual orientation, ethnic background, or disability.

bigorexia An obsession with getting bigger and more muscular, and thinking that your body is never muscular enough.

binge drinking Five or more drinks on the same occasion (at the same time or within a span of a couple of hours) on at least one day in the last two-week period.

binge eating disorder An eating disorder formerly referred to as compulsive overeating disorder; binge eaters use food to cope in the same way that bulimics do and also feel out of control, but do not engage in compensatory purging behavior.

biological air pollutants Living organisms or substances produced by living organisms that cause disease or allergic reactions, including bacteria, molds, mildew, viruses, dust mites, plant pollen, and animal dander, urine, or feces.

biological sexuality Male and female aspects of sexuality.

biological water pollutants Disease-causing organisms that are found in water.

biopsychological model A model that addresses how biological, psychological, and social factors interact and affect psychological health.

bipolar disorder A mood disorder characterized by alternating episodes of depression and mania.

birth control All the methods and procedures that can prevent the birth of a child.

blackout A temporary state of amnesia experienced by a drinker; an inability to remember events that occurred during a period of alcohol use, including things that person said or did during that time.

blastocyst Early stage of the developing life form that embeds itself in the endometrial lining of the uterus.

blood alcohol concentration (BAC) The percentage of alcohol in a measured quantity of blood; BACs can be determined directly through the analysis of a blood sample or indirectly through the analysis of exhaled air.

Bod Pod Body composition system used to measure body fat through air displacement.

body dysmorphic disorder (BDD) A secret preoccupation with an imagined or slight flaw in one's appearance.

body image One's subjective perception of how one's body appears to oneself and others.

body mass index (BMI) A mathematical calculation based on weight and height; used to determine desirable body weight.

bolus theory A theory of nicotine addiction based on the body's response to the bolus (ball) of nicotine delivered to the brain with each inhalation of cigarette smoke.

brand name Specific patented name assigned to a drug by its manufacturer.

bulimia nervosa An eating disorder in which individuals engage in episodes of bingeing—consuming unusually large amounts of food, feeling out of control, and engaging in some compensatory purging behavior to eliminate the food.

c

calcium channel blockers Drugs that prevent arterial spasms; used in the control of blood pressure and the long-term management of angina pectoris.

calendar method A form of periodic abstinence in which the variable lengths of a woman's menstrual cycle are used to calculate her fertile period.

calipers A device used to measure the thickness of a skinfold from which percentage of body fat can be estimated.

caloric balance Caloric intake and caloric expenditure are equal, and body weight remains constant.

calories Units of heat (energy); specifically, 1 calorie is the amount of heat required to raise the temperature of 1 gram of water by 1°C. In common usage, on food labels, and in this book, the term *calorie* is used to refer to a larger energy unit, *kilocalorie* (1,000 calories).

carbohydrates The body's primary source of energy for all body functioning; chemical compounds including sugar, starches, and dietary fibers.

carbon monoxide A gaseous by-product of the incomplete combustion of natural gas, kerosene, heating oil, wood, coal, gasoline, and tobacco; a chemical compound that can "inactivate" red blood cells.

carcinogens Environmental agents, including chemical compounds within cigarette smoke, that stimulate the development of cancerous changes within cells.

cardiac arrest Immediate death resulting from a sudden change in the rhythm of the heart causing loss of heart function.

cardiac muscle Specialized muscle tissue that forms the middle (muscular) layer of the heart wall.

cardiorespiratory endurance The ability of the heart, lungs, and blood vessels to process and transport oxygen required by muscle cells so that they can contract over a period of time.

cardiovascular Pertaining to the heart (*cardio*) and blood vessels (*vascular*).

catabolism The metabolic process of breaking down tissue for the purpose of converting it into energy.

cell-mediated immunity Immunity provided principally by the immune system's T cells, both working alone and in combination with highly specialized B cells; also called *T cell–mediated immunity*.

cerebrovascular occlusions Blockages to arteries supplying blood to the cerebral cortex of the brain; strokes.

cesarean delivery Surgical removal of a fetus through the abdominal wall.

chemical name Name used to describe the molecular structure of a drug.

chemoprevention Cancer prevention using food, food supplements, and medications thought to bolster the immune system and reduce the damage caused by carcinogens.

child maltreatment The act or failure to act by a parent or caregiver that results in abuse or neglect of a child which places the child in imminent risk of serious harm.

chiropractic Manipulation of the vertebral column to relieve misalignments and cure illness.

chlamydia The most prevalent sexually transmitted disease; caused by a nongono-coccal bacterium.

cholesterol A primary form of fat found in the blood; lipid material manufactured within the body and derived from dietary sources.

chronic bronchitis Persistent inflammation and infection of the smaller airways within the lungs.

chronic fatigue syndrome (CFS) An illness that causes severe exhaustion, fatigue, aches, and depression; mostly affects women in their 40s and 50s.

chronic stress Remaining at a high level of physiological arousal for an extended period of time; can also occur when an individual is not able to immediately react to a real or a perceived threat.

cilia (**sill** ee uh) Small, hairlike structures that extend from cells that line the air passages.

circadian rhythms The internal, biological clock that helps coordinate physiological processes with the 24-hour light/dark cycle.

clinical depression A psychological disorder in which individuals experience a lack of motivation, decreased energy level, fatigue, social withdrawal, sleep disturbance, disturbance in appetite, diminished sex drive, feelings of worthlessness, and despair.

cohabitation Sharing of a residence by two unrelated, unmarried people; living together.

coitus (**co** ih tus) Penile-vaginal intercourse.

cold turkey Immediate, total discontinuation of use of a drug; associated with withdrawal discomfort.

colonoscopy (co lun **os** ko py) Examination of the entire length of the colon, using a flexible fiber-optic scope to inspect the structure's inner lining.

compliance Willingness to follow the directions provided by another person.

computed axial tomography (CT) scan An x-ray procedure designed to illustrate structures within the body that would not normally be seen through conventional x-ray procedures.

condom A shield designed to cover the erect penis and retain semen on ejaculation; "rubber." Various types of condoms are available, including latex, polyurethane, lambskin, and female condoms.

congestive heart failure Inability of the heart to pump out all the blood that returns to it; can lead to dangerous fluid accumulations in veins, lungs, and kidneys.

consumer fraud Marketing of unreliable and ineffective services, products, or information under the guise of curing disease or improving health; quackery.

contraception Any method or procedure that prevents fertilization.

contraceptive patch Contraceptive skin patch containing estrogen and progestin; replaced each week for a three-week period.

contraceptive ring A thin, polymer contraceptive device containing estrogen and progestin; placed deep within the vagina for a three-week period.

contraindications Factors that make the use of a drug inappropriate or dangerous for a particular person.

coronary arteries Vessels that supply oxygenated blood to heart muscle tissues.

coronary artery bypass surgery Surgical procedure designed to improve blood flow to the heart by providing new routes for blood to take around points of blockage.

corpus luteum (**kore** pus **loo** tee um) Cellular remnant of the graafian follicle after the release of an ovum.

cremasteric muscles Tiny muscles next to the vasa deferentiae that contract to elevate the testes or relax to lower the testes.

cross-tolerance Transfer of tolerance from one drug to another within the same general category.

cruciferous vegetables Vegetables, such as broccoli, whose plants have flowers with four leaves in the pattern of a cross.

crypts Burial locations generally underneath churches.

cunnilingus (cun uh **ling** gus) Oral stimulation of the vulva or clitoris.

curette A metal scraping instrument that resembles a spoon with a cup-shaped cutting surface on its end.

current use At least one drink in the past 30 days.

cyberstalking The unsolicited contacting, pursuing, or harassing of others, usually through the Internet or e-mail.

D

dehydration Abnormal depletion of fluids from the body; severe dehydration can be fatal.

dendrite (**den** drite) The portion of a neuron that receives electrical stimuli from adjacent neurons; neurons typically have several such branches or extensions.

dependence A physical or psychological need to continue the use of a drug.

desirable weight The weight range deemed appropriate for people, taking into consideration gender, age, and frame size.

diaphragm A soft rubber cup designed to cover the cervix.

diastolic pressure Blood pressure against blood vessel walls when the heart relaxes.

Dietary Reference Intakes (DRIs) Measures that refer to three types of reference values: Estimated Average Requirement, Recommended Dietary Allowance, and Tolerable Upper Intake Level.

dilation Gradual expansion of an opening or passageway, such as the cervix.

dilation and evacuation (D&E) A second-trimester abortion procedure that requires greater dilation, suction, and curettage than first-trimester vacuum aspiration procedures.

dilation and suction curettage (D&C) A surgical procedure in which the cervical canal is dilated to allow the uterine wall to be scraped; vacuum aspiration.

direct (active) euthanasia Intentionally causing death.

dissonance (**dis** son ince) A feeling of uncertainty that occurs when a person believes two equally attractive but opposite ideas.

distillation The process of heating an alcohol solution and collecting its vapors into a more concentrated form.

distress Stress that diminishes the quality of life; commonly associated with disease, illness, and maladaptation.

dose-response curve The size of the effect of a drug on the body related to the amount of the drug administered.

drug Any substance, natural or artificial, other than food, that by its chemical or physical nature alters structure or function in the living organism.

durable power of attorney for health care A legal document that designates who will make health care decisions for people unable to do so.

duration The length of time one needs to exercise at the target heart rate to produce a cardiorespiratory training effect.

dysmenorrhea Abdominal pain caused by muscular cramping during the menstrual cycle.

E

ectopic pregnancy A pregnancy in which the fertilized ovum implants at a site other than the uterus, typically in the fallopian tubes.

embolism A potentially fatal condition in which a circulating blood clot lodges in a smaller vessel.

embryo Developmental stage from the end of the second week after conception until the end of the eighth week.

emergency contraception Contraceptive measures used to prevent pregnancy within five days of unprotected intercourse; also called *postcoital* or *morning-after contraception.*

emotional intelligence The ability to understand others and act wisely in human relations and to measure how well one knows one's emotions, manages one's emotions, motivates oneself, recognizes emotions in others, and handles relationships.

empowerment The nurturing of an individual's or group's ability to be responsible for their own health and well-being.

endocrine-disrupting chemicals A large class of substances that can interact with the system of glands, hormones, and tissues that regulate many physiological processes in humans, including growth, development from fetus to adult, regulation of metabolic rate and blood sugar, function of the reproductive system, and development of the brain and nervous systems.

enriched Foods that have been resupplied with some of the nutritional elements (B vitamins and iron) removed during processing.

environment The physical conditions (temperature, humidity, light, presence of substances) and other living organisms that exist around your body.

environmental tobacco smoke Tobacco smoke, regardless of its source, that stays within a common source of air.

enzymes Organic substances that control the rate of physiological reactions but are not themselves altered in the process.

epidemic A highly significant increase in the number of cases of an infectious illness existing within the same time period in a given geographical area.

epitaph An inscription on a grave marker or monument.

erection The engorgement of erectile tissue with blood; characteristic of the penis, clitoris, nipples, labia minora, and scrotum.

ergogenic aids Supplements that are taken to improve athletic performance.

erotic dreams Dreams whose content elicits a sexual response.

eulogy A composition or speech that praises someone; often delivered at a funeral or memorial service.

euphoria A complex interplay of physical and emotional states that suggest heightened energy, enhanced mood, and greater resistance to pain and discomfort.

eustress Stress that enhances the quality of life.

excitement stage Initial arousal stage of the sexual response pattern.

exercise A subcategory of physical activity; it is planned, structured, repetitive, and purposive in the sense that an improvement or maintenance of physical fitness is an objective.

exhaustion stage The point at which the physical and the psychological resources used to deal with stress have been depleted.

F

false labor Conditions that resemble the start of true labor; may include irregular uterine contractions, pressure, and discomfort in the lower abdomen.

family violence The use of physical force by one family member against another, with the intent to hurt, injure, or harm.

fat density The percentage of a food's total calories that are derived from fat; above 30 percent is considered a high fat density.

FDA Schedule 1 A list of drugs that have a high potential for abuse but no medical use.

fecal coliform bacteria A category of bacteria that live within the intestines of warm-blooded animals; the presence of these bacteria is used as an indicator that water has been contaminated by feces.

fellatio (feh **lay** she oh) Oral stimulation of the penis.

femininity Behavioral expressions traditionally observed in females.

fermentation A chemical process whereby plant products are converted into alcohol by the action of yeast cells on carbohydrate materials.

fertility The ability to reproduce.

fetal alcohol syndrome Characteristic birth defects noted in the children of some women who consume alcohol during their pregnancies.

fetus Developmental stage from the beginning of the ninth week after conception until birth.

fiber Plant material that cannot be digested; found in cereal, fruits, and vegetables.

fight or flight response The physiological response to a stressor that prepares the body for confrontation or avoidance.

fistula An open pathway between the gastrointestinal wall and other internal organs; often caused by Crohn's disease.

flaccid (**fla** sid) Nonerect; the state of erectile tissue when vasocongestion is not occurring.

flexibility The ability of joints to function through an intended range of motion.

follicle-stimulating hormone (FSH) A gonadotropic hormone required for initial development of ova (in the female) and sperm (in the male).

food additives Chemical compounds intentionally added to the food supply to change some aspect of the food, such as its color or texture.

food allergy A reaction in which the immune system attacks an otherwise harmless food or ingredient; allergic reactions can range from mildly unpleasant to life threatening.

food intolerance An adverse reaction to a specific food that does not involve the immune system; usually caused by an enzyme deficiency.

foreplay Activities, often involving touching and caressing, that prepare individuals for sexual intercourse.

frequency The number of exercise sessions per week; for aerobic fitness, three to five days are recommended.

full funeral services All the professional services provided by funeral directors.

functional foods Foods capable of contributing to the improvement/prevention of specific health problems.

G

Gail Score A numerical expression of the risk of developing invasive breast cancer, based on several variables, such as age at first menstrual period, age at first live birth, results of previous biopsies, and a family history of breast cancer. A score of 1.66 percent reflects a high level of risk.

gait Pattern of walking.

gaseous phase The portion of the tobacco smoke containing carbon monoxide and many other physiologically active gaseous compounds.

gateway drug An easily obtainable legal or illegal drug that represents a user's first experience with a mind-altering drug.

gender General term reflecting a biological basis of sexuality; the male gender or the female gender.

gender adoption Lengthy process of learning the behavior that is traditional for one's gender.

gender identification Achievement of a personally satisfying interpretation of one's masculinity or femininity.

gender identity Recognition of one's gender.

gender preference Emotional and intellectual acceptance of one's own gender.

gender roles The cultural expectations for masculine and feminine behaviors and characteristics within a particular society.

general adaptation syndrome (GAS) Sequenced physiological responses to the presence of a stressor, involving the alarm, resistance, and exhaustion stages of the stress response.

generalized anxiety disorder (GAD) An anxiety disorder that involves experiencing intense and nonspecific anxiety for at least six months, in which the intensity and frequency of worry is excessive and out of proportion to the situation.

generic name Common or nonproprietary name of a drug.

genetically modified foods Crops that are bred with genes engineered in labs so the crops are improved, such as being drought, pest, or cold resistant; producing a higher yield; and/or having a higher nutritional content.

genetic predisposition An inherited tendency to develop a disease process if necessary environmental factors exist.

gonads Male or female sex glands; testes produce sperm and ovaries produce eggs.

greenhouse gases A category of gases in the atmosphere that allow solar radiation to pass through the atmosphere to the Earth but then trap the heat that is radiated from the Earth back toward space; greenhouse gases include water vapor, carbon dioxide, methane, nitrous oxide, and tropospheric ozone.

green space Areas of land that are dominated by domesticated or natural vegetation, including rural farmland, city lawns and parks, and nature preserves.

H

habituation The development of psychological dependence on a drug after a period of use.

hallucinogens Psychoactive drugs capable of producing hallucinations (distortions of reality).

health A reflection of the ability to use and apply both the intrinsic and extrinsic resources related to each dimension of our holistic makeup to (1) participate fully in the activities that sustain role fulfillment, (2) foster the mastery of developmental expectations, and (3) experience a sense of well-being as we evaluate our progress through life.

health claims Statements authorized by the FDA as having scientific proof of claims that a food, nutrient, or dietary supplement has an effect on a health-related condition.

health promotion A movement in which knowledge, practices, and values are transmitted to people for use in lengthening their lives, reducing the incidence of illness, and feeling better.

healthy body weight Body weight within a weight range appropriate for a person with an acceptable waist-to-hip ratio.

herbalism An ancient form of healing in which herbal preparations are used to treat illness and disease.

high-density lipoprotein (HDL) The type of lipoprotein that transports cholesterol from the bloodstream to the liver, where it is eventually removed from the body; high levels of HDL are related to a reduction in heart disease.

high-risk health behavior A behavioral pattern, such as smoking, associated with a high risk of developing a chronic illness.

holistic health A view of health in terms of its physical, emotional, social, intellectual, spiritual, and occupational makeup.

homeopathy (hoe mee **op** ah thee) The use of minute doses of herbs, minerals, or other substances to stimulate healing.

homicide The intentional taking of one person's life by another person.

hormone replacement therapy (HRT) Medically administered estrogen and progestin to replace hormones lost as the result of menopause.

hospice care (**hos** pis) An approach to caring for terminally ill patients that maximizes the quality of life and allows death with dignity.

hot flashes Unpleasant, temporary feelings of warmth experienced by women during and after menopause, caused by blood vessel dilation.

human papillomavirus (HPV) Sexually transmitted viruses, some of which are capable of causing precancerous changes in the cervix; causative agent for genital warts.

humoral immunity Immunity responsible for the production of critically important immune system elements known as *antibodies;* also called *B cell–mediated immunity.*

hypothyroidism A condition in which the thyroid gland produces an insufficient amount of the hormone thyroxin.

hypoxia Oxygenation deprivation at the cellular level.

I

identity theft A crime involving the fraudulent use of a person's name, Social Security number, credit line, or other personal, financial, or identifying information.

immune system The system of cellular and chemical elements that protects the body from invading pathogens, foreign protein, and abnormal cells.

indirect (passive) euthanasia Allowing people to die without the use of life-sustaining procedures.

indoor air quality Characteristics of air within homes, workplaces, and public buildings, including the presence and amount of oxygen, water vapor, and a wide range of substances that can have adverse effects on your health.

infatuation A relatively temporary, intensely romantic attraction to another person.

inhalants Psychoactive drugs that enter the body through inhalation.

inhibitions Inner controls that prevent a person from engaging in certain types of behavior.

insulin A pancreatic hormone required by the body for the effective metabolism of glucose (blood sugar).

intensity The level of effort put into an activity.

intentional injuries Injuries that are purposely inflicted, either by the victim or by another person.

interpersonal process therapy A relational approach to psychotherapy that suggests problems are interpersonal in nature and family experiences have a significant impact on one's sense of self and others.

interstitial cell-stimulating hormone (ICSH) (in ter **stish** ul) A gonadotropic hormone of the male required for the production of testosterone.

intervention An organized process that involves encouraging a chemically addicted individual to enter into drug treatment; usually coordinated by family and friends along with a mental health professional.

intimacy Any close, mutual, verbal or nonverbal behavior within a relationship.

intimate partner violence (IPV) Interpersonal violence perpetrated by a current or former spouse, date, or cohabiting partner.

intoxication Dysfunctional and disruptive changes in physiological and psychological functioning, mood, and cognitive processes resulting from the consumption of a psychoactive substance.

intrapsychic stressors Our internal worries, self-criticisms, and negative self-talk.

intrauterine device (IUD) A small, plastic, medicated or unmedicated contraceptive device that prevents pregnancy when inserted into the uterus.

in vitro Outside the living body, in an artificial environment.

ionizing radiation Electromagnetic radiation that is capable of breaking chemical bonds, such as x-rays and gamma rays.

isokinetic exercises Muscular strength training exercises in which machines are used to provide variable resistances throughout the full range of motion at a fixed speed.

isometric exercises Muscular strength training exercises in which the resistance is so great that the object cannot be moved.

isotonic resistance exercises Muscular strength training exercises in which traditional barbells and dumbbells with fixed resistances are used.

L

learned helplessness A theory of motivation explaining how individuals can learn to feel powerless, trapped, and defeated.

learned optimism An attribution style regarding permanence, pervasiveness, and personalization; how people explain both positive and negative events in their lives, accounting for success and failure.

life course The path that people follow through life, or a road map or blueprint of that map.

life expectancy The average number of years that members of a cohort can expect to live.

life fable The "story" of a person's life, as written and directed by that person.

life span The maximum number of years that humans are capable of living.

lifestyle A personalized version of the life course of an individual, cohort, or generation.

living will A legal document that requires physicians or family members to carry out a person's wishes to die naturally, without receiving sustaining treatments.

low-density lipoprotein (LDL) The type of lipoprotein that transports the largest amount of cholesterol in the bloodstream; high levels of LDL are related to heart disease.

luteinizing hormone (LH) (**loo** ten eye zing) A gonadotropic hormone of the female required for fullest development and release of ova; ovulating hormone.

Lyme disease A bacterial infection transmitted by deer ticks.

M

magnetic resonance imaging (MRI) scan An imaging procedure that uses a powerful magnet to generate images of body tissues.

mainstream smoke Smoke inhaled and then exhaled by a smoker.

mania An extremely excitable state characterized by excessive energy, racing thoughts, impulsive and/or reckless behavior, irritability, and proneness to distraction.

manual vacuum aspiration (MVA) The abortion procedure performed in the earliest weeks after a pregnancy is established.

masculinity Behavioral expressions traditionally observed in males.

masturbation Self-stimulation of the genitals.

mausoleum (moz oh **lee** um) An above-ground structure, which frequently resembles a small stone house, into which caskets can be placed for disposition.

medication abortion An abortion caused by the use of prescribed drugs.

menarche (muh **nar** key) Time of a female's first menstrual cycle.

menopause Decline and eventual cessation of hormone production by the female reproductive system.

metabolism The chemical process by which substances are broken down or synthesized in a living organism to provide energy for life.

metabolite A breakdown product of a drug.

metaneeds Secondary concerns, such as spirituality, creativity, curiosity, beauty, philosophy, and justice, that can be addressed only after the basic needs are met.

metastasis (muh **tas** ta sis) The spread of cancerous cells from their site of origin to other areas of the body.

minipills Low-dose progesterone oral contraceptives.

modeling The process of adopting the behavioral patterns of a person one admires or has bonds with.

monogamous (mo **nog** a mus) Paired relationship with one partner.

mononucleosis ("mono") A viral infection characterized by weakness, fatigue, swollen glands, sore throat, and low-grade fever.

morbidity Pertaining to illness and disease.

mortality Pertaining to death.

mucus Clear, sticky material produced by specialized cells within the mucous membranes of the body; mucus traps much of the suspended particulate matter within tobacco smoke.

multiorgasmic capacity Potential to have several orgasms within a single period of sexual arousal.

murmur Atypical heart sound that suggests a backwashing of blood into a chamber of the heart from which it has just left.

muscular endurance The aspect of muscular fitness that deals with the ability of a muscle or muscle group to repeatedly contract over a long period of time.

muscular fitness The ability of skeletal muscles to perform contractions; includes muscular strength and muscular endurance.

muscular strength The component of physical fitness that deals with the ability to contract skeletal muscles to a maximal level; the maximal force that a muscle can exert.

myocardial infarction Heart attack; the death of part of the heart muscle as a result of a blockage in one of the coronary arteries.

N

narcolepsy (nar co **lep** see) A sleep disorder in which a person has a recurrent, overwhelming, and uncontrollable desire to sleep.

narcotics Opiates; psychoactive drugs derived from the Oriental poppy plant. Narcotics relieve pain and induce sleep.

naturally acquired immunity (NAI) A type of acquired immunity resulting from the body's response to naturally occurring pathogens.

nature The innate factors that genetically determine personality traits.

naturopathy (na chur **op** ah thee) A system of treatment that avoids drugs and surgery and emphasizes the use of natural agents, such as sunshine, to correct underlying imbalances.

negative caloric balance Caloric intake is less than caloric expenditure, resulting in weight loss.

neuron (noor on) A nerve cell.

neurotransmitters Chemical messengers that transfer electrical impulses across the synapses between nerve cells.

nicotine A physiologically active, dependence-producing drug found in tobacco.

nocturnal emission Ejaculation that occurs during sleep; "wet dream."

nonionizing radiation Forms of electromagnetic radiation that cannot break chemical bonds but may excite electrons or heat biological materials.

nontraditional-age students An administrative term used by colleges and universities for students who, for whatever reason, are pursuing undergraduate work at an age other than that associated with the traditional college years (18–24).

nurture The effects that the environment, people, and external factors have on personality.

nutrient-dense foods Foods that provide substantial amounts of vitamins and minerals and comparatively few calories.

nutrients Elements in foods that are required for the growth, repair, and regulation of body processes.

O

obesity A condition in which a person's body weight is 20 percent or more above desirable weight as determined by standard height/weight charts.

obsessive-compulsive disorder (OCD) An anxiety disorder characterized by obsessions (intrusive thoughts, images, or impulses causing a great deal of distress)

and compulsions (repetitive behaviors aimed at reducing anxiety or stress that is associated with the obsessive thoughts).

oncogenes Faulty regulatory genes that are believed to activate the development of cancer.

oral contraceptive pill A pill taken orally, composed of synthetic female hormones that prevent ovulation or implantation; "the pill."

orgasmic platform Expanded outer third of the vagina that grips the penis during the plateau phase of the sexual response pattern.

orgasmic stage Third stage of the sexual response pattern; the stage during which neuromuscular tension is released.

osteoarthritis Arthritis that develops with age; largely caused by weight bearing and deterioration of the joints.

osteopathy (os tee **op** ah thee) A system of medical practice in which allopathic principles are combined with specific attention to postural mechanics of the body.

osteoporosis A decrease in bone mass that leads to increased incidence of fracture, primarily in postmenopausal women.

outercourse Sexual activity that does not involve intercourse.

overload principle The principle whereby a person exercises at a level above which he or she is normally accustomed to.

overweight A condition in which a person's excess fat accumulation results in a body weight that exceeds desirable weight by 1–19 percent.

ovolactovegetarian diet (oh voe **lack** toe veg **a ter** ee in) A diet that excludes all meat but does include the consumption of eggs and dairy products.

ovulation The release of a mature egg from the ovary.

oxidation The process that removes alcohol from the bloodstream.

P

pandemic An epidemic that has crossed national boundaries, thus achieving regional or international status (HIV/AIDS is a pandemic).

panic disorder An anxiety disorder characterized by panic attacks, in which individuals experience severe physical symptoms. These episodes can seemingly occur "out of the blue" or be triggered by something and can last for a few minutes or for hours.

Pap test A cancer screening procedure in which cells are removed from the cervix and examined for precancerous changes.

particulate phase The portion of the tobacco smoke composed of small suspended particles.

passively acquired immunity (PAI) A temporary immunity achieved by providing antibodies to a person exposed to a particular pathogen.

pathogen A disease-causing agent.

pelvic inflammatory disease (PID) An acute or chronic infection of the peritoneum or lining of the abdominopelvic cavity and fallopian tubes; associated with a variety of symptoms or none at all, and a potential cause of sterility.

percutaneous coronary intervention (PCI) Any of a group of procedures used to treat patients suffering from an obstruction in an artery; typically involves inserting a slender, balloon-tipped tube into an artery of the heart.

perfectionism A tendency to expect perfection in everything one does, with little tolerance for mistakes.

periodic abstinence Birth control methods that rely on a couple's avoidance of intercourse during the ovulatory phase of a woman's menstrual cycle; also called *fertility awareness, rhythm,* or *natural family planning.*

periodontal disease Destruction of soft tissue and bone that surround the teeth.

peripheral artery disease (PAD) Atherosclerotic blockages that occur in arteries that supply blood to the legs and arms.

peritonitis (pare it ton **eye** tis) Inflammation of the peritoneum, or lining of the abdominopelvic cavity.

permanence The first dimension of learned optimism, related to whether certain events are perceived as temporary or long lasting.

personalization The third dimension of learned optimism, related to whether an individual takes things personally or is more balanced in accepting responsibility for positive and negative events.

personalized medicine Uses the newly established understanding of the human genome and associated technology to identify genetic markers that suggest predispositions for future illnesses.

pervasiveness The second dimension of learned optimism, related to whether events are perceived as specific or general.

pesco-vegetarian diet A vegetarian diet that includes fish, dairy products, and eggs along with plant foods.

phenylpropanolamine (PPA) (**fen** ill **pro** puh **nol** uh meen) An active chemical compound still found in some over-the-counter diet products and associated with increased risk of stroke.

physical activity Any bodily movement produced by skeletal muscles that results in energy expenditure.

physical fitness A set of attributes that people have or achieve that relates to the ability to perform physical activity.

phytochemicals Physiologically active components of foods believed to deactivate carcinogens and to function as antioxidants.

placebo pills Pills that contain no active ingredients.

plateau stage Second stage of the sexual response pattern; a leveling off of arousal immediately before orgasm.

platelet adhesiveness The tendency of platelets to clump together, thus enhancing the speed at which the blood clots.

platonic (pluh **ton** ick) Close association between two people that does not include a sexual relationship.

polycyclic aromatic hydrocarbons (PAHs) Air pollutants from fossil fuel combustion.

positive caloric balance Caloric intake greater than caloric expenditure, resulting in weight gain.

postpartum The period after the birth of a baby, during which the mother's body returns to its prepregnancy state.

potentiated effect (poe **ten** she ay ted) Phenomenon whereby the use of one drug intensifies the effect of a second drug.

preventive/prospective medicine Physician-centered medical care in which areas of risk for chronic illnesses are identified so that they might be lowered.

primary care health providers Health care providers who generally see patients on a routine basis, particularly for preventive health care.

probiotics Living bacteria ("good bugs") that help prevent disease and strengthen the immune system.

problem drinking An alcohol use pattern in which a drinker's behavior creates personal difficulties or difficulties for other people. Also called *alcohol abuse.*

process addictions Addictions in which people compulsively engage in behaviors such as gambling, shopping, gaming, or sexual activity to such an extreme degree that these addictions cause serious financial, emotional, social, and health problems similar to those resulting from drug and alcohol addictions.

procrastination A tendency to put off completing tasks until some later time, sometimes resulting in increased stress.

procreation Reproduction.

prophylactic mastectomy Surgical removal of the breasts to prevent breast cancer in women who are at high risk of developing the disease.

prophylactic oophorectomy Surgical removal of the ovaries to prevent ovarian cancer in women at high risk of developing the disease.

prostate-specific antigen (PSA) test A blood test used to identify prostate-specific antigen, an early indicator that the immune system has recognized and mounted a defense against prostate cancer.

proteins Compounds composed of chains of amino acids; primary components of muscle and connective tissue.

proto-oncogenes (pro toe **on** co genes) Normal regulatory genes that may become oncogenes.

psychoactive drug Any substance capable of altering feelings, moods, or perceptions.

psychological dependence Craving a drug for emotional reasons and to maintain a sense of well-being; also called *habituation.*

psychological health A broadly based concept pertaining to cognitive functioning in conjunction with the way people express their emotions; cope with stress, adversity, and success; and adapt to changes in themselves and their environment.

psychosocial sexuality Masculine and feminine aspects of sexuality.

puberty Achievement of reproductive ability.

pulmonary emphysema An irreversible disease process in which the alveoli are destroyed.

purging Using vomiting, laxatives, diuretics, enemas, or other medications, or means such as excessive exercise or fasting, to eliminate food.

Q

quack A person who earns money by purposely marketing inaccurate health information, unreliable health care, or ineffective health products.

quackery The practice of disseminating or supplying inaccurate health information, unreliable health care, or ineffective health products for the purposes of defrauding another person.

R

radon A naturally occurring radioactive gas that is emitted during the decay of uranium in soil, rock, and water.

refractory phase That portion of the male's resolution stage during which sexual arousal cannot occur.

regenerative medicine Uses stem cell technology to grow replacement body tissues and structures.

regulatory genes Genes that control cell specialization, replication, DNA repair, and tumor suppression.

resistance stage The second stage of the stress response during which the body attempts to reestablish its equilibrium or internal balance.

resolution stage Fourth stage of the sexual response pattern; the return of the body to a preexcitement state.

retinal hemorrhage Uncontrolled bleeding from arteries within the eye's retina.

rheumatic heart disease Chronic damage to the heart (especially heart valves) resulting from a streptococcal infection within the heart; a complication associated with rheumatic fever.

risk factor A biomedical index such as serum cholesterol level or a behavioral pattern such as smoking associated with a chronic illness.

S

salt sensitive Term used to describe people whose bodies overreact to the presence of sodium by retaining fluid and thus experience an increase in blood pressure.

sarcopenia A reduction in the size of the muscle fibers, related to the aging process.

satiety (suh **tie** uh tee) The feeling of no longer being hungry; a diminished desire to eat.

saturated fats Fats that promote cholesterol formation; they are in solid form at room temperature; primarily animal fats.

schizophrenia One of the most severe mental disorders, characterized by profound distortions in one's thought processes, emotions, perceptions, and behavior. Symptoms may include hallucinations, delusions, disorganized thinking, and a rigid posture or motionlessness.

sclerotic changes (skluh **rot** ick) Thickening or hardening of tissues.

seasonal affective disorder (SAD) A type of depression that develops in relation to the changes in the seasons.

self-actualization The highest level of psychological health, at which one reaches his or her highest potential and values truth, beauty, goodness, faith, love, humor, and ingenuity.

self-care movement The trend toward individuals taking increased responsibility for prevention or management of certain health conditions.

self-concept An individual's internal picture of himself or herself; the way one sees oneself.

self-esteem An individual's sense of pride, self-respect, value, and worth.

self-fulfilling prophecy The tendency to make something more likely to happen as a result of one's own expectations and attitudes.

semen Secretion containing sperm and nutrients discharged from the urethra at ejaculation.

set point A genetically programmed range of body weight, beyond which a person finds it difficult to gain or lose additional weight.

sex flush The reddish skin response that results from increasing sexual arousal.

sexting The sharing of sexually explicit photos or messages by cell phone or other digital media device.

sexual fantasies Fantasies with sexual themes; sexual daydreams or imaginary events.

sexuality The quality of being sexual; can be viewed from many biological and psychosocial perspectives.

sexually transmitted diseases (STDs) Infectious diseases that are spread primarily through intimate sexual contact.

shingles Painful fluid-filled skin eruptions along underlying sensory nerve pathways—due to reactivation of once-sequestered herpes zoster (chicken pox) viruses.

shock Profound collapse of many vital body functions; evident during acute alcohol intoxication and other health emergencies.

sidestream smoke Smoke that comes from the burning end of a cigarette, pipe, or cigar.

sigmoidoscopy Examination of the sigmoid colon (lowest section of the large intestine), using a short, flexible fiber-optic scope.

smegma Cellular discharge that can accumulate beneath the clitoral hood and the foreskin of an uncircumcised penis.

social phobia A phobia characterized by feelings of extreme dread and embarrassment in situations in which public speaking or social interaction is involved.

solid waste Pollutants that are in solid form, including nonhazardous household trash, industrial wastes, mining wastes, and sewage sludge from wastewater treatment plants.

spermatogenesis (sper mat oh **jen** uh sis) Process of sperm production.

spermicides Chemicals capable of killing sperm.

spontaneous abortion Any cessation of pregnancy resulting from natural causes; also called a *miscarriage.*

stalking A crime involving repeated visual or physical proximity, nonconsensual communication, or threats that would cause fear in a reasonable person.

static stretching The slow lengthening of a muscle group to an extended stretch; followed by holding the extended position for 15–60 seconds.

stent A device inserted inside a coronary artery during a percutaneous coronary intervention (PCI) to prevent the artery from narrowing at that site.

sterilization Generally permanent birth control techniques that surgically disrupt the normal passage of ova or sperm.

stimulants Psychoactive drugs that stimulate the function of the central nervous system.

stress The physiological and psychological state of disruption caused by the presence of an unanticipated, disruptive, or stimulating event.

stressors Factors or events, real or imagined, that elicit a state of stress.

stress response The physiological and psychological responses to positive or negative events that are disruptive, unexpected, or stimulating.

synapse (**sinn** aps) The location at which an electrical impulse from one neuron is transmitted to an adjacent neuron; also referred to as a *synaptic junction.*

synergistic drug effect (sin er **jist** ick) Heightened, exaggerated effect produced by the concurrent use of two or more drugs.

systolic pressure Blood pressure against blood vessel walls when the heart contracts.

T

tar A chemically rich, syrupy, blackish-brown material obtained from the particulate matter within cigarette smoke when nicotine and water are removed.

target heart rate (THR) The number of times per minute the heart must contract to produce a training effect.

terrorism Any actions intended to harm or kill civilians in order to intimidate a populace or force a government to take some action.

test anxiety A form of performance anxiety that generates extreme feelings of distress in exam situations.

thermic effect of food (TEF) The amount of energy our bodies require for the digestion, absorption, and transportation of food.

thorax The chest; the portion of the torso above the diaphragm and within the rib cage.

threshold dose The least amount of a drug to have an observable effect on the body.

titration (tie **tray** shun) The particular level of a drug within the body; adjusting the level of nicotine by adjusting the rate of smoking.

tolerance An acquired reaction to a drug; continued intake of the same dose has diminished effects.

toxic pollutants Substances known to cause or suspected of causing cancer or other serious health problems.

toxic shock syndrome (TSS) A potentially fatal condition caused by the proliferation of certain bacteria in the vagina that enter the general blood circulation.

trace elements Minerals whose presence in the body occurs in very small amounts; micronutrient elements.

traditional-age students College students between the ages of 18 and 24.

transcervical balloon tuboplasty The use of inflatable balloon catheters to open blocked fallopian tubes; a procedure used for some women with fertility problems.

transient ischemic attack (TIA) Stroke-like symptoms caused by temporary spasm of cerebral blood vessels.

Transtheoretical Model of Health Behavior Change Six predictable stages—precontemplation, contemplation, preparation, action, maintenance, and termination—people go through in establishing new habits and patterns of behavior.

trimester A three-month period of time; human pregnancies encompass three trimesters.

tropospheric ozone Ozone comprises three oxygen atoms that are bound into a single molecule; tropospheric ozone refers to this substance as it occurs in the lower layer of the atmosphere, close to the ground.

tumor Mass of cells; may be cancerous (malignant) or noncancerous (benign).

U

underweight A condition in which the body is below the desirable weight.

unintentional injuries Injuries that occur without anyone's intending that harm be done.

urethra (yoo **ree** thra) The passageway through which urine leaves the urinary bladder.

V

vasectomy Surgical procedure in which the vasa deferentia are cut to prevent the passage of sperm from the testicles; the most common form of male sterilization.

vegan vegetarian diet (vee gun or **vay** gun**)** A vegetarian diet that excludes all animal products, including eggs and dairy products.

virulent (**veer** yuh lent) Capable of causing disease.

vitamins Organic compounds that facilitate the action of enzymes.

volatile organic compounds (VOCs) A wide variety of chemicals that contain carbon and readily evaporate into the air.

W

wellness A process intended to aid individuals in unlocking their full potential through the development of an overall wellness lifestyle.

Wernicke-Korsakoff syndrome A syndrome that results from vitamin B_1 deficiency, often the result of alcoholism.

Symptoms include impaired short-term memory, psychosis, impaired coordination, and abnormal eye movements.

withdrawal Uncomfortable, perhaps toxic response of the body as it attempts to maintain homeostasis in the absence of a drug; also called *abstinence syndrome*.

withdrawal (coitus interruptus) A contraceptive practice in which the erect penis is removed from the vagina before ejaculation.

Y

Yerkes-Dodson Law A bell-shaped curve demonstrating that there is an optimal level of stress for peak performance; this law states that too little or too much stress is not helpful, whereas a moderate level of stress is positive and beneficial.

Z

zero-tolerance laws Laws that severely restrict the right to operate motor vehicles for underage drinkers who have been convicted of driving under any influence.

zygote A fertilized ovum.

Chapter 1
Page 1: Dynamic Graphics Group /IT Stock Free /Alamy; **3:** Lifesize/Getty Images; **7:** ERproductions Ltd/Blend Images LLC; **13:** William Ryall 2010; **14:** © Brand X Pictures/PunchStock.

Chapter 2
Page 29: Polka Dot Images /JupiterImages; **36:** © BananaStock/JupiterImages; **44:** © The McGraw-Hill Companies, Inc./Gary He, photographer.

Chapter 3
Page 50: Jack Hollingsworth/Getty Images; **55:** Ingram Publishing; **58:** © The McGraw-Hill Companies, Inc./Andrew Resek, photographer; **59:** © Radius Images /Alamy; **66:** © Royalty-Free/Corbis.

Chapter 4
Page 73: Corbis /JupiterImages; **76:** © The McGraw-Hill Companies, Inc./Gary He, photographer; **80:** Courtesy of Leonard Kaminsky; **83:** © The McGraw-Hill Companies, Inc./Andrew Resek, photographer; **85:** © The McGraw-Hill Companies, Inc./Lars A. Niki, photographer; **87 (left):** Photodisc/Getty Images; **87 (right):** Getty Images; **92, 93 all:** Courtesy of Stewart Halperin.

Chapter 5
Page 94: Ariel Skelley/Blend Images LLC; **98:** © The McGraw-Hill Companies, Inc./Andrew Resek, photographer; **106:** © Rubberball Production/Getty Images; **111:** © Mitch Hrdlicka/Getty Images; **115:** Comstock Images; **119:** UpperCut Images/Getty Images.

Chapter 6
Page 125: Blend Images/Getty Images; **127:** © The McGraw-Hill Companies, Inc./John Flournoy, photographer; **132:** © Lars A. Niki; **137 (left):** © The McGraw-Hill Companies, Inc./John Flournoy, photographer; **137 (right):** © Royalty-Free/Corbis; **142:** © The McGraw-Hill Companies, Inc./Jill Braaten, photographer; **145:** © BananaStock/PunchStock.

Chapter 7
Page 154: Ingram Publishing; **156:** © The McGraw-Hill Companies, Inc./Gary He, photographer; **165:** © U.S. Drug Enforcement Administration; **169:** © The McGraw-Hill Companies, Inc./Jill Braaten, photographer; **174:** Image Source/Getty Images.

Chapter 8
Page 186: Ingram Publishing; **189:** Dave Moyer; **191:** © The McGraw-Hill Companies, Inc./Gary He, photographer; **194:** © BananaStock/PunchStock; **201 (both):** Courtesy of Wayne Jackson; **202:** © The McGraw-Hill Companies, Inc./Christopher Kerrigan, photographer; **203:** © 1996 Copyright IMS Communications Ltd./Capstone Design. All Rights Reserved; **206:** © Royalty-Free/Corbis; **212:** © Stockbyte/JuniperImages.

Chapter 9
Page 216: The McGraw-Hill Companies, Inc./John Flournoy, photographer; **222:** © BananaStock/PunchStock; **227:** © Keith Brofsky/Getty Images; **228:** © The McGraw-Hill Companies, Inc./Rick Brady, photographer.

Chapter 10
Page 238: Photo provided by Ball Memorial Hospital, Muncie, IN; **245 (both):** © The Skin Cancer Foundation, www.skincancer.org; **247:** Kerry-Edwards 2004, Inc./Sharon Farmer, photographer; **258:** © National Cancer Institute/Bill Branson, photographer; **260:** Photo provided by Ball Memorial Hospital, Muncie, IN.

Chapter 11
Page 271: © Steve Allen/Getty Images; **282:** © PhotoAlto; **288:** © The McGraw-Hill Companies, Inc./Christopher Kerrigan, photographer; **290:** © F. Schussler/PhotoLink/Getty Images; **293:** Image Source Pink/Alamy; **294:** © Steven J. Nussenblatt/Custom Medical Stock Photo; **295:** © Custom Medical Stock Photo.

Chapter 12
Page 302: Jose Luis Pelaez Inc/Blend Images LLC; **305:** Brand X Pictures/JupiterImages; **316, 320:** © Ryan McVay/Getty Images; **323:** ThinkStock; **324:** © Buccina Studios/Getty Images.

Chapter 13
Pages 328, 334, 336: The McGraw-Hill Companies, Inc./Kristan Price, photographer; **337:** Courtesy of Stewart Halperin; **341 (left):** Courtesy of Organon USA; **341 (right):** © The McGraw-Hill Companies, Inc./Christopher Kerrigan, photographer; **348:** © Science Photo Library/Photo Researchers; **351:** © E. Dygas/Getty Images.

Chapter 14
Page 357: Rubberball/Mike Kemp/Getty Images; **365:** © Creata/PunchStock; **372:** © Kent Knudson/PhotoLink/Getty Images.

Chapter 15
Page 384: Scott T. Baxter/Getty Images; **387:** ©Tom Grill/Corbis; **396 (top):** © The McGraw-Hill Companies, Inc./Jill Braaten, photographer; **396 (bottom):** © Purestock/PunchStock; **399:** Photodisc/Getty Images.

Chapter 16
Page 407: Don Mason/Blend Images RF/Photolibrary; **411:** © Alex L. Fradkin/Getty Images; **420:** Jocelyn Augustino/FEMA; **421:** © Royalty-Free/Corbis.

Chapter 17
Page 434: Rubberball/Getty Images; **437, 444:** © Royalty-Free/Corbis; **448 (left):** © Melba Photo Agency/PunchStock; **488 (right):** © D. Normark/PhotoLink/Getty Images.

Page numbers in italics indicate photos or captions. Those ending with an italic *f* indicate figures, and those ending with an italic *t* indicate tables.

index